Handbook of Evidence-Based Radiation Oncology

3rd Edition

Handbook of Evidence-Based Radiation Oncology

3rd *Edition*

Eric K. Hansen, MD
The Oregon Clinic
Radiation Oncology
Providence St. Vincent Medical Center
Portland, OR
USA

Mack Roach III, MD, FACR, FASTRO
Professor
Radiation Oncology and Urology
Director
Particle Therapy Research Program & Outreach
Department of Radiation Oncology
UCSF Helen Diller Family Comprehensive Cancer Center
San Francisco, CA
USA

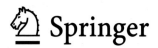 Springer

Editors
Eric K. Hansen
The Oregon Clinic
Providence St. Vincent Medical Center
Portland, OR,
USA

Mack Roach III
University of California
San Francisco, CA,
USA

ISBN 978-3-319-62641-3   ISBN 978-3-319-62642-0   (eBook)
https://doi.org/10.1007/978-3-319-62642-0

Library of Congress Control Number: 2018932328

Printed on acid-free paper

This Springer imprint is published by the registered company Springer International Publishing AG part of Springer Nature.
The registered company address is: Gewerbestrasse 11, 6330 Cham, Switzerland

To our patients – thank you for your trust, sharing, and the daily lessons you teach us. You keep us inspired.

Preface to the 3rd Edition

In his 1901 textbook, The Roentgen Rays in Medicine and Surgery, Dr. Francis Williams wrote in his preface, "The following pages are rather a report of progress than a final presentation on a growing subject." Never has that been more true. From 2010 to 2016, over 50,000 articles were published with "radiotherapy" in the title or abstract. Medical knowledge is expanding more rapidly than our ability to keep up and apply it to patient care, research, and education. To cope, we must identify the essential core of best practices for our specialty. Clinical expertise also requires easy access to well-organized knowledge.

In the third edition of Handbook of Evidence-Based Radiation Oncology, we strive to meet these demands. We have kept the same concise format to meet our aim of a practical quick reference guide. All chapters have been carefully revised and include the latest key trials, studies, and techniques. We encourage readers to continue to refer to primary literature for updates on the myriad subtopics not discussed herein.

We are pleased that our third edition is the first radiation oncology text to include the newly published eighth edition of AJCC Cancer Staging Manual. Because most of the literature published in the last 6 years refers primarily to the seventh edition of AJCC Cancer Staging Manual, we include it as well.

Importantly, we appreciate that experienced physicians are very capable of weighing evidence and individualizing care based on it. All patients are unique, so our treatment algorithms and recommendations are not to be considered edicts. Rather, consider our book a framework upon which you build a personalized treatment plan for each patient.

We are extremely grateful to the contributing authors for all their hard work and dedication. We believe Handbook of

Evidence-Based Radiation Oncology will continue to be an invaluable resource for students, resident physicians, fellows, and other practitioners of radiation oncology.

Finally, we owe special thanks to our families for their patience, understanding, and good humor during our many hours of work on this new edition. A round of applause for them!

Eric K. Hansen   Portland, OR, USA
Mack Roach III   San Francisco, CA, USA

Contents

Contributors

Mekhail Anwar, MD, PhD
Department of Radiation Oncology, University of California San Francisco, San Francisco, CA, USA

Eleanor A. Blakely, BA, MS, PhD
Biological System Engineering, Lawrence Berkeley National Laboratory, Berkeley, CA, USA

Lauren Boreta, MD
Department of Radiation Oncology, University of California San Francisco, San Francisco, CA, USA

Steve E. Braunstein, MD, PhD
Department of Radiation Oncology, University of California San Francisco, San Francisco, CA, USA

Jason Chan, MD
Department of Radiation Oncology, University of California San Francisco, San Francisco, CA, USA

Albert J. Chang, MD, PhD
Department of Radiation Oncology, University of California, San Francisco, San Francisco, CA, USA

Jennifer S. Chang, MD, PhD
Department of Radiation Oncology, University of California San Francisco, San Francisco, CA, USA
Marin General Hospital, Greenbrae, CA, USA

Christopher H. Chapman, MD, MS
Department of Radiation Oncology, University of California San Francisco, San Francisco, CA, USA

Serah Choi, MD, PhD
Department of Radiation Oncology, University of California San Francisco, San Francisco, CA, USA

Hans T. Chung, MD, FRCPC
Department of Radiation Oncology, Sunnybrook Odette Cancer Centre, University of Toronto, Toronto, ON, Canada

Michael A. Garcia, MD, MS
Department of Radiation Oncology, University of California San Francisco, San Francisco, CA, USA

Adam Garsa, MD
Radiation Oncology, University of Southern California, Los Angeles, CA, USA

Alexander R. Gottschalk, MD, PhD
Department of Radiation Oncology, University of California San Francisco, San Francisco, CA, USA

Matthew A. Gubens, MD, MS
Department of Medicine, University of California San Francisco, San Francisco, CA, USA

Daphne A. Haas-Kogan, MD
Department of Radiation Oncology, Brigham and Women's Hospital, Dana-Farber Cancer Institute; Boston Children's Hospital, Harvard Medical School, Boston, MA, USA

Eric K. Hansen, MD
The Oregon Clinic, Radiation Oncology, Providence St. Vincent Medical Center, Portland, OR, USA

I-Chow J. Hsu, MD
Department of Radiation Oncology, University of California San Francisco, San Francisco, CA, USA

Kavita K. Mishra, MD, MPH
Department of Radiation Oncology, University of California San Francisco, San Francisco, CA, USA

John Murnane, PhD
Department of Radiation Oncology, University of California San Francisco, San Francisco, CA, USA

Jean L. Nakamura, MD
Department of Radiation Oncology, University of California San Francisco, San Francisco, CA, USA

Catherine C. Park, MD
Department of Radiation Oncology, UCSF Helen Diller Family Comprehensive Cancer, San Francisco, CA, USA

Anna K. Paulsson, MD
Department of Radiation Oncology, University of California San Francisco, San Francisco, CA, USA

David R. Raleigh, MD, PhD
Department of Radiation Oncology, University of California San Francisco, San Francisco, CA, USA

Mack Roach III, MD, FACR, FASTRO
Radiation Oncology and Urology, Particle Therapy Research Program & Outreach, Department of Radiation Oncology, UCSF Helen Diller Family Comprehensive Cancer Center, San Francisco, CA, USA

Tracy Sherertz, MD
Department of Radiation Oncology, University of California San Francisco, San Francisco, CA, USA

Lisa Singer, MD, PhD
Radiation Oncology, University of Texas, MD Anderson Cancer Center, Houston, TX, USA

Michael Wahl, MD, MS
Department of Radiation Oncology, University of California San Francisco, San Francisco, CA, USA

Sue S. Yom, MD, PhD, MAS
Department of Radiation Oncology, University of California San Francisco, San Francisco, CA, USA

Yao Yu, MD
Department of Radiation Oncology, University of California San Francisco, San Francisco, CA, USA

PART I
Skin

Chapter I
Skin Cancer

Lisa Singer and Sue S. Yom

PEARLS

- Skin is composed of 3 layers: epidermis (melanocytes), dermis (hair follicles, sweat glands), and subcutis.
- Skin cancers can be divided into melanoma and non-melanoma skin cancers; sun/UV exposure is a major cause for both subtypes.
- Skin cancers can also be associated with immunosuppression, chronic irritation, and certain genetic disorders (Jaju, J Am Acad Dermatol 2016):
  - Gorlin syndrome (basal cell nevus syndrome, *PTCH* mutations): autosomal dominant, associated with multiple BCCs, rhabdomyosarcomas, fibrosarcomas, palmar/plantar pits
  - Xeroderma pigmentosum: X-linked, increased sensitivity to UV radiation, 1000× increased risk of skin cancer
- Non-melanoma skin cancers are the most common malignancies in the USA, with millions diagnosed each year, but true incidence is unknown as cases are not required to be reported to cancer registries (Siegel, CA Cancer J Clin 2015).
- Major subtypes of non-melanoma skin cancers include basal cell carcinoma (BCC), squamous cell carcinoma (SCC), and Merkel cell carcinoma (MCC):

© Springer International Publishing AG, part of Springer Nature 2018   **3**
Eric K. Hansen and M. Roach III (eds.), *Handbook of Evidence-Based Radiation Oncology*, https://doi.org/10.1007/978-3-319-62642-0_1

BCC
- 80% of non-melanoma skin cancers; common in sun-exposed areas.
- >90% of cases associated with abnormal hedgehog pathway signaling (Lacouture, Oncologist 2016).
- Pathologic subtypes: nodular (most common, papule); superficial (scaly macule); morpheaform (sclerosing, can have PNI); infiltrative (Veness and Howle 2016).
- Only 0.1% have perineural spread; most common affected CN are V and VII.
- <1% metastasize (Ganti, Cancer Manag Res 2013).

SCC
- Common in sun-exposed areas.
- Actinic keratosis (AK) is a premalignant lesion that can develop into SCC, with multiple AKs, 6–10% chance of invasive SCC in 10 years.
- Pathologic subtypes: SCC in situ (*Bowen's disease*), superficial, spindle cell (may require IHC for diagnosis) (Veness and Howle 2016)
- More frequently metastasizes than BCC: about 5%.

MCC
- Rare, aggressive neuroendocrine cancer of the skin with more frequent local, regional, and distant recurrence rates than other cutaneous carcinomas.
- Cell of origin is Merkel cell (aka Tastzellen or touch cell), a tactile neuroendocrine epithelial cell, first described by Friedrich Sigmund Merkel in 1875 (Erovic and Erovic 2013).
- Merkel cell virus (MCV): polyomavirus, found to be pathogenic factor in 60–80% MCC (Feng, Science 2008).

Cutaneous Melanoma
- Rising incidence.
- Melanoma once viewed as radioresistant, but this is not supported by data.
- "ABCDE" mnemonic raises awareness of suspicious lesions (A = asymmetry, B = borders not smooth, C = color change/variegation, D = diameter > pencil eraser, E = evolving) (Chair, J Am Acad Dermatol 2015).

، Pathologic subtypes: superficial spreading, nodular, lentigo maligna (best prognosis; Hutchinson's freckle involves epidermis only), acral lentiginous (usually presents on soles, palms), desmoplastic (recurs locally).

، 85% of patients (pts) present with localized disease with 5-yr survival >90% for pts with tumor ≤1 mm thick vs 50–90% for pts with primary >1 mm thick depending on thickness, ulceration, and mitotic rate.

، LN status: most prognostic factor for recurrence and survival. In the absence of risk factors, there is <5–7% risk of +SLN if primary <1 mm thick.

، About 10% of pts present with regional disease, with 5-yr. survival 20–70% depending primarily on nodal burden.

، Historically, long-term survival was <10% for stage IV disease, but some pts have a distinct indolent course, and emerging effective systemic therapies have made long-term remission possible in more pts.

، Other prognostic factors: ulceration, thickness, anatomic site (trunk worse), gender (male worse), age (older worse), #LN involved, and mitotic rate.

WORK-UP

، H&P. Describe the primary lesion (see Table 1.1); identify lesion number, location/distribution, borders, color, shape (linear, round, etc.), and any secondary features (scale, induration, erosion, ulceration, etc.). Palpate for the deep edge of the tumor. For head/neck lesions, do a cranial nerve exam. Palpate for lymph node involvement.

، Biopsy the lesion and suspicious lymph nodes.

، Breslow thickness = measured depth of lesion.

Table 1.1 Primary lesion characteristics

Primary lesion characteristics	Size <0.5 cm	Size >0.5 cm
Flat, non-palpable	Macule	Patch
Elevated	Papule	Nodule (plaque is >1 cm, flat topped)
Fluid filled	Vesicle	Bullae
Pus filled	Pustule	Abscess

ˌ Clark level = related to histologic level of dermis (I = epidermis only, II = invasion of papillary dermis, III = filling papillary dermis compressing reticular dermis, IV = invading reticular dermis, V = invades subcutaneous tissues).

ˌ SLN biopsy is typically performed in clinically node-negative patients with MCC or with >0.75 mm thick melanoma.

ˌ Additional imaging: MRI if PNI suspected and for lesions of medial/lateral canthi, to rule out orbit involvement. CT is useful to rule out suspected bone invasion.

ˌ Melanoma: imaging to work-up suspected sites of additional disease.

ˌ PET/CT often ordered for melanoma and MCC due to high rates of metastasis.

BASAL CELL CARCINOMA AND SQUAMOUS CELL CARCINOMA

STAGING

Editors' note: All TNM stage and stage groups referred to elsewhere in this chapter reflect the 2010 AJCC staging nomenclature unless otherwise noted as the new system below was published after this chapter was written (Tables 1.2, 1.3, 1.4, and 1.5).

Table 1.2 (AJCC 7TH ED., 2010)

Primary tumor (T)*	
TX:	Primary tumor cannot be assessed
T0:	No evidence of primary tumor
Tis:	Carcinoma in situ
T1:	Tumor 2 cm or less in greatest dimension with less than two high-risk features**
T2:	Tumor greater than 2 cm in greatest dimension or tumor any size with two or more high-risk features*
T3:	Tumor with invasion of maxilla, mandible, orbit, or temporal bone
T4:	Tumor with invasion of skeleton (axial or appendicular) or perineural invasion of skull base

Note: Excludes cSCC of the eyelid
**High-risk features for the primary tumor (T) staging
Depth/invasion: >2 mm thickness, Clark level ≥ IV, perineural invasion
Anatomic location: primary site ear, primary site non-hair-bearing lip
Differentiation: poorly differentiated or undifferentiated

Regional lymph nodes (N)

NX: Regional lymph nodes cannot be assessed

N0: No regional lymph node metastases

N1: Metastasis in a single ipsilateral lymph node, 3 cm or less in greatest dimension

N2: Metastasis in a single ipsilateral lymph node, more than 3 cm but not more than 6 cm in greatest dimension; or in multiple ipsilateral lymph nodes, not more than 6 cm in greatest dimension; or in bilateral or contralateral lymph nodes, not more than 6 cm in greatest dimension

N2a: Metastasis in a single ipsilateral lymph node, more than 3 cm but not more than 6 cm in greatest dimension

N2b: Metastasis in multiple ipsilateral lymph nodes, not more than 6 cm in greatest dimension

N2c: Metastasis in bilateral or contralateral lymph nodes, not more than 6 cm in greatest dimension

N3: Metastasis in a lymph node, more than 6 cm in greatest dimension

Distant metastasis (M)

M0: No distant metastases

M1: Distant metastases

Anatomic stage/prognostic groups

0: Tis N0 M0

I: T1 N0 M0

II: T2 N0 M0

III: T3 N0 M0, T1–T3 N1 M0

IV: T1–T3 N2 M0, T any N3 M0, T4 N any M0, T any N any M1

Used with the permission from the American Joint Committee on Cancer (AJCC), Chicago, Illinois. The original source for this material is the *AJCC Cancer Staging Manual*, Seventh Edition (2010), published by Springer Science + Business Media

Table 1.3 (AJCC 8TH ED., 2017)

Definitions of AJCC TNM	
Definition of primary tumor (T)	
T category	**T criteria**
TX	Primary tumor cannot be identified
Tis	Carcinoma in situ
Tl	Tumor smaller than 2 cm in the greatest dimension
T2	Tumor 2 cm or larger but smaller than 4 cm in the greatest dimension
T3	Tumor 4 cm or larger in maximum dimension or minor bone erosion or perineural invasion or deep invasion*
T4	Tumor with gross cortical bone/marrow, skull base invasion, and/or skull base foramen invasion
T4a	Tumor with gross cortical bone/marrow invasion
T4b	Tumor with skull base invasion and/or skull base foramen involvement

*Deep invasion is defined as invasion beyond the subcutaneous fat or> 6 mm (as measured from the granular layer of the adjacent normal epidermis to the base of the tumor); perineural invasion for T3 classification is defined as tumor cells within the nerve sheath of a nerve lying deeper than the dermis or measuring 0.1 mm or larger in caliber or presenting with clinical or radiographic involvement of named nerves without skull base invasion or transgression

DEFINITION OF REGIONAL LYMPH NODE (N) CLINICAL N (CN)

Table 1.4 (AJCC 8TH ED., 2017)

N category	N criteria
NX	Regional lymph nodes cannot be assessed
NO	No regional lymph node metastasis
Nl	Metastasis in a single ipsilateral lymph node, 3 cm or smaller in the greatest dimension and ENE(-)
N2	Metastasis in a single ipsilateral node larger than 3 cm but not larger than 6 cm in the greatest dimension and ENE(-)
	Metastases in multiple ipsilateral lymph nodes, not larger than 6 cm in the greatest dimension and ENE(-),*or* in bilateral or contralateral lymph nodes, not larger than 6 cm in the greatest dimension and ENE(-)
N2a	Metastasis in a single ipsilateral node larger than 3 cm but not larger than 6 cm in the greatest dimension and ENE(-)
N2b	Metastasis in multiple ipsilateral nodes, not larger than 6 cm in the greatest dimension and ENE(-)
N2c	Metastasis in bilateral or contralateral lymph nodes, not larger than 6 cm in the greatest dimension and ENE(-)
N3	Metastasis in a lymph node larger than 6 cm in the greatest dimension and ENE(-) *or* metastasis in any node(s) and clinically overt ENE [ENE(+)]
N3a	Metastasis in a lymph node larger than 6 cm in the greatest dimension and ENE(-)
N3b	Metastasis in any node(s) and ENE(+)

Note: A designation of "U" or "L" may be used for any N category to indicate metastasis above the lower border of the cricoid (U) or below the lower border of the cricoid (L) Similarly, clinical and pathological ENE should be recorded as ENE(-) or ENE(+)

PATHOLOGICAL N (PN)

Table 1.5 (AJCC 8TH ED., 2017)

N category	N criteria
NX	Regional lymph nodes cannot be assessed
N0	No regional lymph node metastasis
Nl	Metastasis in a single ipsilateral lymph node, 3 cm or smaller in the greatest dimension and ENE(-)
N2	Metastasis in a single ipsilateral lymph node, 3 cm or smaller in the greatest dimension and ENE(+), *or* larger than 3 cm but not larger than 6 cm in the greatest dimension and ENE(-), *or* metastases in multiple ipsilateral lymph nodes, not larger than 6 cm in the greatest dimension and ENE(-), *or* in bilateral or contralateral lymph nodes, not larger than 6 cm in the greatest dimension, ENE(-)
N2a	Metastasis in single ipsilateral or contralateral node 3 cm or smaller in the greatest dimension and ENE(+) *or* a single ipsilateral node larger than 3 cm but not larger than 6 cm in the greatest dimension and ENE(-)
N2b	Metastasis in multiple ipsilateral nodes, not larger than 6 cm in the greatest dimension and ENE(-)
N2c	Metastasis in bilateral or contralateral lymph nodes, not larger than 6 cm in the greatest dimension and ENE(-)
N3	Metastasis in a lymph node larger than 6 cm in the greatest dimension and ENE(-) *or* in a single ipsilateral node larger than 3 cm in the greatest dimension and ENE(+) *or* multiple ipsilateral, contralateral, or bilateral nodes, any with ENE(+)
N3a	Metastasis in a lymph node larger than 6 cm in the greatest dimension and ENE(-)
N3b	Metastasis in a single ipsilateral node larger than 3 cm in the greatest dimension and ENE(+) *or* multiple ipsilateral, contralateral, or bilateral nodes, any with ENE(+)

Note: A designation of "U" or "L" may be used for any N category to indicate metastasis above the lower border of the cricoid (U) or below the lower border of the cricoid (L) Similarly, clinical and pathological ENE should be recorded as ENE(-) or ENE(+)

DEFINITION OF DISTANT METASTASIS (M)

Table 1.6 (AJCC 8TH ED., 2017)

M category	M criteria
M0	No distant metastasis
M1	Distant metastasis

AJCC PROGNOSTIC STAGE GROUPS

Table 1.7   (AJCC 8TH ED., 2017)

When T is...	And N is...	And M is...	Then the stage group is...
Tis	N0	M0	0
T1	N0	M0	I
T2	N0	M0	II
T3	N0	M0	III
T1	N1	M0	III
T2	N1	M0	III
T3	N1	M0	III
T1	N2	M0	IV
T2	N2	M0	IV
T3	N2	M0	IV
Any T	N3	M0	IV
T4	Any N	M0	IV
Any T	Any N	M1	IV

Used with permission from the American Joint Committee on Cancer (AJCC), Chicago, Illinois. The original and primary source for this information is the *AJCC Cancer Staging Manual,* Eighth Edition (2017) published by Springer International Publishing

Table 1.8   NCCN BCC and SCC risk factors for recurrence

High risk	Location (regardless of size): mask areas (central face, eyelids, eyebrows, periorbital, nose, lips, chin, mandible, preauricular, postauricular, temple), genitalia, hands, feet. If >1 cm: cheek, forehead, scalp, neck, pretibia. If >2 cm: trunk, extremities
	Border: poorly defined
	Recurrent
	Immunosuppression
	Site of prior RT or chronic inflammation
	BCC subtype: morpheaphorm, basosquamous, sclerosing, micronodular features
	SCC subtype: adenoid, adenosquamous, desmoplastic, metaplastic
	SCC: rapidly growing. Neurologic symptoms. >2 mm depth or Clark level IV–V. PNI or LVSI.
Low risk	None of above

Table 1.9   TREATMENT RECOMMENDATIONS

Localized, low risk	If surgical candidate: curettage and electrodessication (not used for hair-bearing areas), surgical excision, or Mohs micrographic surgery (staged resection with micrographic examination of each horizontal and deep margin), with re-resection for positive margin. Recommended margin: BCC 2–4 mm, SCC 4–6 mm
	RT: if not surgical candidate due to poor functional/cosmetic outcome with resection or re-resection for close/+ margin(s)
	Relative RT contraindications include postradiation recurrence, area prone to repeated trauma such as bony prominences, poor blood supply, high occupational sun exposure, exposed cartilage/bone, Gorlin's, CD4 count <200
	RT contraindicated for xeroderma pigmentosum, basal cell nevus syndrome, scleroderma

Table 1.9 (continued)

Localized, high risk	If surgical candidate: WLE or Mohs. Recommended margin: BCC 4–10 mm, SCC ≥10 mm
	Post-op RT indications: positive margin(s), extensive PNI, or involvement of large-caliber nerves (≥0.1 mm)
	Definitive RT: if not surgical candidate
	Relative RT contraindications as above
Node-positive BCC or SCC	Resection with lymph node dissection
	Post-op RT indicated as above for primary lesions or for nodal ECE or multiple nodes involved. Consider post-op RT vs surveillance for 1 LN involved if <3 cm without ECE
	Inoperable: RT with or without systemic therapy (typically regimens used for head and neck SCC primaries are used) – Results much better for BCC than SCC
Systemic therapy	BCC: Vismodegib and sonidegib are small molecule inhibitors of hedgehog pathway; FDA approved for metastatic BCC and in BCC patients who are not candidates for surgery or RT (Lacouture, Oncologist 2016). About 30–65% response rate with median response duration 7–10 months
	SCC: TROG 05.01 post-op RT +/− concurrent carboplatin, results pending. Cetuximab may sometimes produce tumor regression with unresectable or metastatic SCC. Biochemotherapy or chemotherapy as used in head/neck cancer (e.g., cisplatin or cisplatin/5FU) may be considered

Other topical therapies:

- Imiquimod: topical immunomodulator FDA approved for <2 cm trunk/extremity superficial BCC (5× weekly for 6 weeks) or actinic keratosis (2× weekly for 16 weeks) (Hanna, Int J Dermatol 2016).
- Topical 5-fluorouracil: can be used for superficial BCC or AKs (Moore, J Dermatolog Treat 2009).

STUDIES
IDENTIFYING POINTS THAT MAY BENEFIT FROM POST-OP RT

- Review of 1818 cutaneous SCC cases identified 4 risk factors for recurrence: size ≥2 cm, poorly differentiated, PNI (≥0.1 mm nerves), and tumor invasion beyond fat. 10-yr. local recurrence: 0 factors = 0.6%, 1 factor = 5%, 2–3 factors = 21%, 4 factors or bone invasion = 67%. 10-yr nodal mets: 0 factors = 0.1%, 1 factor = 3%, 2–3 factors = 21%, 4 factors or bone invasion = 67% (Karia, JCO 2014).
- 122 pts with cutaneous SCC of head and neck with cervical LN involvement. Post-op RT reduced LRR (23% vs 55%) and improved DFS (74% vs 34%) and OS (66% vs 27%) (Wang, Head Neck 2011).

- Multi-institutional retrospective review of SCC found that immunocompromised status was associated with higher locoregional recurrence (Manyam, IJROBP 2016).

MULTIPLE RETROSPECTIVE STUDIES REPORT EXCELLENT LC WITH RT

- 389 patients with BCC were included in a retrospective study at Washington University in St. Louis; excellent outcomes were achieved for RT alone (LC >90% for tumors <=3 cm treated with SRT and >80% for tumors <=3 cm treated with electrons; for tumors >5 cm treated w/electrons, LC was 100% w/margins >2 cm, 67% for margins 1.1–2 cm, and 80% for margins <=1 cm) (Locke, IJROBP 2001).
- 604 BCCs and 106 SCCs treated with RT. 97% of lesions involved face and head. 18% of lesions were recurrent. 5/15-yr. LC: BCC 94%/85%, SCC 93%/79%. Tumor size >1 cm and nasolabial fold location were independent predictors for BCC recurrence. Recurrent SCC had higher recurrence risk (Hernández-Machin, Int J Dermatol 2007).
- 129 eyelid and 857 lesions overlying nasal cartilage treated with RT, 98% BCC, 2% SCC. 5-yr. LC eyelid 96%, nose 92% (Caccialanza, G Ital Dermatol Venereol 2013).
- 712 BCCs and 994 SCCs treated with RT. 5-yr. LC: BCC 96%, SCC 94%. Tumors >2 cm had increased recurrence risk (Cognetta, J Am Acad Dermatol 2012).

OTHER STUDIES

- *Vismodegib*: ERIVANCE was a single-arm phase II study of vismodegib; of the 33 patients in the study with metastatic BCC, 30% responded; of the 63 with locally advanced BCC, 43% responded (response was defined as a decrease of at least 30% in the externally visible or radiographic dimension of the lesion or complete resolution of ulceration) (Sekulic, NEJM 2012).
- *p16 status*: positive in 31% of SCC but not prognostic in an Australian study of 143 patients with cutaneous SCC of the head and neck (McDowell, Cancer 2016).

RADIATION TECHNIQUES
SIMULATION AND FIELD DESIGN

- Most skin cancers are treated with superficial radiation therapy (SRT) (50–100 kVp), orthovoltage (150–300 kVp), or with megavoltage electrons (McDermott and Orton 2010).
- SRT advantages (vs electrons): less margin (electrons require additional margin at skin surface), less expensive, maximum dose at surface (vs electrons which have built up and require bolus) (Cognetta and Mendenhall 2013); disadvantages: SRT not appropriate for >1 cm deep lesion.
- For SRT a photon energy is selected, so tumor is encompassed by 90% depth dose (90% IDL: 50 kV [0.7 mm Al] ~1 mm; 100 kV [4–7 mm Al] ~5 mm; 150 kV [0.52 mm Cu] ~1.0 cm).
- At energies below 300 kV, photoelectric effect is dominant, varying with Z^3; bone is high Z due to calcium, and therefore f-factor, or Roentgen to rad conversion, is important (note that cartilage is not similar to bone in terms of absorption) (Atherton, Clin Oncol 1993).
- Lead shields should be used to block the lens, cornea, nasal septum, oral cavity, etc.; backscattered electrons/photons can lead to conjunctival/mucosal irritation; therefore, for eyelids, thin coating of wax or porcelain can be used over lead.
- Margins
  - Orthovoltage: Tumor size <2 cm = 0.5–1.0 cm horizontal margin; tumor size >2 cm = 1.5–2 cm horizontal margin. Deep margin should be at least 0.5 cm deeper than the suspected depth of tumor.
  - Electron margins: Add additional 0.5 cm margin at skin surface due to lateral constriction of isodose curves in deep portion of tumor volume, respecting adjacent normal tissues such as orbit.
  - Recurrent and morpheaform BCCs are more infiltrative, requiring 0.5–1.0 cm additional margin at skin surface.
  - High-risk SCC: Add 2 cm margin around tumor if possible.

- Gross or extensive PNI: consider IMRT to cover named nerve from the primary to skull base.
  - Recommend careful review of target volumes following cranial nerves V and/or VII as appropriate (Anwar, Pract Radiat Oncol 2016; Gluck, IJROBP 2009).
- Elective nodal treatment should be considered for recurrences after surgery and is indicated for poorly differentiated, >3 cm tumors, and/or large infiltrative-ulcerative SCC.
- Irradiation of a *graft* should not begin until after it is well healed; entire graft should be included in the target volume.

DOSE PRESCRIPTIONS

- For SRT or orthovoltage prescribe to surface $D_{max.}$
- For electrons, prescribe to 90% to account for lower RBE.
- Fractionation
  - Size <2 cm: 64 Gy/32 fx, 55 Gy/20 fx, 45–51 Gy/15–17 fx, 40–44 Gy/10 fx, 35 Gy/5 fx.
  - Size >2 cm and no cartilage involvement: 55 Gy at 2.5 Gy/fx.
  - Size >2 cm and cartilage involved: 64–66 Gy at 2 Gy/fx.
  - While treating cartilage, always keep daily dose <3 Gy/fx.
  - Hypofractionation reduces long-term cosmesis but is an option for selected patients or for palliative treatment.
  - Elective LN (high-risk SCC; rarely BCC): 50 Gy/25 fx.
  - Grossly involved LN 66–70 Gy at 2 Gy/fx:
    - Post-op adjuvant
    - Primary negative margins: 60 Gy/30 fx or 50 Gy/20 fx
    - Primary, +margin: as primary definitive
  - LN: 50–56 Gy at 2 Gy/fx if no ECE; 60 Gy if ECE.
- Electronic surface brachytherapy: 5 Gy/fraction given twice a week to 40 Gy.

DOSE LIMITATIONS

- Cartilage: Chondritis rare if fraction size <3 Gy.
- Skin: Larger volumes of tissue require smaller daily fractions; moist desquamation is expected for larger surface areas.

COMPLICATIONS

, Telangiectasias, skin atrophy, hypopigmentation, alopecia, loss of sweat glands, skin necrosis (~3%), osteoradionecrosis (~1%), chondritis/cartilage necrosis (rare if fx <3Gy)

FOLLOW-UP (BASED ON NCCN GUIDELINES)

, BCC: H&P every 6–12 months for life with sun protection education

, Localized SCC: H&P every 3–12 months × 2 years, then every 6–12 months × 3 years, then annually; sun protection education

, Regionally metastatic SCC: H&P every 1–3 months × 1 year, then every 2–4 months × 1 year, then every 4–6 months × 3 years, then every 6–12 months long term; sun protection education

MERKEL CELL CARCINOMA (MCC)

Table 1.10 Staging (AJCC 7TH ED., 2010): Merkel cell carcinoma

Primary tumor (T)	
TX:	Primary tumor cannot be assessed
T0:	No evidence of primary tumor (e.g., nodal/metastatic presentation without associated primary)
Tis:	In situ primary tumor
T1:	Less than or equal to 2 cm maximum tumor dimension
T2:	Greater than 2 cm, but not more than 5 cm maximum tumor dimension
T3:	Over 5 cm maximum tumor dimension
T4:	Primary tumor invades bone, muscle, fascia, or cartilage

Table 1.10 (continued)

Regional lymph nodes (N)	
NX:	Regional lymph nodes cannot be assessed
N0:	No regional lymph node metastasis
cN0:	Nodes negative by clinical exam* (no pathologic node exam performed)
pN0:	Nodes negative by pathologic exam
N1:	Metastasis in regional lymph node(s)
N1a:	Micrometastasis**
N1b:	Macrometastasis***
N2:	In-transit metastasis****

*Note: Clinical detection of nodal disease may be via inspection, palpation, and/or imaging
**Micrometastases are diagnosed after sentinel or elective lymphadenectomy
***Macrometastases are defined as clinically detectable nodal metastases confirmed by therapeutic lymphadenectomy or needle biopsy
****In-transit metastasis: a tumor distinct from the primary lesion and located either (1) between the primary lesion and the draining regional lymph nodes or (2) distal to the primary lesion

Table 1.11 (AJCC 7TH ED., 2010)

Distant metastasis (M)	
M0:	No distant metastasis
M1:	Metastasis beyond regional lymph nodes
M1a:	Metastasis to skin, subcutaneous tissues, or distant lymph nodes
M1b:	Metastasis to lung
M1c:	Metastasis to all other visceral sites

ANATOMIC STAGE/PROGNOSTIC GROUPS

Patients with primary Merkel cell carcinoma with no evidence of regional or distant metastases (either clinically or pathologically) are divided into two stages: Stage I for primary tumors ≤2 cm in size and stage II for primary tumors >2 cm in size. Stages I and II are further divided into A and B substages based on the method of nodal evaluation

Patients who have pathologically proven node-negative disease (by microscopic evaluation of their draining lymph nodes) have improved survival (substaged as A) compared with those who are only evaluated clinically (substaged as B). Stage II has an additional substage (IIC) for tumors with extracutaneous invasion (T4) and negative node status, regardless of whether the negative node status was established microscopically or clinically. Stage III is also divided into A and B categories for patients with microscopically positive and clinically occult nodes (IIIA) and macroscopic nodes (IIIB). There are no subgroups of stage IV Merkel cell carcinoma

Table 1.12 (AJCC 7TH ED., 2010)

0:	Tis N0 M0
IA:	T1 pN0 M0
IB:	T1 cN0 M0
IIA:	T2/T3 pN0 M0
IIB:	T2/T3 cN0 M0
IIC:	T4 N0 M0
IIIA:	Any T N1a M0
IIIB:	Any T N1b/N2 M0
IV:	Any T Any N M1

Used with the permission from the American Joint Committee on Cancer (AJCC), Chicago, Illinois. The original source for this material is the AJCC Cancer Staging Manual, Seventh Edition (2010), published by Springer Science + Business Media

Table 1.13 (AJCC 8TH ED., 2017)

Definitions of AJCC TNM	
Definition of primary tumor (T)	
T category	**T criteria**
TX	Primary tumor cannot be assessed (e.g., curetted)
T0	No evidence of primary tumor
Tis	In situ primary tumor
T1	Maximum clinical tumor diameter ≤ 2 cm
T2	Maximum clinical tumor diameter > 2 but ≤ 5 cm
T3	Maximum clinical tumor diameter > 5 cm
T4	Primary tumor invades the fascia, muscle, cartilage, or bone

DEFINITION OF REGIONAL LYMPH NODE (N) CLINICAL (N)

Table 1.14 (AJCC 8TH ED., 2017)

N category	**N criteria**
NX	Regional lymph nodes cannot be clinically assessed (e.g., previously removed for another reason or because of body habitus)
N0	No regional lymph node metastasis detected on clinical and/or radiologic examination
N1	Metastasis in regional lymph node(s)
N2	In-transit metastasis (discontinuous from primary tumor; located between primary tumor and draining regional nodal basin or distal to the primary tumor) *without* lymph node metastasis
N3	In-transit metastasis (discontinuous from primary tumor; located between primary tumor and draining regional nodal basin or distal to the primary tumor) *with* lymph node metastasis

PATHOLOGICAL (PN)

Table 1.15 (AJCC 8TH ED., 2017)

pN category	pN criteria
pNX	Regional lymph nodes cannot be assessed (e.g., previously removed for another reason or *not* removed for pathological evaluation)
pN0	No regional lymph node metastasis detected on pathological evaluation
pNl	Metastasis in regional lymph node(s)
pNla(sn)	Clinically occult regional lymph node metastasis identified only by sentinel lymph node biopsy
pNla	Clinically occult regional lymph node metastasis following lymph node dissection
pNlb	Clinically and/or radiologically detected regional lymph node metastasis, microscopically confirmed
pN2	In-transit metastasis (discontinuous from primary tumor; located between primary tumor and draining regional nodal basin, or distal to the primary tumor) *without* lymph node metastasis
pN3	In-transit metastasis (discontinuous from primary tumor; located between primary tumor and draining regional nodal basin or distal to the primary tumor) *with* lymph node metastasis

DEFINITION OF DISTANT METASTASIS (M)
CLINICAL (M)

Table 1.16 (AJCC 8TH ED., 2017)

M category	M criteria
M0	No distant metastasis detected on clinical and/or radiologic examination
M1	Distant metastasis detected on clinical and/or radiologic examination
M1a	Metastasis to the distant skin, distant subcutaneous tissue, or distant lymph node(s)
M1b	Metastasis to the lung
M1c	Metastasis to all other visceral sites

PATHOLOGICAL (M)

Table 1.17 (AJCC 8TH ED., 2017)

M category	M criteria
M0	No distant metastasis detected on clinical and/or radiologic examination
pM1	Distant metastasis microscopically confirmed
pM1a	Metastasis to the distant skin, distant subcutaneous tissue, or distant lymph node(s), microscopically confirmed
pM1b	Metastasis to the lung, microscopically confirmed
pM1c	Metastasis to all other distant sites, microscopically confirmed

AJCC PROGNOSTIC STAGE GROUPS
CLINICAL STAGE GROUP (CTNM)

Table 1.18 (AJCC 8TH ED., 2017)

When T is...	And N is...	And M is...	Then the stage group is...
Tis	N0	M0	0
T1	N0	M0	I
T2-3	N0	M0	IIA
T4	N0	M0	IIB
T0-4	N1-3	M0	III
T0-4	Any N	M1	IV

PATHOLOGICAL STAGE GROUP (PTNM)

Table 1.19 (AJCC 8TH ED., 2017)

When T is...	And N is...	And M is...	Then the stage group is...
Tis	N0	M0	0
T1	N0	M0	I
T2-3	N0	M0	IIA
T4	N0	M0	IIB
T1-4	N1a(sn) or N1a	M0	IIIA
T0	N1b	M0	IIIA
T1-4	N1b-3	M0	IIIB
T0-4	Any N	M1	IV

Used with permission from the American Joint Committee on Cancer (AJCC), Chicago, Illinois. The original and primary source for this information is the AJCC Cancer Staging Manual, Eighth Edition (2017) published by Springer International Publishing

TREATMENT RECOMMENDATIONS

- cN0: Wide local excision with 1–2 cm margin and sentinel lymph node biopsy (SLNB) followed always by adjuvant RT to primary site.
  - If SLN negative, elective nodal RT should be considered due to higher false-negative SLNB rates for head and neck regions, prior surgery, failure to perform ICH on sentinel node, immunosuppression, or SLNB operator concerns.
  - Post-op nodal RT always indicated for multiple involved LN or ECE.

, cN+: Node dissection or nodal RT is indicated.
, Chemotherapy is not routinely recommended but may be considered on a case-by-case basis, such as cisplatin or carboplatin +/− etoposide.
, M1: clinical trial, chemotherapy (cisplatin or carboplatin +/− etoposide, topotecan, cyclophosphamide, doxorubicin, vincristine), immunotherapy (pembrolizumab, atezolizumab), and/or palliative RT.

RADIATION TECHNIQUES

, At UCSF, adjuvant radiation therapy for Merkel cell carcinoma (MCC) is as follows:
  , Primary site is covered, as well as in-transit lymphatics, regional LN with wide margins.
    , May consider eliminating regional LN RT if primary small with negative SLN or if regional lymph node dissection is performed and patient cN0.
  , Margins on primary site: ≥2 cm in head and neck, 3–5 cm elsewhere (Lok, Cancer 2012).
  , Dose (at 1.8–2 Gy/fx):
    , Tumor bed, negative margins: 50–56 Gy.
    , Tumor bed, positive margins: 56–60 Gy.
    , Gross residual and/or gross nodal disease: 60–66 Gy.
    , Clinically N0 nodes: 45–50 Gy.
    , Negative nodal post-op bed: 46–50 Gy.
    , Nodal bed with multiple nodes or ECE: 50–60 Gy.
    , Inoperable: 60–66 Gy.
    , Palliation: 30 Gy/10 fx.

STUDIES

, *SLN biopsy*: In a study at University of Michigan, no subgroup of clinically node-negative patients had less than 15–20% likelihood of +SLN; thus, SLNB is advised for all patients (Swartz, JCO 2011).
, *Adjuvant RT*:
  , In a randomized study, 83 stage I patients receiving WLE and primary site post-op RT were randomized to

adjuvant nodal RT. Regional RT reduced regional recurrence (0% vs 17%) but did not improve PFS or OS. Study terminated early due to decline in accrual due to increasing use of SLNB (Jouary, Ann Oncol 2012).

, In a retrospective SEER study of 1665 stage I–III cases, adjuvant RT improved MS for all patients (63 vs 45 mo), including <1 cm (93 vs 48 mo), 1–2 cm (86 vs 52 mo), and >2 cm (50 vs 21 mo) (Mojica, JCO 2007).

, In a NCDB study of 4815 pts with head/neck MCC, post-op RT or chemoRT improved 5-yr. OS (43–48% vs 39%) (Chen, JAMA Otolaryngol Head Neck Surg 2015).

, In a systematic review of 34 studies with 4475 pts, post-op RT or chemoRT improved 3-yr. LC (65–67% vs 20%) and OS (70–73% vs 56%) (Hasan, Frontiers Oncol 2013).

, *Margins:* In a retrospective study of RT failures, 5 locoregional failures were identified, and 2 were at the field edge with margin >2 cm; margins > > 2 cm were therefore suggested when feasible (Lok, Cancer 2012).

, *MCV Antibodies*: Higher MCV antibody titers have been found to be associated with better PFS; titers are expected to decline after completion of treatment (Touzé, JCO 2011).

FOLLOW-UP (BASED ON NCCN GUIDELINES)
, H&P every 3–6 months × 3 years, then every 6–12 months; cross-sectional imaging for high-risk patients

MELANOMA

STAGING
Editors' note: All TNM stage and stage groups referred to elsewhere in this chapter reflect the 2010 AJCC staging nomenclature unless otherwise noted as the new system below was published after this chapter was written (Table 1.8).

Table 1.20   (AJCC 7TH ED., 2010)

Primary tumor (T)	
TX:	Primary tumor cannot be assessed (e.g., curettaged or severely regressed melanoma)
T0:	No evidence of primary tumor
Tis:	Melanoma in situ
T1:	Melanomas 1.0 mm or less in thickness
T2:	Melanomas 1.01–2.0 mm
T3:	Melanomas 2.01–4.0 mm
T4:	Melanomas more than 4.0 mm

Note: a and b subcategories of T are assigned based on ulceration and number of mitoses per mm^2 as shown below.

Table 1.21   (AJCC 7TH ED., 2010)

T classification	Thickness (mm)	Ulceration status/mitoses
TI	≤1.0	(a) Without ulceration and mitosis <1/mm^2
		(b) With ulceration or mitoses ≥1/mm^2
T2	1.01–2.0	(a) Without ulceration
		(b) With ulceration
T3	2.01–4.0	(a) Without ulceration
		(b) With ulceration
T4	>4.0	(a) Without ulceration
		(b) With ulceration

REGIONAL LYMPH NODES (N)

Table 1.22

NX:	Patients in whom the regional nodes cannot be assessed (e.g., previously removed for another reason)
N0:	No regional metastases detected
N1–3:	Regional metastases based upon the number of metastatic nodes and presence or absence of intralymphatic metastases (in-transit or satellite metastases)

Note: N1–3 and a–c subcategories assigned as shown below

Table 1.23

N classification	Number of metastatic nodes	Nodal metastatic mass
N1	1 node	Micrometastasis*
		Macrometastasis**
N2	2–3 nodes	Micrometastasis*
		Macrometastasis**
		In-transit met(s)/satellite(s) without metastatic nodes
N3	4 or more metastatic nodes, or matted nodes, or in-transit met(s)/satellite(s) with metastatic node(s)	

*Micrometastases are diagnosed after sentinel lymph node biopsy and completion of lymphadenectomy (if performed)
***Macrometastases are defined as clinically detectable nodal metastases confirmed by therapeutic lymphadenectomy or when nodal metastasis exhibits gross extracapsular extension

DISTANT METASTASIS (M)

Table 1.24

M0:	No detectable evidence of distant metastases
M1a:	Metastases to skin, subcutaneous, or distant lymph nodes
M1b:	Metastases to lung
M1c:	Metastases to all other visceral sites or distant metastases to any site combined with an elevated serum LDH

Note: Serum LDH is incorporated into the M category as shown below

Table 1.25

M classification	Site	Serum LDH
M1a	Distant skin, subcutaneous, or nodal mets	Normal
M1b	Lung metastases	Normal
M1c	All other visceral metastases	Normal
	Any distant metastasis	Elevated

ANATOMIC STAGE/PROGNOSTIC GROUPS

Table 1.26

Clinical staging*				Pathologic staging**			
Stage 0	Tis	N0	M0	0	Tis	N0	M0
Stage IA	T1a	N0	M0	IA	T1a	N0	M0
Stage IB	T1b	N0	M0	IB	T1b	N0	N0
	T2a	N0	M0		T2a	N0	M0
Stage IIA	T2b	N0	M0	IIA	T2b	N0	M0
	T3a	N0	M0		T3a	N0	M0
Stage IIB	T3b	N0	M0	IIB	T3b	N0	M0
	T4a	N0	M0		T4a	N0	M0
Stage IIC	T4b	N0	M0	IIC	T4b	N0	M0
Stage III	Any T	≥N1	M0	IIIA	T1–4a	N1a	M0
					T1–4a	N2a	M0
				IIIB	T1–4b	N1a	M0
					T1–4b	N2a	M0
					T1–4a	N1b	M0
					T1–4a	N2b	M0
					T1–4a	N2c	M0
				IIIC	T1–4b	N1b	M0
					T1–4b	N2b	M0
					T1–4b	N2c	M0
					T1–4b	N3	M0
					Any T	N3	M0
Stage IV	Any T	Any N	M1	IV	Any T	Any N	M1

*Clinical staging includes microstaging of the primary melanoma and clinical/radiologic evaluation for metastases. By convention, it should be used after complete excision of the primary melanoma with clinical assessment for regional and distant metastases

**Pathologic staging includes microstaging of the primary melanoma and pathologic information about the regional lymph nodes after partial or complete lymphadenectomy. Pathologic stage 0 or stage IA patients are the exception; they do not require pathologic evaluation of their lymph nodes
Used with the permission from the American Joint Committee on Cancer (AJCC), Chicago, Illinois. The original source for this material is the AJCC Cancer Staging Manual, Seventh Edition (2010), published by Springer Science + Business Media

Table 1.27 (AJCC 8TH ED., 2017)

Definitions of TNM

Definition of primary tumor (T)

T category	Thickness	Ulceration status
TX: primary tumor thickness cannot be assessed (e.g., diagnosis by curettage)	Not applicable	Not applicable
T0: no evidence of primary tumor (e.g., unknown primary or completely regressed melanoma)	Not applicable	Not applicable
Tis (melanoma in situ)	Not applicable	Not applicable
T1	≤1.0 mm	Unknown or unspecified
T1a	<0.8 mm	Without ulceration
T1b	<0.8 mm 0.8–1.0 mm	With ulceration With or without ulceration
T2	>1.0-2.0 mm	Unknown or unspecified
T2a	>1.0–2.0 mm	Without ulceration
T2b	>1.0–2.0 mm	With ulceration
T3	>2.0–4.0 mm	Unknown or unspecified
T3a	>2.0–4.0 mm	Without ulceration
T3b	>2.0–4.0 mm	With ulceration
T4	>4.0 mm	Unknown or unspecified
T4a	>4.0 mm	Without ulceration
T4b	>4.0 mm	With ulceration

DEFINITION OF REGIONAL LYMPH NODE (N)

Table 1.28

Extent of regional lymph node and/or lymphatic metastasis		
N category	Number of tumor-involved regional lymph node	Presence of in-transit, satellite, and/or microsatellite metastases
NX	Regional nodes not assessed (e.g., SLN biopsy not performed, regional nodes previously removed for another reason). Exception: pathological N category is not required for T1 melanomas, use cN	No
N0	No regional metastases detected	No
N1	One tumor-involved node or in-transit, satellite, and/or microsatellite metastases with no tumor-involved nodes	
N1a	One clinically occult (i.e., detected by SLN biopsy)	No
N1b	One clinically detected	No
N1c	No regional lymph node disease	Yes
N2	Two or three tumor-involved nodes or in-transit, satellite, and/or microsatellite metastases with one tumor-involved node	

N2a	Two or three clinically occult (i.e., detected by SLN biopsy)	No
N2b	Two or three, at least one of which was clinically detected	No
N2c	One clinically occult or clinically detected	Yes
N3	Four or more tumor-involved nodes or in-transit, satellite, and/or microsatellite metastases with two or more tumor-involved nodes or any number of matted nodes without or with in-transit, satellite, and/or microsatellite metastases	
N3a	Four or more clinically occult (i.e., detected by SLN biopsy)	No
N3b	Four or more, at least one of which was clinically detected, or the presence of any number of matted nodes	No
N3c	Two or more clinically occult or clinically detected and/or presence of any number of matted nodes	Yes

DEFINITION OF DISTANT METASTASIS (M)

Table I.29

| M category | M criteria | |
	Anatomic site	LDH level
		Not applicable
M0	No evidence of distant metastasis	
M1	Evidence of distant metastasis	See below
M1a	Distant metastasis to the skin, soft tissue including muscle, and/or nonregional lymph node	Not recorded or unspecified
M1a(0)		Not elevated
M1a(l)		Elevated
M1b	Distant metastasis to the lung with or without Mia sites of disease	Not recorded or unspecified
M1b(0)		Not elevated
M1b(l)		Elevated
M1c	Distant metastasis to non-CNS visceral sites with or without Mia or M1b sites of disease	Not recorded or unspecified
M1c(0)		Not elevated
M1c(1)		Elevated
M1d	Distant metastasis to CNS with or without Mia, M1b, or M1c sites of disease	Not recorded or unspecified
M1d(0)		Normal
M1d(1)		Elevated

Suffixes for M category: (0) LDH not elevated, (1) LDH elevated. No suffix is used if LDH is not recorded or is unspecified

CLINICAL (CTNM)

Table 1.30

When T is...	And N is...	And M is...	Then the clinical stage group is...
Tis	N0	M0	0
T1a	N0	M0	IA
T1b	N0	M0	IB
T2a	N0	M0	IB
T2b	N0	M0	IIA
T3a	N0	M0	IIA
T3b	N0	M0	IIB
T4a	N0	M0	IIB
T4b	N0	M0	IIC
Any T, Tis	≥N1	M0	III
Any T	Any N	M1	IV

Used with the permission from the American Joint Committee on Cancer (AJCC), Chicago, Illinois. The original and primary source for this information is the AJCC Cancer Staging Manual, Eighth Edition (2017) published by Springer International Publishing

TREATMENT RECOMMENDATIONS

PRIMARY THERAPY FOR LOCALIZED DISEASE

- cN0: SLN biopsy and WLE, with completion LND if SLN+.
- Minimal surgical margins are Tis = 5–10 mm, T1 = 1 cm, T2 = 1-2 cm, and T3–4 = 2 cm.
- SLNB improves staging to identify pts who may need completion node dissection and/or adjuvant therapy. SLNB improved DSS for pts with intermediate thickness (1.2–3.5 mm) primary who had microscopic (vs subsequent macroscopic) nodal involvement in MSLT-I trial (Morton, NEJM 2014).
- Elective lymph node dissection (ELND) is controversial as multiple RCTs report no survival benefit to ELND vs observation with delayed LND (Balch, Ann Surg Oncol 2000; Cascinelli, Lancet 1998; Sim, Mayo Clin Proc 1986; Veronesi, Cancer 1982).
- Clinically N+: therapeutic nodal dissection and WLE.
- Primary RT is rarely indicated with the exception of lentigo maligna melanomas on the face that would cause severe cosmetic/functional deficits with surgery. These can be treated with a 1.5 cm margin with 50–100 Gy/10–20fx with 100–250 kV photons. For

medically inoperable patients, hyperthermia can improve response and local control, especially for tumors >4 cm (Overgaard, Lancet 1995).

ADJUVANT SYSTEMIC THERAPY
, See NCCN guidelines.
  , For node-negative early stage: observation or clinical trial
  , For node-negative IIB–IIC: observation vs clinical trial vs high-dose IFN
  , For node positive: observation, clinical trial, interferon alfa, ipilimumab, or other biochemotherapy agents

ADJUVANT RT
, Adjuvant primary site RT is considered to reduce LRR for deep desmoplastic melanoma with narrow margins, extensive neurotropism, or locally recurrent disease.
, Adjuvant nodal radiotherapy indications:
  , Parotid LN: extracapsular extension (ECE) and/or ≥ 1 involved LN
  , Cervical LN: ECE, node >3 cm, ≥ 2 involved LN, or recurrent disease
  , Axillary nodes: ECE, node >3–4 cm, ≥ 2–4 involved LN, recurrent disease
  , Groin/pelvic nodes: higher threshold for elective nodal RT due to morbidity of lymphedema
    , BMI <25 kg/m^2: presence of any 1 of the following: ECE, >3–4 involved lymph nodes, recurrent disease, node >3–4 cm
    , BMI >25 kg/m^2: presence of ECE and 1 of the following: >3–4 involved lymph nodes, node >3–4 cm
, Consider elective nodal RT in high-risk pts unable to undergo completion surgery due to medical comorbidities

METASTATIC DISEASE
, Biopsy for genetic analysis (e.g., BRAF mutation, c-KIT).
, Consider resection of limited resectable metastasis.
, Disseminated metastases: clinical trial, systemic therapy, palliative resection, or RT:

- Immunotherapy: interferon alfa-2b, interleukin-2, anti-CTLA4 (ipilimumab), anti PD-1 (pembrolizumab, nivolumab), injectable oncolytic virus (talimogene laherparepvec).
- Targeted therapy: BRAF (dabrafenib, vemurafenib), MEK (trametinib, cobimetinib).
- Chemotherapy: dacarbazine, temozolomide (for brain metastases).

RADIOTHERAPY STUDIES

- ANZMTG 01.02/TROG 02.01: 250 pts with nonmetastatic palpable LN at diagnosis or isolated palpable LN relapse treated with lymphadenectomy randomized to adjuvant RT (48 Gy/20 fx) or observation. RT reduced 5-yr. LN relapse (18% vs 33%) but did not improve RFS or OS (Henderson, Lancet Oncol 2015).
- 615 pts had therapeutic lymphadenectomy and were at high risk of regional recurrence due to ECE and multiple or enlarged nodes. Adjuvant RT reduced 5-yr. regional recurrence (10% vs 41%) (Agrawal, Cancer 2009).
- LRC control is similar with hypofractionated RT or standard fractionated RT.
  - In data from University of Florida, 82 high-risk pts were treated with surgery and adjuvant RT, 47% with hypofractionated RT (mostly 30 Gy in 5 fx at 2 fx per week) or conventional fractionation. No significant difference in 5-yr. LRC (87% hypofx vs 78% conventional fx) (Mendenhall, Am J Otolaryngol 2013).
- MDACC has the largest published experience with 30 Gy/5 fx over 2.5 wks hypofractionation, reporting regional control 88–94% (Ballo, Cancer 2003; Beadle, IJROBP 2009).
- In a retrospective study of 277 pts with nonmetastatic desmoplastic melanoma, 41% received adjuvant RT. Adjuvant RT improved 5-yr. LC (95% vs 76%) especially for +margin or pts with negative margin and high-risk features (head and neck location, depth > 4 mm, Clark level V) (Strom, Cancer 2014).

˒ RTOG 8305 was a prospective study randomizing 137 patients to 32 Gy in 4 fx once weekly or 50 Gy in 20 fx. No difference in response rate between arms: 23.8% complete remission and 34.9% partial remission. Study included large tumors (56% were ≥5 cm) (Sause, IJROBP 1991).

˒ Patients with recurrent/metastatic melanoma randomized to 24 or 27 Gy in 3 fx over 8 days +/− hyperthermia (43 °C for 60 min). LC was improved with HT (26 vs 46%; LC was 25% vs 56% with 24 vs 27 Gy (Overgaard, Lancet 1995).

˒ RT may optimize systemic antitumor immune response induced by immunotherapy (Chandra, Oncoimmunology 2015; Grimaldi, Oncoimmunology 2014).

RADIATION TECHNIQUES
SIMULATION AND FIELD DESIGN

˒ Treatment setup
  ˒ Head and neck: supine or open neck position; depending on tumor location, bolus can be used to reduce dose to temporal lobe, larynx, ear canal.
  ˒ Axilla: supine with treatment arm akimbo, AP/PA.
  ˒ Groin: unilateral frog-leg position.
˒ Target volume for primary lesion: primary site +2–4 cm margin.
˒ Nodal target volume depends on primary site:
  ˒ H&N: preauricular, postauricular LN for facial and posterior scalp primaries, and ipsilateral cervical LN levels I through V, including ipsilateral supraclavicular fossa, for tumors at high risk.
  ˒ Axilla: levels I through III; for bulky high axillary disease, include supraclavicular fossa and low cervical LN.
  ˒ Groin: include entire scar and regions with confirmed nodal disease. Can include external iliac LNs for cases with positive inguinal lymphadenopathy, but toxicity will increase.

DOSE PRESCRIPTIONS

꜕ Dose recommendations for SCC/BCC can be followed, but hypofractionation approaches are well tolerated and more convenient.

꜕ If hypofractionating, adjuvant RT is 30 Gy in 5 fractions twice weekly; if microscopic residual disease is present in the H&N, 1 boost fraction is added to total dose 36 Gy.

DOSE LIMITATIONS

꜕ Hypofractionation: spinal cord or small bowel Dmax <24 Gy over 5 fractions

COMPLICATIONS

꜕ Site dependent:

꜕ Most sites: erythema, tanning, dry or moist desquamation

꜕ Late complications: thinning of subcutaneous fat; mild to moderate fibrosis

꜕ Postoperative lymphedema, particularly in patients with high body mass index or treated with adjuvant RT to groin

꜕ Other late effects: osteitis, fracture, joint stiffness, and neuropathy

FOLLOW-UP (BASED ON NCCN GUIDELINES)

꜕ Stage IA–IIA: H&P every 6–12 months × 5 years, then annually; LN US considered in patients who did not undergo successful SLNB or if +SLNB and no LND.

꜕ Stage IIB–IV: H&P every 3–6 months × 2 years, every 3–12 months × 3 years, then annually for life; if NED, imaging can be considered every 3–12 months to screen for recurrence; additionally, LN US can be considered in patients who did not undergo successful SLNB or if +SLNB and no LND.

Acknowledgment We thank Tania Kaprealian, MD, James Rembert, MD, and Lawrence W. Margolis, MD, for their work on prior editions of this chapter.

REFERENCES

Agrawal S, Kane JM, Guadagnolo BA, Kraybill WG, Ballo MT. The benefits of adjuvant radiation therapy after therapeutic lymphadenectomy for clinically advanced, high-risk, lymph node-metastatic melanoma. Cancer (Wiley Subscription Services, Inc., A Wiley Company). 2009;115(24):5836–44.

Anwar M, Yu Y, Glastonbury CM, El-Sayed IH, Yom SS. Delineation of radiation therapy target volumes for cutaneous malignancies involving the ophthalmic nerve (cranial nerve V-1) pathway. Pract Radiat Oncol. 2016;6(6):e277–81.

Ganti AK, Macha M, Batra S. Profile of vismodegib and its potential in the treatment of advanced basal cell carcinoma. CMAR (Dove Press). 2013;5:197–203.

Atherton P, Townley J, Glaholm J. Cartilage: the "F-"factor fallacy. Clin Oncol. 1993;5(6):391–2.

Balch CM, Soong S, Ross MI, Urist MM, Karakousis CP, Temple WJ, et al. Long-term results of a multi-institutional randomized trial comparing prognostic factors and surgical results for intermediate thickness melanomas (1.0 to 4.0 mm). Intergroup melanoma surgical trial. Ann Surg Oncol. 2000;7(2):87–97.

Ballo MT, Bonnen MD, Garden AS, Myers JN, Gershenwald JE, Zagars GK, et al. Adjuvant irradiation for cervical lymph node metastases from melanoma. Cancer (Wiley Subscription Services, Inc., A Wiley Company). 2003;97(7):1789–96.

Beadle BM, Guadagnolo BA, Ballo MT, Lee JE, Gershenwald JE, Cormier JN, et al. Radiation therapy field extent for adjuvant treatment of axillary metastases from malignant melanoma. Int J Radiat Oncol Biol Phys (Elsevier). 2009;73(5):1376–82.

Caccialanza M, Piccinno R, Gaiani F, Contini D. Relevance of dermatologic radiotherapy in the therapeutic strategy of skin epithelial neoplasms: excellent results in the treatment of lesions localized on eyelids and skin overlying the cartilage of the nose. G Ital Dermatol Venereol. 2013;148(1):83–8.

Cascinelli N, Morabito A, Santinami M, MacKie RM, Belli F. Immediate or delayed dissection of regional nodes in patients with melanoma of the trunk: a randomised trial. WHO Melanoma Programme. Lancet. 1998;351(9105):793–6.

American Academy of Dermatology Ad Hoc Task Force for the ABCDEs of Melanoma, Tsao H, Olazagasti JM, Cordoro KM, Brewer JD, Taylor SC, Bordeaux JS, Chren MM, Sober AJ, Tegeler C, Bhushan R, Begolka WS. Early detection of melanoma: reviewing the ABCDEs. J Am Acad Dermat (Elsevier). 2015;72(4):717–23.

Chandra RA, Wilhite TJ, Balboni TA, Alexander BM, Spektor A, Ott PA, et al. A systematic evaluation of abscopal responses following radiotherapy in patients with metastatic melanoma treated with ipilimumab. Oncoimmunology (Taylor & Francis). 2015;4(11):e1046028.

Chen MM, Roman SA, Sosa JA, Judson BL. The role of adjuvant therapy in the management of head and neck merkel cell carcinoma: an analysis of 4815 patients. JAMA Otolaryngol Head Neck Surg (American Medical Association). 2015;141(2):137–41.

Cognetta AB, Howard BM, Heaton HP, Stoddard ER, Hong HG, Green WH. Superficial x-ray in the treatment of basal and squamous cell carcinomas: a viable option in select patients. J Am Acad Dermatol. 2012;67(6):1235–41.

Cognetta AB, Mendenhall WM. In: Cognetta AB, Mendenhall WM, editors. Radiation therapy for skin cancer. New York: Springer Science & Business Media; 2013.

Erovic I, Erovic BM. Merkel cell carcinoma: the past, the present, and the future. J Skin Cancer. 2013;2013(1):1–6.

Feng H, Shuda M, Chang Y, Moore PS. Clonal integration of a polyomavirus in human Merkel cell carcinoma. Science. 2008;319(5866):1096–100.

Gluck I, Ibrahim M, Popovtzer A, Teknos TN, Chepeha DB, Prince ME, et al. Skin cancer of the head and neck with perineural invasion: defining the clinical target volumes based on the pattern of failure. Int J Radiat Oncol Biol Phys. 2009;74(1):38–46.

Grimaldi AM, Simeone E, Giannarelli D, Muto P, Falivene S, Borzillo V, et al. Abscopal effects of radiotherapy on advanced melanoma patients who progressed after ipilimumab immunotherapy. Oncoimmunology. 2014;3(5):e28780.

Hanna E, Abadi R, Abbas O. Imiquimod in dermatology: an overview. Int J Dermatol. 2016;55(8):831–44.

Hasan S, Liu L, Triplet J, Li Z, Mansur D. The role of postoperative radiation and chemoradiation in merkel cell carcinoma: a systematic review of the literature. Front Oncol (Frontiers). 2013;3:276.

Henderson MA, Burmeister BH, Ainslie J, Fisher R, Di Iulio J, Smithers BM, et al. Adjuvant lymph-node field radiotherapy versus observation only in patients with melanoma at high risk of further lymph-node field relapse after lymphadenectomy (ANZMTG 01.02/ TROG 02.01): 6-year follow-up of a phase 3, randomised controlled trial. Lancet Oncol (Elsevier). 2015;16(9):1049–60.

Hernández-Machin B, Borrego L, Gil-García M, Hernández BH. Office-based radiation therapy for cutaneous carcinoma: evaluation of 710 treatments. Int J Dermatol (Blackwell Publishing Ltd). 2007;46(5):453–9.

Jaju PD, Ransohoff KJ, Tang JY, Sarin KY. Familial skin cancer syndromes: Increased risk of nonmelanotic skin cancers and extracutaneous tumors. J Am Acad Dermatol. 2016;74(3):437–51. quiz452–4

Jouary T, Leyral C, Dreno B, Doussau A, Sassolas B, Beylot-Barry M, et al. Adjuvant prophylactic regional radiotherapy versus observation in stage I Merkel cell carcinoma: a multicentric prospective randomized study. Ann Oncol. 2012;23(4):1074–80.

Karia PS, Jambusaria-Pahlajani A, Harrington DP, Murphy GF, Qureshi AA, Schmults CD. Evaluation of American joint committee on cancer, International Union against Cancer, and Brigham and Women's Hospital tumor staging for cutaneous squamous cell carcinoma. J Clin Oncol (American Society of Clinical Oncology). 2014;32(4):327–34.

Lacouture ME, Dréno B, Ascierto PA, Dummer R, Basset-Seguin N, Fife K, et al. Characterization and management of hedgehog pathway inhibitor-related adverse events in patients with advanced basal cell carcinoma. Oncologist. 2016;21(10):1218–29.

Locke J, Karimpour S, Young G, Lockett MA, Perez CA. Radiotherapy for epithelial skin cancer. Radiat Oncol Biol. 2001;51(3):748–55.

Lok B, Khan S, Mutter R, Liu J, Fields R, Pulitzer M, et al. Selective radiotherapy for the treatment of head and neck Merkel cell carcinoma. Cancer (Wiley Subscription Services, Inc., A Wiley Company). 2012;118(16):3937–44.

Manyam B, Garsa AA, Chin RI, Reddy CA, Gastman B, Vidimos AT, et al. A multi-institutional comparison of outcomes of immunocompromised and immunocompetent patients treated with surgery and radiation therapy for cutaneous squamous cell carcinoma of the head and neck. Int J Radiat Oncol Biol Phys. 2016;94(4):–948.

McDermott PN, Orton CG. The physics & technology of radiation therapy. Madison: Medical Physics Publishing Corporation; 2010.

McDowell LJ, Young RJ, Johnston ML, Tan T-J, Kleid S, Liu CS, et al. p16-positive lymph node metastases from cutaneous head and neck squamous cell carcinoma: no association with high-risk human papillomavirus or prognosis and implications for the workup of the unknown primary. Cancer. 2016;122(8):1201–8.

Mendenhall WM, Shaw C, Amdur RJ, Kirwan J, Morris CG, Werning JW. Surgery and adjuvant radiotherapy for cutaneous melanoma considered high-risk for local-regional recurrence. Am J Otolaryngol (Elsevier). 2013;34(4):320–2.

Mojica P, Smith D, Ellenhorn JDI. Adjuvant radiation therapy is associated with improved survival in Merkel cell carcinoma of the skin. J Clin Oncol (American Society of Clinical Oncology). 2007;25(9):1043–7.

Morton DL, Thompson JF, Cochran AJ, Mozzillo N, Nieweg OE, Roses DF, et al. Final trial report of sentinel-node biopsy versus nodal observation in melanoma. N Engl J Med (Massachusetts Medical Society). 2014;370(7):599–609.

I

Overgaard J, Gonzalez Gonzalez D, Hulshof MC, Arcangeli G, Dahl O, Mella O, et al. Randomised trial of hyperthermia as adjuvant to radiotherapy for recurrent or metastatic malignant melanoma. European Society for Hyperthermic Oncology. Lancet. 1995;345(8949):540–3.

Sause WT, Cooper JS, Rush S, Ago CT, Cosmatos D, Coughlin CT, et al. Fraction size in external beam radiation therapy in the treatment of melanoma. Radiat Oncol Biol. 1991;20(3):429–32.

Sekulic A, Migden MR, Oro AE, Dirix L, Lewis KD, Hainsworth JD, et al. Efficacy and safety of vismodegib in advanced basal-cell carcinoma. N Engl J Med. 2012;366(23):2171–9.

Siegel RL, Miller KD, Jemal A. Cancer statistics, 2015. CA Cancer J Clin. 2015;65(1):5–29.

Sim FH, Taylor WF, Pritchard DJ, Soule EH. Lymphadenectomy in the management of stage I malignant melanoma: a prospective randomized study. Mayo Clin Proc. 1986;61(9):697–705.

Strom T, Caudell JJ, Han D, Zager JS, Yu D, Cruse CW, et al. Radiotherapy influences local control in patients with desmoplastic melanoma. Cancer (7 ed.). 2014;120(9):1369–78.

Swartz JL, Griffith KA, Lowe L, et al. Features predicting sentinel lymph node positivity in Merkel cell carcinoma. J Clin Oncol. 2011;29(8):1036–41.

Touzé A, Le Bidre E, Laude H, Fleury MJJ, Cazal R, Arnold F, et al. High levels of antibodies against merkel cell polyomavirus identify a subset of patients with merkel cell carcinoma with better clinical outcome. J Clin Oncol (American Society of Clinical Oncology). 2011;29(12):1612–9.

Veness MJ, Howle J. Cutaneous carcinoma. In: Gunderson LL, Tepper JE, editors. Clinical radiation oncology. 4th ed. Philadelphia: Clinical Radiation Oncology; 2016. p. 763–776.e2.

Veronesi U, Adamus J, Bandiera DC, Brennhovd O, Caceres E, Cascinelli N, et al. Delayed regional lymph node dissection in stage I melanoma of the skin of the lower extremities. Cancer. 1982;49(11):2420–30.

Wang JT, Palme CE, Morgan GJ, Gebski V, Wang AY, Veness MJ. Predictors of outcome in patients with metastatic cutaneous head and neck squamous cell carcinoma involving cervical lymph nodes: improved survival with the addition of adjuvant radiotherapy. Head Neck (Wiley Subscription Services, Inc., A Wiley Company). 2011;34(11):1524–8.

Moore AY. Clinical applications for topical 5-fluorouracil in the treatment of dermatological disorders. J Dermatol Treat. 2009;20(6):328–35.

PART II

Central Nervous System

Chapter 2
Central Nervous System

Yao Yu, Steve E. Braunstein, Daphne A. Haas-Kogan, and Jean L. Nakamura

ANATOMY

- Meninges: dura mater, arachnoid mater, pia mater
- Precentral gyrus: primary motor strip
- Postcentral gyrus: primary somatosensory cortex
- Broca's area: dominant frontal lobe. Injury leads to expressive aphasia
- Wernicke's area: dominant temporal lobe. Injury leads to receptive aphasia
- Ventricular structures: foramen of Monroe, 3rd ventricle, aqueduct of Sylvius, 4th ventricle, foramen of Magendie, foramina of Lushka
- Cavernous sinus contents: CN III, IV, V1, V2, VI and internal carotid artery. Cavernous involvement commonly produces CN VI palsy
- Tumors with propensity for CSF spread: pineoblastoma, medulloblastoma, primitive neuroectodermal tumors (PNET), CNS lymphoma, germ cell tumors, ATRT.
- CN exits:
  - Superior orbital fissure = CN III, IV, VI, V1
  - Foramen rotundum = V2
  - Foramen ovale = V3
  - Foramen spinosum = middle meningeal artery and vein
  - Internal auditory meatus = CN VII, VIII

© Springer International Publishing AG, part of Springer Nature 2018   **37**
Eric K. Hansen and M. Roach III (eds.), *Handbook of Evidence-Based Radiation Oncology*, https://doi.org/10.1007/978-3-319-62642-0_2

- Jugular foramen = CN IX, X, XI
- Hypoglossal canal = CN XII
- Lateral plain film.
  - Hypothalamus = 1 cm superior to sellar floor.
  - Optic canal = 1 cm superior and 1 cm anterior to the hypothalamus.
  - Pineal body (supratentorial notch) = 1 cm posterior and 3 cm superior to external acoustic meatus.
  - Lens = 1 cm posterior to anterior eyelid, 8 mm posterior to line connecting lateral canthus. Median globe size = 2.5 cm.
  - Location of cribriform plate cannot always be correctly identified with lateral plain film alone (Gripp IJROBP 2004).
- Spinal cord.
  - Thirty-one pairs of spinal nerves: 8 cervical, 12 thoracic, 5 lumbar, 5 sacral, 1 coccygeal.
  - Spinal cord white matter is peripheral and gray matter is central.
  - Pia mater covers cord and condenses into dentate ligaments.
  - Arachnoid contains CSF (normal pressure 70–200 mm H_2O lying down, 100–300 mm H_2O sitting or standing, ~150 mg total volume).
  - Dura ends at S2.
  - Cord ends at L1 in adults, conus medullaris ends at ~L2 in adults; cord ends ~L3–4 in newborns.

EPIDEMIOLOGY

- US Incidence: 77,670 primary brain tumors, including 24,790 malignant and 52,880 non-malignant brain tumors per year. 16,616 deaths attributable to malignant brain tumors. (Ostrom Neuro Oncol 2015)
- Malignant tumors comprise ~40% of all primary brain/CNS tumors.
- Adult primary CNS tumors: 30–35% meningioma, 20% GBM, 10% pituitary, 10% nerve sheath, 5% low-grade glioma, <5% anaplastic astrocytoma, <5% primary CNS lymphoma.
- Of adult gliomas, ~80% are high-grade and ~20% are low-grade.
- Children: 20% of all pediatric tumors (second to ALL). Twenty percent pilocytic astrocytoma, 15–20% malignant

glioma/GBM, 15% medulloblastoma, 5–10% pituitary, 5–10% ependymoma, <5% optic nerve glioma.
, Possible etiologic associations: rubber compounds, polyvinyl chloride, N-nitroso compounds, and polycyclic hydrocarbons.
, Prior ionizing RT has been associated with new meningiomas, gliomas, and sarcomas (~2% at 20-years).

GENETIC SYNDROMES

, NF-1: von Recklinghausen, chromosome 17q11.2, 1/3500 live births, *NF1* encodes neurofibromin, autosomal dominant, 50% germline, 50% de novo, peripheral nerve sheath neurofibromas, café au lait spots, optic and intracranial gliomas, and bone abnormalities.
, NF-2: chromosome 22, 1/50,000 live births, *NF2* encodes merlin, autosomal dominant, bilateral acoustic neuromas, gliomas, ependymomas, and meningiomas.
, von Hippel-Lindau: chromosome 3, autosomal dominant, renal clear cell carcinoma, pheochromocytoma, hemangioblastoma, pancreatic tumors, and renal cysts.
, Tuberous sclerosis (Bourneville's disease): TSC1 on chromosome 9, TSC2 on chromosome 16, autosomal dominant, subependymal giant cell astrocytoma, retinal and rectal hamartomas.
, Retinoblastoma: Rb tumor suppressor gene, chromosome 13.
, Li-Fraumeni syndrome: germline p53 mutation.
, Turcot's syndrome: primary brain tumors with colorectal CA.
, Neuroblastoma: *MYCN* amplification commonly seen and serves as a prognostic factor.

IMAGING

, Common MRI sequences: T1 pre- and postgadolinium, T2, fluid attenuation inversion recovery (FLAIR), diffusion-weighted imaging (DWI), diffusion tensor imaging (DTI), perfusion, dynamic contrast enhanced (DCE), Spectroscopy.

, Enhancement with gadolinium is indicative blood–brain barrier (BBB) disruption.

, Acute blood is bright on T1 pregadolinium.

, Postop MRI with DWI should be completed within 48 h. Devascularized normal tissue at the resection cavity border can exhibit reduced diffusion and can enhance on subsequent scans. Must take caution to distinguish this enhancement from tumor recurrence or treatment effect.

RADIATION TECHNIQUE

FRACTIONATED EBRT

, Simulate patient with head mask.

, 3DCRT or IMRT for most lesions. 3DCRT provides better dose homogeneity, fewer hot spots. Inverse planning may allow greater sparing of critical structures and/or deliver hot spots in center of (hypoxic) tumor. Must be determined on a case-by-case basis.

, Fuse planning CT and MRI (preop vs. postop) to help delineate target volume. Postop MRs are better than preop MRs in most cases.

, Fetal dose from cranial RT = 0.05–0.1% of total dose (<0.1 Gy).

, Individual patient dose constraints should be determined based on physicians' clinical judgment and experience.

Table 2.1 Dose tolerance guidelines

EBRT using 1.8–2.0 Gy/fx	SRS single fraction max point dose
Whole brain 50 Gy	Brainstem 12 Gy
Partial brain 60 Gy	Visual pathway 12 Gy
Brainstem 54 Gy (Small volumes may receive up to 60 Gy)	Pituitary (mean dose) 12 Gy
Spinal cord 45 Gy	Infundibulum 12 Gy
Chiasm 50–54 Gy	Cochlea (mean) 4 Gy, max 8 Gy
Retina 45 Gy	Optic nerve and chiasm 8 Gy
Lens 10 Gy	
Inner ear 30 Gy (increasing risk of hearing deficit with increasing dose)	
Pituitary 30 Gy	
Hypothalamus 30 Gy	
Epilation 20–30 Gy	
Lacrimal gland: 30 Gy transient, 60 Gy permanent	

POSSIBLE RADIATION COMPLICATIONS

II

- *Acute*: alopecia, radiation dermatitis, fatigue, transient worsening of symptoms due to edema, nausea, and vomiting (particularly with brainstem [area postrema] and posterior fossa [PF] radiation), and otitis externa. Mucositis, esophagitis, and myelosuppression are associated with craniospinal irradiation and subside within 4–6 weeks after radiation (dose-related).
- *Subacute* (6 weeks to 6 months after RT): somnolence syndrome, fatigue, neurologic deterioration, perhaps caused by changes in capillary permeability and transient demyelination.
- *Late* (6 months to many years after RT): radiation necrosis, diffuse leukoencephalopathy (especially with chemo, but not necessarily correlated with clinical symptoms), hearing loss, retinopathy, cataract, visual changes, endocrine abnormalities (if hypothalamic-pituitary axis is irradiated), cerebrovascular accidents, cavernous malformations, Moyamoya syndrome, decreased new learning ability, short-term memory, and problem solving skills.

FUNCTIONAL STATUS

See Appendix A.

HIGH GRADE GLIOMA

PEARLS
- Most common primary malignant CNS tumor in adults.
- IDH mutant GBMs (6%), or secondary GBMs, have improved prognosis compared with IDH wild-type primary GBMs. (Sanson, JCO 2009; Yan, NEJM 2009)
- Multicentric tumors in <5% of cases.

- Incidence rises with age, peaks at 45–55 years (bimodal based on primary vs. transformation).
- Presentation: headache (50%), seizures (20%).
- Clinical prognostic factors: age, histology, KPS, extent of surgery, duration of symptoms (see RPA below)
- Molecular prognostic factors (favorable): IDH1/2 mutation, 1p/19q codeletion, ATRX loss, TP53 wt., TERT promoter wt., MGMT promoter hypermethylation.
- ATRX and TERT promotor mutations provide mechanism for telomere lengthening via alternative lengthening of telomeres and telomerase, respectively. ATRX is mutually exclusive with 1p/19q codeletion. (Abedalthagafi Modern Path 2013; Eckel-Passow NEJM 2015)
- Molecular characteristics have been integrated into pathologic diagnostic criteria. (Louis Acta Neuropath 2016)

IMAGING

- MR spectroscopy: Tumors have high choline, decreased creatine and NAA (neuronal marker). Necrosis has high lactate, decreased choline, creatine, and NAA.
- Dynamic MR perfusion: Astrocytomas have high CBV, increasing with grade. Oligodendrogliomas have high CBV due to hypervascularity. Radiation necrosis and tumefactive demyelinating lesions have low CBV.

PATHOLOGY

- Updated WHO diffuse glioma classification (2016)
  - Oligodendroglioma grade 2 or anaplastic oligodendroglioma grade 3: IDH mutant and 1p/19q codeleted (MS >8–10 yrs)
  - Diffuse astrocytoma grade 2 or anaplastic astrocytoma grade 3: IDH mutant, 1p/19q intact (MS 6–8 yrs)
  - IDH wild-type diffuse astrocytoma grade 2 is uncommon (review carefully to avoid misdiagnosis of lower grade lesions such as ganglioglioma)
  - IDH wild-type anaplastic astrocytoma grade 3 is rare with MS similar to glioblastoma IDH wild-type
  - Oligoastrocytoma diagnosis is discouraged because nearly all can be classified as oligodendroglioma or astrocytoma by genetic testing

ˌ Glioblastoma, IDH mutant (~10% of cases, secondary GBM, MS 2.6 yrs)
ˌ Glioblastoma, IDH wild-type (~90% of cases, de novo GBM, MS 15 mo)
ˌ Diffuse midline glioma H3 K27 M mutant (primarily in children, but sometimes adults too, includes brainstem, thalamic, spinal cord locations)
ˌ Astrocytoma grading (AMEN) = nuclear atypia, mitoses, endothelial proliferation, necrosis.

Table 2.2 TREATMENT RECOMMENDATIONS

High grade glioma (AA/AO, GBM)	Maximal safe resection, followed by one of the following: GBM/AA: RT (60 Gy/30 fx) + concurrent and adjuvant TMZ (EORTC/NCIC, RTOG 9813, EORTC 26951, CATNON) MGMT hypermethylation is predictive of response to TMZ-based chemoRT; TMZ should not be withheld for nonhypermethylated patients. AO/STR/Age ≥ 40: RT (60 Gy/30 fx) + concurrent and adjuvant TMZ (EORTC 26951, RTOG 9402, RTOG 9802; efficacy of TMZ vs. Nitrosurea-based chemo compared in NOA-04) AO/GTR/Age < 40: RT (54–60 Gy/30 fx) + concurrent and adjuvant TMZ (extrapolating from EORTC 26951, RTOG 9402, RTOG 9802, CODEL). We favor combined RT + TMZ over TMZ alone. NOA-04 showed RT alone and TMZ alone have similar outcomes, and RTOG 9802 showed low-grade oligodendrogliomas benefit from RT/PCV over RT alone. Randomized data comparing chemo alone vs. chemoRT are not mature; however, the TMZ alone arm of the CODEL clinical trial was closed due to inferior PFS and OS compared with the RT arms.
Elderly high grade glioma	Maximal safe resection, followed by one of the following: RT (40 Gy/15 fx or 60 Gy/30 fx) + concurrent and adjuvant TMZ (NCIC CE.6, EORTC/NCIC)
Poor performance status	Patients who are not eligible for combined modality therapy: MGMT hypermethylated: TMZ alone (NOA-04/NOA-08) MGMT not hypermethylated: RT alone 25/5 or 40/15 (NOA-04/NOA-08/IAEA) Very poor performance status: Best supportive care Best supportive care may be appropriate in selected patients with very poor performance status
Recurrence	Resectable and/or symptomatic: surgery. Consider adjuvant chemo or RT Unresectable, localized: Chemo and/or highly conformal RT (30–35 Gy/ 10 fx, 25 Gy/5 fx) or SRS Diffuse recurrence: chemo + best supportive care

STUDIES
PROGNOSIS

- *MGMT Promotor methylation* (Hegi NEJM 2005): 206 patients with GBM from the EORTC/NCIC trial (see below). Among MGMT-methylated cases, MS was 21.7 vs. 15.3 mo for chemoRT vs. RT alone. This effect may be dependent upon IDH status. (Wick Neurology 2013)
- *IDH mutation* (Yan NEJM 2009, Sanson JCO 2009): Mutations in IDH1 and IDH2 are common in gliomas, alter enzymatic function, and confer good prognosis. These mutations can be found in both oligodendrogliomas and in astrocytomas, indicative of an early genomic change.
- *RTOG-RPA Recalibration* (Mirimanoff JCO 2006): Recalibration and validation of the RTOG RPA classification using the EORTC/NCIC clinical trial (see below). Addition of TMZ to radiation improved survival in classes III and IV, but was of borderline significance for patients in class V. Median survival was 21, 16, and 10 months for patients in classes III, IV, and V treated with RT/TMZ.
- *EORTC/NCIC Nomogram* (Gorlia Lancet Oncol 2008): Nomogram using patient level data from the EORTC/NCIC clinical trial (see below). MGMT methylation status, age, performance status, extent of resection, MMSE, and baseline corticosteroid use were prognostic factors.

RT VERSUS OBSERVATION

- *BTSG 6901* (Walker JNS 1978): Phase III. 222 patients with HGG (90% GBM) treated with surgery. Patients were randomized adjuvant BCNU vs. WBRT vs. WBRT + BCNU or no therapy. RT was WB to 50 Gy, then boost to 60 Gy. RT ± BCNU improved MS by 3–6 months vs. observation or BCNU alone.
- *BTSG Meta-analysis* (Walker IJROBP 1979): Pooled analysis with 621 patients enrolled on 3 BTSG protocols of adjuvant radiation and/or chemotherapy. Median survival increased with radiation dose: Reported MS of 18, 13.5, 28, 36, 42 weeks for no RT, ≤45, 50, 55, 60 Gy, respectively.
- *Keime-Guibert* (NEJM 2007): Phase III. 81 patients >70 years with GBM and KPS >70 after surgery (~50%

biopsy only, ~30% GTR) randomized to best supportive care ± RT (50.4 Gy/28 fx to enhancing tumor +2 cm). Trial stopped early because RT improved MS (4.3 vs. 7.3 mo; 53% risk reduction for mortality) and MPFS (1.4 vs. 3.7 mo) independent of the extent of surgery, with no difference in QOL and cognitive evaluations.

DOSE ESCALATION/SRS BOOST

, *BTSG Meta-analysis* (Walker JIROBP 1979): See above

, *RTOG 74-01* (Nelson NCI Monogr 1988): Phase III, 626 patients randomized to 1) WBRT 60 Gy, 2) WBRT 60 Gy + 10 Gy boost, 3) WBRT 60 Gy + BCNU, 4) WBRT 60 Gy + semustine/dacarbazine. No benefit to RT dose escalation. Chemotherapy improved 2-yr. survival for patients age 40–60.

, *MRC* (Bleehen, Br J Cancer 1991): Phase II, 474 patients randomized to 45 Gy/20 fx vs. 60 Gy/30 fx. No adjuvant chemo. MS 9 vs. 12 mo favoring high dose arm ($p = 0.007$).

, *Michigan* (Chan JCO 2002): Single arm, patterns of failure. 34 patients treated to 90 Gy with 3D-CRT. Median survival 11.7 mo. 78% of failures central, 13% in field, 2% marginal, and 0% distant.

, *RTOG 9305* (Souhami IJROBP 2004): Phase III, 203 resected patients randomized to EBRT (60 Gy) + BCNU ± SRS. Dose of radiosurgery dependent on tumor size (range 15–24 Gy). No difference in survival (MS 13.5 months) or patterns of failure.

ELDERLY/SHORT COURSE

, Bauman (IJROBP 1994): Single arm prospective study of short-course radiation for poor-prognosis GBM. Twenty-nine patients age ≥ 65 or KPS ≤50 treated with WBRT (30 Gy/10 fx). Median survival 6 months.

, *NCIC* (Roa JCO 2004): Phase III trial of 100 patients with GBM age ≥ 60 and KPS ≥50 randomized to 60 Gy/30 fx vs. 40 Gy/15 fx. No difference in MS (5.1 vs. 5.6 mo). Fewer patients in the short course RT arm required increased steroids (23 vs. 49%). Not a non-inferiority trial.

, *Nordic* (Malmström Lancet Oncol 2012): 291 patients, age > 60, randomized to TMZ alone, HFX-RT (34 Gy/10 fx), or ST-RT (60 Gy/30 fx); of these, 51 patients were randomized between TMZ and HFX-RT. Median survival was 8.3 vs. 7.5 vs. 6.0 mo, respectively; in pairwise comparisons, MS was better with TMZ than ST-RT (HR 0.7, p = 0.01). For patients aged > 70, survival was better for TMZ (HR 0.3) or HFX-RT (HR 0.59) than ST-RT.

- *IAEA* (Roa JCO 2015): Phase III non-inferiority trial of 98 patients with resected GBM who were either elderly (age ≥ 65), frail (KPS 50–70%), or both, randomized to 25 Gy/5 fx vs. 40 Gy/15 fx. No difference in overall survival (median survival 7.9 mo vs. 6.4 mo), progression-free survival (4.2 vs. 4.2 mo), or quality of life (at 4 weeks and 8 weeks).

- *NCIC CTG CE.6* (Perry, NEJM 2017): Phase III trial of 562 patients age ≥ 65, ECOG 0–2, randomized to short-course RT (40 Gy/15 fx) +/– 21 days concurrent and 12 months adjuvant TMZ. Adding TMZ improved MS (9.3 vs. 7.6 mo) and median PFS (5.3 vs. 3.9 mo). Among MGMT methylated patients, median survival was 13.5 vs. 7.7 mo favoring chemoRT (p = 0.0001). Among MGMT unmethylated patients, median survival was 10 vs. 7.9 mo, p = 0.055. TMZ resulted in more nausea, vomiting, and constipation.

CHEMORT (GBM)

- *BTSG 7201* (Walker NEJM 1980): Phase III, 476 patients (84% GBM, 11% AA) randomized to postop MeCCNU vs. RT alone vs. RT + MeCCNU vs. RT + BCNU. RT was WB 60 Gy/30–35 fx. RT ± chemo increased MS compared to chemo alone (37–43 vs. 31 weeks). No difference between MeCCNU and BCNU.

- *EORTC/NCIC* (Stupp NEJM 2005, Lancet Oncol 2009): Phase III, 573 patients with newly diagnosed glioblastoma (16% biopsy only, 40% GTR, 44% STR) randomized to RT vs. RT + concurrent and adjuvant temozolomide. RT was 60 Gy/30 fx. Temozolomide was concurrent daily (75 mg/m²/day) and adjuvant (150–200 mg/m²/day × 5 days) q4 weeks × 6 months. Concurrent and adjuvant temozolomide significantly improved MS (14.6 vs. 12.1 mo) and 5-year OS (9.8 vs. 1.9%). MGMT gene promoter methylation was the strongest predictor for outcome and benefit from temozolomide.

NOA-08 (Wick Lancet Oncol 2012): Phase III non-inferiority, 412 elderly patients with AA or GBM (89% GBM), age > 65, KPS ≥60, randomized to postop (40% bx only) TMZ vs. RT. 25% non-inferiority margin. MS (8.6 vs. 9.6 mo, $p_{non-inferiority} = 0.033$) and Median EFS (3.3 vs. 4.7 mo, $p_{non-inferiority} = 0.043$). MGMT status was available in 209 patients (53% hypermethylated). Unplanned subset analysis showed MGMT status was predictive of response to TMZ, but not RT. Hypermethylated patients had longer OS and EFS with TMZ than RT; nonhypermethylated patients did better with RT. Grade 2–4 toxicity more common in TMZ arm. Criticism: did not compare with TMZ + RT.

CHEMORT (GRADE III)

RTOG 9402 (Cairncross JCO 2013): Phase III, 291 patients with grade 3 AO/AOA (43% 1p/19q codeleted) randomized to postop PCV followed by RT vs. RT alone. Pathology confirmed by central review. No difference in MS (4.9 vs. 4.7 yrs), but PCV chemo improved PFS (2.6 vs. 1.7 years). Patients with 1p/19q codeletion had longer PFS and OS. Benefit of PCV only observed for PFS in codeleted tumors.

EORTC 26951 (van den Bent JCO 2013): Phase III, 368 patients with AO/AOA (22% 1p/19q codeleted) randomized to postop RT followed by PCV vs. RT alone. No central pathology review. Median OS (40 vs. 31 mo, $p = 0.23$), PFS (23 vs. 13mo, $p = 0.002$). 1p/19q loss was associated with better PFS and OS. In codeleted tumors, MS not reached vs. 112 mo). In contrast to RTOG 9402, PFS and OS benefit seen in both codeleted and non-codeleted tumors; benefit of PCV greater in codeleted tumors.

NOA-04 (Wick JCO 2009, Neuro Oncol 2016): Phase III, 318 patients with grade 3 AA/AO/AOA randomized to postop RT (arm A) vs. chemo (arm B). Chemotherapy was randomized to PCV (B1) vs. TMZ (B2). At 1st progression, patients in the RT arm (arm A) were randomized to receive PCV or TMZ, with cross over to the alternate chemo at 2nd progression. Patients in the chemo arm (arm B), received RT at 1st progression with cross over to alternate chemo at 2nd progression. Extent of resection, MGMT status, and IDH1 mutation were prognostic. TTF, PFS, and OS similar between arms. No difference between TMZ and PCV in arm B, but study not powered for this analysis.

˻ *RTOG 9813* (Chang ASCO 2015, Bell ASCO 2016): Phase III, closed due to accrual. 196 patients with AA randomized to chemoRT with TMZ vs. Nitrosurea (NU). Oncologic outcomes were similar (MS 3.9 vs. 3.8 yrs), PFS and TTP were similar. TMZ was better tolerated. Post hoc multivariate analysis of mutational status showed IDH1 and ATRX mutations were favorable prognostic factors for PFS and OS. There was a trend for worse outcomes with TERT promotor mutations.

˻ *CODEL* (Jaeckle AAN 2016): Phase III, 1p/19q codeleted anaplastic gliomas. This trial has undergone several modifications. The original trial had four arms: RT alone, RT/adjuvant PCV, RT/concurrent and adjuvant TMZ, TMZ alone. The RT alone arm closed after RTOG 9402/EORTC 26951. On interim analysis, the TMZ alone arm showed inferior PFS (2.5 vs. not reached, $p < 0.001$) and OS (HR 9.2, $p = 0.048$). The TMZ alone arm was closed, and the trial continued with 2 arms: RT + PCV vs. RT + concurrent and adjuvant TMZ, and eligibility was opened to grade 2 tumors.

˻ *CATNON* (van den Bent ASCO 2016): Phase III, 1p/19q noncodeleted anaplastic gliomas randomized to RT alone, RT/concurrent TMZ, RT/adjuvant TMZ, RT/concurrent and adjuvant TMZ. Preliminary results (ASCO 2016) show a survival benefit for adjuvant TMZ. Results for concurrent TMZ are pending.

REIRRADIATION

˻ *Germany* (Combs JCO 2005): 172 previously radiated patients with recurrent gliomas (71 Grade II, 42 Grade III, 59 Grade IV) were treated at recurrence with reirradiation in 2 Gy/fx to median 36 Gy.

˻ *Jefferson* (Fogh JCO 2010): 147 previously radiated (median 60 Gy) patients with recurrent high grade gliomas (71% GBM) were treated at recurrence with reirradiation in 3.5 Gy/fx to median 35 Gy. 57% were re-resected prior to recurrence. Median interval to retreatment was 8 months. MS 11 and 10 mo for grade III and grade IV patients. Reirradiation was well-tolerated. One patient experienced grade 3 late CNS toxicity. No subsequent surgeries were performed for symptomatic radionecrosis; all subsequent surgeries showed evidence of disease progression.

TUMOR TREATING FIELDS

, *TTF at recurrence* (Stupp Eur J Cancer 2012): Phase III, 237 patients with recurrent GBM randomized to TTF vs. chemotherapy (clinician discretion). Median two prior treatments. MS 6.6 vs. 6.0 months ($p = 0.27$), 5-yr. PFS 21 vs. 15% ($p = 0.13$). Responses similar in both arms (14 vs. 9.6%). Severe adverse events in 6 and 16% ($p = 0.022$), favoring TTF.

, *Maintenance TTF* (Stupp JAMA 2015): Phase III, interim analysis of 310 initial patients (695 enrolled) with newly diagnosed GBM treated with surgery and chemoradiotherapy (60 Gy, TMZ), randomized to adjuvant TMZ ± TTF. PFS (7.1 vs. 4.0 mo, $p = 0.001$) and MS (20.5 vs. 15.6 mo, $p = 0.004$) favored addition of TTF.

BEVACIZUMAB

, *RTOG 0825* (Gilbert NEJM 2014): Phase III, randomized, placebo controlled, 637 patients with supratentorial glioblastoma treated with RT (60 Gy/30 fx), concurrent and adjuvant TMZ ± bevacizumab, followed by maintenance bevacizumab until progression or unacceptable toxicity. Median PFS 10.7 vs. 7.3 mo, favoring bevacizumab. Median survival was 15.7 vs. 16.1 mo (NS). Increased symptom burden and declines in HR-QOL and neurocognitive function in bevacizumab arm.

, *AVAglio* (Chinot NEJM 2014): Phase III, randomized, placebo controlled, 458 patients with supratentorial glioblastoma treated with RT (60 Gy/30 fx), concurrent and adjuvant TMZ ± bevacizumab, followed by maintenance bevacizumab until progression or unacceptable toxicity. Industry sponsored. Median PFS 10.6 vs. 6.2 mo, favoring bevacizumab. Median survival was 16.8 vs. 16.7 mo (NS). Maintenance of HR-QOL was longer in the bevacizumab arm.

DOSE/VOLUME

- UCSF:
  - 1.8–2 Gy/fx to 59.4–60 Gy to enhancing and mass-like FLAIR +1.5–2 cm.
- RTOG:
  - 1.8–2 Gy/fx to 45–46 Gy followed by boost to 59.4–60 Gy
  - GTV1 = T1 enhancement + T2/FLAIR. CTV1 = GTV1 + 2 cm margin
  - Boost: GTV2 = T1 enhancement. CTV2 = GTV2 + 2 cm
- PTV = CTV + 0.3–0.5 cm

FOLLOW-UP

- MRI 2–6 weeks after RT and then every 2–3 months.
- Pseudoprogression can occur in 15–30% of patients treated with chemoRT. Advanced imaging, clinical correlation, and prognostic factors can help differentiate true progression for pseudoprogression. (Taal Cancer 2008)

LOW GRADE GLIOMA

PEARLS

- Ten percent of primary intracranial tumors, 20% of gliomas.
- Age of onset: 30–40 for Grade II gliomas and 10–20 for pilocytic astrocytomas.
- Presentation: seizures (60–70%, better prognosis) > headache > paresis.
- Favorable prognostic factors: age < 40 years, good KPS, GTR, low proliferative indices, oligodendroglioma (IDH1 mutant, 1p/19q codeleted), absence of neurologic symptoms, size <6 cm.
- LGGs are often nonenhancing
- Pathology: See WHO 2016 revised classification above in High Grade Glioma section

Table 2.3 **TREATMENT RECOMMENDATIONS**

Pilocytic astrocytoma, subependymoma	GTR/STR, followed by observation.
Subependymal Giant Cell Astrocytoma (SEGA)	Surgery and mTOR inhibitors
Adult low-grade gliomas	Maximal safe resection (GTR or STR) Low-Risk (eg. IDHmut, 1p/19q codeleted, GTR): Observation vs. chemoRT vs. chemo High-Risk (eg. IDHwt, STR, Age ≥ 45): ChemoRT vs. chemo Refractory Seizures: chemoRT Treatment of adult low grade gliomas is controversial, and standards of care with regard to new molecular classifications have yet to be established. Based upon RTOG 9802, addition of chemotherapy to radiation should be strongly considered for every subgroup. PCV was used in 9802; however, TMZ is an acceptable alternative based upon NOA-04 and RTOG 9813. Results from ongoing trials will further clarify management. For patients who wish to delay radiation, chemotherapy alone may be a reasonable alternative for asymptomatic grade 2 gliomas. Timing of chemotherapy and radiation is the subject of an ongoing trial.

STUDIES
TIMING OF RT

　EORTC 22845 "Non-Believers" (Karim IJROBP 2002, van den Bent Lancet 2005): Phase III. 311 patients (WHO 1–2, 51% A, 14% O, 13% OA) treated with surgery (42% GTR, 19% STR, 35% Bx) randomized to observation vs. postop RT (54 Gy). RT improved median progression-free survival (5.3 vs. 3.4 yrs), 5-year PFS (55 vs. 35%), but not OS (68 vs. 66%). 65% of patients in the observation arm received salvage RT. No difference in rate of malignant transformation (66–72%). Seizures were better controlled at 1-year in the radiation arm.

　RTOG 9802 Low-Risk Arm (Shaw JNS 2008): Phase II. 111 patients with supratentorial LGG age < 40, GTR (determined by neurosurgeon) who were observed after surgery. 5-year OS and PFS were 93% and 48%. Poor prognostic factors included initial size ≥4 cm, A/OA histology, residual ≥1 cm on MRI review.

- *EORTC 22033* (Baumert Lancet Oncol 2016, Reijneveld Lancet Oncol 2016): Phase III. 477 patients with previously-untreated high-risk low-grade glioma (age > 40, radiographic progression, tumor size >5 cm, tumor crossing midline, or neurologic symptoms) randomized to RT alone 50.4 Gy or TMZ up to 12 cycles. Median FU 4 yrs. Median PFS overall: RT 51 mo, TMZ 40 mo. IDH1/2 mutation and 1p19q codeletion status are prognostic factors. Median PFS IDH mutated and codeleted: RT 62 mo, TMZ 55 mo. Median PFS IDH mutated & noncodeleted: RT 55 mo, TMZ 36 mo. Median PFS IDH wild type: RT 19 mo, TMZ 24 mo. No difference in 3 yr. HRQOL or cognitive dysfunction by MMSE. Criticism: RT alone arm has similar PFS to the RT alone arm of RTOG 9802, but is clearly inferior to the RTOG 9802 chemoRT arm.

DOSE

- *EORTC 22844 "Believers"* (Karim IJROBP 1996): Phase III. 343 patients (WHO 1–2, astro., oligo. and mixed) treated with surgery (25% GTR, 30% STR, 40% biopsy) randomized to postop RT 45 Gy vs. 59.4 Gy (shrinking fields). No difference in OS (59%) or PFS (49%). 5-year OS was better with oligo histology (75 vs. 55), and age < 40 (80 vs. 60%). Age < 40, oligo histology, small tumor size, GTR, and good neurologic status are prognostic factors.
- *INTERGROUP* (Shaw JCO 2002): Phase III. 203 patients (WHO I–II, astro, oligo, mixed) treated with surgery (14% GTR, 35% STR, 51% Bx) randomized to postop RT 50.4 Gy vs. 64.8 Gy. No difference in 5-year OS (72% low dose vs. 64% high dose). Best survival in patients age < 40, tumor <5 cm, oligo histology and GTR. Increased Grade 3–5 toxicities (2.5 vs. 5%) with higher dose. Pattern of failure: 92% in field, 3% within 2 cm of RT field.

CHEMORT

- *RTOG 9802 High-Risk Arm* (Buckner NEJM 2016): Phase III. 251 patients with high-risk (age ≥ 40 or STR/biopsy)

LGG randomized to postop RT alone vs. RT → PCV × 6 cycles. RT 54 Gy to FLAIR +2 cm margin. PFS and OS curves diverged with long-term follow-up. OS (7.8 vs. 13.3 yrs) and PFS (4.0 vs. 10.4 yrs) favored the RT-PCV arm. 10-year PFS and OS were 21% vs. 51%, and 40% vs. 60%, respectively. On post hoc analysis, PFS was improved for oligodendrogliomas, oligoastrocytomas ($P < 0.05$), and a trend was observed in astrocytomas ($p = 0.06$), and IDH R132H mutants with chemoRT. OS was improved for oligodendrogliomas, oligoastrocytomas, and R132H mutants ($p \leq 0.05$), but the finding was not significant for astrocytomas.

RTOG 0424 (Fisher IJROBP 2015): Phase II. 129 patients with high-risk LGG (≥3 risk factors: age ≥ 40, astrocytoma, bihemispheric, tumor ≥6 cm, neurologic function status >1) treated with TMZ, concurrent and adjuvant TMZ. 3-year OS was 73.1%, which was higher than the prespecified historical control ($p < 0.001$). Stratification by molecular subtype not yet reported.

MOLECULAR SUBTYPE

TCGA (NEJM 2015): Exome, DNA copy number, DNA methylation, mRNA expression, microRNA expression, targeted protein expression profiling for 293 lower-grade gliomas. Three groups identified based upon IDH, 1p/19q, and TP53 status. IDHmut 1p/19q codeleted tumors have the most favorable prognosis, followed by IDHmut 1p/19q intact, which are associated with TP53 mutations and ATRX loss. IDHwt low-grade gliomas behave similarly to primary GBM.

Mayo-UCSF (Eckel-Passow NEJM 2015): Genomic analysis of 1087 gliomas was performed from 3 different data sets (Mayo Clinic, UCSF, TCGA). Tumors were classified based upon IDH, 1p/19q codeletion, and TERT promotor mutations. 5 subtypes were identified. Subtype correlated with prognosis in grade II/III gliomas; patients with glioblastomas had poor prognosis regardless of subtype.

DOSE

EBRT: 1.8 Gy/fx to 50.4–54 Gy.
GTV = T1 enhancement and mass-like FLAIR.
CTV = GTV + 1–2 cm margin.
PTV = CTV + 0.3–0.5 cm.

FOLLOW-UP
- MRI 2–6 weeks after RT, then every 6 months for 5 years, then annually.

CNS LYMPHOMA

PEARLS
- Approximately 2% of intracranial tumors.
- EBV present in 60–70% of immunodeficient, and 15% immunocompetent patients.
- Median age: 55 years in immunocompetent, and 31 years in immunocompromised patients.
- Multifocal tumors: 25–50% of immunocompetent, and 60–80% of immunodeficient patients.
- MRI: single or multiple periventricular masses, intensely enhancing.
- In AIDS patients, smaller lesions may demonstrate ring enhancement. Differential diagnosis includes toxoplasmosis.
- Leptomeningeal involvement in 1/3 of patients.
- Retinal and vitreous seeding in 15–20% of patients.
- In primary intraocular lymphoma, 80% develop CNS involvement within 9 months.
- Histology: 90% are DLBCL.
- Presentation: focal deficits, seizures, headache, lethargy, confusion. Neck or back pain (spinal cord involvement). Blurred vision or floaters (ocular involvement, which presents in ~20% of patients).
- Workup: MRI brain and spine, biopsy, ophthalmologic exam, CXR, CSF cytology, CBC, EBV titer, HIV serology. CT chest, abdomen, and pelvis and bone marrow biopsy, testicular ultrasound, PET scan. Hold steroids, if possible, prior to diagnostic procedures
- Systemic or intrathecal methotrexate given with RT has synergistic neurotoxicity.

Table 2.4 TREATMENT RECOMMENDATIONS

Surgery	Biopsy for tissue diagnosis. Extensive resection does not improve OS
steroids	Should be withheld until after biopsy. Ninety percent have clinical response. Forty percent have shrinkage. Ten percent have complete resolution on imaging. Response is short-lived and tumor recurs weeks after steroid discontinuation
General management	If KPS ≥40 and acceptable renal function → high-dose methotrexate-based regimen followed by WBRT 24–36 Gy at 1.8–2-Gy/fx, If PR → boost gross disease to 45 Gy. If CSF positive or spinal MRI positive, consider intrathecal chemotherapy. If eye exam positive, intraocular chemotherapy or RT to globe
	If KPS <40 or renal dysfunction → WBRT. If CSF positive or spinal MRI positive, consider intrathecal chemotherapy and focal spinal RT. If eye exam positive, RT to globe. Consider non-methotrexate chemo alternatives
	For patients >60, may omit WBRT if CR to chemo and reserve RT for recurrence
	For leptomeningeal spread, use intrathecal chemo or CSI to 39.6 Gy with additional 5.4–10.8 Gy to gross disease
	See Chap. 3 regarding ocular lymphoma

STUDIES

- *RTOG 8315* (Nelson IJROBP 1992): Phase II. 41 patients with CNS lymphoma treated with 40 Gy WBRT +20 Gy boost to tumor bed. 88% of recurrences were within the boost field. MS 12.2 months. 2-year OS 28%. Better survival in patients with KPS >70 and Age < 60.

- *RTOG 8806* (Schultz JCO 1996): Phase I/II. 51 patients with HIV-negative CNS lymphoma treated with CHOD × 2 (cytoxan, adriamycin, vincristine, dexamethasone) → WB to 41.4 Gy and boost to 59.4 Gy. No difference in MS when compared with RTOG 83–15.

- *RTOG 9310* (DeAngelis JCO 2002): Phase II. 102 HIV-negative CNS lymphoma patients treated with chemo × 5 (IV/IT MTX, vincristine, procarbazine) → WBRT 45 Gy → high-dose cytarabine. 58% CR, 36% PR, MPFS 24 months, MS 36.9 months. 15% with severe delayed neurotoxicity. Better survival in patients aged < 60 (50 vs. 22 months, $p < 0.001$).

- *MSKCC* (Gavrilovic, JCO 2006): 57 patients treated with high-dose MTX ± RT. Five-year OS 74% for patients aged < 60 treated with RT, but no difference in MS for patients aged > 60 with or without RT (29 months). 25%

neurotoxicity for patients aged < 60 with RT vs. 75% for those aged > 60 with RT vs. 3% if no RT.

, *G-PCNSL-SG-1* (Thiel Lancet Oncol 2010, Korfel Neurology 2015): Phase III. 409 patients with primary CNS lymphoma treated with HD-MTX + ifosfamide, randomized to treatment with or without WBRT (45 Gy/30 fx). Patients randomized to no RT received cytarabine for < CR after HD-MTX + ifosfamide. WBRT improved PFS (15.4 vs. 9.9) by ITT, but did not prolong OS (32.4 vs. 36.1 mo). 74 patients in the non-RT arm received RT at salvage.

SURVIVAL

, RT alone MS 12 months, 2-year OS 20–30%.
, Chemo (high-dose MTX-based) + WBRT MS 30–60 months, 2-year OS 55–75%.
, Survival recursive partitioning analysis from MSKCC, confirmed with RTOG data. (Abrey JCO 2006)
  , I: Age < 50: MS 8 years, failure-free survival (FFS) 2 years.
  , II: Age ≥ 50 and KPS ≥70: MS 3 years, FFS 1.8 years.
  , III: Age ≥ 50 and KPS <70: MS 1 years, FFS 0.6 years.

PEDIATRIC GLIOMAS

DIFFUSE INTRINSIC PONTINE GLIOMA (DIPG)

, Incidence peaks between ages 4 and 6 years
, Diagnosis often established based on imaging. Biopsy often omitted due to concerns regarding toxicity, but recently biopsy is undertaken more frequently for molecular characterization.
, Molecular subgroups have been described (Sturm Nat Rev Cancer 2014, Gajjar JCO 2015) and stratified clinical trials are ongoing.
, On pathology, 70–80% of DIPGs are high-grade gliomas. Grade (grades II-IV) is not prognostic for DIPGs.
, Mutations in H3-K27 M are common in DIPGs and other midline gliomas.(Gajjar JCO 2015)
, RT (54 Gy at 1.8 Gy/day) remains the standard treatment as altered fractionation and systemic agents have failed to

improve outcomes. (Hargrave Lancet Oncol 2006, Jansen Cancer Treat Rev 2012) Hypofractionated RT remains investigational. (Negretti JNO 2011, Zaghloul Radiother Oncol 2014)

, Symptomatic improvement is seen in >75% of patients and radiographic improvement is seen in ~50% of patients. (Hargrave Lancet Oncol 2006, Jansen Cancer Treat Rev 2012)

, Median survival ~12 months.

OPTIC PATHWAY GLIOMAS

, Commonly diagnosed in pediatric patients, and associated with NF-1. Patients with NF-1 have a favorable prognosis compared with sporadic optic pathway gliomas.

, May involve the optic nerves, chiasm, hypothalamus, anterior 3rd ventricle

, Most commonly pilocytic or fibrillary astrocytomas; both diffuse and circumscribed growth patterns have been described.

, Diagnosis can be established based upon imaging characteristics for prechiasmatic lesions. Suprasellar, and hypothalamic lesions may require pathologic diagnosis to differentiate from other suprasellar tumors.

, Treatment with radiation can result in durable control, but must be balanced against potential long-term toxicities.

, Patients aged 7 and younger are often treated with chemotherapy and deferred radiation.

, Long-term PFS is 60–90%, and OS is 90–100%.

, Chiasmatic/hypothalamic gliomas have long-term OS 50–80%.

LOW GRADE GLIOMAS

, Histologies include pilocytic astrocytoma, pleomorphic xanthoastrocytoma, subependymal giant cell astrocytoma, and diffuse astrocytoma.

, Pilocytic astrocytomas (previously juvenile pilocytic astrocytoma) have excellent prognosis after resection, and observation is often recommended, especially after gross total resection.

- These tumors are commonly found in the posterior fossa, tectum, or involving the optic pathway.
- Alterations in the Raps-Raf-MEK-ERK pathway are common, often occurring via mutations in NF1 or KIAA1549-BRAF gene fusion.
- Pleomorphic xanthoastrocytomas commonly have BRAF V600E mutations and CDKN2A inactivation.
- Patients with tuberous sclerosis are at risk for development of subependymal giant cell astrocytomas (SEGAs).
  - Typically identified prior to the age of 25.
  - Observation is typically recommended for asymptomatic tumors.
  - Symptomatic tumors may be treated with surgery and/or mTOR inhibitors.
  - Radiation may be associated with increased risk for secondary malignancy.
- Gangliogliomas have astrocytic and neuronal features on histology, and commonly present with seizures. EFS with surgery alone is excellent. (Luyken Cancer 2004)
- In contrast to adult low grade gliomas, mutations in IDH are infrequent among pediatric low grade gliomas. (Gajjar JCO 2015)
- Epigenetic and genetic profiling has revealed multiple molecular subtypes, termed K27, G32, IDH, RTK-1, Mesenchymal, and PXA-like. Mutations in H3.1 and H3.3 at the K27 locus are enriched in pediatric midline gliomas, including DIPGs. (Sturm Nat Rev Cancer 2014, Gajjar JCO 2015)

HIGH GRADE GLIOMAS

- Treatment typically includes maximal safe resection, followed by combination chemo-radiotherapy.
- Addition of chemotherapy (prednisone, nitrosurea, vincristine) to adjuvant radiation improves survival (CCG 943); however, trials with TMZ have not shown benefit. The optimal adjuvant therapy regimen is under investigation. Clinical trial enrollment is encouraged.
- High dose chemotherapy with autologous stem cell rescue that delays or omits radiation has demonstrated favorable durable control rates, at the cost of treatment-related morbidity and mortality.

Table 2.5 **TREATMENT RECOMMENDATIONS**

Diffuse brainstem glioma	Conventionally fractionated radiation (54 Gy at 1.8 – 2 Gy/day) Hypofractionated radiation may be appropriate in selected patients.(Janssens IJROBP 2013, Zaghloul Radiother Oncol 2014) Alternative fractionation schemes and chemotherapy have not proven effective. Improved understanding of the biology of these tumors has led to development of new trials using targeted therapies. Clinical trial enrollment is encouraged
Optic pathway gliomas	Biopsy is not required for diagnosis, but can be helpful for suprasellar lesions and in patients without NF-1. Asymptomatic: Observation NF-1, mildly symptomatic tumors can be closely observed as progression is uncommon, even after diagnosis. NF-1, symptomatic patients should be treated with surgery and/or chemotherapy. Radiation should be deferred as long as possible and can often be avoided. Young patients (age < 7) with sporadic, symptomatic tumors can be treated with debulking and/or chemotherapy. Radiation is typically reserved for progressive disease. Older patients (age > 10) can be treated with chemotherapy or radiation Treatment with surgery is effective, but must be balanced against the risks to vision, cognition, and neuroendocrine function.
Grade I gliomas	Pilocytic astrocytoma: Surgery + observation. Radiation reserved for salvage Subependymal Giant Cell Tumor: Surgery and/or mTOR inhibitors Gangliogliomas: Surgery + observation.
Low grade gliomas	Maximal safe resection, followed by: Chemotherapy vs. Observation Radiation should be delayed and reserved for progressive disease to reduce neurocognitive effects.
High grade gliomas	Surgery + adjuvant radiation and chemotherapy The benefit of chemoRT over RT alone was demonstrated in CCG 943. The optimal chemotherapy regimen remains under investigation.
Very young children (age < 3 years)	Children <3 years of age can be treated with systemic therapy alone and deferred radiation.

STUDIES
OPTIC PATHWAY GLIOMAS

₃ *Pittsburgh* (Flickinger Cancer 1988): 36 patients with optic pathway glioma, including 25 patients treated with radiation. At 5, 10, and 15 years, OS was 96%, 90%, and 90%, respectively and PFS was 87%. A dose response was observed for PFS; and a recommendation for 45–50Gy was recommended.

, *Institute Curie* (Bataini IJROBP 1991): 57 patients with optic pathway gliomas were treated with radiation (40–60 Gy over 5–7 weeks). 37% were confined to the chiasm, and 63% extended beyond the chiasm. 5- and 10-year OS was 83.5%. 15%, 46%, and 22% had complete response, partial response, stable disease. 94% had stabilization or improvement of vision

, *Joint Center* (Tao IJROBP 1997): 42 patients with optic pathway gliomas, including 29 treated with radiation. Among radiated patients, 18, 38, and 46% of patients had ≥50% radiographic response at 24, 48, and 60 months. 10-year FFP and OS were 100% and 89%. Stable or improved vision observed in 81%.

LOW-GRADE GLIOMAS

Pilocytic Astrocytomas

, *Zürich* (Burkhard JNS 2003): Registry analysis, 55 patients with pilocytic astrocytoma. 40% cerebellar, 35% supratentorial, 11% optic pathway/hypothalamus, 9% brainstem. 10-year OS 96%. Seven patients treated with postoperative radiation, which did not impact survival.

, *NCCTG/RTOG* (Brown IJROBP 2004): 20 adults with pilocytic astrocytomas treated with RT after biopsy (3 patients), or observation after GTR (11 patients) or STR (6 patients). With median follow-up of 10 years, 5-year PFS was 95%. Close observation sufficient for adult patients with resected pilocytic astrocytomas; insufficient evidence for tumors treated with stereotactic biopsy only.

, *Multi-institutional* (Tihan Am J Surg Path 2012): 116 pilocytic astrocytomas treated at 4 institutions. Median age 6 years. Age ≥ 3 years, gross total resection, and treating institution prognostic factors. 10-year PFS (35% vs. 90%) favored GTR.

Gangliogliomas

, *Germany* (Luyken Cancer 2004): 184 patients with gangliogliomas treated at a single center. 97% presented with long-term seizures, 80% of tumors were located in the temporal lobe. 93% of tumors were WHO grade I, and

GTR was achieved in 80%. 84% of patients with epilepsy had durable seizure relief, and the 7.5 year recurrence rate was 97%.

Subependymal Giant Cell Astrocytoma

- *Everolimus* (Krueger Neurology 2013): 28 patients with Tuberous Sclerosis and SEGA were treated with everolimus. Median follow-up was 34 months, and 25 patients remained on treatment at the time of report. 65–79% of patients experienced ≥30% tumor volume reduction.

Low Grade Glioma

- *Conformal Radiation* (Merchant JCO 2009): Phase II trial of conformal radiation for LGGs. 78 pediatric patients with low grade gliomas (50 pilocytic astrocytomas, 13 optic pathway gliomas, 3 gangliogliomas, 1 pleomorphic xanthoastrocytoma, and 11 grade 2 gliomas). RT was 54 Gy/30 fx, with a 1 cm CTV margin and a 0.5 cm PTV margin. At 10-years, EFS was 77% for grade I tumors and 64% for grade 2 tumors. Adverse events were carefully documented. Incidence of vasculopathy at 6-years was 5%. Caveat: predominantly WHO grade I tumors.
- *Packer Regimen* (Packer JCO 1993, JNS 1997): 78 patients, mean age 3, with newly diagnosed LGGs (astro, oligo, oligo-astro, mixed low-grade tumor, ganglioglioma) treated with surgery (≤50% debulking) and chemotherapy (carboplatin/vincristine). 2- and 3-year PFS were 75% and 68%. Younger patients (age ≤ 5) fared better (74 vs. 39%).
- *UCSF* (Prados JNO 1997): 42 patients (median age 5) with LGGs treated with chemotherapy. Eligible histologies included astros (fibrillary or pilocytic), oligos, oligoastros, and ganglioglioma. Patients had either newly diagnosed or progressive tumors, but prior chemotherapy or radiation was excluded. Chemotherapy consisted of 6-thioguanine, procarbazine, dibromodulcitol, lomustine, and vincristine.
- *COG A9952* (Ater JCO 2012): 274 patients (age < 10) with previously untreated low grade gliomas with progressive or residual disease randomized to treatment

with one of two treatment regimens: carboplatin/vincristine (CV) vs. thioguanine/procarbazine/lomustine/vincristine (TPCV). 5-year EFS and OS were 45% and 86% for all patients. 5-year EFS was 39% in the CV group, vs. 52% in the TPCV group (log-rank $p = 0.10$). Young age, tumor size >3 cm, and thalamic location were poor prognostic factors.

HIGH GRADE GLIOMAS

- *CCG 943* (Sposto JNO 1989): Prospective randomized trial of 58 patients with high grade astrocytoma, randomized to surgery followed by RT ± chemo (nitrosurea, vincristine, prednisone). 5-year EFS was improved with chemoRT (18 vs. 36%). EFS ($p = 0.026$) and PFS ($p = 0.067$) were improved with chemoRT.
- *CCG 945* (Finlay JCO 1995): 172 patients (median age 10) with high grade gliomas (33% GBM, 48% AA, 19% other) outside the brainstem or spinal cord, treated with radiation and concurrent chemotherapy. Patients were randomized between two chemotherapy regimens: lomustine/vincristine/prednisone vs. eight-in-one chemotherapy (vincristine/CCNU/procarbazine/hydroxyurea/ cisplatin/mannitol/cytarabine/dacarbazine/methylprednisolone). 5-year PFS and OS were 33% and 36%, respectively. There was no difference in PFS between regimens. 8-in-1 chemo was more toxic.
- *ACNS 0126* (Cohen Neuro Oncol 2011): Single-arm prospective trial of RT vs. RT + concurrent and adjuvant TMZ for patients with high grade gliomas and diffuse intrinsic pontine gliomas. Among 107 patients with anaplastic astrocytoma, glioblastoma, or gliosarcoma, 90 patients were eligible. 3-year EFS and OS were 11% and 22%, respectively. TMZ did not improve EFS or OS. MGMT overexpression was correlated with worse survival.
- *HIT-GBM-C* (Wolff Cancer 2010): Single-arm prospective study of 97 patients with DIPG or HGG treated with fractionated radiation and concurrent and adjuvant chemotherapy. Chemotherapy included 1 cycle of cisplatin/etoposide/vincristine (PEV), weekly vincristine, and 1 cycle of cisplatin/etoposide/ifosfamide (PEI). Adjuvant

PEI and valproic acid was given. OS was 19% at 5 years, similar to historical controls. Among patients with GTR, 5-year survival was 63%, compared with 17% (historical control, p = 0.003).

VERY YOUNG CHILDREN
- See section in medulloblastoma
- Head Start II/III HGG (Espinoza Pediatr Blood Cancer 2016): 32 patients with AA (n = 19), GBM (n = 11), or other HGG (n = 2), excluding patients with predominantly brainstem gliomas, were treated with induction chemotherapy, marrow-ablative chemotherapy, followed by autologous hematopoietic cell rescue. 5-year EFS and OS was 25% and 36%, respectively.

EPENDYMOMA

PEARLS
- Ependymal cells form the lining of the ventricular system and the central spinal canal.
- 2nd most common group of primary pediatric brain tumor (10%)
- Among pediatric patients, 90% of tumors are intracranial, 60% arise in the posterior fossa. Among adults, tumors predominantly arise in the spine. 10–30% of 4th ventricular tumors extend through the foramen magnum.
- Increased frequency of spinal cord ependymomas in patients with NF2.
- Less than 7% incidence of CSF spread at diagnosis, up to 15% ultimately, rare without local progression. More common with infratentorial and high grade tumors.
- Extent of resection and age are important prognostic factors.(Merchant Lancet Oncol 2009)
- Molecular subtypes have recently been identified, which may aid in risk stratification. (Witt Cancer Cell 2011, Pajtler Cancer Cell 2015)

Table 2.6 TREATMENT RECOMMENDATIONS

Subependymoma	Maximal safe resection and observation
Spinal cord ependymoma	Maximal safe resection GTR: Observation STR: Adjuvant RT (50.4 Gy)
Pilomyxoid ependymoma (commonly in the filum terminale)	Maximal safe resection GTR: Observation STR: Adjuvant RT (50.4–54 Gy) can improve local control. Lower doses can be used for spinal cord lesions
Grade II/III, gross total resection	Maximal safe resection M0: Adjuvant conformal RT (54–60 Gy) Spine MRI/CSF+: CSI (30–36 Gy) + Focal boost (54–60 Gy for local disease, 45 Gy for spine)
Grade II/III, subtotal resection	Maximal safe resection Adjuvant chemotherapy, followed by second look surgery and conformal RT (54–60 Gy) Spine MRI/CSF+: CSI (30–36 Gy) + Focal boost (54–60 Gy for local disease, 45 Gy for spine)
Recurrence	Maximal surgical resection Radiation if no prior RT; consider SRS Chemotherapy, best supportive care
Very young children (age < 3 years)	Maximal safe surgical resection Chemotherapy alone with delayed radiation

STUDIES

- *Molecular Subtype* (Witt Cancer Cell 2011, Pajtler Cancer Cell 2015): 9 molecular subtypes were identified across 3 anatomic compartments: supratentorial, posterior-fossa, and spinal cord. Pediatric posterior fossa ependymomas predominantly fall into two categories: EPN_A and EPN_B. Among supratentorial ependymomas, 3 subgroups were identified, including subgroups characterized by YAP1-fusion and RELA-fusion. The RELA-fusion subtype was recently incorporated into the 2016 revised WHO criteria.

- *Conformal Radiation* (Merchant Lancet Oncol 2009): 153 patients (median age 2.9 years) with localized ependymomas (85 anaplastic, 122 infratentorial) treated with surgery (125 GTR, 17 NTR, 11 STR) followed by definitive radiation (59.4 Gy or 54 Gy) with 1 cm CTV margin. At 7-years, local control was 87%, EFS was 69%, and OS was 81%. Cumulative incidences of local and distant failure were 16% and 11%.

- *Extent of Resection* (Ramaswamy JCO 2016): Molecular subtype was retrospectively evaluated in 4 independent cohorts of 820 patients. Molecular subtype is a strong prognostic factor. Extent of resection remains a prognostic factor after controlling for subtype. Patients with EPN_PFA had poor prognosis, particularly after subtotal resection. Patients with EPN_PFB had excellent prognosis after surgery, even with delayed radiation; these patients may be candidates for clinical trials with delayed radiation.

- *Chemo with Deferred RT* (Grundy Lancet Oncol 2007): 89 patients age 3 or younger with intracranial ependymomas. Patients were treated with 1 year of chemotherapy following maximal safe resection, reserving RT for progression. 50 of 80 patients with localized disease progressed. 5-year freedom from radiation was 42%. 5-year EFS and OS for nonmetastatic patients was 41.8% and 63.4%, respectively. Among patients who progressed, median time to progression was 1.6 years.
- *Myxopapillary Ependymoma* (Weber Neuro Oncol 2015): 183 patients treated with surgery ± radiation. 10-year OS and PFS were 92.4 and 61.2%. Poor prognostic factors included age < 36 years (10-year PFS 40% vs. 85%), surgery alone (<40% vs. 70% for patients treated with surgery + RT), and extent of resection. Dose ≥50.4 Gy was associated with improved local and distant control on univariate analysis. 3.3% patients developed secondary cancers, only half of which received radiation. Other series have shown 10% recurrence risk after GTR. (Sonneland Cancer 1985)
- *Spinal Cord Ependymomas* (Abdel-Wahab IJROBP 2006): 183 patients with spinal cord gliomas, including 120 patients with ependymomas. 15-year PFS and OS were 35 and 75%, respectively. Young age and subtotal resection were poor prognostic factors. Postoperative radiation did not improve outcomes on multivariate analysis, but this may have been due to selection bias.

FOLLOW-UP
- MRI brain and spine (if initially positive) every 3–4 months for the first year, every 4–6 months for the second year, then every 6–12 months.

PINEAL TUMORS

PEARLS

- Adults: 1% of primary brain tumors. 30–40% percent are germinomas and 10–20% NGGCTs.
- Children: 5% of pediatric brain CA. Fifty percent are germ-cell tumors and 25–33% pineal parenchymal tumors. Incidence peaks at age 10–12 years. M:F 3:1.
- Nongerminomatous germ-cell tumors (NGGCTs) include embryonal carcinoma (produces both β-HCG and AFP), endodermal sinus tumor (elevated AFP), choriocarcinoma (elevated β-HCG), and malignant teratoma.
- High risk of CSF dissemination among pineoblastomas (up to 50%), and NGGCTs.
- Presenting symptoms: sellar (visual field cut), suprasellar (endocrinopathies), and pineal (hydrocephalus, Parinaud's syndrome).
- Parinaud's syndrome: paralysis of upward gaze, pseudo-Argyll Robertson pupil, convergence-retraction nystagmus, Collier's sign, sun-setting sign.
- Classic triad: diabetes insipidus, precocious or delayed sexual development, visual deficits.
- Workup: MRI brain and spine, baseline ophthalmologic exam, CSF and serum markers (β-HCG and AFP), and CSF cytology.
- A whole ventricular radiation (WVI) radiation atlas is available on the QARC website.

PINEAL PARENCHYMAL TUMORS

- Pineal parenchymal tumors include a spectrum of histologies, ranging from pineocytomas, grade 2 pineoparenchymal tumors of intermediate differentiation (PPTID), grade 3 PPTID, and pineoblastomas.
- Pineoblastomas are WHO grade IV tumor, similar to PNETs.
  - Associated with germline RB mutations and bilateral retinoblastoma (trilateral retinoblastoma).
  - Rates of craniospinal dissemination are high (~50%). Craniospinal imaging and prophylactic CSI is recommended.

GERMINOMAS

- Similar to seminoma in men, dysgerminoma in women
- MRI: hypodense, well-circumscribed, homogeneous enhancement
- AFP must be undetectable
- Historically, treatment with CSI (30–36 Gy) + local boost (45–50 Gy) has yielded 10-year survival ~90%. Current protocols (ACNS 1123) aim to reduce the dose and volume of RT via addition of chemotherapy.
- Elevated HCG may be a poor prognostic indicator. Patients with HCG > 100 or disseminated disease are considered high-risk and treated per the NGGCT stratum in ACNS 1123.

NONGERMINOMATOUS GERM CELL TUMOR

- Elevated serum or CSF AFP and marked elevated B-HCG
- Surgery and neoadjuvant chemotherapy improve survival compared with RT alone
- Second look surgery is recommended for patients with partial response as mature teratoma and nonviable scar can present as residual disease on imaging. (Weiner Neurosurg 2002, Souweidane JNS 2010)

TREATMENT RECOMMENDATIONS AND OUTCOME

Pineoblastoma	Maximal safe resection, CSI (23.4–36 Gy) + local boost to 54–55.8 Gy, and chemo. Radiosurgery boost possible for gross residual.
Pineocytoma	Maximal safe resection. GTR: observation STR: Postop RT can be considered
Mature teratoma	Maximal safe resection + observation

Germinoma (ACNS 1123)	Localized disease: (omit CSI)
	    Tissue diagnosis, followed by induction chemotherapy (carboplatin/etoposide)
	    CR/CCR: reduced dose RT (18 Gy WVI + 12 Gy Boost)
	    PR/SD: second look surgery
	    PD or residual disease on 2nd look surgery: RT (off protocol)
	    PR/SD with limited residual: RT (24 Gy WVI + 12 Gy boost)
	Metastatic disease:
	    RT (24 Gy CSI + 16–20 Gy boost)

continued

NGGCT (ACNS 1123)	Localized disease
	Tissue diagnosis (unless elevated AFP), followed by induction chemotherapy (carboplatin/etoposide, ifosfamide/etoposide)
	CR/PR: RT (30.6 Gy WVI + 23.4 Gy boost)
	PR/SD/PD:
	Normalized markers: 2nd look surgery
	Positive markers: Surgery, Chemotherapy, or RT
	Metastatic disease (per ACNS 0112)
	Tissue diagnosis, followed by induction chemotherapy (carboplatin/etoposide, ifosfamide/etoposide)
	Non-responders: Consider thiotepa + etoposide/ autologous peripheral blood stem cell rescue
	All patients: RT (36 Gy CSI + 18 Gy local boost, 9 Gy boost to mets).

STUDIES
INTRACRANIAL GERM CELL TUMORS

- *ACNS 1123* (Ongoing): Phase II trial of response-based radiation for localized intracranial germ cell tumors.
  - Patients with NGGCTs are treated with induction chemotherapy, followed by RT (30.6 Gy WVI + 23.4 Gy boost) for patients with complete or partial response. Nonresponders with normalized markers treated with second-look surgery.
  - Patients with germinomas are treated with induction chemotherapy. Patients with CR/CCR are treated with dose-reduced RT (18 Gy WVI + 12 Gy boost), those with PR or SD with residual disease (0.5–1.5 suprasellar or 1–1.5 cm pineal) treated with standard-dose RT (24 Gy WVI + 12 Gy boost). Patients who have second-look and who have no viable tumor may have reduced-dose RT; those with viable tumor or progressive disease treated off-protocol.
- *UCSF/Stanford* (Haas-Kogan IJROBP 2003): 93 patients intracranial GCTs (49 germinomas, 16 NGGCTs, 28 no biopsy). Of 6 patients with NCCTG treated without CSI, only 1 failure occurred, which was salvaged. Of 35 germinomas treated without CSI, no isolated spinal cord relapses occurred. Of 21 patients with localized germinomas, no local recurrences occurred among 18 patients

treated with WVI. CSI for GCTs; WVI recommended over WBRT.

- *COG* (Kretschmar Pediatr Blood Cancer 2007): Phase II trial. 12 patients with germinomas and 14 patients with NGGCTs were treated with induction chemotherapy, followed by response-based RT. 91% of germinomas and 55% of NGGCTs responded to induction chemotherapy with promising outcomes.

GERMINOMAS

- *MAKEI 83/86/89* (Bamberg JCO 1999): 60 patients with germinoma treated with RT alone, including 49 patients treated with reduced-dose RT (30 Gy CSI + 15 Gy boost). 5-year EFS 91%, OS 93.7%. Moderately reduced-dose radiation associated with excellent outcomes.
- *SIOP CNS GCT 96* (Calaminus Neuro Oncol 2013): 235 patients (190 localized, 45 metastatic) with germinoma. Localized disease was treated with reduced-dose RT (24 Gy CSI + 16 Gy boost) or induction chemo (carboplatin/etoposide) + local RT (40 Gy). Metastatic patients with or without induction chemo, followed by CSI (24 Gy CSI + 16 Gy boost). For local disease, no difference in 5-year OS, but PFS was lower in the local RT arm (97 vs. 88%). The pattern of failure was predominantly ventricular, outside the RT field. Metastatic patients had 5-year EFS and OS of 98%.

NGGCTS

- *ACNS 0122* (Goldman JCO 2015): 102 patients (median age 12 years) with NGGCTs treated with induction chemotherapy ± second look surgery for partial responders. Patients with PR or CR underwent RT (36 Gy CSI + local boost to 54 Gy, 45 Gy to sites of metastatic disease). Patients with less than CR underwent high-dose consolidation with thiotepa and etoposide, followed by autologous peripheral blood stem cell rescue, prior to the same RT. 5-year EFS and OS were 84% and 93%. No therapy-related deaths.

MEDULLOBLASTOMA

PEARLS

- Twenty percent of pediatric CNS tumors, 40% of all PF tumors.
- The second most common pediatric CNS tumor: low-grade glioma 35–50%, medulloblastoma 20%, brainstem glioma 10–15%, high-grade glioma 10%.
- M: F = 2:1. Varies according to molecular subgroup.
- Median age 5–6 years in children and 25 years in adults.
- 30–40% of patients have CSF spread at the time of diagnosis.
- Poor prognostic factors: male, age < 5, M1 disease.
- At diagnosis, 2/3 of patients are standard risk and 1/3 are high risk.
- Common presentation: vomiting, nausea, ataxia, headaches, papilledema, CN palsy, and motor weakness.
- Differential diagnosis of Posterior Fossa (PF) mass: medulloblastoma, ependymoma, astrocytoma/glioma, and metastasis.
- PF syndrome = difficulty swallowing, truncal ataxia, mutism, respiratory failure in 10–15% of children after PF craniotomy for medulloblastoma.
- Extent of residual disease has been considered a dominant prognostic factor, and used for risk stratification in clinical trials. (Chang Radiology 1969) This has been challenged in the era of molecular subgroups. (Thompson Lancet Oncol 2016)

WORKUP

- H&P
- MRI of the brain (preop and postop within 24–48 h after surgery)
- MRI of the spine to rule out leptomeningeal spread
- CSF cytology
- Bilateral bone marrow biopsy
- Consider bone scan and CXR
- Baseline audiometry, IQ, TSH, CBC, and growth measurements

STAGING

M0	No metastases
M1	Microscopic cells in CSF
M2	Gross Nodular seeding in cerebellar, cerebral subarachnoid space, third or lateral ventricles
M3	Gross Nodular seeding in spinal subarachnoid space
M4	Extraneuraxial metastasis

RISK CATEGORIES

Standard risk: age > 3 years and GTR/STR with <1.5 cm^2 residual and M0

High risk: age < 3 years or >1.5 cm^2 residual, or M+, anaplasia

SURVIVAL

Standard-risk DFS 60–90%

High-risk DFS 20–40%, increased to 50–85% with adjuvant chemo

MOLECULAR SUBGROUPS (NORTHCOTT JCO 2011, NAT REV CANCER 2012)

WNT: 10% of medulloblastoma. 95% 5-year OS, 5–10% M+ at dx

SHH: 30% of medulloblastoma. 75% 5-year OS, 15–20% M+ at dx

Group 3: 25% of medulloblastoma. 50% 5-year OS, 40–45% M+ at dx

Group 4: 35% of medulloblastoma. 75% 5-year OS, 35–50% M+ at dx

Table 2.7 TREATMENT RECOMMENDATIONS

General management	Hydrocephalus and increased ICP: steroids and VP shunt before attempting resection
Standard risk	Surgical resection → CSI 23.4 Gy at 1.8-Gy/fx with boost to the tumor bed (IFRT) to 54 Gy with concurrent vincristine → PCV chemo. DFS ~ 80%
High risk	Surgical resection → postop CSI 36–39 Gy at 1.8-Gy/fx, with entire PF and mets >1 cm boosted to 54 Gy with concurrent vincristine → PCV chemo. DFS ~ 60%
Very young children (age < 3 years)	Surgery → intensive chemo/HCT. Reserve RT for salvage. DFS ~ 30–40%

The next generation of clinical trials will stratify patients according to molecular subgroup.

STUDIES
ROLE OF CHEMOTHERAPY

- *CCSG/RTOG* (Evans JNS 1990): Phase III. 233 patients with medulloblastoma → surgery → randomized to postop RT vs. postop chemoRT followed by chemo × 1 year. RT was CSI 35–40 Gy with PF boost to 50–55 Gy + spinal mets to 50 Gy. Chemo was concurrent vincristine, adjuvant vincristine, CCNU, and prednisone ×1 year. 5-year OS 65% in both arms. Chemo improved EFS in T3–4, M1–3 (46% for chemoRT vs. 0% for RT alone).

- *SIOP I* (Tait Eur J Cancer 1990): Phase III. 286 patients with medulloblastoma → surgery → randomized to postop RT vs. postop chemoRT followed by chemo × 1 year. RT was CSI 30–35 Gy/PF boost to 50–55 Gy. 5/10-year OS 53/45%. Initial DFS and OS benefit of chemo disappeared with longer F/U secondary to late failures in chemo arm. Subgroups T3–4 and gross residual disease still benefited from chemo.

- *PNET 3* (Taylor JCO 2003, Bull JCO 2007): Phase III. 217 patients with M0–1 medulloblastoma → surgery → randomized to postop RT vs. postop chemoRT. Chemo was vincristine/etoposide/carboplatin/cyclophosphamide. Patients age 3–16 received CSI 35 Gy + 20 Gy PF boost. Trial closed early due to low accrual in RT-alone arm. 5-year OS 71%. 5-year EFS significantly better for chemoRT arm (74 vs. 60%, $p = 0.04$). Follow-up QOL paper reported poorer outcomes in behavior and quality of life for chemoRT arm.

TIMING OF CHEMOTHERAPY

- *SIOP II* (Bailey Med Ped Onc 1995): 364 patients with low-risk (GTR/STR, no brainstem involvement, M0) and high-risk (gross residual, brainstem invasion, or M+) medulloblastoma. All low-risk patients randomized to surgery + chemo → RT vs. surgery → RT. Chemo was vincristine, procarbazine, and methotrexate. RT was randomized to either standard dose 35 Gy CSI + 20 Gy PF boost vs. low-dose 25 Gy CSI + 30 Gy PF boost. All high-risk patients received 35 Gy CSI + adjuvant vincristine and CCNU. Results: preRT chemo did not improve 5-year

EFS (58% with chemo and 60% without chemo). For low-risk, no difference with RT alone for 35 vs. 25 Gy (5-year EFS 75 vs. 69%).

STANDARD/AVERAGE/LOW RISK

- *POG8631/CCG923* (Thomas JCO 2000): 88 low-risk (age 3–21, Chang T1–3a, residual <1.5 cm, M0) medulloblastoma → randomized to CSI 23.4 Gy/PF 54 Gy vs. CSI 36 Gy/PF 54 Gy. No chemo. A trend toward improved outcome with 36 Gy. However, overall EFS is suboptimal in the absence of chemo.

- *POG A9961* (Packer JCO 2006, Neuro Oncol 2013): 379 average-risk medulloblastoma patients (age 3–21, no disseminated disease, residual <1.5 cm) → CSI 23.4 Gy/PF 55.8 Gy randomized one of two adjuvant chemotherapy regimens (CCNU, cisplatin, vincristine vs. CPM, cisplatin, vincristine). No difference between chemo arms. 5 and 10-year EFS were 81% and 75.8%, respectively. 5 and 10-year OS were 87% and 81%. The cumulative incidence of secondary malignancies at 10-years was 4% (primarily gliomas).

- *St. Jude* (Merchant IJROBP 2008): 86 newly diagnosed, average-risk medulloblastoma. RT began within 28 days of definitive surgery, and consisted of CSI (23.4 Gy), conformal RT to PF tumor bed (36 Gy), and primary site RT (55.8 Gy). 5-year EFS 83%, comparable to historical CSI + PF RT.

- *ACNS 0331* (Abstract IPSNO 2016): Phase III randomized noninferiority trial for standard risk medulloblastoma. Patients age 3–7 underwent double-randomization to standard (23.4 Gy) vs. reduced dose (18 Gy) CSI, and posterior fossa (PFRT) boost (54 Gy total) vs. tumor bed (IFRT) boost (54 Gy total). Children 8 years and older received standard dose CSI, but underwent randomization for boost field size. All children received weekly vincristine concurrently with radiation, and 9 cycles of maintenance chemotherapy. 5-year OS and EFS for PFRT vs. IFRT were 84.8 vs. 84.7% and 80.5 vs. 82.4%, respectively. 5-year OS and EFS for standard vs. reduced dose CSI were 85.3 vs. 78.2% and 82.1 and 71.4%, respectively. Conclusions support IFRT noninferior to PFRT, but reduced dose CSI was inferior to standard dose.

HIGH-RISK

- *CCG 921* (Zeltzer JCO 1999): high-risk patients (age 1.5–21, or M1–4, or T3–4, or residual >1.5 cm^2) randomized between 2 arms. Arm 1: CSI 36 Gy/PF 54 Gy/spinal mets 50.4–54 Gy (age < 3 received CSI 23.4 Gy/PF 45 Gy) with concurrent vincristine, followed by VCP × 8. Arm 2: "8 in 1" chemo × 2 → RT → "8 in 1" chemo × 8. "8 in 1" chemo was vincristine, prednisone, lomustine, hydroxyurea, procarbazine, cisplatin, cyclophosphamide, and cytarabine. Better 5-year PFS with VCP (63 vs. 45%, p = 0.006). Seventy-eight percent 5-year PFS for M0, age > 3, ≤1.5 cm^2 residual.
- *POG 9031* (Tarbell JCO 2013): 226 high-risk patients. Randomized to chemo1 → RT → chemo2 vs. RT → chemo1 → chemo2. Chemo1 was cisplatin/etoposide × 7 weeks. Chemo2 was vincristine/cyclophosphamide. RT was CSI 35.2–44 Gy/PF 53.2–56.8 Gy. Results: no difference in 5-year EFS (70 vs. 66%) or OS (73 vs. 76%).
- *St. Jude Medullo-96* (Gajjar Lancet Oncol 2006): 134 patients (age 3–21). Low-risk patients received CSI (23.4 Gy)/PF (36 Gy)/primary bed (55.8). High-risk patients received CSI 39.6 Gy/boost to 55.8 Gy. All patients received dose-intensive chemo × 4 cycles. Low-risk 5-year EFS 83%; high risk 70%.
- *CCG 99701* (Jakacki JCO 2012): 81 patients with high-risk medulloblastoma were treated with 36 Gy CSI with concurrent carboplatin + vincristine, followed by adjuvant chemotherapy (cyclophosphamide, vincristine ± cisplatin). 5-year OS and PFS were 82% and 71%.
- See ACNS 0332

VERY YOUNG CHILDREN

There is a high risk for neurocognitive impairment with radiation for children < 36 months old. Clinical trials have focused on chemotherapy to delay or omit radiation for this age group.

- *POG* (Duffner NEJM 1993): 102 patients, single arm. This study addressed whether postop chemo can delay RT until after 36 mo. Patients <36 months old with malignant brain tumors (including medulloblastoma, glioma, ependymoma, PNET, etc.) underwent surgery, and chemotherapy (24 vs. 12 mo, depending on age), followed by delayed RT. Chemo was cyclophosphamide, vincristine, cisplatin, etoposide. RT was CSI 35.2 Gy/PF 54 Gy (reduced to 24 Gy/50 Gy if complete response after surgery/chemo). 39% CR after the first 2 cycles of chemo. No difference in 2-year PFS (39 vs. 33%) and OS (53 vs. 55%) between age groups (<2 vs. >2 years). 34% PFS and 46% OS for medulloblastoma at 2 years. These results suggest that postop chemotherapy can safely delay radiation until after 36 months.

, *German BTSG* (Rutkowski NEJM 2005). Phase II: 43 patients (age < 3) with medulloblastoma treated with surgery (40% GTR, 32% STR, and 28% macro mets) and intensive chemo alone. Chemo was cyclophosphamide, vincristine, methotrexate, carboplatin, etoposide, and intrathecal methotrexate. RT was reserved for salvage. 5-year PFS was 82 vs. 50 vs. 33% and 5-year OS was 93 vs. 56 vs. 38% for GTR vs. STR vs. macro mets. For M0 patients, 5-year PFS and OS were 68% and 77%, respectively. 62% chemo response rate in patients with measurable disease after surgery. Age > 2, desmoplastic histology and M0 were good prognostic factors. Mean IQ after treatment higher than those who received RT.

, *CCG 9921* (Geyer JCO 2005): 284 patients <36 months-old with malignant brain tumors treated with surgery (167 < 1.5 cm residual, 117 > 1.5 cm residual) were randomized to two chemo regimens (no difference in response or EFS). Patients with residual disease after chemo or with M+ at presentation received RT (tumor +1.5 cm margin or CSI, respectively) at age 3 (18 months for medullo or supra PNET) or after 8 cycles chemo. 5-year EFS 27%, OS 43%. 58% of patients alive at 5-years spared RT. 5-year EFS for medullo and supra-PNET were 32% and 17%.

, *Head Start I/II Medulloblastoma* (Mason JCO 1998, Dhall Pediatr Blood Cancer 2008): The Head Start protocols established the feasibility of surgery followed by intensive chemotherapy with autologous bone-marrow transplant for young patients with brain tumors, avoiding radiation in ~70% of medulloblastoma cases. Head Start I/II have been completed, and Head Start III/IV are ongoing. 21 patients <36 mo of age with nonmetastatic medulloblastoma were treated on Head Start protocols I and II. Patients received surgery, followed by induction chemo, myeloablative chemo, and

ABMR. Radiation was reserved for relapse. 5-year EFS and OS were 52% and 70% for all patients. 70% of patients avoided radiation. 20% treatment related mortality.

, *P9934* (Ashley JCO 2012): 74 patients 8–36 mo of age were treated with induction chemotherapy, followed by age/response adjusted CRT (18 vs. 23.4 Gy CSI, 50.4 vs. 54 Gy PF boost). 4-yr. EFS and OS were 50% and 69%, which compared favorably to POG 9233. Neurocognitive outcomes were assessed via telephone.

, See ACNS 0334

ONGOING TRIALS

, *ACNS0332*: Phase III randomized trial for other than average risk medulloblastoma. Patients were treated with surgery, postoperative chemoradiotherapy, and adjuvant systemic therapy. Patients were randomized to chemoRT with vincristine ± carboplatin, and standard maintenance chemotherapy ± isoretinoin.

, *ACNS0334:* Phase III randomized trial for children age < 36 months with high-risk medulloblastoma or PNET. Trial designed to evaluate the addition of high-dose methotrexate to the four drug induction chemo regimen of vincristine, etoposide, cyclophosphamide, cisplatin. Patients then undergo second surgery, followed by consolidation and PBSC rescue. RT at discretion of individual institution.

TREATMENT PLANNING
TRADITIONAL PRONE TECHNIQUE

, Simulate patient prone, hyperextend the neck to avoid PA beam exiting through mouth. Head mask for immobilization. Use CT for treatment planning. Anesthesia may be required for patients unable to cooperate.

, Simulate the spine field first.

, Superior border: C2 without exiting through mouth (slight neck hyperextension may help minimize exit through mouth).

- Inferior border: bottom of S2 or lowest level of the thecal sac as seen on MRI.
- Lateral borders: 1 cm lateral to the lateral edge of pedicles, increase by 1–2 cm in sacrum to cover spreading of neural foramen inferiorly.
- Field length < 35 cm, use 100 cm SSD; >35 cm, use 120 cm SSD.
- In some patients, two adjacent spinal fields may be required to encompass the spine. When two spinal fields are used, match at depth of mid spinal cord.
- Use CT or MRI to determine depth of spinal cord.
- Simulate the cranial field second. Two parallel-opposed lateral fields.
  - Superior border flashes the skin. Inferior border 0.5–1 cm on cribriform plate, 1 cm on middle cranial fossa. One cm anterior to the vertebral bodies, 2–2.5 cm posterior to eye markers. May angle gantry to align eyelid markers to avoid radiation to the lens.
- *Collimator angle* (of the cranial field) to match diverging spinal fields = arctan(1/2 length superior spine field/SSD).
- *Couch angle* (of the spinal field) to match diverging cranial fields = arctan(1/2 length cranial field/SAD). The foot of couch is rotated toward the side treated. Alternative to couch angle is to beam split lower border of the cranial field to avoid any overlaps at any depth with upper border of the spinal field.
- Various beam-split techniques may be utilized to avoid overlaps at depth (see Fig. 2.1).
- *Gap shift* = For every 9 Gy, extend the cranial field inferiorly by 1 cm, shift the upper spine field inferiorly by 1 cm, and shorten the lower spine field by 1 cm. Need to recalculate couch angle each time.
- *PF boost*: use 3DCRT and CT/MRI for planning. CTV consisting of PF tumor bed +2 cm anatomically confined margin is favored over entire PF boost.

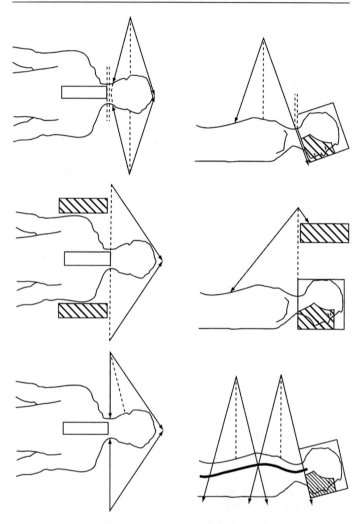

Fig. 2.1 Various techniques of craniospinal irradiation

ALTERNATIVE DELIVERY METHODS

- Protons may be employed to reduce exit dose and toxicity, particularly the risk for secondary malignancy
- Tomotherapy may avoid the need to match fields, but greater whole body dose exposure
- VMAT may be used to increase conformality and reduce toxicity

CRANIOPHARYNGIOMA

PEARLS

, Benign, partially cystic, epithelial tumors.

, Arise from Rathke's pouch in the sellar region.

, Histologic subtypes: adamantinomatous, squamous papillary.

, Five to ten percent of pediatric intracranial tumors, ages 5–14.

, Bimodal distribution: 55% occur in children and 45% are over age 20 with another peak between ages 55 and 65.

, Present with neuroendocrine deficits such as diabetes insipidus or growth failure, visual field cuts, decreased acuity, increased ICP, cognitive, and behavioral changes.

, MRI: solid nodule (calcified and contrast enhancing) with cystic component filled lipoid, cholesterol laden fluid ("crankcase oil").

, Cysts can reaccumulate during RT. During treatment, imaging every 1–2 weeks is recommended to avoid geometric miss due to cyst enlargement.

, May develop invaginations into adjacent brain, causing a glial reaction.

, Limited surgery with postoperative radiation results in similar local control as radical surgery with a more favorable toxicity profile. (Merchant IJROBP 2002)

, Radiation can be delayed, particularly for pediatric patients, and is effective at salvage. (Stripp IJROBP 2004)

, Papillary tumors are associated with BRAF V600E mutations, and adamantinomatous tumors are associated with beta-catenin mutations, although these are not mutually exclusive. (Oikonomou JNO 2005, Brastianos Nat Genetics 2014, Larkin Acta Neuropath 2014)

, There are case reports of response to BRAF inhibitors. (Brastianos JNCI 2016)

STUDIES

, *British Columbia* (Lo IJROBP 2014): 123 patients, including 39% treated with STR + RT, 28% with STR alone, and 11% treated with cyst drainage + RT. 10-year PFS was ~82% for STR or cyst drainage followed by RT. Toxicities included visual deterioration (27%), hormonal deficiency (76%), diabetes insipidus (45%), seizures (16%), and CVE

(11%). CVE was particularly common among patients who received intralesional bleomycin.

ʒ *St. Jude's* (Merchant IJROBP 2002): 30 patients treated with radical surgery or limited surgery + RT. Patients with radical surgery had inferior neurocognitive outcomes (loss of 9.8 vs. 1.25 IQ points), and more frequent neurologic, visual, and endocrine complications. Local control was similar.

ʒ *CHOP* (Stripp IJROBP 2004): 76 patients with craniopharyngioma treated with surgery ± radiation. Adjuvant postoperative radiation improved 10-year local control (42 vs. 84%). Radiation was routinely used at salvage; patients treated with salvage vs. adjuvant RT had similar survival and local control.

TREATMENT RECOMMENDATIONS

ʒ Maximal safe resection

ʒ If GTR → observation (LC 85–100%).

ʒ If STR → postop EBRT to 54 Gy at 1.8-Gy/fx (LC 75–90%), or observation (LC 30%).

ʒ Cyst decompression for unresectable lesions prior to RT may ease sparing of critical structures and sometimes may be required during the course of RT.

ʒ SRS: for small primaries or recurrent tumors.

ʒ Intralesional bleomycin and intracavitary injection of radioactive colloid are effective in shrinking and fibrosing cysts, although data are limited.

ʒ Treatment toxicity can mimic disease progression with multiple endocrinopathies, visual loss, seizures, other cranial neuropathies, motor neuropathies, and neurocognitive deficits.

ʒ For children age < 3, limited surgery and close follow-up, defer RT.

SURVIVAL

ʒ Long-term event-free survival 80–100%.

CHOROID PLEXUS TUMORS

II

PEARLS

- Less than 2% of all glial tumors.
- Most common location: lateral ventricles in children, the fourth ventricle in adults.
- Benign (WHO grade I) = choroid plexus papilloma, 60–80%, papillary formation, lack of mitosis, and normal tissue invasion.
- Malignant (WHO grade III) = choroid plexus carcinoma, 20–40%, nuclear atypia, pleomorphism, frequent mitoses, and invasion of subependymal brain tissue.
- Most commonly present with hydrocephalus due to CSF overproduction and flow obstruction.
- Up to 30% of children present with metastatic disease at diagnosis.
- Workup: MRI brain and spine, CSF cytology.

SURVIVAL

- Choroid plexus papilloma 5-year OS 90–100%.
- Choroid plexus carcinoma 5-year OS 20–30%.

Table 2.8 TREATMENT RECOMMENDATIONS

General management	Maximal safe resection is first-line therapy for both choroid plexus papilloma and carcinoma
Choroid plexus papilloma	GTR and spine negative → observation
	STR and spine negative → RT to postop bed 50–54 Gy
	STR and spine positive (rare!) → CSI 36 Gy + LF boost 54 Gy and boost to mets 45–54 Gy
	No role for chemotherapy
Choroid plexus carcinoma	GTR and spine negative → observation, consider RT
	STR and spine negative → RT to postop bed to 54 Gy
	STR and spine positive → CSI 36 Gy + LF boost 54 Gy and boost to mets 45–54 Gy
	Consider chemotherapy

MENINGIOMA

PEARLS

- 30% of primary intracranial neoplasms
- Most common benign intracranial tumor in adults

- 25,110 annual cases in the US in 2015 (Ostrom Neuro Oncol 2015)
- Incidence increases with age, into the 8th decade of life (Ostrom Neuro Oncol 2015)
- F:M = 2:1 for all meningiomas and 1:1 for anaplastic meningiomas (rhabdoid and papillary)
- Risk factors: ionizing radiation and NF2 are known risk factors. Estrogen/Progesterone are controversial risk factors: a significant proportion of meningiomas express progesterone/estrogen receptors, however epidemiologic data is conflicting. (Wiemels JNO 2010)
- Pathology:
  - WHO grade I: ~75% of meningiomas, not meeting criteria for higher grade
  - WHO grade II: Includes atypical, clear cell, or chordoid subtypes. Atypical meningiomas characterized by either 4–19 mitotic figures/10 HPF, brain invasion, or ≥3 of the following: high cellularity, high N:C ratio, prominent nucleoli, sheeting, focal necrosis. (Brain invasion is a new criterion in the WHO 2016 revision)
  - WHO grade III: Includes anaplastic, papillary, or rhabdoid subtypes. Anaplastic meningiomas are characterized by ≥20 mitoses/HPF, carcinoma/sarcoma/melanoma features, multifocal necrosis, abundant mitoses with atypical forms.
- 70% of meningiomas express progesterone; however, trials with hormone manipulation have not proven effective. (Goodwin JNO 1993, Ji JCO 2015)
- Molecular characterization has identified NF2, AKT1 and SMO as oncogenic driver mutations. (Brastianos Nat Genetics 2013, Clark Science 2013) Targeted agents are currently being tested.

WORKUP

- H&P: historically, most common presentation was headaches > personality change/confusion > paresis. Cranial neuropathies can occur with base of skull involvement.
- CT: extra-axial, well-circumscribed and smooth, with moderate to intense homogenous enhancement with contrast. Bony changes may reflect hyperostosis due to tumor involvement in 15–20%. Calcification associated with slow growth.

- MRI: isointense on T1 and T2, intensely enhancing with gadolinium. Edema is uncommon. Brain invasion is uncommon, except with malignant meningiomas.
- Dural tail sign: linear thickening and enhancement adjacent to extra-axial mass, reported in 60% of meningiomas.
- Symptomatic improvement is achieved in approximately 40–70% of patients; however, significant radiographic responses are uncommon. (Rogers JNS 2015)
- Rapid radiographic response may indicate the tumor is a hemangiopericytoma.
- There is concern regarding malignant degeneration after radiation; however, this has not been proven.
- The WHO redefined grade II meningiomas in 2000, which has expanded this category to ~20% of meningiomas. (Smith Br J Neurosurg 2007)

STUDIES
SYSTEMIC THERAPY
- ALLIANCE (Currently Enrolling): Phase II trial of SMO/AKT/NF2 inhibitors (NCT02523014). Patients with SMO mutations will be treated with vismodegib until progression. Patients with NF2 mutations will be treated with GSK2256098 (FAK kinase inhibitor). The small molecule inhibitor for AKT mutations is not available, so this arm remains closed.

OBSERVATION
- *Japan* (Yano JNS 2006): Study of 1434 patients with meningioma treated from 1989–2003. Of 603 asymptomatic meningiomas, 58% were treated with observation alone. For 171 patients with short-term follow-up ($\geq$1 year), 6.4% became asymptomatic, all of whom had tumors $\geq$3 cm at diagnosis. For 67 patients with long-term follow-up, ($\geq$5 yrs), tumor growth occurred in 37.3% (crude). Postoperative morbidity approached 10% for patients aged $\geq$ 70. Tumors grew at a rate of ~2 mm per year.
- *Karolinska* (Jadid Acta Neurochir 2015): Study of 65 patients with initially asymptomatic meningiomas treated with initial observation, with minimum follow-up of

10 years. Progression was observed in 35% of patients, yielding 10-year actuarial progression in 50%.

POSTOP EBRT

With surgery alone, GTR yields approximately 5-year local control of 90%, 50–60%, and 20–30% for WHO grade I, II, and III tumors (Stafford Mayo Clin Proc 1998, Dziuk JNO 1998; Aghi Neurosurg 2009). STR yields approximately 5-year local control of 40–50%, 20–30% and 0% for the same groups, respectively (Stafford Mayo Clin Proc 1998, Dziuk *JNO* 1998, Goyal IJROBP 2000). RT is commonly used to improve control for subtotally resected grade II and all grade III meningiomas. (Rogers JNS 2015)

- *UCSF* (Goldsmith JNS 1994): 140 patients from USCF with STR + postop RT for benign (84%) and malignant (16%) meningiomas. 5-year OS 85% for benign, 58% for malignant. Improved PFS in patients who received >52 Gy (95 vs. 65% benign, 65 vs. 15% malignant). No benefit to aggressive STR vs. biopsy alone if postop RT given. Benign tumors treated after 1980 had better 5-year PFS compared to those treated before 1980 (98 vs. 77%, *p* = 0.002).
- *UCSF* (Sughrue JNS 2010): 63 patients with malignant meningioma, including 34 patients who had received their initial surgery at UCSF. Primary tumors treated at UCSF uniformly received postoperative EBRT. 5- and 10-year RFS were 57% and 40%.
- *RTOG 0539* (Rogers ASTRO 2015, Rogers ASTRO 2016): 65 low-risk patients with WHO grade I meningioma, 92% s/p GTR (Simpson I-III) and 8% STR (Simpson IV-V) observed. 5-yr. PFS 86%, local failure 12.5% overall (9% after GTR, 2/5 40% after STR). 52 intermediate-risk patients, 69% with WHO grade II s/p GTR or 31% with recurrent grade I tumors received postop RT 54 Gy/30 fx. 5-yr. PFS 84%, local failure 14%. High-risk patients with WHO grade III, recurrent WHO grade II, or grade II s/p STR treated with 60 Gy/30 fx.

SRS

, *Pittsburgh* (Kondziolka Neurosurg 2008): 1045 meningiomas among 972 patients. 49% of patients had received prior surgery, 5% had received prior fractionated radiotherapy. Tumor control was 97% for image-defined meningiomas, 93% for WHO grade I meningiomas, 50 and 17% for WHO grade II and III meningiomas, respectively.

, Multi-institutional (Santacroce Neurosurg 2012): 3768 meningiomas treated at 15 centers in Europe with SRS. 92.5% control rate. 5- and 10-year PFS of 95.2 and 88.6%. Control better for image-defined tumors than grade I meningiomas, female patients, sporadic meningiomas, and skull base tumors. 6.6% permanent morbidity rate with long-term follow-up.

, *UCSF* (Kaprealian JNO 2016): 264 patients with 406 eligible tumors were treated with SRS. 5-year freedom from progression was 97% for presumed meningioma, 87% for grade I, 56% for grade II, and 47% for grade III tumors. Patients treated at recurrence after surgery and recurrence after RT had 5-year FFP of 86 and 38%, respectively, compared with 97% in the up-front setting.

DOSES

, EBRT: 54 Gy for benign, 54–60 Gy for atypical, 60 Gy for anaplastic/malignant.

, SRS or FSRT: 12–15 Gy/1fx or 25 Gy/5 fx for benign. 16–20 Gy for atypical.

Table 2.9 TREATMENT RECOMMENDATIONS

Benign-appearing, completely resectable	Surgery (± preop angiography, embolization) Definitive RT or SRS may achieve symptom relief and durable control for patients Observation can be considered for small, asymptomatic tumors
Postop	WHO grade I GTR/STR: Observation. Consider RT if significant residual or symptomatic. WHO grade II GTR: Radiation vs. observation Grade II STR: 54–60 Gy/30 fx WHO grade III 60 Gy/30 fx
Inoperable	RT alone or SRS alone
Recurrent, not previously radiated	Surgery Adjuvant RT or SRS

⌕ Dose, fractionation, and technique should take volume, location, and prior treatment history into account. Careful target delineation and setup error management is needed for conformal treatment.

OUTCOMES
⌕ WHO I: 5-year LC for GTR ~90%, STR ~40–60%, and STR + RT ~95%.
⌕ WHO II: 5-year LC for GTR ~50–60%, GTR + RT ~60–90%, STR ~20–30%, STR + RT ~50–60%.
⌕ WHO III: Surgery + RT, 5-year RFS 50%. (Rogers JNS 2015)

FOLLOW-UP
⌕ MRI every 4 months for 1 year, every 6 months for 2 years, then annually.

ACOUSTIC NEUROMA

PEARLS
⌕ 6% of intracranial tumors
⌕ Arise from Schwann cells of myelin sheath of peripheral nerves.
⌕ Sporadic (unilateral, age 40–50) or associated with NF 2 (bilateral).
⌕ Slow growing, well-circumscribed, expansile, displace adjacent nerves.
  ⌕ 50% of tumors demonstrate little to no growth (<1 mm annually). 40% grow 1–3 mm annually, and 10% grow >3 mm annually.
⌕ Symptoms: progressive sensorineuronal hearing loss, ataxia, tinnitus. May affect CN VII function. Cerebellopontine angle involvement can lead to CN V deficits.
⌕ Screening: pure tone and speech audiometry (selective loss of speech discrimination common).
⌕ 50/50 rule: pure-tone average > 50 dB and speech discrimination <50% indicates limited useful hearing
⌕ 3 surgical approaches: retromastoid, translabyrinthine (for large tumors, no hearing preservation), middle-fossa

approach (hearing preservation). Surgical sequelae include headaches, CN VII palsy, hearing loss, CSF leak, lower cranial nerve palsies. Operative mortality ~1%. (Ryzenman Laryngoscope 2005, Samii Neurosurg 1997)

, Thin slice, gadolinium-enhanced MRI through the cerebellopontine angle is the imaging modality of choice.

, Suspected NF should have neuraxis imaging.

, Radiation for patients with NF2 is controversial due to concerns regarding secondary malignancy, malignant transformation, and delayed hearing loss. (Evans J Med Genetics 2006, Lunsford JNS 2013, Sun JNS 2014)

, Transient posttreatment tumor enlargement can occur that often resolves with conservative management. (Pollock Neurosurg 2006)

STUDIES

, Pittsburgh (Kondziolka NEJM 1998, Lunsford JNS 2013): 827 patients treated with GKRS for vestibular schwannoma at the University of Pittsburgh. Initial marginal doses of 18–20 Gy achieved excellent control with high morbidity (20% CN VII toxicity, 27% CN V toxicity, 50% hearing preservation). At 6 years, patients treated with 12–13 Gy (margin) had 98.6% local control, 100% CN VII preservation, 95% CN V preservation, 70% unchanged hearing, and 78% useful hearing preservation. Small intracanalicular tumors were associated with 90% hearing preservation.

TREATMENT RECOMMENDATIONS

, *Observation*: In selected patients, observation can be recommended. Approximately 50% have little to no growth with serial imaging. 10% grow >3 mm per year and 20% eventually require treatment. (Smouha Laryngoscope 2005, Bakkouri JNS 2009)

, *Surgery*: 90% are total or near-total resection (<5% LF) (Samii Neurosurg 1997). STR without postop RT (15% LF) vs. STR with postop RT (6% LF). Operative morbidity is variable.

, *SRS*: >95% LC for selected tumors. Dose 12–13 Gy single fraction, increased complications with >14 Gy. (Kondziolka NEJM 1998, Lunsford JNS 2013) Similar outcome with fractionated and single session SRS. CN V and CN VII preserved in >95%. Preop hearing preserved in 84%, testable hearing retained in 97%. 73% of patients had tumor regression and 25% had stable disease. Hearing preservation possible in up to 90% for patients with intracanalicular tumors at 5 years, but continues to decline with follow-up. (Lunsford JNS 2013)

, *FSRT*: Can be used for larger tumors or tumors abutting the brainstem. 25 Gy/5 fx.
, *EBRT*: 50.4–54 Gy/1.8 Gy fx. Preservation of CN VII function >95%. Preservation of useful hearing ~75%. Preservation of CN V function ~95%. (Kapoor IJROBP 2011)

PITUITARY TUMORS

PEARLS

, Ten to fifteen percent of primary brain tumors.
, 2.5: 1 incidence (female to male).
, Long natural history with insidious onset of symptoms; often slow (or no) detectable radiologic progression.
, The pituitary gland is bordered by the anterior and posterior clinoids; superiorly by anterior cerebral arteries, the optic nerves, and chiasm; laterally by cavernous sinuses (CN III, IV, V1, V2, VI, internal carotid artery); inferiorly by sphenoid sinus.
, Nearly all pituitary tumors arise from the anterior lobe, which is derived from Rathke's pouch (an evagination of ectodermal tissue from NPX).
, Anterior lobe produces GH, PRL, ACTH, TSH, FSH, LH controlled by hypothalamic portal system hormones. Posterior lobe produces ADH and oxytocin.
, 75% functional, 25% nonfunctional.
, Tumors secreting prolactin are the most common secreting tumors (30%), followed by GH (25%) → ACTH → TSH (rare).
, Macroadenomas: ≥1 cm; microadenomas: <1 cm.
, MEN-1: autosomal dominant, pituitary, parathyroid, pancreatic island cell tumors.

- Mass effect on stalk (infundibulum) causes mild increased PRL (~20 ng/ml). A similar effect after radiation of the stalk can be observed with persistent PRL elevation.
- Immunohistochemistry to identify subtype.
- After radiation therapy, prolactin and growth hormone levels normalize over several years. ACTH usually normalizes within 1 year.
- Nonrandomized data suggest radiation response may be lower while patients are on suppressive medications. (Sheehan JNS 2011) Discontinuation of suppressive medications several weeks prior to radiation is a reasonable precaution.

WORKUP
- H&P: headache, visual field testing (bitemporal hemianopsia, superior temporal deficits, homonymous hemianopsia, central scotoma, etc.), CN deficits (involvement of cavernous sinus), sleep/appetite/behavior changes (compression of hypothalamus), growth abnormalities, cold or heat intolerance.
- Imaging: MRI (thin cuts with contrast, coronal) or CT (look for bone destruction), skeletal survey when indicated.
- Complete endocrine evaluation.
  - Prolactin
  - Basal GH, IGF-1, glucose suppression, insulin tolerance, TRH stimulation
  - Serum ACTH, 24-h urine 17-hydroxycorticosteroids and free cortisol, dexamethasone suppression
  - Gonadal: LH, FSH, plasma estradiol, testosterone
  - Thyroid: TSH, T3, T4
  - Basal plasma or urinary steroids; cortisol response to insulin-induced hypoglycemia and plasma ACTH response to metyrapone
- Acromegaly = headache, changes in facial/skull/hand bones, heat intolerance, wt. gain. Dx = GH >10 ng/mL, not suppressed by glucose, or elevated IGF-1.
- Prolactinoma = amenorrhea, infertility, decreased libido, impotence galactorrhea, PRL >20 ng/mL.
- Cushing's disease = bilateral adrenal hyperplasia, central obesity, HTN, glucose intolerance, hirsutism, easy

bruising, osteoporosis. Diagnosis = elevated cortisol, not suppressed with low-dose dexamethasone, partially suppressed with high-dose dexamethasone, normal or moderately elevated plasma ACTH. In adrenal tumors, ACTH is depressed.

TREATMENT RECOMMENDATIONS

Table 2.10 TREATMENT MODALITIES

Medical management	Bromocriptine or cabergoline for prolactinomas, somatostatin analogs and pegvisomant (GH receptor antagonist) for GH-secreting tumors, and ketoconazole, metyrapone, mitotane for ACTH-secreting tumors may be used Frequent relapse when discontinued Provide temporary control of remission while awaiting response to RT
Surgery	Immediate decompression Microadenomas Maximal safe resection even for unresectable tumors, which may result in better normal tissue sparing by making SRS feasible
Radiation	Indications: medically inoperable (especially with hypopituitarism), STR with persistent postop hypersecretion, or large tumor with extrasellar extension. SRS or FSRT can be considered for small tumors not abutting the optic nerves/chiasm. EBRT can be used for larger tumors, or tumors abutting the optic nerves/chiasm.

Table 2.11 TREATMENT AND OUTCOME BY TUMOR TYPE

Nonfunctioning pituitary tumors	Surgery → (observation or RT) vs. definitive RT alone. 10-year DFS 90% (S + RT) vs. 80% (RT alone)
GH-secreting	Surgery → observation → RT 45–50 Gy for recurrent GH elevation. Or, RT alone 45–50 Gy for inoperable patients. 10-year DFS 70–80% (S + RT) vs. 60–70% (RT alone)
Prolactin-secreting	Observation vs. medical management vs. surgery vs. RT, individualize treatment based on symptoms, side effect profile, and patient preferences. Ten-year DFS 80–90%
ACTH-secreting	Surgery → observation → RT 45–50 Gy for recurrent ACTH elevation. RT alone 45–50 Gy for inoperable patients. Surgery results in more rapid normalization of hormones than RT alone. Ten-year remission rate 50–60%
TSH-secreting	Aggressive, always treat with postop RT
Histiocytosis X	5–15 Gy in 3–8 fx

DOSE

- 1.8 Gy/fx to 45–50 Gy for nonfunctioning, or 50.4–54 Gy for functioning.
- No more than 5% of dose inhomogeneity in tumor volume.
- 1.8–54 Gy for TSH and to 50.4 Gy for ACTH-secreting tumors.
- Radiosurgery: dose prescribed to the tumor margin: 12–20 Gy for nonfunctioning tumors, 15–30 Gy for functioning adenomas. Keep optic chiasm dose <8 Gy.

SURVIVAL

- No difference in OS between surgery, surgery + RT, or RT alone; best therapy based on minimizing side effects.

FOLLOW-UP

- PostRT contrast-enhanced MRI every 6 months ×1 year, then annually.
- Endocrine testing every 6 months – 1 year. Assess hormonal response and monitor gonadal, thyroid, and adrenal function for hypopituitarism.
- Formal visual field testing before RT for baseline and annually.

PRIMARY SPINAL CORD TUMORS

PEARLS

- Primary spinal cord tumors account for 4% of all CNS tumors overall, and 6% of CNS tumors in children.
- 2/3 extramedullary, 1/3 intramedullary.
- Intramedullary = astrocytoma (most common), ependymoma, and oligodendroglioma.
- Intradural-extramedullary = meningioma, ependymoma, nerve sheath tumors.

- Extradural = metastasis, bone osteogenic sarcoma, chondrosarcoma, chordoma, myeloma, epidural hemangiomas, lipomas, extradural meningiomas, and lymphomas.
- Astrocytomas are more common in C/T spine and frequently associated with cysts.
- Ependymomas are more common in L/S spine.
- Presentation: focal pain, segmental or nerve root weakness, sensory deficit in dermatomal distribution, incontinence.
- Brown-Séquard Syndrome = ipsilateral loss of motor function and fine touch sensation, and contralateral loss of pain and temperature sensation.
- Workup: MRI spine, CSF cytology, MRI brain for ependymoma, lymphoma, AA, metastases and GBM, CT chest for sarcomas, no LP before MRI.
- MRI: nearly all spinal cord tumors enhance with gadolinium, including low-grade gliomas.
- CSF: increased protein, possible xanthochromia (with extradural compression).

Table 2.12 TREATMENT RECOMMENDATIONS

Low-grade glioma, GTR	Observation	5-year OS 60–90% 5-year DFS 40%
Low-grade glioma, STR	RT to 50–54 Gy	5-year OS 60–90% 5-year DFS 40%
High-grade glioma	RT to 54 Gy. Consider adjuvant chemo	5-year OS 0–30% MS 6–24 months
Ependymoma	RT to 50–54 Gy ± CSI (for documented neuraxis dissemination)	5-year OS 60–100% 5-year DFS 60–90% Low-grade OS: 85–100% High-grade OS: 25–70%
Meningioma, GTR	Observation	
Meningioma, STR	Observation, or RT to 50–54 Gy or SBRT	
Spinal cord sarcomas, vertebral body chondrosarcomas, chordomas, osteogenic sarcomas	SBRT or charged particle beams	
Recurrent tumor	Surgical resection or reirradiation	

ARTERIOVENOUS MALFORMATION

PEARLS

- Median age at diagnosis: 30
- Annual rate of spontaneous hemorrhage ~2–4% with morbidity 20–30% per bleed and mortality 1%/year or 10–15% per bleed.
- There is a period of decreased risk of hemorrhage during latent interval after SRS treatment before complete angiographic resolution.
- After angiographic obliteration, lifetime risk of hemorrhage is ≤1%.
- SRS produces progressive thickening of the vascular wall and luminal thrombosis, and obliteration takes years.
- Obliteration rate at 2-year for lesions <2 cm is 90–100% and for >2 cm is 50–70%.
- For lesions with low surgical risk, surgery is favored due to rapid reduction in hemorrhage risk. SRS is a good alternative for small, deep lesions that are considered to have high risk of surgical morbidity.
- For large, unresectable lesions, staged radiosurgery can be safe and effective. (Seymour JNS 2015)
- The Spetzler-Martin grading scale can be used to assess surgical risk. (Spetzler JNS 1986, Starke JNS 2013)
- The role of preSRS embolization is controversial due to procedural risk, potential for recanalization, and potential difficulties with postembolization target delineation. We do not routinely employ preSRS embolization at UCSF.
- Target delineation based upon day-of-treatment angiography and time-of-flight MRI

STUDIES

- Maruyama (NEJM 2005): 500 patients treated with SRS that was followed with serial exams, MRI and/or angiography. Mean dose 21 Gy. Cumulative 4- and 5-year obliteration rates were 81% and 91%. Hemorrhage risk reduced by 54% during latency period and by 88% after obliteration compared to before SRS.

, ARUBA (Mohr Lancet 2014): Phase III international trial, closed early by the data safety monitoring board. Patients with unruptured AVMs were randomized to medical management with intervention (neurosurgery, embolization, SRS, combination) per investigator choice, or medical management alone. 223 patients were enrolled. The primary endpoint was death or symptomatic stroke. Death or stroke occurred in 10% of the medical management arm vs. 30% of the intervention arm. Criticisms include short follow-up (33 mo) for disease with long natural history; risk is accepted early for intervention groups vs. medical management alone; poor outcomes with interventions compared with historical controls; inclusion of low enrollment centers; all interventions included per investigator choice.

TREATMENT RECOMMENDATIONS

, Observation, microsurgical resection ± pretreatment embolization, and SRS/staged SRS are treatment options.
, Treat entire nidus, but not feeding arteries or draining veins.
, Tailor dose (15–25Gy) according to volume and location. Careful retrospective analyses by the Pittsburgh group identified a dose response curve, with obliteration rates of ~50% at 14 Gy and ~90% at ≥18 Gy. (Flickinger IJROBP 1996, Prog Neuro Surg 2013) Obliteration rates are likely modified by AVM size, architecture, and clinical factors.
, Volume-staged radiosurgery can be considered for lesions too large to treat in a single session.
, Targets in the brainstem and thalamus may be at increased risk of radiation injury.

FOLLOW-UP

, F/U: MRI every 6 months × 1–3 years, then annually.
, Once MRI shows obliteration, obtain angiogram to confirm (gold standard).

TRIGEMINAL NEURALGIA

PEARLS

- Disorder of the sensory nucleus of CN V causing episodic, paroxysmal, severe pain lasting seconds to minutes, followed by a pain free period in the distribution of one or more of its divisions.
- Peak age 60. F:M 2:1.
- Often precipitated by stimulation (e.g., shaving, brushing teeth, wind).
- Obtain MRI to rule-out neoplasm in cerebellopontine angle.
- Medical management is standard treatment (carbamazepine, gabapentin, antidepressants, etc.).
- Surgical options include nerve blocks, partial sensory rhizotomy, balloon decompression of the Gasserian ganglion, microvascular decompression, and peripheral nerve ablation (radiofrequency, neurectomy, cryotherapy).
- Patients who have symptoms refractory to medical management may be considered for SRS. (Gronseth Neurology 2008)
- Median time to pain relief with SRS is ~1 month. Approximately 50–60% become pain free, ~10–20% have decreased severity or frequency of pain, and ~5–10% have slight improvement only. Less than 10% developed facial numbness.
- Anesthesia dolorosa is a rare complication following Gamma Knife radiosurgery.

STUDIES

- University of Virginia (Sheehan JNS 2005): 151 patients with trigeminal neuralgia were treated with Gamma Knife radiosurgery. 50–90 Gy, 2–4 mm from the pons. 47% were pain free at 1 year, and 90% achieved improvement in pain. 35% were pain free at 3 years, and 70% had improved pain.

TREATMENT RECOMMENDATIONS

- Initial treatment: Gamma Knife radiosurgery, 80 Gy max dose, delivered to the proximal trigeminal root.

Acknowledgment We thank Charlotte Dai Kubicky MD, PhD, Linda W. Chan MD, Stuart Y. Tsuji MD, PhD, and David A. Larson MD, PhD for their work on the prior edition of this chapter.

REFERENCES

Abdel-Wahab M, Etuk B, Palermo J, et al. Spinal cord gliomas: a multi-institutional retrospective analysis. Int J Radiat Oncol Biol Phys. 2006;64:1060–71.

Abedalthagafi M, Phillips JJ, Kim GE, et al. The alternative lengthening of telomere phenotype is significantly associated with loss of ATRX expression in high-grade pediatric and adult astrocytomas: a multi-institutional study of 214 astrocytomas. Mod Pathol. 2013;26:1425–32.

Abrey LE, Ben-Porat L, Panageas KS, et al. Primary central nervous system lymphoma: the Memorial Sloan-Kettering Cancer Center prognostic model. J Clin Oncol. 2006;24:5711–5.

Aghi MK, Carter BS, Cosgrove GR, et al. Long-term recurrence rates of atypical meningiomas after gross total resection with or without post-operative adjuvant radiation. Neurosurgery. 2009;64:56–60.

Ashley DM, Merchant TE, Strother D, et al. Induction chemotherapy and conformal radiation therapy for very young children with nonmetastatic medulloblastoma: Children's Oncology Group study P9934. J Clin Oncol. 2012;30:3181–6.

Ater JL, Zhou T, Holmes E, et al. Randomized study of two chemotherapy regimens for treatment of low-grade glioma in young children: a report from the Children's Oncology Group. J Clin Oncol. 2012;30:2641–7.

Bailey CC, Gnekow A, Wellek S, et al. Prospective randomised trial of chemotherapy given before radiotherapy in childhood medulloblastoma. International Society of Paediatric Oncology (SIOP) and the (German) Society of Paediatric Oncology (GPO): SIOP II. Med Pediatr Oncol. 1995;25:166–78.

Bakkouri WE, Kania RE, Guichard J-P, et al. Conservative management of 386 cases of unilateral vestibular schwannoma: tumor growth and consequences for treatment. J Neurosurg. 2009;110:662–9.

Bamberg M, Kortmann RD, Calaminus G, et al. Radiation therapy for intracranial germinoma: results of the German cooperative prospective trials MAKEI 83/86/89. J Clin Oncol. 1999;17:2585–92.

Bataini JP, Delanian S, Ponvert D. Chiasmal gliomas: results of irradiation management in 57 patients and review of literature. Int J Radiat Oncol Biol Phys. 1991;21:615–23.

Bauman GS, Gaspar LE, Fisher BJ, et al. A prospective study of short-course radiotherapy in poor prognosis glioblastoma multiforme. Int J Radiat Oncol Biol Phys. 1994;29:835–9.

Baumert BG, Hegi ME, van den Bent MJ, et al. Temozolomide chemotherapy versus radiotherapy in high-risk low-grade glioma (EORTC 22033-26033): a randomised, open-label, phase 3 intergroup study. Lancet Oncol. 2016.; epub ahead of print

Bell EH, McElroy JP, Fleming J, et al. Comprehensive mutation analysis in NRG Oncology/RTOG 9813: a phase III trial of RT + TMZ + RT + nu for anaplastic astrocytoma and mixed anaplastic oligoastrocytoma (Astrocytoma Dominant). J Clin Oncol.2016; 34(suppl; abstr 2016).

Bleehen NM, Girling DJ, Gregor A, et al. A Medical Research Council phase II trial of alternating chemotherapy and radiotherapy in small-cell lung cancer. The Medical Research Council Lung Cancer Working Party. Br J Cancer. 1991;64:775–9.

Brastianos PK, Horowitz PM, Santagata S, et al. Genomic sequencing of meningiomas identifies oncogenic SMO and AKT1 mutations. Nat Genet. 2013;45:285–9.

Brastianos PK, Shankar GM, Gill CM, et al. Dramatic Response of BRAF V600E Mutant Papillary Craniopharyngioma to Targeted Therapy. J Natl Cancer Inst. 2016;108

Brastianos PK, Taylor-Weiner A, Manley PE, et al. Exome sequencing identifies BRAF mutations in papillary craniopharyngiomas. Nat Genet. 2014;46:161–5.

Brown PD, Buckner JC, O'Fallon JR, et al. Adult patients with supratentorial pilocytic astrocytomas: a prospective multicenter clinical trial. Int J Radiat Oncol Biol Phys. 2004;58:1153–60.

Buckner JC, Shaw EG, Pugh SL, et al. Radiation plus procarbazine, CCNU, and vincristine in low-grade glioma. N Engl J Med. 2016;374:1344–55.

Bull KS, Spoudeas HA, Yadegarfar G, et al. Reduction of health status 7 years after addition of chemotherapy to craniospinal irradiation for medulloblastoma: a follow-up study in PNET 3 trial survivors on behalf of the CCLG (formerly UKCCSG). J Clin Oncol. 2007;25:4239–45.

Burkhard C, Di Patre P-L, Schüler D, et al. A population-based study of the incidence and survival rates in patients with pilocytic astrocytoma. J Neurosurg. 2003;98:1170–4.

Cairncross G, Wang M, Shaw E, et al. Phase III trial of chemoradiotherapy for anaplastic oligodendroglioma: long-term results of RTOG 9402. J Clin Oncol. 2013;31:337–43.

Calaminus G, Kortmann R, Worch J, et al. SIOP CNS GCT 96: final report of outcome of a prospective, multinational nonrandomized trial for children and adults with intracranial germinoma, comparing craniospinal irradiation alone with chemotherapy followed by focal primary site irradiation for patients with localized disease. Neuro-Oncology. 2013;15:788–96.

Cancer Genome Atlas Research Network, Brat DJ, Verhaak RGW, et al. Comprehensive, integrative genomic analysis of diffuse lower-grade gliomas. N Engl J Med. 2015;372:2481–98.

Chan JL, Lee SW, Fraass BA, et al. Survival and failure patterns of high-grade gliomas after three-dimensional conformal radiotherapy. J Clin Oncol. 2002;20:1635–42.

Chang CH, Housepian EM, Herbert C. An operative staging system and a megavoltage radiotherapeutic technic for cerebellar medulloblastomas. Radiology. 1969;93:1351–9.

Chang S, Zhang P, Cairncross G et al. ATCT-12, Results of NRG oncology/RTOG 9813: a phase III randomized study of radiation therapy (RT) and temozolomide (TMZ) versus RT and nitrosourea (NU) therapy for anaplastic astrocytoma (AA). J Clin Oncol. 201533(suppl; abstr 2002).

Chinot OL, Wick W, Mason W, et al. Bevacizumab plus radiotherapy–temozolomide for newly diagnosed glioblastoma. N Engl J Med. 2014;370:709–22.

Clark VE, Erson-Omay EZ, Serin A, et al. Genomic analysis of non-NF2 meningiomas reveals mutations in TRAF7, KLF4, AKT1, and SMO. Science. 2013;339:1077–80.

Cohen KJ, Pollack IF, Zhou T, et al. Temozolomide in the treatment of high-grade gliomas in children: a report from the Children's Oncology Group. Neuro-Oncology. 2011;13:317–23.

Combs SE, Thilmann C, Edler L, et al. Efficacy of fractionated stereotactic reirradiation in recurrent gliomas: long-term results in 172 patients treated in a single institution. J Clin Oncol. 2005;23:8863–9.

DeAngelis LM, Seiferheld W, Schold SC, et al. Combination chemotherapy and radiotherapy for primary central nervous system lymphoma: Radiation Therapy Oncology Group Study 93-10. J Clin Oncol. 2002;20:4643–8.

Dhall G, Grodman H, Ji L, et al. Outcome of children less than three years old at diagnosis with non-metastatic medulloblastoma treated with chemotherapy on the "Head Start" I and II protocols. Pediatr Blood Cancer. 2008;50:1169–75.

Duffner PK, Horowitz ME, Krischer JP, et al. Postoperative chemotherapy and delayed radiation in children less than three years of age with malignant brain tumors. N Engl J Med. 1993;328:1725–31.

Dziuk TW, Woo S, Butler EB, et al. Malignant meningioma: an indication for initial aggressive surgery and adjuvant radiotherapy. J Neuro-Oncol. 1998;37:177–88.

Eckel-Passow JE, Lachance DH, Molinaro AM, et al. Glioma 'groups based on 1p/19q, IDH, and TERT promoter mutations in tumors. N Engl J Med. 2015;372:2499–508.

Espinoza JC, Haley K, Patel N, et al. Outcome of young children with high-grade glioma treated with irradiation-avoiding intensive chemotherapy regimens: Final report of the Head Start II and III trials. Pediatr Blood Cancer. 2016;63:1806–13.

Evans AE, Jenkin RD, Sposto R, et al. The treatment of medulloblastoma. Results of a prospective randomized trial of radiation therapy with and without CCNU, vincristine, and prednisone. J Neurosurg. 1990;72:572–82.

Evans DGR, Birch JM, Ramsden RT, et al. Malignant transformation and new primary tumours after therapeutic radiation for benign disease: substantial risks in certain tumour prone syndromes. J Med Genet. 2006;43:289–94.

Finlay JL, Boyett JM, Yates AJ, et al. Randomized phase III trial in childhood high-grade astrocytoma comparing vincristine, lomustine, and prednisone with the eight-drugs-in-1-day regimen. Childrens Cancer Group. J Clin Oncol. 1995;13:112–23.

Fisher BJ, Hu C, Macdonald DR, et al. Phase 2 study of temozolomide-based chemoradiation therapy for high-risk low-grade gliomas: preliminary results of Radiation Therapy Oncology Group 0424. Int J Radiat Oncol Biol Phys. 2015;91:497–504.

Flickinger JC, Kano H, Niranjan A, et al. Dose selection in stereotactic radiosurgery. Prog Neurol Surg. 2013;27:49–57.

Flickinger JC, Pollock BE, Kondziolka D, et al. A dose-response analysis of arteriovenous malformation obliteration after radiosurgery. Int J Radiat Oncol Biol Phys. 1996;36:873–9.

Flickinger JC, Torres C, Deutsch M. Management of low-grade gliomas of the optic nerve and chiasm. Cancer. 1988;61:635–42.

Fogh SE, Andrews DW, Glass J, et al. Hypofractionated stereotactic radiation therapy: An effective therapy for recurrent high-grade gliomas. J Clin Oncol. 2010;28:3048–53.

Gajjar A, Bowers DC, Karajannis MA, et al. Pediatric brain tumors: innovative genomic information is transforming the diagnostic and clinical landscape. J Clin Oncol. 2015;33:2986–98.

Gajjar A, Chintagumpala M, Ashley D, et al. Risk-adapted craniospinal radiotherapy followed by high-dose chemotherapy and stem-cell rescue in children with newly diagnosed medulloblastoma (St Jude Medulloblastoma-96): long-term results from a prospective, multicentre trial. Lancet Oncol. 2006;7:813–20.

Gavrilovic IT. Long-term follow-up of high-dose methotrexate-based therapy with and without whole brain irradiation for newly diagnosed primary CNS lymphoma. J Clin Oncol. 2006;24:4570–4.

Geyer JR, Sposto R, Jennings M, et al. Multiagent chemotherapy and deferred radiotherapy in infants with malignant brain tumors: a report from the Children's Cancer Group. J Clin Oncol. 2005;23:7621–31.

Gilbert MR, Dignam JJ, Armstrong TS, et al. A randomized trial of bevacizumab for newly diagnosed glioblastoma. N Engl J Med. 2014;370:699–708.

Goldman S, Bouffet E, Fisher PG, et al. Phase II trial assessing the ability of neoadjuvant chemotherapy with or without second-look surgery to eliminate measurable disease for nongerminomatous germ cell tumors: a Children's Oncology Group Study. J Clin Oncol. 2015;33:2464–71.

Goldsmith BJ, Wara WM, Wilson CB, et al. Postoperative irradiation for subtotally resected meningiomas. J Neurosurg. 1994;80:195–201.

Goodwin JW, Crowley J, Eyre HJ, et al. A phase II evaluation of tamoxifen in unresectable or refractory meningiomas: a Southwest Oncology Group study. J Neuro-Oncol. 1993;15:75–7.

Gorlia T, van den Bent MJ, Hegi ME, et al. Nomograms for predicting survival of patients with newly diagnosed glioblastoma: prognostic factor analysis of EORTC and NCIC trial 26981-22981/CE.3. Lancet Oncol. 2008;9:29–38.

Goyal LK, Suh JH, Mohan DS, et al. Local control and overall survival in atypical meningioma: a retrospective study. Int J Radiat Oncol Biol Phys. 2000;46:57–61.

Gripp S, Kambergs J, Wittkamp M, et al. Coverage of anterior fossa in whole-brain irradiation. Int J Radiat Oncol Biol Phys. 2004;59:515–20.

Gronseth G, Cruccu G, Alksne J, et al. Practice parameter: the diagnostic evaluation and treatment of trigeminal neuralgia (an evidence-based review): report of the Quality Standards Subcommittee of the American Academy of Neurology and the European Federation of Neurological Societies. Neurology. 2008;71:1183–90.

Grundy RG, Wilne SA, Weston CL, et al. Primary postoperative chemotherapy without radiotherapy for intracranial ependymoma in children: the UKCCSG/SIOP prospective study. Lancet Oncol. 2007;8:696–705.

Haas-Kogan DA, Missett BT, Wara WM, et al. Radiation therapy for intracranial germ cell tumors. Int J Radiat Oncol Biol Phys. 2003;56:511–8.

Hargrave D, Bartels U, Bouffet E. Diffuse brainstem glioma in children: critical review of clinical trials. Lancet Oncol. 2006;7:241–8.

Hegi ME, Diserens A-C, Gorlia T, et al. MGMT gene silencing and benefit from temozolomide in glioblastoma. N Engl J Med. 2005;352:997–1003.

Jadid KD, Feychting M, Höijer J, et al. Long-term follow-up of incidentally discovered meningiomas. Acta Neurochir. 2015;157:225–30.

Jaeckle K, Vogelbaum M, Ballman K, et al. CODEL (Alliance-N0577; EORTC-26081/22086; NRG-1071; NCIC-CEC-2): Phase III Randomized Study of RT vs. RT+TMZ vs. TMZ for Newly Diagnosed 1p/19q-Codeleted Anaplastic Oligodendroglial Tumors. Analysis of Patients Treated on the Original Protocol Design (PL02.005). Neurology 2016.

Jakacki RI, Burger PC, Zhou T, et al. Outcome of children with metastatic medulloblastoma treated with carboplatin during craniospinal radiotherapy: a Children's Oncology Group Phase I/II study. J Clin Oncol. 2012;30:2648–53.

Jansen MHA, van Vuurden DG, Vandertop WP, et al. Diffuse intrinsic pontine gliomas: a systematic update on clinical trials and biology. Cancer Treat Rev. 2012;38:27–35.

Janssens GO, Jansen MH, Lauwers SJ, et al. Hypofractionation vs conventional radiation therapy for newly diagnosed diffuse intrinsic pontine glioma: a matched-cohort analysis. Int J Radiat Oncol Biol Phys. 2013;85:315–20.

Ji Y, Rankin C, Grunberg S, et al. Double-blind phase III randomized trial of the antiprogestin agent mifepristone in the treatment of unresectable meningioma: SWOG S9005. J Clin Oncol. 2015;33:4093–8.

Kapoor S, Batra S, Carson K, et al. Long-term outcomes of vestibular schwannomas treated with fractionated stereotactic radiotherapy: an institutional experience. Int J Radiat Oncol Biol Phys. 2011;81:647–53.

Kaprealian T, Raleigh DR, Sneed PK, et al. Parameters influencing local control of meningiomas treated with radiosurgery. J Neuro-Oncol. 2016;128:357–64.

Karim AB, Maat B, Hatlevoll R, et al. A randomized trial on dose-response in radiation therapy of low-grade cerebral glioma: European Organization for Research and Treatment of Cancer (EORTC) Study 22844. Int J Radiat Oncol Biol Phys. 1996;36:549–56.

Karim AB, Afra D, Cornu P, et al. Randomized trial on the efficacy of radiotherapy for cerebral low-grade glioma in the adult: European Organization for Research and Treatment of Cancer Study 22845 with the Medical Research Council study BRO4: an interim analysis. Int J Radiat Oncol Biol Phys. 2002;52:316–24.

Keime-Guibert F, Chinot O, Taillandier L, et al. Radiotherapy for glioblastoma in the elderly. N Engl J Med. 2007;356:1527–35.

Kondziolka D, Lunsford LD, McLaughlin MR, et al. Long-term outcomes after radiosurgery for acoustic neuromas. N Engl J Med. 1998;339:1426–33.

Kondziolka D, Mathieu D, Lunsford LD, et al. Radiosurgery as definitive management of intracranial meningiomas. Neurosurgery. 2008;62:53–8.

Korfel A, Thiel E, Martus P, et al. Randomized phase III study of whole-brain radiotherapy for primary CNS lymphoma. Neurology. 2015;84:1242–8.

Kretschmar C, Kleinberg L, Greenberg M, et al. Pre-radiation chemotherapy with response-based radiation therapy in children with central nervous system germ cell tumors: a report from the Children's Oncology Group. Pediatr Blood Cancer. 2007;48:285–91.

Krueger DA, Care MM, Agricola K, et al. Everolimus long-term safety and efficacy in subependymal giant cell astrocytoma. Neurology. 2013;80:574–80.

Larkin SJ, Preda V, Karavitaki N, et al. BRAF V600E mutations are characteristic for papillary craniopharyngioma and may coexist with CTNNB1-mutated adamantinomatous craniopharyngioma. Acta Neuropathol. 2014;127:927–9.

Lo AC, Howard AF, Nichol A, et al. Long-term outcomes and complications in patients with craniopharyngioma: the British Columbia Cancer Agency experience. Int J Radiat Oncol Biol Phys. 2014;88:1011–8.

Louis DN, Perry A, Reifenberger G, et al. The 2016 World Health Organization Classification of Tumors of the Central Nervous System: a summary. Acta Neuropathol. 2016;131:803–20.

Lunsford LD, Niranjan A, Flickinger JC, et al. Radiosurgery of vestibular schwannomas: summary of experience in 829 cases. J Neurosurg. 2013;119(Suppl):195–9.

Luyken C, Blümcke I, Fimmers R, et al. Supratentorial gangliogliomas: histopathologic grading and tumor recurrence in 184 patients with a median follow-up of 8 years. Cancer. 2004;101:146–55.

Malmström A, Grønberg BH, Marosi C, et al. Temozolomide versus standard 6-week radiotherapy versus hypofractionated radiotherapy in patients older than 60 years with glioblastoma: the Nordic randomised, phase 3 trial. Lancet Oncol. 2012;13:916–26.

Maruyama K, Kawahara N, Shin M, et al. The risk of hemorrhage after radiosurgery for cerebral arteriovenous malformations. N Engl J Med. 2005;352:146–53.

Mason WP, Grovas A, Halpern S, et al. Intensive chemotherapy and bone marrow rescue for young children with newly diagnosed malignant brain tumors. J Clin Oncol. 1998;16:210–21.

Merchant TE, Kiehna EN, Sanford RA, et al. Craniopharyngioma: the St. Jude Children's Research Hospital experience 1984-2001. Int J Radiat Oncol Biol Phys. 2002;53:533–42.

Merchant TE, Kun LE, Krasin MJ, et al. Multi-institution prospective trial of reduced-dose craniospinal irradiation (23.4 Gy) followed by conformal posterior fossa (36 Gy) and primary site irradiation (55.8 Gy) and dose-intensive chemotherapy for average-risk medulloblastoma. Int J Radiat Oncol Biol Phys. 2008;70:782–7.

Merchant TE, Kun LE, Wu S, et al. Phase II trial of conformal radiation therapy for pediatric low-grade glioma. J Clin Oncol. 2009a;27:3598–604.

Merchant TE, Li C, Xiong X, et al. Conformal radiotherapy after surgery for paediatric ependymoma: a prospective study. Lancet Oncol. 2009b;10:258–66.

Michalski J, Vezina G, Burger P, et al. Preliminary results of COG ACNS0331: a phase III trial of Involved Field Radiotherapy (IFRT) and Low Dose Craniospinal Irradiation (LD-CSI) with chemotherapy in average risk medulloblastoma: a report from the Children's Oncology Group. Neuro-Oncology. 2016;18(suppl_3):iii122.

Mirimanoff R-O, Gorlia T, Mason W, et al. Radiotherapy and temozolomide for newly diagnosed glioblastoma: recursive partitioning analysis of the EORTC 26981/22981-NCIC CE3 phase III randomized trial. J Clin Oncol. 2006;24:2563–9.

Mohr JP, Parides MK, Stapf C, et al. Medical management with or without interventional therapy for unruptured brain arteriovenous malformations (ARUBA): a multicentre, non-blinded, randomised trial. Lancet. 2014;383:614–21.

Negretti L, Bouchireb K, Levy-Piedbois C, et al. Hypofractionated radiotherapy in the treatment of diffuse intrinsic pontine glioma in children: a single institution's experience. J Neuro-Oncol. 2011;104:773–7.

Nelson DF, Diener-West M, Horton J, et al. Combined modality approach to treatment of malignant gliomas--re-evaluation of RTOG 7401/ECOG 1374 with long-term follow-up: a joint study of the Radiation Therapy Oncology Group and the Eastern Cooperative Oncology Group. NCI Monogr. 1988:279–84.

Nelson DF, Martz KL, Bonner H, et al. Non-Hodgkin's lymphoma of the brain: can high dose, large volume radiation therapy improve survival? Report on a prospective trial by the Radiation Therapy Oncology Group (RTOG): RTOG 8315. Int J Radiat Oncol Biol Phys. 1992;23:9–17.

Northcott PA, Jones DTW, Kool M, et al. Medulloblastomics: the end of the beginning. Nat Rev Cancer. 2012;12:818–34.

Northcott PA, Korshunov A, Witt H, et al. Medulloblastoma comprises four distinct molecular variants. J Clin Oncol. 2011;29:1408–14.

Oikonomou E, Barreto DC, Soares B, et al. Beta-catenin mutations in craniopharyngiomas and pituitary adenomas. J Neuro-Oncol. 2005;73:205–9.

Ostrom QT, Gittleman H, Fulop J, et al. CBTRUS statistical report: primary brain and central nervous system tumors diagnosed in the United States in 2008–2012. Neuro-Oncology. 2015;17 Suppl 4:iv1–iv62.

Packer RJ, Ater J, Allen J, et al. Carboplatin and vincristine chemotherapy for children with newly diagnosed progressive low-grade gliomas. J Neurosurg. 1997;86:747–54.

Packer RJ, Gajjar A, Vezina G, et al. Phase III study of craniospinal radiation therapy followed by adjuvant chemotherapy for newly diagnosed average-risk medulloblastoma. J Clin Oncol. 2006;24:4202–8.

Packer RJ, Lange B, Ater J, et al. Carboplatin and vincristine for recurrent and newly diagnosed low-grade gliomas of childhood. J Clin Oncol. 1993;11:850–6.

Packer RJ, Zhou T, Holmes E, et al. Survival and secondary tumors in children with medulloblastoma receiving radiotherapy and adjuvant chemotherapy: results of Children's Oncology Group trial A9961. Neuro-Oncology. 2013;15:97–103.

Pajtler KW, Witt H, Sill M, et al. Molecular classification of ependymal tumors across all CNS compartments, histopathological grades, and age groups. Cancer Cell. 2015;27:728–43.

Perry JR, Laperriere N, O'Callaghan CJ, et al. Short-course radiation plus temozolomide in elderly patients with glioblastoma. NEJM. 2017;376(11):1027–37.

Pollock BE. Management of vestibular schwannomas that enlarge after stereotactic radiosurgery: treatment recommendations based on a 15 year experience. Neurosurgery. 2006;58:241–8.

Prados MD, Edwards MS, Rabbitt J, et al. Treatment of pediatric low-grade gliomas with a nitrosourea-based multiagent chemotherapy regimen. J Neuro-Oncol. 1997;32:235–41.

Ramaswamy V, Hielscher T, Mack SC, et al. Therapeutic impact of cytoreductive surgery and irradiation of posterior fossa ependymoma in the molecular era: a retrospective multicohort analysis. J Clin Oncol. 2016;34:2468–77.

Reijneveld JC, Taphoorn MJB, Coens C, et al. Health-related quality of life in patients with high-risk low-grade glioma (EORTC 22033-26033): a randomised, open-label, phase 3 intergroup study. Lancet Oncol. 2016;17(11):1533–42.

Roa W, Brasher PMA, Bauman G, et al. Abbreviated course of radiation therapy in older patients with glioblastoma multiforme: a prospective randomized clinical trial. J Clin Oncol. 2004;22:1583–8.

Roa W, Kepka L, Kumar N, et al. International atomic energy aency randomized phase III study of radiation therapy in elderly and/or frail patients with newly diagnosed glioblastoma multiforme. J Clin Oncol. 2015;33:4145–50.

Rogers L, Barani I, Chamberlain M, et al. Meningiomas: knowledge base, treatment outcomes, and uncertainties. A RANO review. J Neurosurg. 2015a;122:4–23.

Rogers L, Zhang P, Vogelbaum MA, et al. Intermediate-risk meningioma: initial outcomes from NRG oncology/RTOG-0539. Int J Radiat Oncol Biol Phys. 2015b;93:S139–40.

Rogers L, Zhang P, Vogelbaum MA, et al. Low-risk meningioma: initial outcomes from NRG oncology/RTOG 0539. Int J Radiat Oncol Biol Phys. 2016;96:939–40.

Rutkowski S, Bode U, Deinlein F, et al. Treatment of early childhood medulloblastoma by postoperative chemotherapy alone. N Engl J Med. 2005;352:978–86.

Ryzenman JM, Pensak ML, Tew JM. Headache: a quality of life analysis in a cohort of 1,657 patients undergoing acoustic neuroma surgery, results from the acoustic neuroma association. Laryngoscope. 2005;115:703–11.

Samii M, Matthies C. Management of 1000 vestibular schwannomas (acoustic neuromas): surgical management and results with an emphasis on complications and how to avoid them. Neurosurgery. 1997;40:11–21.

Sanson M, Marie Y, Paris S, et al. Isocitrate dehydrogenase 1 codon 132 mutation is an important prognostic biomarker in gliomas. J Clin Oncol. 2009;27:4150–4.

Santacroce A, Walier M, Régis J, et al. Long-term tumor control of benign intracranial meningiomas after radiosurgery in a series of 4565 patients. Neurosurgery. 2012;70:32–9.

Schultz C, Scott C, Sherman W, et al. Preirradiation chemotherapy with cyclophosphamide, doxorubicin, vincristine, and dexamethasone for primary CNS lymphomas: initial report of radiation therapy oncology group protocol 88-06. J Clin Oncol. 1996;14:556–64.

Seymour ZA, Sneed PK, Gupta N, et al. Volume-staged radiosurgery for large arteriovenous malformations: an evolving paradigm. J Neurosurg. 2015:1–12.

Shaw E, Arusell R, Scheithauer B, et al. Prospective randomized trial of low- versus high-dose radiation therapy in adults with supratentorial low-grade glioma: initial report of a North Central Cancer Treatment Group/Radiation Therapy Oncology Group/Eastern Cooperative Oncology Group study. J Clin Oncol. 2002;20:2267–76.

Shaw EG, Berkey B, Coons SW, et al. Recurrence following neurosurgeon-determined gross-total resection of adult supratentorial low-grade glioma: results of a prospective clinical trial. J Neurosurg. 2008;109:835–41.

Sheehan J, Pan H-C, Stroila M, et al. Gamma knife surgery for trigeminal neuralgia: outcomes and prognostic factors. J Neurosurg. 2005;102:434–41.

Sheehan JP, Pouratian N, Steiner L, et al. Gamma Knife surgery for pituitary adenomas: factors related to radiological and endocrine outcomes. J Neurosurg. 2011;114:303–9.

Smith SJ, Boddu S, Macarthur DC. Atypical meningiomas: WHO moved the goalposts? Br J Neurosurg. 2007;21:588–92.

Smouha EE, Yoo M, Mohr K, et al. Conservative management of acoustic neuroma: a meta-analysis and proposed treatment algorithm. Laryngoscope. 2005;115:450–4.

Sonneland PR, Scheithauer BW, Onofrio BM. Myxopapillary ependymoma. A clinicopathologic and immunocytochemical study of 77 cases. Cancer. 1985;56:883–93.

Souhami L, Seiferheld W, Brachman D, et al. Randomized comparison of stereotactic radiosurgery followed by conventional radiotherapy with carmustine to conventional radiotherapy with carmustine for patients with glioblastoma multiforme: Report of Radiation Therapy Oncology Group 93-05 protocol. Int J Radiat Oncol Biol Phys. 2004;60:853–60.

Souweidane MM, Krieger MD, Weiner HL, et al. Surgical management of primary central nervous system germ cell tumors: proceedings from the Second International

Symposium on Central Nervous System Germ Cell Tumors. J Neurosurg Pediatr. 2010;6:125–30.

Spetzler RF, Martin NA. A proposed grading system for arteriovenous malformations. J Neurosurg. 1986;65:476–83.

Sposto R, Ertel IJ, Jenkin RD, et al. The effectiveness of chemotherapy for treatment of high grade astrocytoma in children: results of a randomized trial. A report from the Childrens Cancer Study Group. J Neuro-Oncol. 1989;7:165–77.

Stafford SL, Perry A, Suman VJ, et al. Primarily resected meningiomas: outcome and prognostic factors in 581 Mayo Clinic patients, 1978 through 1988. Mayo Clin Proc. 1998;73:936–42.

Starke RM, Yen C-P, Ding D, et al. A practical grading scale for predicting outcome after radiosurgery for arteriovenous malformations: analysis of 1012 treated patients. J Neurosurg. 2013;119:981–7.

Stripp DCH, Maity A, Janss AJ, et al. Surgery with or without radiation therapy in the management of craniopharyngiomas in children and young adults. Int J Radiat Oncol Biol Phys. 2004;58:714–20.

Stupp R, Hegi ME, Mason WP, et al. Effects of radiotherapy with concomitant and adjuvant temozolomide versus radiotherapy alone on survival in glioblastoma in a randomised phase III study: 5-year analysis of the EORTC-NCIC trial. Lancet Oncol. 2009;10:459–66.

Stupp R, Mason WP, van den Bent MJ, et al. Radiotherapy plus concomitant and adjuvant temozolomide for glioblastoma. N Engl J Med. 2005;352:987–96.

Stupp R, Taillibert S, Kanner AA, et al. Maintenance therapy with tumor-treating fields plus temozolomide vs temozolomide alone for glioblastoma: a randomized clinical trial. JAMA. 2015;314:2535–43.

Stupp R, Wong ET, Kanner AA, et al. NovoTTF-100A versus physician's choice chemotherapy in recurrent glioblastoma: a randomised phase III trial of a novel treatment modality. Eur J Cancer. 2012;48:2192–202.

Sturm D, Bender S, Jones DTW, et al. Paediatric and adult glioblastoma: multiform (epi) genomic culprits emerge. Nat Rev Cancer. 2014;14:92–107.

Sughrue ME, Sanai N, Shangari G, et al. Outcome and survival following primary and repeat surgery for World Health Organization Grade III meningiomas. J Neurosurg. 2010;113:202–9.

Sun S, Liu A. Long-term follow-up studies of Gamma Knife surgery for patients with neurofibromatosis Type 2. J Neurosurg. 2014;121(Suppl):143–9.

Taal W, Brandsma D, de Bruin HG, et al. Incidence of early pseudo-progression in a cohort of malignant glioma patients treated with chemoirradiation with temozolomide. Cancer. 2008;113:405–10.

Tait DM, Thornton-Jones H, Bloom HJ, et al. Adjuvant chemotherapy for medulloblastoma: the first multi-centre control trial of the International Society of Paediatric Oncology (SIOP I). Eur J Cancer. 1990;26:464–9.

Tao ML, Barnes PD, Billett AL, et al. Childhood optic chiasm gliomas: radiographic response following radiotherapy and long-term clinical outcome. Int J Radiat Oncol Biol Phys. 1997;39:579–87.

Tarbell NJ, Friedman H, Polkinghorn WR, et al. High-risk medulloblastoma: a pediatric oncology group randomized trial of chemotherapy before or after radiation therapy (POG 9031). J Clin Oncol. 2013;31:2936–41.

Taylor RE, Bailey CC, Robinson K, et al. Results of a randomized study of preradiation chemotherapy versus radiotherapy alone for nonmetastatic medulloblastoma: the International Society of Paediatric Oncology/United Kingdom Children's Cancer Study Group PNET-3 Study. J Clin Oncol. 2003;21:1581–91.

Thiel E, Korfel A, Martus P, et al. High-dose methotrexate with or without whole brain radiotherapy for primary CNS lymphoma (G-PCNSL-SG-1): a phase 3, randomised, non-inferiority trial. Lancet Oncol. 2010;11:1036–47.

Thomas PR, Deutsch M, Kepner JL, et al. Low-stage medulloblastoma: final analysis of trial comparing standard-dose with reduced-dose neuraxis irradiation. J Clin Oncol. 2000;18:3004–11.

Thompson EM, Hielscher T, Bouffet E, et al. Prognostic value of medulloblastoma extent of resection after accounting for molecular subgroup: a retrospective integrated clinical and molecular analysis. Lancet Oncol. 2016;17:484–95.

Tihan T, Ersen A, Qaddoumi I, et al. Pathologic characteristics of pediatric intracranial pilocytic astrocytomas and their impact on outcome in 3 countries: a multi-institutional study. Am J Surg Pathol. 2012;36:43–55.

van den Bent MJ, Afra D, de Witte O, et al. Long-term efficacy of early versus delayed radiotherapy for low-grade astrocytoma and oligodendroglioma in adults: the EORTC 22845 randomised trial. Lancet. 2005;366:985–90.

van den Bent MJ, Brandes AA, Taphoorn MJB, et al. Adjuvant procarbazine, lomustine, and vincristine chemotherapy in newly diagnosed anaplastic oligodendroglioma: long-term follow-up of EORTC Brain Tumor Group Study 26951. J Clin Oncol. 2013;31:344–50.

van den Bent MJ, Erridge S, Vogelbaum MA, et al. Results of the interim analysis of the EORTC randomized phase III CATNON trial on concurrent and adjuvant temozolomide in anaplastic glioma without 1p/19q co-deletion: an Intergroup trial. J Clin Oncol 2016; 34(suppl; abstr LBA2000).

Walker MD, Alexander E Jr, Hunt WE, et al. Evaluation of BCNU and/or radiotherapy in the treatment of anaplastic gliomas. J Neurosurg. 1978;49:333–43.

Walker MD, Green SB, Byar DP, et al. Randomized comparisons of radiotherapy and nitrosoureas for the treatment of malignant glioma after surgery. N Engl J Med. 1980;303:1323–9.

Walker MD, Strike TA, Sheline GE. Analysis of dose-effect relationship in the radiotherapy of malignant gliomas. Int J Radiat Oncol Biol Phys. 1979;5:1725–31.

Weber DC, Wang Y, Miller R, et al. Long-term outcome of patients with spinal myxopapillary ependymoma: treatment results from the MD Anderson Cancer Center and institutions from the Rare Cancer Network. Neuro-Oncology. 2015;17:588–95.

Weiner HL, Lichtenbaum RA, Wisoff JH, et al. Delayed surgical resection of central nervous system germ cell tumors. Neurosurgery. 2002;(50):727–33–discussion733–4.

Wick W, Hartmann C, Engel C, et al. NOA-04 randomized phase III trial of sequential radiochemotherapy of anaplastic glioma with procarbazine, lomustine, and vincristine or temozolomide. J Clin Oncol. 2009;27:5874–80.

Wick W, Meisner C, Hentschel B, et al. Prognostic or predictive value of MGMT promoter methylation in gliomas depends on IDH1 mutation. Neurology. 2013;81:1515–22.

Wick W, Platten M, Meisner C, et al. Temozolomide chemotherapy alone versus radiotherapy alone for malignant astrocytoma in the elderly: the NOA-08 randomised, phase 3 trial. Lancet Oncol. 2012;13:707–15.

Wick W, Roth P, Hartmann C, et al. Long-term analysis of the NOA-04 randomized phase III trial of sequential radiochemotherapy of anaplastic glioma with PCV or temozolomide. Neuro-Oncology. 2016;18(11):1529–37.

Wiemels J, Wrensch M, Claus EB. Epidemiology and etiology of meningioma. J Neuro-Oncol. 2010;99:307–14.

Witt H, Mack SC, Ryzhova M, et al. Delineation of two clinically and molecularly distinct subgroups of posterior fossa ependymoma. Cancer Cell. 2011;20:143–57.

Wolff JEA, Driever PH, Erdlenbruch B, et al. Intensive chemotherapy improves survival in pediatric high-grade glioma after gross total resection: results of the HIT-GBM-C protocol. Cancer. 2010;116:705–12.

Yan H, Parsons DW, Jin G, et al. IDH1and IDH2Mutations in gliomas. N Engl J Med. 2009;360:765–73.

Yano S, Kuratsu J-I, Kumamoto Brain Tumor Research Group. Indications for surgery in patients with asymptomatic meningiomas based on an extensive experience. J Neurosurg. 2006;105:538–43.

Zaghloul MS, Eldebawy E, Ahmed S, et al. Hypofractionated conformal radiotherapy for pediatric diffuse intrinsic pontine glioma (DIPG): a randomized controlled trial. Radiother Oncol. 2014;111:35–40.

Zeltzer PM, Boyett JM, Finlay JL, et al. Metastasis stage, adjuvant treatment, and residual tumor are prognostic factors for medulloblastoma in children: conclusions from the Children's Cancer Group 921 randomized phase III study. J Clin Oncol. 1999;17:832–45.

II

PART III
Head and Neck

III

Chapter 3
Malignant and Benign Diseases of the Eye and Orbit

Jason Chan and Kavita K. Mishra

GENERAL PEARLS

- All eye/orbit malignancies are uncommon: ACS estimates for 2016 approximately 2810 new cases and 280 deaths.
- Percentage of malignant tumors increases with age, due to increases in primary orbital lymphoma (OL) and metastatic lesions in the elderly (both in the choroid and in the orbit).
- Most common intraocular malignancy in adults: choroidal metastasis, usually adenocarcinoma, especially from the lung, breast, and prostate.
  - Palliative RT (30 Gy/10 fx, 40 Gy/20 fx, or shorter course) can offer up to 70% symptomatic stability or improvement, >80% local control.
- Most common primary eye malignancy in adults: uveal melanoma.
- Most common primary eye malignancy in children: retinoblastoma (see Chap. 41).
- Most common primary orbital malignancy in adults: lymphoma.
- Most common primary orbital malignancy in children: rhabdomyosarcoma (see Chap. 41).

- Ocular/orbital RT risks (Jeganathan, IJROBP 2011):
  - Eyelashes: loss at >20 Gy at 1.5–2 Gy/fx.
  - Dry eye (xerophthalmia) from RT to lacrimal gland/Meibomian glands: 1/3–1/2 pts after 24–25.5 Gy at 1.5–2 Gy/fx, sharp increase at >50 Gy, permanent at >60 Gy.
  - Chronic skin effects or eyelid changes can occur after >50 Gy at 1.5–2 Gy/fx.
  - Conjunctivitis: acute after >30 Gy, chronic after >50 Gy, permanent conjunctival scarring after >60 Gy.
  - Corneal ulceration: >60 Gy at conventional fractionation, late corneal decompensation at >50 Gy.
  - Late iritis: >70 Gy with conventional fractionation.
  - Cataracts: 1/3 after 2.5–6.5 Gy with 8-year latent period; 2/3 after 6.5–11.5 Gy with 4-year latent period.
  - Late retinopathy: 0 at <24 Gy, TD 5/5 45–50 Gy, TD 50/5 55 Gy, 85% at 70–80 Gy.
  - Late optic neuropathy: near 0 at <50 Gy, rare with Dmax <55 Gy at <2 Gy/fx, 3–7% at 55–60 Gy, 7–20% at >60 Gy. For SRS, very low <8 Gy, increases at 8–12 Gy, >10% at 12–15 Gy.
  - Neovascular glaucoma up to 20% of pts treated in the eye with multiple risk factors, little dose volume data.
  - Ocular implants can also affect external beam dosimetry or backscatter.

UVEAL MELANOMA

PEARLS

- Most common primary intraocular malignancy in adults.
- Ocular melanomas represent ~3–5% of all melanomas, of which 85% are uveal, 5% conjunctival, and 10% others.
- In the USA, ~1500–2000 cases/year.
- Thought to arise from melanocytes of the uveal tract (pigmented layer of the eye that includes the iris, ciliary body, and choroid).
- Average age at diagnosis is 60 years (peak incidence 60–79).
- Male-to-female ratio is 1.3:1.

- Risk factors: light eyes, melanocytosis in affected eye, arc welding, history of sun/snow burn.
- Xeroderma pigmentosum, oculodermal melanocytosis, and dysplastic nevus syndrome may predispose to melanoma.
- Histologic subtypes: spindle cell (grade 1), mixed cell (grade 2), epithelioid cell (grade 3).
- Presentation: ~1/3 asymptomatic, found on exam; patient reports visual distortion, field loss, floaters, scotomas, flashing lights, unilateral cataract, pain.
- Patterns of spread: (1) intraocular spread, including vitreous seeding; (2) extrascleral extension (15% of pts); (3) metastasis may occur after a prolonged disease-free interval, typically the liver (~90%) and also the skin and lung; brain mets are rare.
- Poor prognostic factors include larger tumor diameter, greater thickness, ciliary body invasion, near fovea/macula, scleral penetration, optic nerve invasion, mixed/epithelioid cell type, high mitotic rate, Ki-67+, pleomorphic nucleoli, lymphocytic infiltration, monosomy of chromosome 3, gene expression profiling, and older age.
- Collaborative Ocular Melanoma Study (COMS) 3-arm study:
    - Small melanomas followed clinically on registry: 1–3 mm thick and 5–16 mm in largest dimension. 5 yr tumor-related mortality 0–2.5%.
    - Medium-sized melanomas randomized to enucleation or brachytherapy: 2.5–10 mm thick and ≤16 mm in largest dimension. 5 yr tumor-related mortality 7–13%.
    - Large melanomas randomized to enucleation +/− pre-op EBRT 20 Gy: >10 mm thick and/or >16 mm in largest dimension. 5 yr tumor-related mortality 22–32%.

WORKUP
- H&P includes measurement of tumor diameter/thickness, location, geometry, and tumor coloration.
- Labs: CBC, LFTs, LDH.
- Imaging: fundus photography, fluorescein angiography, ocular ultrasound (Kretz A&B), and MRI. CT of chest/abdomen if LFTs are elevated.

STAGING: UVEAL MELANOMA

Editors' note: All TNM stage and stage groups referred to elsewhere in this chapter reflect the 2010 AJCC staging nomenclature unless otherwise noted as the new system below was published after this chapter was written.

Table 3.1 (AJCC 7TH ED., 2010)

Primary tumor (T)

All uveal melanomas

TX: Primary tumor cannot be assessed

T0: No evidence of primary tumor

Iris

T1: Tumor limited to the iris

T1a: Tumor limited to the iris not more than 3 clock hours in size

T1b: Tumor limited to the iris more than 3 clock hours in size

T1c: Tumor limited to the iris with secondary glaucoma

T2: Tumor confluent with or extending into the ciliary body, choroid, or both

T2a: Tumor confluent with or extending into the ciliary body, choroid, or both, with secondary glaucoma

T3: Tumor confluent with or extending into the ciliary body, choroid, or both, with scleral extension

T3a: Tumor confluent with or extending into the ciliary body, choroid, or both, with scleral extension and secondary glaucoma

T4: Tumor with extrascleral extension

T4a: Tumor with extrascleral extension less than or equal to 5 mm in diameter

T4b: Tumor with extrascleral extension more than 5 mm in diameter

Ciliary body and choroid

  Primary ciliary body and choroidal melanomas are classified according to the four tumor size categories below:

T1: Tumor size category 1

T1a: Tumor size category 1 without ciliary body involvement and extraocular extension

T1b: Tumor size category 1 with ciliary body involvement

T1c: Tumor size category 1 without ciliary body involvement, but with extraocular extension less than or equal to 5 mm in diameter

T1d: Tumor size category 1 with ciliary body involvement and extraocular extension less than or equal to 5 mm in diameter

T2: Tumor size category 2

T2a: Tumor size category 2 without ciliary body involvement and extraocular extension

T2b: Tumor size category 2 with ciliary body involvement

T2c: Tumor size category 2 without ciliary body involvement, but with extraocular extension less than or equal to 5 mm in diameter

T2d: Tumor size category 2 with ciliary body involvement and extraocular extension less than or equal to 5 mm in diameter

Table 3.1 (continued)

T3:	Tumor size category 3
T3a:	Tumor size category 3 without ciliary body involvement and extraocular extension
T3b:	Tumor size category 3 with ciliary body involvement
T3c:	Tumor size category 3 without ciliary body involvement, but with extraocular extension less than or equal to 5 mm in diameter
T3d:	Tumor size category 3 with ciliary body involvement and extraocular extension less than or equal to 5 mm in diameter
T4:	Tumor size category 4
T4a:	Tumor size category 4 without ciliary body involvement and extraocular extension
T4b:	Tumor size category 4 with ciliary body involvement
T4c:	Tumor size category 4 without ciliary body involvement, but with extraocular extension less than or equal to 5 mm in diameter
T4d:	Tumor size category 4 with ciliary body involvement and extraocular extension less than or equal to 5 in diameter
T4e:	Any tumor size category with extraocular extension more than 5 mm in diameter

Regional lymph nodes (N)

NX:	Regional lymph nodes cannot be assessed
N0:	No regional lymph node metastasis
N1:	Regional lymph node metastasis

Distant metastasis (M)

M0:	No distant metastasis
M1:	Distant metastasis
M1a:	Largest diameter of the largest metastasis 3 cm or less
M1b:	Largest diameter of the largest metastasis 3.1–8.0 cm
M1c:	Largest diameter of the largest metastasis 8 cm or more

Anatomic stage/prognostic groups

I:	T1a N0 M0
IIA:	T1b–d N0 M0
	T2a N0 M0
IIB:	T2b N0 M0
	T3a N0 M0
IIIA:	T2c–d N0 M0
	T3b–c N0 M0
	T4a N0 M0
IIIB:	T3d N0 M0
	T4b–c N0 M0
IIIC:	T4d–e N0 M0
IV:	Any T N1 M0
	Any T Any N M1a–c

Used with the permission from the American Joint Committee on Cancer (AJCC), Chicago, Illinois. The original source for this material is the AJCC Cancer Staging Manual, Seventh Edition (2010), published by Springer Science + Business Media

Table 3.2 (AJCC 8TH ED., 2017)

Classification of ciliary body and choroid uveal melanoma based on thickness and diameter

Thickness (mm)						
>15.0				4	4	4
12.1–15.0			3	3	4	4
9.1–12.0	3	3	3	3	3	4
6.1–9.0	2	2	2	2	3	3	4
3.1-6.0	1	1	1	2	2	3	4
≤3.0	1	1	1	1	2	2	4
	≤3.0	3.1–6.0	6.1–9.0	9.1–12.0	12.1–15.0	15.1–18.0	>18.0

Largest basal diameter (mm)

DEFINITION OF PRIMARY TUMOR (T) IRIS MELANOMAS

T category	T criteria
T1	Tumor limited to the iris
T1a	Tumor limited to the iris, not more than 3 clock hours in size
T1b	Tumor limited to the iris, more than 3 clock hours in size
T1c	Tumor limited to the iris with secondary glaucoma
T2	Tumor confluent with or extending into the ciliary body, choroid, or both
T2a	Tumor confluent with or extending into the ciliary body, without secondary glaucoma
T2b	Tumor confluent with or extending into the ciliary body and choroid, without secondary glaucoma
T2c	Tumor confluent with or extending into the ciliary body, choroid, or both, with secondary glaucoma
T3	Tumor confluent with or extending into the ciliary body, choroid, or both, with scleral extension
T4	Tumor with extrascleral extension
T4a	Tumor with extrascleral extension ≤5 mm in largest diameter
T4b	Tumor with extrascleral extension >5 mm in largest diameter

Note: Iris melanomas originate from, and are predominantly located in, this region of the uvea. If less than half the tumor volume is located within the iris, the tumor may have originated in the ciliary body, and consideration should be given to classifying it accordingly

CHOROIDAL AND CILIARY BODY MELANOMAS

T category	T criteria
T1	Tumor size category 1
T1a	Tumor size category 1 without ciliary body involvement and extraocular extension
T1b	Tumor size category 1 with ciliary body involvement
T1c	Tumor size category 1 without ciliary body involvement but with extraocular extension ≤5 mm in largest diameter

T1d	Tumor size category 1 with ciliary body involvement and extraocular extension ≤5 mm in largest diameter
T2	Tumor size category 2
T2a	Tumor size category 2 without ciliary body involvement and extraocular extension
T2b	Tumor size category 2 with ciliary body involvement
T2c	Tumor size category 2 without ciliary body involvement but with extraocular extension ≤5 mm in largest diameter
T2d	Tumor size category 2 with ciliary body involvement and extraocular extension ≤5 mm in largest diameter
T3	Tumor size category 3
T3a	Tumor size category 3 without ciliary body involvement and extraocular extension
T3b	Tumor size category 3 with ciliary body involvement
T3c	Tumor size category 3 without ciliary body involvement but with extraocular extension <5 mm in largest diameter
T3d	Tumor size category 3 with ciliary body involvement and extraocular extension ≤5 mm in largest diameter
T4	Tumor size category 4
T4a	Tumor size category 4 without ciliary body involvement and extraocular extension
T4b	Tumor size category 4 with ciliary body involvement
T4c	Tumor size category 4 without ciliary body involvement but with extraocular extension ≤5 mm in largest diameter
T4d	Tumor size category 4 with ciliary body involvement and extraocular extension ≤5 mm in largest diameter
T4e	Any tumor size category with extraocular extension >5 mm in largest diameter

Notes:
1. Primary ciliary body and choroidal melanomas are classified according to the four tumor size categories above
2. In clinical practice, the largest tumor basal diameter may be estimated in optic disc diameters (DD; average, 1 DD = 1.5 mm), and tumor thickness may be estimated in diopters (average, 2.5 diopters = 1 mm). Ultrasonography and fundus photography are used to provide more accurate measurements
3. When histopathologic measurements are recorded after fixation, tumor diameter and thickness may be underestimated because of tissue shrinkage

DEFINITION OF REGIONAL LYMPH NODE (N)

N category	N criteria
N1	Regional lymph node metastases or discrete tumor deposits in the orbit
N1a	Metastasis in one or more regional lymph node(s)
N1b	No regional lymph nodes are positive, but there are discrete tumor deposits in the orbit that are not contiguous to the eye

DEFINITION OF DISTANT METASTASIS (M)

M category	M criteria
M0	No distant metastasis by clinical classification
M1	Distant metastasis
M1a	Largest diameter of the largest metastasis ≤3.0 cm
M1b	Largest diameter of the largest metastasis 3.1–8.0 cm
M1c	Largest diameter of the largest metastasis ≥8.1 cm

AJCC PROGNOSTIC STAGE GROUPS CHOROIDAL AND CILIARY BODY MELANOMAS

When T is...	And N is...	And M is...	Then the stage group is...
T1a	N0	M0	I
T1b–d	N0	M0	IIA
T2a	N0	M0	IIA
T2b	N0	M0	IIB
T3a	N0	M0	IIB
T2c–d	N0	M0	IIIA
T3b–c	N0	M0	IIIA
T4a	N0	M0	IIIA
T3d	N0	M0	IIIB
T4b–c	N0	M0	IIIB
T4d–e	N0	M0	IIIC
Any T	N1	M0	IV
Any T	Any N	M1a–c	IV

Used with permission of the American Joint Committee on Cancer (AJCC), Chicago, Illinois. The original and primary source for this information is the AJCC Cancer Staging Manual, Eighth Edition (2017) published by Springer International Publishing

STUDIES
NATURAL HISTORY

- Observation
  - COMS (three-part multicenter randomized study) small tumors (Arch Ophthalmol 1997): 204 pts with small/T1 nonprogressive tumors enrolled for observational study with treatment only if progression documented. Five-year OS 94%, 8-year OS 85%, 5-year DSS 99%, 8-year DSS 96%. No apparent loss of survival and good preservation of vision with *close* follow-up of small lesions.
  - COMS medium tumors no treatment (Straatsma Am J Ophthalmol 2003): 42 pts with medium-sized tumors eligible for COMS trial either declined (20) or deferred

treatment until later date (22) were followed for natural history. Five-year OS was only 70%, suggesting upfront treatment is preferred for medium-sized tumors.

- Metastatic progression: *COMS 26* (Diener-West Arch Ophthalmol 2005): COMS medium and large trial pts were followed prospectively for metastatic progression. Metastatic melanoma rate at 5 years 25%, 10 years 34%, with increased tumor size as poor prognostic factor. MS (median survival) ~ 6 months. Most common sites included ~90% liver, 30% lung, 20% bone.

ENUCLEATION VS. RT

- COMS medium tumors/T2 (Arch Ophthalmol 2006): 1317 pts with selected T2 tumors (not abutting optic disk) randomized to brachytherapy (*n* = 657) vs. enucleation (*n* = 660). No difference in 5-year OS (81–82%). Approximately 60% pts who died had DM at death. Visual acuity declined over time with brachytherapy plaque pts 5-year LF ~ 10%, 5-year eye retention ~85%. Twelve-year update: OS 57–59%, 12-year CSS 79–83%.

Table 3.3 TREATMENT RECOMMENDATIONS

Stage	Recommended treatment
Small, indeterminate pigmented lesions	Serial observation (COMS showed no difference in survival with early treatment, and vision preserved longer with observation). ~2/3 do not grow If growth, then consider surgery, laser, protons/charged particles, plaque, or SRS

Medium-sized lesions (T2)	Options:
	  Surgery: enucleation, orbital exenteration, local resection ± adjuvant RT
	  Proton radiotherapy, helium, or SRS
	  I-125 brachytherapy (other isotopes also used)

Large-sized lesions (T3+)	Select large tumors, consider eye-conserving options or surgery as above

Recurrent lesion without metastases	Options:
	  Surgical salvage: enucleation
	  Re-irradiation

ENUCLEATION +/− PRE-OP RT

  ˌ COMS large tumors (Am J Ophthalmol 2004): 1003 pts with large-sized tumors randomized to enucleation vs. pre-op 20 Gy EBRT + enucleation. No OS difference (5-year OS ~60%, 5-year DSS 73%). Ten-year update: OS 39%, CSS 55–60%.

PLAQUE BRACHYTHERAPY

  ˌ UCSF (Quivey IJROBP 1993): 449 pts treated with I-125; ~13% recurred locally; increased local failure with smaller tumor height, closer proximity to fovea/disk and optic nerve, larger diameter, lower radiation dose.

  ˌ Wills Eye Hospital (Shields, Arch Ophthalmol 2000). 1300 consecutive pts treated with plaque brachy. Long-term visual acuity depends on initial visual acuity, age, tumor size, location, subretinal fluid, final tumor control. At 10 yrs 68% of pts have poor visual acuity. Visual acuity most effectively preserved for small tumors >5 mm from optic disk and foveola.

PROTON THERAPY

  ˌ Systematic review (Verma, Clin Oncol 2016). Updated review of protons for uveal melanoma including 14 large series describing tumor factors, proton dose and fractionation, oncologic and ophthalmological outcomes. More recent studies use 50–60 CGE. Excluding smaller series 5-yr LC over 94% with sustained LC through 10–15 yrs, 5-yr OS 70–85%, 5-yr DM-free survival 75–90%. 5-yr enucleation 7–10%, visual acuity stabilizes or improves in 30–40%, deteriorates in 30–40%. Variable complication rates due to tumor size/location and dosimetry: glaucoma 7–30%, cataract 20–62%, vitreous bleeding 9–14%, retinopathy 23–67%, optic neuropathy 7–33%.

CHARGED PARTICLES VS. PLAQUE BRACHYTHERAPY

  ˌ Only randomized study of plaques vs. particles: UCSF/Berkeley (Mishra IJROBP 2015a, Char, Opthal 1993): 184 pts with T2/T3 lesions randomized to 70 GyE with helium vs. I-125 plaque. 5y LC 100% He vs. 84% I-125;

12y LC 98% He vs. 79% I-125. 12y enucleation rate 17% He vs. 37% plaque. No overall survival difference. Different toxicities: more dry eye, epiphora, neovascular glaucoma with He vs. temporary strabismus unique to brachytherapy.

˒ Meta-analysis (Chang & McCannel, B J Ophthal 2013): brachytherapy pts (n = 3868) and particle pts (n = 7043) treatment. 5 yr LF 9.5% brachy vs. 4.2% particle studies.

III

STEREOTACTIC RADIOSURGERY (SRS)/STEREOTACTIC RADIOTHERAPY (SRT)

˒ Muller (Radiother Oncol 2012)(2): 102 pts with T1–T4 lesions, median tumor thickness 6 mm. 50 Gy in 5 fx given. Median FU 32 months. LC 96%, subsequent enucleation 14.7% (crude).

RADIATION TECHNIQUES
PROTON/CHARGED PARTICLE THERAPY

˒ Surgical placement of tantalum rings for tumor localization purpose: perilimbal incision made and rectus muscles isolated with suture slings; melanoma localized with transillumination and 3–5 marker rings sutured in position around the tumor base.

˒ Treatment planning: use EYEPLAN software with around the tumor base tantalum ring coordinates, ultrasound measurements, surgeon's mapping, fundus photo, MRI to build model of patient eye, tumor, and normal structures.

˒ Field design: 2–2.5 mm margin on tumor. Optimize gaze angle, field collimation, and beam depth and width of Bragg peak to ensure tumor coverage and minimize dose to critical structures (ON, disk, macula, lens, ciliary body, etc.).

˒ Dose prescription: 56 GyE in five fractions (GyE = gray equivalent = dose in Gy × RBE of protons 1.1). Typical treatment duration 1–2 min/fx. Other dose regimens include 56–70 GyE in 4–5 fractions. See PTCOG-OPTIC guidelines (Hrbacek IJROBP 2016).

EPISCLERAL PLAQUE

- See ABS Ophthalmic Oncology Task Force guidelines (Brachytherapy 2014)
  - Relative contraindication: Pts with peripapillary and subfoveal or exudative retinal detachment typically have poor resultant vision and LC.
  - Contraindications: T4 extraocular extension with basal diameter exceeding limit of brachy, blind painful eyes, pts with no light perception.
- Field design: tumor + margin to include scleral thickness (1 mm) + 1–2 mm around tumor.
- One millimeter spacer (or contact lens) used to minimize hot spots over individual seeds.
- Surgical placement with general or local anesthesia, and as above, localize melanoma with transillumination. Suture dummy plaque into place, and verify position. Then suture radioactive plaque, irrigate eye with antibiotic solution, close conjunctiva, and place lead eye shield.
- Patient usually discharged in 24 h, return for plaque removal in 4–7 days.
- Dose prescription: minimum tumor I-125 dose 85 Gy; dose rate 0.60–1.05 Gy/h.

STEREOTACTIC RADIOSURGERY (SRS)

- Treatment planning, dose prescription/homogeneity, and method of eye fixation/monitoring vary for typical duration of each treatment fraction of up to 1 h (concerns of corneal dryness and fatigue). Doses include 25–40 Gy single fx to 50% isodose line; 48–70 Gy multifraction.
- SRS/SRT generally deliver higher doses to normal structures (i.e., ipsilateral lacrimal gland, contralateral eye, thyroid, and peripheral organs) and has greater tumor inhomogeneity compared with either proton therapy or plaque (Weber et al. 2005; Zytkovicz et al. 2007).

OUTCOMES

- LC higher for charged particles/protons vs. plaques in prospective randomized and retrospective data. Five-year LC particles ~92–99%. Five-year LC plaque ~81–96%.
- Need RCT and longer follow-up to evaluate relative outcomes and toxicity for SRS.

, Overall survival rates are comparable between surgery and radiation techniques of plaque and charged particles.

COMPLICATIONS

, Episcleral plaque: RT retinopathy up to 43% (Nomogram – Aziz et al. JAMA Ophthalmol 2016), optic atrophy, cystoid macular edema, cataracts, vitreous hemorrhage, neovascular glaucoma, central retinal vein occlusion, scleral necrosis, secondary strabismus (5%).

, Proton/helium: increased anterior complications from entrance beam including epiphora, dry eye, lash loss, neovascular glaucoma, cataract, telangiectasias, hemorrhage, maculopathy, retinopathy, and optic neuropathy.

, Need for enucleation for complications or tumor recurrence.

, Vision loss variable; depends on initial visual acuity, tumor location/size, distance/dose to macula, disk, and nerve.

FOLLOW-UP

, H&P including ocular ultrasound and fundus photo every 3–6 months initially, then annually for life (Lane JAMA Ophthalmol 2015). LFTs or abdominal imaging (Choudhary JAMA Ophthalmol 2016) ± CXR annually.

ORBITAL LYMPHOMA

PEARLS

, Includes lymphoid malignancies of the conjunctiva, lacrimal apparatus, eyelids, uvea, and intraconal and extraconal retrobulbar areas.

, In contrast to IOL, OL is generally an indolent disease.

, Most lesions are low-grade B-cell lymphomas.

, Most common histology: extranodal marginal zone B-cell lymphoma or mucosa-associated lymphoid tissue (MALT).

, Common presentations: orbital mass, proptosis, eye swelling, diplopia, salmon colored conjunctival mass, and increased tearing.

, Most pts present in seventh decade of life.

WORKUP

- ˒ H&P includes fundoscopy and measurement of tumor including exophthalmometer if proptosis.
- ˒ Labs: CBC, LFTs.
- ˒ Imaging: fine cut orbit CT and MRI. Brain MRI. Rule out systemic lymphoma with CT chest, abdomen, and pelvis.
- ˒ Tissue diagnosis: biopsy of lesion with immunohistochemistry and flow cytometry analysis; also bone marrow biopsy for systemic workup (Tables 3.4 and 3.5).

Table 3.4 STAGING (AJCC 7TH ED., 2010): ORBITAL LYMPHOMA

Primary tumor (T)

TX: Lymphoma extent not specified

T0: No evidence of lymphoma

T1: Lymphoma involving the conjunctiva alone without orbital involvement

T1a: Bulbar conjunctiva only

T1b: Palpebral conjunctiva ± fornix ± caruncle

T1c: Extensive conjunctival involvement

T2: Lymphoma with orbital involvement ± any conjunctival involvement

T2a: Anterior orbital involvement (± conjunctival involvement)

T2b: Anterior orbital involvement (± conjunctival involvement + lacrimal involvement)

T2c: Posterior orbital involvement (± conjunctival involvement ± anterior involvement and ± any extraocular muscle involvement)

T2d: Nasolacrimal drainage system involvement (± conjunctival involvement but not including nasopharynx)

T3: Lymphoma with preseptal eyelid involvement (defined above)16 ± orbital involvement ± any conjunctival involvement

T4: Orbital adnexal lymphoma extending beyond orbit to adjacent structures such as bone and brain

T4a: Involvement of nasopharynx

T4b: Osseous involvement (including periosteum)

T4c: Involvement of maxillofacial, ethmoidal, and/or frontal sinuses

T4d: Intracranial spread

Regional lymph node (N)

NX: Involvement of lymph nodes not assessed

N0: No evidence of lymph node involvement

N1: Involvement of ipsilateral regional lymph nodes*

N2: Involvement of contralateral or bilateral regional lymph nodes*

N3: Involvement of peripheral lymph nodes not draining ocular adnexal region

N4: Involvement of central lymph nodes

*Note: The regional lymph nodes include preauricular(parotid), submandibular, and cervical.

continued

Table 3.4 (continued)

Distant metastasis (M)
M0: No evidence of involvement of other extranodal sites
M1a: Noncontiguous involvement of tissues or organs external to the ocular adnexa (e.g., parotid glands, submandibular gland, lung, liver, spleen, kidney, breast, etc.)
M1b: Lymphomatous involvement of the bone marrow
M1c: Both M1a and M1b involvement

Used with the permission from the American Joint Committee on Cancer (AJCC), Chicago, Illinois. The original source for this material is the AJCC Cancer Staging Manual, Seventh Edition (2010), published by Springer Science+Business Media.

Table 3.5 STAGING (AJCC 8TH ED., 2017)

Definitions of AJCC TNM

Definition of primary tumor (T)

T category	T criteria
TX	Lymphoma extent not specified
T0	No evidence of lymphoma
T1	Lymphoma involving the conjunctiva alone without eyelid or orbital involvement
T2	Lymphoma with orbital involvement with or without conjunctival involvement
T3	Lymphoma with preseptal eyelid involvement with or without orbital involvement and with or without conjunctival involvement
T4	Orbital adnexal lymphoma and extraorbital lymphoma extending beyond the orbit to adjacent structures, such as the bone, maxillofacial sinuses, and brain

DEFINITION OF REGIONAL LYMPH NODE (N)

N category	N criteria
NX	Involvement of lymph nodes not assessed
N0	No evidence of lymph node involvement
N1	Involvement of lymph node region or regions draining the ocular adnexal structures and superior to the mediastinum (preauricular, parotid, submandibular, and cervical nodes)
N1a	Involvement of a single lymph node region superior to the mediastinum
N1b	Involvement of two or more lymph node regions, superior to the mediastinum
N2	Involvement of lymph node regions of the mediastinum
N3	Diffuse or disseminated involvement of peripheral and central lymph node regions

DEFINITION OF DISTANT METASTASIS (M)

M category	M criteria
M0	No evidence of involvement of other extranodal sites
M1a	Noncontiguous involvement of tissues or organs external to the ocular adnexa (e.g., parotid glands, submandibular gland, lung, liver, spleen, kidney, breast)
M1b	Lymphomatous involvement of the bone marrow
M1c	Both Mia and Mlb involvement

Used with permission of the American Joint Committee on Cancer (AJCC), Chicago, Illinois. The original and primary source for this information is the AJCC Cancer Staging Manual, Eighth Edition (2017) published by Springer International Publishing

- Ann Arbor staging system often used as for other lymphomas (see Chap. 35).
- Working Formulation and REAL classifications of NHL used to characterize low-grade vs. intermediate-/high-grade lesions for management decisions.

STUDIES
RT VS. SURGERY VS. CHEMO

- Esik (Radiother Oncol 1996): review of 37 pts with OL treated with RT after biopsy (17 pts), surgery alone (13 pts), or chemo (7 pts). Median RT dose 34.8 Gy. Ten-year local RFS was 100% with RT, 0% with surgery alone, and 42% with chemo. Twenty-year CSS was 100% with RT, 67% with surgery alone, and 0% with chemo.

LOW-GRADE DISEASE

- Several series report excellent LC 94–100% with RT. Optimal dose remains uncertain. Involved site RT appropriate.
- Woolf (Clin Oncol 2015). 81 pts with orbital lymphoma treated with median 30 Gy in 15 fx. LC 100%. 5% developed distant failure.

Table 3.6 TREATMENT RECOMMENDATIONS

Extent of disease	Treatment options
Low-grade, limited disease	Best results seen with RT alone, typically 24–30.6 Gy at 1.5–1.8 Gy/fx. For select indolent pts may consider reducing dose as low as 4 Gy in 2 fx
Intermediate-/high-grade or systemic disease with orbital involvement	Combine systemic chemo (e.g., CHOP) and RT to orbit (30–36 Gy). For CD20+, add rituximab

- Stanford (Le IJROBP 2002): series of 31 pts with MALT lymphoma treated with 30–40 Gy (mean 34 Gy) using 9–20 MeV electrons for conjunctival lesions, 6 MV photons for retrobulbar; lens shielded. 10-yr LC 100%, freedom from relapse 71% with most failures extranodal mucosa. No difference with dose ≤34 vs. >34 Gy. Two pts had retinal damage >34 Gy.

- Fasola (IJROBP 2013): 20 pts with 27 lesions treated with 2 Gy x 2. Median FU 26 months. Overall response rate 96%, CR 85% and PR 11%. Only 1 out of field ipsilateral relapse at two years salvaged with additional 4 Gy with CR at additional 42 months of follow-up.

- Pfeffer (IJROBP 2004): 23 pts with OL were retrospectively reviewed. Twelve pts with limited disease were treated to partial orbital volumes and 11 pts with more extensive disease received whole orbit RT. Dose was 20–30 Gy for low-grade lymphoma and 24–40 Gy for intermediate- to high-grade lymphoma. All pts had complete response to RT. Four pts (33%) treated with partial orbital RT had intraorbital recurrence in previously uninvolved regions not covered in the initial target volume. These pts were salvaged with RT or surgery. No intraorbital recurrences seen in pts treated with whole orbit RT.

INTERMEDIATE-/HIGH-GRADE DISEASE

- Increased risk of distant failure, so include systemic therapy. See Chapter 36.

RADIATION TECHNIQUES
EBRT

- Follow ILROG guidelines for ISRT (Illidge, IJROBP 2014).
- Set up patient supine, immobilize head with thermoplastic mask.
- Place radio-opaque markers at lateral canthus or radio-opaque contact lens to help define fields.
- For anterior lesions involving eyelid or bulbar conjunctiva, use electron beam 6–9 MeV with 0.5–1.0 cm bolus.
- Lens shield used if tumor coverage is not compromised. Lens block can be placed directly on the cornea after topical anesthetic if mounted on a Lucite conformer. Daily placement of block should carefully place it within the

limbus. Hanging blocks provide less reliable shielding when using electron beams.

, Lacrimal lesions as well as those involving intra- or extra-conal spread benefit from more sophisticated planning techniques: obtain CT for 3D CRT/IMRT planning.

, Dose prescription:

   , Low grade: 24–30 Gy in 1.5–2 Gy fx.

   , DLBCL: CR after chemo – 30 Gy; PR after chemo 30–36 Gy; residual GTV after chemo: 40–45 Gy depending on volume and proximity to critical structures.

COMPLICATIONS

, Acute: mild skin erythema.

, Late: depends on technique and shielding; includes cataracts, possibly dry eye.

FOLLOW-UP

, H&P every 3 months for 1 year, every 4 months for second year, every 6 months for third and fourth years, then annually.

INTRAOCULAR LYMPHOMA

PEARLS

, Very rare: a subset of primary CNS lymphomas, which account for 1–2% extranodal lymphomas.

, Confined to neural structures; distinguished from OLs, which involve the uvea and ocular adnexa of the orbit, lacrimal gland, and conjunctiva.

, Histology: usually diffuse large B-cell non-Hodgkin's lymphoma.

, Median age of onset in immunocompetent pts is late 50s–60s.

, More common in men.

, Of the pts who develop primary intraocular lymphoma (PIOL), 60–80% will go on to develop CNS disease within 3 years.

, Conversely, 25% of pts with primary CNS lymphoma without initial eye involvement will develop IOL.

- Common presentations: blurred vision, floaters; less common: red eye, photophobia, ocular pain, uveitis; ocular disease is bilateral in ~80% cases.
- Recurs in 50% of cases.
- No universal staging system.
- Optimum treatment remains unclear.

WORKUP

- H&P includes fundoscopy, slit lamp examination, measurement of tumor; thorough CNS evaluation.
- Labs: CBC, LFTs, ESR, lumbar puncture – CSF for cytology, chemistry, cytokine analysis; immunohistochemistry and flow cytometry of lymphoma cells from CSF/vitrectomy/biopsy.
- Brain/orbit MRI. Consider stereotactic brain biopsy for suspicious brain lesions, fluorescein angiography, and ocular ultrasound.
- Systemic workup (CT chest, abdomen, pelvis, and bone marrow biopsy).
- Tissue diagnosis: diagnostic vitrectomy, vitreous aspiration needle tap. Pts suspected of having IOL with no lesion on imaging should have diagnostic vitrectomy on eye with more severe vitreitis/worse visual acuity.
- If vitrectomy is nondiagnostic, consider chorioretinal biopsy or enucleation.

TREATMENT RECOMMENDATIONS

- Due to its rarity, literature mainly consists of small case series so no definitive treatment recommendations are available.
- Optimal initial therapy definitely includes local treatment, typically RT 36 Gy or may consider intraocular methotrexate.
- Most pts have pathologic or clinical suspicion of bilateral ocular involvement, but may consider treating only involved eye when no suspicion of contralateral involvement.
- ILROG (Illidge, IJROBP 2014): CTV = globe(s), optic nerve(s) to level of chiasm. PTV = 5 mm. Dose 36 Gy. If treat bilaterally with opposed laterals, set isocenter at posterior border to reduce divergence in case need salvage

whole brain RT. If treat unilaterally, use conformal RT or IMRT.
- May consider CNS prophylaxis (WBRT or intrathecal chemo) vs. salvage therapy for CNS relapse.
- Systemic therapy generally recommended due to predominance of high-grade histology.

STUDIES
- Berenbom (Eye 2007): 12 pts with 21 eyes diagnosed with PIOL retrospectively reviewed. Six pts were treated with RT and chemotherapy, 4 pts chemotherapy alone, 1 patient RT alone, and 1 patient no treatment. No relapses seen in pts treated with RT compared with two relapses in pts who did not receive RT.
- Grimm (Ann Oncol 2007). 83 HIV negative pts with primary intraocular lymphoma. 23 received focal ocular treatment alone (17 with RT), 53 received more extensive treatment with chemo, intrathecal chemo, and/or whole brain RT. Pattern of relapse: 47% brain, 30% eyes, 15% both, systemic 8%. Focal only therapy did not increase risk of brain relapse. Median PFS 30 mo, OS 58 mo.
- Teckie (Leukemia Lymphoma 2014). 18 pts with primary intraocular lymphoma. 12 treated with RT alone, 6 with chemo then RT. Median dose 36 Gy/20 fx. Of RT alone pts, 7/12 pts controlled, 3 recurred in the brain, 2 in the eye and were effectively salvaged with chemo +/− RT. 2 yr OS 94% overall, 83% with upfront chemo, 100% with RT alone.

THYROID OPHTHALMOPATHY

PEARLS
- Usually in association with Graves' disease but can arise in association with Hashimoto's thyroiditis.
- Histopathology: T-cell predominant lymphocytic infiltration of orbital tissues; also glycosaminoglycans in periorbital fat and extraocular muscles.
- Present with exophthalmos, impaired extraocular muscle involvement, diplopia, blurred vision, periorbital edema,

chemosis (conjunctival edema), lid retraction, and compressive optic neuropathy.

WORKUP
- H&P includes measurement of proptosis with Hertel exophthalmometer.
- Labs: CBC, chemistries, thyroid function tests.
- Imaging: orbit CT, MRI.

TREATMENT RECOMMENDATIONS
- If stable, no threat of impending visual loss, begin with treatment of underlying thyroid disorder.
- If moderate symptomatic, progressive, or refractory to thyroid treatment, options include orbital RT ± systemic immunosuppressive agents (IV or oral corticosteroids, cyclosporine, others).
- For visual loss unresponsive to corticosteroids (loss of color vision, a key symptom of optic nerve compression), decompressive surgery.
- EBRT: 20 Gy in 10 fx, 50–80% response rate.

STUDIES
- UPenn Study (Prummel Lancet 1993): 56 pts with moderately severe Graves' ophthalmopathy (no corneal involvement or loss of visual acuity) euthyroid for at least 2 months, randomized to 3 months oral prednisone + sham RT vs. retrobulbar RT to 20 Gy + placebo capsules. Results: same rate of responders/no change/failures (RT 46/40/14%, prednisone 50/36/14%), but steroid therapy had much higher minor, moderate, and major complication rates. Note that 75% of all pts (71% RT, 79% prednisone) ultimately needed decompressive/squint/rehabilitation surgery, regardless of treatment.
- Prummel (J Clin Endocrinol Metabol 2004): double-blind RCT. 44 pts received orbital RT and 44 pts received sham RT. RT-treated pts had significant improvement in eye motility and diplopia. RT may not be associated with improvement in quality of life.

, Stanford series (Lanciano IJROBP 1990): 311 pts treated from 1968 to 1988, most with 20 Gy. Some pts treated from 1979 to 1983 received 30 Gy, but no benefit was noted from increased dose. Results: improved or complete resolution of soft tissue changes 80%, proptosis 51%, eye muscle impairment 61%, visual acuity 61%. Of 1/3 pts who were on steroids when starting RT, 76% were able to discontinue use. Treatment well-tolerated with 10% acute toxicity.

, Bradley (Ophthalmology 2008): literature review of five observational studies and nine RCTs regarding orbital RT for Graves' ophthalmopathy. Three of the RCTs were sham controlled and none showed that RT was better than sham for improving proptosis, lid fissure, or soft tissue changes (i.e., eyelid swelling). Two of the 3 RCTs had improved vertical range of motion in RT-treated subjects compared to controls. Risk of radiation retinopathy is 1–2% within 10 years of RT.

RADIATION TECHNIQUES

, Set up patient supine; immobilize head with thermoplastic mask. Highly recommend cutting out around eyes to allow verification of clinical setup.

, Place radio-opaque markers at lateral canthus or radio-opaque contact lens to define fields.

, Targets: Both orbits including entire extraocular muscles.

, Place the beam split anterior field border 11–12 mm behind the cornea to spare lens (Fig. 3.1).

, Fields: usually lateral opposed, although angled opposed beams needed for marked asymmetry of proptosis, extending from just behind the lens of the globe to the anterior clinoids with superior and inferior margins defined by the bony orbit; general range of 4 × 4 to 5.5 × 5.5 cm with appropriate shielding.

, Techniques to minimize divergence into contralateral lens:

  , Half beam block anterior edge of field (preferred).

  , Alternatively, angle lateral fields 5° posteriorly (can use CT scan to ensure the optimal beam angle is selected).

, Dose prescription: 20 Gy in 2 Gy fx.

, Dose limitation: lens < 10 Gy.

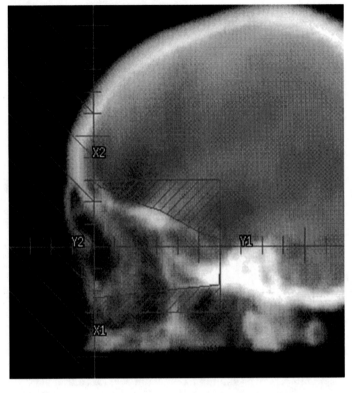

Fig. 3.1 Lateral DRR of a field used to treat thyroid ophthalmopathy

ORBITAL PSEUDOTUMOR/ LYMPHOID HYPERPLASIA/ PSEUDOLYMPHOMA

PEARLS
- Very rare benign orbital mass lesions in which mature lymphocytes (polyclonal) are noted.
- Usually present with soft tissue swelling, orbital pain, proptosis, extraocular muscle involvement, and less common decreased visual acuity.

WORKUP

- A diagnosis of exclusion: need to rule out lymphoma, metastatic carcinoma, sarcoma, and infectious causes of orbital inflammation.
- H&P exam includes measurement of tumor diameter, location, and geometry.
- Labs: CBC, LFTs, ESR, lumbar puncture – CSF for cytology, chemistry, and cytokine analysis.
- Imaging: brain/orbit CT, MRI.
- Tissue diagnosis: biopsy to rule out malignancy; may analyze with flow cytometry for clonality and immunohistochemistry.

TREATMENT RECOMMENDATIONS

- First line: corticosteroids; ~50% pts have durable complete response.
- If contraindications to steroid therapy, unacceptable toxicities with steroids, or refractory/recurrent: EBRT most commonly 20 Gy in 10 fx.
- Local control rates with radiation, 74–100% for doses 380–3600 cGy.

STUDIES

- Lanciano (IJROBP 1990): series of 26 orbits in 23 patients with orbital pseudotumor, of whom 87% had a trial of corticosteroids before RT (20 Gy/10 fx). 66% durable CR; 11% had local relapse and went on to achieve CR with more treatment or spontaneously. PR 11%. Only 11% had no response.
- Prabhu (IJROBP 2013). 20 pts with 26 affected orbits treated with RT. Median dose 27 Gy (25.2–30.6 Gy). 80% IMRT. 85% RR: 35% PR, 5% complete symptom resolution with reduced steroids, 45% complete symptom resolution and complete steroid taper.

RADIATION TECHNIQUES

- Simulation and field design: typically bilateral orbital involvement as per thyroid ophthalmopathy. Unilateral treatment with IMRT or a single lateral field +/− AP field, weighted more heavily laterally.
- Dose prescription: 20 Gy in 2 Gy fxs.

COMPLICATIONS
- Acute: mild skin erythema.
- Late: depends on technique and shielding; includes cataracts.

III

FOLLOW-UP
- H&P every 3 months for 1 year, every 4 months/ Pseudolymphoma for second year, every 6 months for third and fourth years, then annually.

Acknowledgment We thank Tania Kaprealian MD, Alice Wang-Chesebro MD, and Jeanne Marie Quivey MD, FACR, for their work on the prior edition of this chapter.

REFERENCES

Akpek E, et al. Intraocular-central nervous system lymphoma: clinical features, diagnosis, and outcomes. Ophthalmology. 1999;106:1805–10.

Aziz HA, Singh N, Bena J, Wilkinson A, Singh AD. Vision loss following episcleral brachytherapy for uveal melanoma: development of a vision prognostication tool. JAMA ophthalmology. 2016;134(6):615–20.

Bell D, et al. Choroidal melanoma: natural history and management options. Cancer Control. 2004;11(5):296–303.

Berenbom A, Davila RM, Lin H-S, et al. Treatment outcomes for primary intraocular lymphoma: implications for external beam radiotherapy. Eye. 2007;21: 1198–201.

Bhatia S, et al. Curative radiotherapy for primary orbital lymphoma. Int J Radiat Oncol Biol Phys. 2002;54:818–21.

Bolek T, et al. Radiotherapy in the management of orbital lymphoma. Int J Radiat Oncol Biol Phys. 1999;44:31–6.

Bradley EA, Gower EW, Bradley DJ, et al. Orbital radiation for graves ophthalmopathy. Ophthalmology. 2008;115:398–409.

Chan C, Wallace D. Intraocular lymphoma: update on diagnosis and management. Cancer Control. 2004;11(5):285–95.

Chang MY, McCannel TA. Local treatment failure after globe- conserving therapy for choroidal melanoma. Br J Ophthalmol. 2013;97:804–11.

Char D, et al. Primary intraocular lymphoma (ocular reticulum cell sarcoma) diagnosis and management. Ophthalmology. 1988;95:625–30.

Char D, Quivey J, et al. Helium ions versus I-125 brachytherapy in management of uveal melanoma. A prospective, dynamically balanced trial. Ophthalmology. 1993;100:1547–54.

Choudhary MM, Gupta A, Bena J, Emch T, Singh AD. Hepatic ultrasonography for surveillance in pts with uveal melanoma. JAMA Ophthalmol. 2016;134(2):174–80.

COMS. Mortality in pts with small choroidal melanoma. COMS report no. 4. Arch Ophthalmol. 1997;115:886.

COMS. The COMS randomized trial of pre-enucleation radiation of large choroidal melanoma: IV. Ten-year mortality findings and prognostic factors. COMS report no 24. Am J Ophthalmol. 2004;138(6):936.

COMS. The COMS randomized trial of iodine 125 brachytherapy for choroidal melanoma: V. Twelve-year mortality rates and prognostic factors: COMS report no. 28. Arch Ophthalmol. 2006;124:1684.

Daftari I, et al. Newer radiation modalities for choroidal tumors. Int Ophthal Clin. 2006;46:69.

Diener-West M, et al. Screening for metastasis from choroidal melanoma: the COMS group report 23. J Clin Oncol. 2004;22:2438–44.

Diener-West M, et al. Development of metastatic disease after enrollment in the COMS trials for treatment of choroidal melanoma: COMS report no. 26. Arch Ophthalmol. 2005;123(12):1639.

Egger E, et al. Maximizing local tumor control and survival after proton beam radiotherapy of uveal melanoma. Int J Radiat Oncol Biol Phys. 2001;51:138.

Esik O, et al. Retrospective analysis of different modalities for treatment of primary orbital non-Hodgkin's lymphomas. Radiother Oncol. 1996;38:13–8.

Fasola CE, Jones JC, Huang DD, Le QT, Hoppe RT, Donaldson SS. Low-dose radiation therapy (2 Gy× 2) in the treatment of orbital lymphoma. Int J Radiat Oncol Biol Phys. 2013;86(5):930–5.

Force, Task, and ABS–OOTF Committee. The American brachytherapy society consensus guidelines for plaque brachytherapy of uveal melanoma and retinoblastoma. Brachytherapy. 2014;13(1):1–14.

Gragoudas ES. Proton beam irradiation of uveal melanomas: the first 30 years. Invest Ophthalmol Vis Sci. 2006;47:4666–73.

Gragoudas ES, et al. A randomized controlled trial of varying radiation doses in the treatment of choroidal melanoma. Arch Ophthalmol. 2000;118:773.

Grimm SA, et al. Primary intraocular lymphoma: an international primary central nervous system lymphoma collaborative group report. Ann Oncol. 2007;18:1851–5.

Hoffman PM, et al. Intraocular lymphoma: a series of 14 pts with clinicopathological features and treatment outcomes. Eye. 2003;17:513–21.

Hrbacek J, Mishra KK, Kacperek A, et al. Practice patterns analysis of ocular proton therapy centers: the international OPTIC survey. Int J Radiat Oncol Biol Phys. 2016;95:336–43.

Illidge T, Specht L, Yahalom J, Aleman B, Berthelsen AK, Constine L, Dabaja B, Dharmarajan K, Ng A, Ricardi U, Wirth A. Modern radiation therapy for nodal non-hodgkin lymphoma—target definition and dose guidelines from the international lymphoma radiation oncology group. Int J Radiat Oncol Biol Phys. 2014;89(1):49–58.

Jeganathan V, Swetha E, Wirth A, MacManus MP. Ocular risks from orbital and periorbital radiation therapy: a critical review. Int J Radiat Oncol Biol Phys. 2011;79(3):650–9.

Kath R, et al. Prognosis and treatment of disseminated uveal melanoma. Cancer. 1993;72(7):2219–23.

Kujala E, et al. Very long term prognosis of pts with malignant uveal melanoma. Invest Ophthalmol Vis Sci. 2003;44:4651–9.

Lanciano R, et al. The results of radiotherapy for orbital pseudotumor. Int J Radiat Oncol Biol Phys. 1990;18:407.

Lane AM, Kim IK, Gragoudas ES. Long-term risk of melanoma-related mortality for pts with uveal melanoma treated with proton beam therapy. JAMA Ophthalmol. 2015;133(7):792–6.

Le Q, et al. Primary radiotherapy for localized orbital malt lymphoma. Int J Radiat Oncol Biol Phys. 2002;52:657–63.

Marucci L, Lane AM, Li W, et al. Conservation treatment of the eye: conformal proton reirradiation for recurrent uveal melanoma. Int J Radiat Oncol Biol Phys. 2006;64:1018–22.

Mishra KK, Quivey JM, Daftari IK, Weinberg V, Cole T, Patel K, Castro JR, Phillips TL, Char DH. Long-term results of the UCSF-LBNL randomized trial: charged particle with helium ion versus iodine-125 plaque therapy for choroidal and ciliary body melanoma. Int J Radiat Oncol Biol Phys. 2015a;92(2):376–83.

Muller K, Naus N, Nowak PJCM, Schmitz PIM, De Pan C, Van Santen CA, et al. Fractionated stereotactic radiotherapy for uveal melanoma, late clinical results. Radiother Oncol. 2012;102:219–24.

Nag S, et al. The American brachytherapy society recommendations for brachytherapy of uveal melanomas. Int J Radiat Oncol Biol Phys. 2003;56:544.

Nathan P, et al. Uveal melanoma UK national guidelines. Eur J Cancer. 2015;51(16):2404–12.

Nguyen LN, Ang K. The orbit. In: Cox J, Ang K, editors. Radiation oncology. 8th ed. St. Louis: Mosby; 2003. p. 282–92.

Pelloski CE, et al. Clinical stage IEA-IIEA orbital lymphomas: outcomes in the era of modern staging and treatment. Radiother Oncol. 2001;59:145–51.

Peterson IA, et al. Prognostic factors in the radiotherapy of graves' ophthalmopathy. Int J Radiat Oncol Biol Phys. 1990;19:259–64.

Peterson K, et al. The clinical spectrum of ocular lymphoma. Cancer. 1993;72:843–9.

Pfeffer MR, Rabin T, Tsvang L, et al. Orbital lymphoma: is it necessary to treat the entire orbit? Int J Radiat Oncol Biol Phys. 2004;60:527–30.

Prabhu RS, Kandula S, Liebman L, Wojno TH, Hayek B, Hall WA, Shu HK, Crocker I. Association of clinical response and long-term outcome among patients with biopsied orbital pseudotumor receiving modern radiation therapy. Int J Radiat Oncol Biol Phys. 2013;85(3):643–9.

Prummel M, et al. Randomized double-blind trial of prednisone versus radiotherapy in graves' ophthalmopathy. Lancet. 1993;342:949–54.

Prummel MF, Terwee CB, Gerding MN, et al. A randomized controlled trial of orbital radiotherapy versus sham irradiation in pts with mild graves' ophthalmopathy. J Clin Endocrinol Metab. 2004;89:15–20.

Quivey J, Char D, et al. High intensity 125-iodine (125I) plaque treatment of uveal melanoma. Int J Radiat Oncol Biol Phys. 1993;26(4):613–8.

Rosenthal S. Benign disease. In: Leibel SA, Phillips TL, editors. Textbook of radiation oncology. 2nd ed. Philadelphia: Saunders; 2004. p. 1525–43.

Shields C, Shields J. Diagnosis and management of retinoblastoma. Cancer Control. 2004;11(5):317–27.

Shields CL, et al. Plaque radiotherapy for uveal melanoma: long-term visual outcome in 1106 consecutive patients. Arch Ophthalmol. 2000;118(9):1219–28.

Shields J, et al. Survey of 1264 pts with orbital tumors and simulating lesions. Ophthalmology. 2004;111:997–1008.

Stafford SL, et al. Orbital lymphoma: radiotherapy outcome and complications. Radiother Oncol. 2001;59:139–44.

Straatsma BR, Diener-West M, Caldwell R, Engstrom RE. Mortality after deferral of treatment or no treatment for choroidal melanoma. Am J Ophthalmol. 2003;136(1):47–54.

Teckie S, Yahalom J. Primary intraocular lymphoma: treatment outcomes with ocular radiation therapy alone. Leuk Lymphoma. 2014;55(4):795–801.

Verma V, Mehta MP. Clinical outcomes of proton radiotherapy for uveal melanoma. Clin Oncol. 2016;28(8):e17–27.

Weber DC, Bogner J, Verwey J, et al. Proton beam radiotherapy versus fractionated stereotactic radiotherapy for uveal melanomas: a comparative study. Int J Radiat Oncol Biol Phys. 2005;63:373–84.

Woolf DK, et al. Outcomes of primary lymphoma of the ocular adnexa (orbital lymphoma) treated with radiotherapy. Clin Oncol. 2015;27(3):153–9.

Zytkovicz A, et al. Peripheral dose in ocular treatments with cyberknife and gamma knife radiosurgery compared to proton radiotherapy. Phys Med Biol. 2007;52(19):5957.

III

Chapter 4
Cancer of the Ear

Jason Chan and Sue S. Yom

III

PEARLS

- The external ear consists of the pinna (auricle), external auditory canal (EAC), tympanic membrane.
- The middle ear contains the auditory ossicles and communicates with the pharynx via the Eustachian tube.
- The inner ear is in the petrous portion of the temporal bone and consists of the bony and membranous labyrinth.
- The University of Florida published a contouring atlas of the middle and inner ear (Pacholke, Am J Clin Oncol 2005).
- Primary middle ear and temporal bone tumors are rare, but external ear cutaneous malignancies may involve these structures.
- BCC >> SCC for malignancies of the external ear, but SCC accounts for 85% of EAC, middle ear, and mastoid tumors.
- Nodal metastases occur in <15% with lymphatic drainage to parotid > cervical > postauricular nodes.

WORKUP

- H&P with otoscopy and careful LN exam. CBC, chemistries, BUN/Cr. CT, MRI. Biopsy.
- Audiologic testing includes measuring pure tone threshold with both air and bone conduction, speech reception threshold, word discrimination score, and impedance audiometry.

© Springer International Publishing AG, part of Springer Nature 2018   **137**
Eric K. Hansen and M. Roach III (eds.), *Handbook of Evidence-Based
Radiation Oncology*, https://doi.org/10.1007/978-3-319-62642-0_4

STAGING

, No site-specific AJCC/UICC staging system exists; may use histology appropriate staging (e.g. skin, Table 4.1).
, Several proposed staging systems for EAC and middle ear; modified University of Pittsburgh system often cited (Hirsch, Arch Otolaryngol Head Neck Surg 2002).

Table 4.1

T-stage	AJCC staging criteria for cutaneous carcinomas	Pittsburgh staging system for temporal bone carcinomas
T1	<2 cm in greatest dimension	Limited to EAC without bony or soft-tissue extension
T2	≥2 cm, <5 cm	Limited (not full thickness) EAC bony erosion or radiographic limited (<0.5 cm) soft-tissue involvement
T3	>5 cm	Eroding osseous EAC (full thickness) with limited (<0.5 cm) soft-tissue involvement or tumor involving middle ear and/or mastoid or p/w facial paralysis
T4	Invading deep extra dermal structures (i.e., cartilage, bone, muscle)	Eroding cochlea, petrous apex, medial wall of middle ear, carotid canal, jugular foramen or dura, or with extensive (> 0.5 cm) soft-tissue involvement

TREATMENT RECOMMENDATIONS

, Tumors of the external ear may be treated with surgery or RT (either EBRT or IS brachytherapy). Surgery is used if the lesion has invaded the cartilage or extends medially into the auditory canal. Advanced lesions or close/+ margins require post-op RT. Treatment of the lymphatics may be indicated for tumors >4 cm or for cartilage invasion.
, Tumors of the middle ear or temporal bone may be treated with surgery or RT. Facial nerve paralysis at presentation is considered a negative prognostic feature. Surgery may

require mastoidectomy or subtotal or total temporal bone resection. Lateral temporal bone resection is often indicated for T1–2 cases and en bloc subtotal or total temporal bone resection for T3–4 tumors. Post-op RT is generally required for close/+ margin or T2–4 disease to increase LRC.

, LC depends on the extent of disease, and ranges from 40 to 100% across multiple small published case series (owing to rarity of condition).

, Preoperative RT or chemo-RT has also been advocated as an alternative to post-op RT for selected cases (Nakagawa, Otol Neurotol 2006).

STUDIES

, Madsen (Head Neck 2008): 68 primary cancers of EAC and middle ear in Denmark. Five years LRC rates for surgery, RT, or surgery + RT were 55.6%, 47.4%, and 45.3%, respectively. Of 28 recurrences, 24 were purely local.

, Pfreundner (IJROBP 1999): 27 primary carcinomas of EAC and middle ear. Five-year OS 61%. Five-year LC 50%. Five-year OS by stage: T1–T2 86%, T3 50%, T4 41%. Complete resection and clear margins were prognostic. All patients with dural invasion died.

, Ogawa (IJROBP 2007). 87 pts with EAC SCC, 61% treated with surgery and post-op RT, 39% with RT alone. 5-yr DFS with surgery and post-op RT: T1 75%, T2 75%, T3 46%. 5-yr DFS with RT alone: T1 83%, T2 45%, T3 0%. T-stage and margins prognostic.

, Yin (Auris Nasus Larynx 2006). 95 SCC cases of middle ear and EAC. 14% had regional LN metastasis. 5-yr OS: stage I/II 100%, stage III 67%, stage IV 30%. Stage, completeness of resection with negative margin, recurrence, and metastasis influence survival.

, Clark (J Plastic Reconstr Aesthet Surg 2008): Meta-analysis of LN metastases from auricular SCC. Metastatic rate is 11.2%, commonly to parotid and upper cervical chain. Usually develops within 12 months and half will die.

RADIATION TECHNIQUES

SIMULATION AND FIELD DESIGN

- Definitive RT (usually considered for early-stage or inoperable advanced-stage pts).
  - Superficial tumors of the pinna may be treated with electrons or orthovoltage photons. For small tumors, 1 cm margins are adequate, but for larger lesions, 2–3 cm margins are required (see Chap. 1).
  - Advanced or unresectable EAC or middle ear tumors may be treated definitively with high energy electrons (energy appropriate for tumor depth) alone or mixed with photons, or with 3DCRT/IMRT if coverage of nodal volumes is desired.
    - GTV: clinical and radiographic gross disease.
    - CTV1: GTV + 0.3–0.5 cm margin; 66–70 Gy at 2.0 Gy per fraction.
    - CTV2: CTV1 + 0.5–0.7 cm margin, including ipsilateral preauricular and postauricular nodes, and upper level II nodes, and parotid gland (if involved); 63 Gy at 1.8 Gy per fraction.
    - CTV3 (considered for more advanced and aggressive tumors): ipsilateral level III and IV, contralateral level II; 56 Gy at 1.6 Gy per fraction.
    - PTV: CTV + 0.3–0.5 cm margin.
- Postoperative treatment.
  - CTV1: original tumor, surgical bed, soft-tissue invasion, areas with possible residual disease; 60–66 Gy at 2 Gy per fraction (62–70 Gy at 2–2.2 Gy per fraction for gross residual disease).
  - CTV2: CTV1 + 0.5–0.7 cm margin, depending on anatomy include ipsilateral level II and parotid; 54–60 Gy at 1.8 Gy per fraction.
  - CTV3: ipsilateral level III and IV ± contralateral level II; 50–54 Gy at 1.6 Gy per fraction.

- ˌ PTV: CTV + 0.3–0.5 cm margin.
- ˌ Care should be taken to cover the glenoid fossa of the TMJ and periauricular soft tissue as marginal misses have been identified in these locations with IMRT (Chen, IJROBP 2012).
- ˌ Immobilization with a thermoplastic mask is necessary.
- ˌ Use wax bolus to fill EAC and surrounding concha for pinna tumors to decrease complications and improve homogeneity and superficial dose delivery.
- ˌ In carefully selected pts at experienced centers, post-op intracavitary brachy boost may be considered (Badakh, J Cancer Res Ther 2014).

DOSE PRESCRIPTIONS

- ˌ Tumors of the pinna may be treated with 1.8–2 Gy per fraction to 50 Gy for small, thin lesions <1.5 cm, 55 Gy for larger tumors, 60 Gy for minimal or suspected cartilage or bone invasion, or 65 Gy for large lesions with bone or cartilage invasion.
- ˌ Tumors of the auditory canal or temporal bone: postoperative, 54–66 Gy; definitive, 66–70 Gy, and may consider chemo-RT.

DOSE LIMITATIONS

- ˌ Limit temporal bone to ≤70 Gy to minimize risk of osteoradionecrosis (~10% for doses >65 Gy) (Fig 4.1).

COMPLICATIONS

- ˌ Cartilage necrosis of the pinna and/or temporal bone necrosis is possible if careful planning is not used.
- ˌ Neurosensory: hearing compromise or loss.
- ˌ Chronic otitis media.
- ˌ Xerostomia.

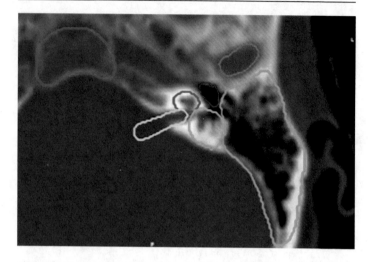

Fig. 4.1 Organs at risk delineated on planning CT: cochlea (*magenta*), vestibular apparatus (*cyan*), middle ear (*red*), CN VIII (*yellow*), clivus (*blue*), temporomandibular joint (*teal*), temporal bone/mastoid air cells (*green*)

FOLLOW-UP

＞ Frequent H&P with otoscopy every 3–4 months for 1–2 years, then every 6 months for 1–2 years, then annually.

Acknowledgment We thank Fred Y. Wu MD, PhD, and Eric K. Hansen MD for their work on the prior edition of this chapter.

REFERENCES

Badakh DK, Grover AH. To analyze the impact of intracavitary brachytherapy as boost radiation after external beam radiotherapy in carcinoma of the external auditory canal and middle ear: A retrospective analysis. J Cancer Res Ther. 2014;10(2):342.

Chen WY, Kuo SH, Chen YH, et al. Postoperative intensity-modulated radiotherapy for squamous cell carcinoma of the external auditory canal and middle ear: treatment outcomes, marginal misses, and perspective on target delineation. Int J Radiat Oncol Biol Phys. 2012;82(4):1485–93.

Clark RR, Soutar DS. Lymph node metastases from auricular squamous cell carcinoma. A systematic review and meta-analysis. J Plast Reconstr Aesthet Surg. 2008;61(10):1140–7.

Gal T, Futran N, Bartels L, et al. Auricular carcinoma with temporal bone invasion: outcome analysis. Otolaryngol Head Neck Surg. 1999;121:62–5.

Hirsch BE. Staging system revision. Arch Otolaryngol Head Neck Surg. 2002;128:93–4.

Jereczek-Fossa B, Zarowski A, Milani F, et al. Radiotherapy-induced ear toxicity. Cancer Treat Rev. 2003;29:417–30.

Lin R, Hug E, Schaefer R, et al. Conformal proton radiation therapy of the posterior fossa: a study comparing protons with three-dimensional planned photons in limiting dose to auditory structures. IJROBP. 2000;48:1219–26.

Osborne R, Shaw T, Zandifar H, et al. Elective parotidectomy in the management of advanced auricular malignancies. Laryngoscope. 2008;118:2139–45.

Madsen A, Gundgaard M, Hoff C, et al. Cancer of the external auditory canal and middle ear in Denmark from 1992 to 2001. Head Neck. 2008;30:1332–8.

Nakagawa T, Kumamoto Y, Natori Y, et al. Squamous cell carcinoma of the external auditory canal and middle ear: an operation combined with preoperative chemoradiotherapy and a free surgical margin. Otol Neurotol. 2006;27:242–8.

Ogawa K, Nakamura K, Hatano K, et al. Treatment and prognosis of squamous cell carcinoma of the external auditory canal and middle ear: a multi-institutional retrospective review of 87 patients. Int J Radiat Oncol Biol Phys. 2007;68(5):1326–34.

Pacholke HD, Amdur RJ, Schmalfuss IM, et al. Contouring the middle and inner ear on radiotherapy planning scans. Am J Clin Oncol. 2005;28(2):143–7.

Pfreundner L, Schwager K, Willner J, et al. Carcinoma of the external auditory canal and middle ear. Int J Radiat Oncol Biol Phys. 1999;44:777–88.

Wang TJC, Chao KSC. Ear. In: Perez CA, Wazer DE, Brady LW, Halperin EC, et al., editors. Principles and practice of radiation oncology. 6th ed. Philadelphia: Lippincott Williams & Wilkins; 2013. p. 711–7.

Yin M, Ishikawa K, Honda K, et al. Analysis of 95 cases of squamous cell carcinoma of the external and middle ear. Auris Nasus Larynx. 2006;33(3):251–7.

III

Chapter 5
Nasopharyngeal Cancer

III

Jason Chan and Sue S. Yom

PEARLS

- Epidemiology
  - Rare in the USA (<1 in 100,000) but endemic in SE Asia (25–50 in 100,000)
  - #1 most common HN cancer and #6 in cancer deaths in SE Asia
  - Two peak ages: 15–25 and 50–60; males > females (2:1)
- Histology
  - WHO I: Keratinizing; tobacco-associated; poor LRC
  - WHO IIA/IIB: Non-keratinizing/undifferentiated; endemic, EBV-associated; high DM
  - Lymphoepithelioma = with high lymphoid component; better LRC but same OS due to increased DM
  - Other nasopharynx tumors: lymphoma, minor salivary gland, plasmacytoma, melanoma, chordoma, rhabdomyosarcoma

© Springer International Publishing AG, part of Springer Nature 2018   145
Eric K. Hansen and M. Roach III (eds.), *Handbook of Evidence-Based Radiation Oncology*, https://doi.org/10.1007/978-3-319-62642-0_5

Table 5.1 ANATOMY

Border	Structure(s)	Pattern of spread	Significance
Lateral	Eustachian tube, torus tubarius, fossa of Rosenmuller, superior pharyngeal constrictors, medial pterygoid plate	Parapharyngeal space	Fossa of Rosenmuller is the most common site for NPC. Retroparotid space syndrome = involvement of CN IX–XII and cervical sympathetics
		Masticator space	Trismus
Anterior	Posterior nasal septum/choanae	Pterygopalatine fossa (PPF) via sphenopalatine foramen from nasal cavity	Tumors can extend proximally along V2 from PPF to cavernous sinus
Posterior	Clivus and C1–2	Retropharyngeal (RP) nodes and prevertebral space	>75% of patients are cN+, 90% have subclinical nodes, and 40–50% have bilateral nodes. Level 2 and lateral RP nodes are the first echelon
Superior	Sphenoid bone/sinus	Skull base	Foramen ovale (CN V3) and foramen lacerum commonly involved. True intracranial extension is uncommon (<10%). Petrosphenoidal syndrome = extension through foramen lacerum to cavernous sinus
Inferior	Roof of soft palate	Hard palate (oropharynx)	Infrequent compared to anterior, superior, or lateral spread

WORKUP

, *H&P.* Common signs/symptoms include hearing loss, otitis media, neck mass, nasal obstruction, epistaxis, headache, diplopia, and trismus. Perform fiberoptic nasopharyngolaryngoscopy and thorough oropharyngeal and neck exam. Also perform otoscopy. Thorough CN exam is critical.

, Labs: CBC, LFTs, BUN/Cr, baseline TSH, EBV IgA/DNA titer.

, MRI ± CT head/neck with contrast. CT optimally demonstrates cortical bone and MRI, medullary bone. A normal-appearing basisphenoid (clivus) on CT may demonstrate marked tumor infiltration on MRI.
, For Stage III/IV, consider CT of chest and abdomen + bone scan or PET/CT scan.
, Pre-RT dental, nutritional, speech and swallow, and audiology evaluations.

STAGING: NASOPHARYNGEAL CANCER

Editors' note: All TNM stage and stage groups referred to elsewhere in this chapter reflect the 2010 AJCC staging nomenclature unless otherwise noted as the new system below was published after this chapter was written.

Table 5.2 (AJCC 7TH ED., 2010)

Primary tumor (T)

TX:	Primary tumor cannot be assessed
T0:	No evidence of primary tumor
Tis:	Carcinoma in situ
T1:	Tumor confined to the nasopharynx, or tumor extends to oropharynx and/or nasal cavity without parapharyngeal extension
T2:	Tumor with parapharyngeal extension*
T3:	Tumor involves bony structures of skull base and/or paranasal sinuses
T4:	Tumor with intracranial extension and/or involvement of cranial nerves, hypopharynx, and orbit or with extension to the infratemporal fossa/masticator space

*Note: Parapharyngeal extension denotes posterolateral infiltration of tumor

Regional lymph nodes (N)

NX:	No regional lymph node metastasis can be assessed
N0:	No regional lymph node metastasis
N1:	Unilateral metastasis in cervical lymph node(s), 6 cm or less in greatest dimension, above the supraclavicular fossa, and/or unilateral or bilateral, retropharyngeal lymph nodes, 6 cm or less, in greatest dimension*
N2:	Bilateral metastasis in cervical lymph node(s), 6 cm or less in greatest dimension, above the supraclavicular fossa*

continued

Table 5.2 (continued)

N3:	Metastasis in a lymph node(s)** >6 cm and/or to supraclavicular fossa*
N3a:	Greater than 6 cm in dimension
N3b:	Extension to the supraclavicular fossa*

Note: Midline nodes are considered ipsilateral nodes
**Note*: Supraclavicular zone or fossa is relevant to the staging of nasopharyngeal carcinoma and is the triangular region originally described by Ho. It is defined by three points: (1) the superior margin of the sternal end of the clavicle, (2) the superior margin of the lateral end of the clavicle, and (3) the point where the neck meets the shoulder (Fig. 4.2). Note that this would include caudal portions of levels IV and VB. All cases with lymph nodes (whole or part) in the fossa are considered N3b

Distant metastasis (M)	
MX:	Distant metastasis cannot be assessed
M0:	No distant metastasis
Stage grouping	
0:	TisN0M0
I :	T1N0M0
II:	T1N0M0, T2N0-1M0
III:	T1-2N2M0, T3N0-2M0
IVA:	T4N0-2M0
IVB:	Any T, N3, M0
IVC:	Any T, any N, M1

Used with the permission from the American Joint Committee on Cancer (AJCC), Chicago, Illinois. The original source for this material is the AJCC Cancer Staging Manual, Seventh Edition (2010), published by Springer Science + Business Media

Table 5.3 (AJCC 8TH ED., 2017)

Definitions of AJCC TNM	
Definition of Primary Tumor (T)	
T category	**T criteria**
TX	Primary tumor cannot be assessed
T0	No tumor identified but there is EBV-positive cervical node involvement
T1	Tumor confined to the nasopharynx or extension to the oropharynx and/or nasal cavity without parapharyngeal involvement
T2	Tumor with extension to parapharyngeal space and/or adjacent soft tissue involvement (medial pterygoid, lateral pterygoid, prevertebral muscles)
T3	Tumor with infiltration of bony structures at the skull base, cervical vertebra, pterygoid structures, and/or paranasal sinuses
T4	Tumor with intracranial extension; involvement of cranial nerves, hypopharynx, orbit, and parotid gland; and/or extensive soft tissue infiltration beyond the lateral surface of the lateral pterygoid muscle

DEFINITION OF REGIONAL LYMPH NODE (N)

N category	N criteria
NX	Regional lymph nodes cannot be assessed
N0	No regional lymph node metastasis
N1	Unilateral metastasis in the cervical lymph node(s) and/or unilateral or bilateral metastasis in the retropharyngeal lymph node(s), 6 cm or smaller in greatest dimension, above the caudal border of the cricoid cartilage
N2	Bilateral metastasis in cervical lymph node(s), 6 cm or smaller in the greatest dimension, above the caudal border of cricoid cartilage
N3	Unilateral or bilateral metastasis in cervical lymph node(s), larger than 6 cm in the greatest dimension, and/or extension below the caudal border of cricoid cartilage

DEFINITION OF DISTANT METASTASIS (M)

M category	M criteria
M0	No distant metastasis
M1	Distant metastasis

AJCC PROGNOSTIC STAGE GROUPS

When T is...	And N is...	And M is...	Then the stage group is...
Tis	N0	M0	Stage 0
T1	N0	M0	Stage I
T1, T0	N1	M0	Stage II
T2	N0	M0	Stage II
T2	N1	M0	Stage II
T1, T0	N2	M0	Stage III
T2	N2	M0	Stage III
T3	N0	M0	Stage III
T3	N1	M0	Stage III
T3	N2	M0	Stage III
T4	N0	M0	Stage IVA
T4	N1	M0	Stage IVA
T4	N2	M0	Stage IVA
Any T	N3	M0	Stage IVA
Any T	Any N	M1	Stage IVB

Used with permission of the American Joint Committee on Cancer (AJCC), Chicago, Illinois. The original and primary source for this information is the AJCC Cancer Staging Manual, Eighth Edition (2017) published by Springer International Publishing

TREATMENT RECOMMENDATIONS

Table 5.4 TREATMENT RECOMMENDATIONS

2010 AJCC stage	Recommended treatment
Stage I	RT alone (70/2 Gy)
Stages II–IVB	Concurrent chemo-RT followed by adjuvant chemo 70/2 Gy + cisplatin 100 mg/m² on days 1, 21, and 42 → cisplatin/5-FU × 3c Neck dissection for persistent/recurrent neck nodes IMRT may improve LRC and reduces severe xerostomia 80% → 35–40% Neoadjuvant chemo (platinum/5FU +/− taxane) is under investigation
Stage IVC	Platinum-based combination chemo; if CR, definitive RT, otherwise palliative RT dose to metastatic sites
Local recurrence	Re-irradiation with IMRT, SRS, or brachytherapy. Cumulative dose is limited with respect to surrounding normal tissue tolerance. Alternative, surgery
Pediatric	Per COG ARAR 0331 protocol: Stage I: RT alone (61.2/1.8 Gy for Stage I; 66.6/1.8 Gy for Stage IIa) with daily amifostine Stage ≥ II: Cisplatin/5-FU × 3c → RT (CR/PR to chemo 61.2/1.8 Gy, SD to chemo 70.2/1.8 Gy) with daily amifostine and concurrent cisplatin ×3c 36–46/2–3 Gy to unresectable metastases

STUDIES

RT ± CHEMOTHERAPY

- *Int 0099* (Al Sarraf JCO 1998). 147 patients with Stage III–IV disease randomized to RT (2/70 Gy) vs. chemo-RT (2/70 Gy + concurrent cisplatin (100 mg/m²) × 3 → adjuvant cisplatin/5-FU × 3 cycles). Used old staging, so many Stage II would now be included. Chemo-RT improved 3-year OS (47 → 78%) and PFS (24 → 69%). Trial stopped early due to OS benefit. Criticized because of poor LRC and OS for RT alone group and high % of WHO I tumors (rare outside the USA).
- Wee (JCO 2005). Confirmed Int 0099 results with 221 patients from Singapore with Stage III–IV disease and same randomization. Chemo-RT improved 2-year OS (78 → 85%), DFS (57 → 75%) and DM (30 → 13%).

, Chan (IJROBP & JNCI 2005a, b). Phase III study showing benefit of weekly, low-dose (40 mg/m^2) cisplatin with RT vs. RT alone in 350 patients. No adjuvant chemotherapy. Cisplatin-RT improved 5-year OS (59 → 70%) with main benefits seen in T3/T4. Relatively low toxicity compared to Int 0099 chemo.

, MAC-NPC meta-analysis (Blanchard, Lancet Oncol 2015). 19 trials with 4806 pts. 5-yr OS benefit for concurrent and adjuvant chemo (12.4%) or concurrent chemo alone (9.4%), but not adjuvant chemo alone or induction chemo alone. Concurrent/adjuvant and concurrent alone improved PFS, LRC, and DM too.

CONCURRENT ± ADJUVANT CHEMOTHERAPY

, Chen (Lancet Oncol 2012): 251 Stage III of IV (except T3-4N0) patients randomized to concurrent chemo-RT + adjuvant chemotherapy versus concurrent chemo-RT alone. At median follow-up of 38 months, 2-year FFS is not significantly different (86% vs. 84%). The authors do not recommend adjuvant cisplatin/5FU outside of clinical trials given no clear benefit, but this is a controversial issue.

NEOADJUVANT CHEMOTHERAPY

, Numerous older studies reported no OS advantage with neoadjuvant chemo + RT vs. RT alone including using cisplatin/5-FU (Chan IJROBP 1995), cisplatin-epirubicin-bleomycin (INCSG IJROBP 1996), cisplatin-epirubicin (Chua et al. 1998), and cisplatin-bleomycin-5-FU (Ma et al. 2001).

, Lee (Cancer 2015). 706 patients randomized into 6-arm trial: 1) induction-concurrent versus concurrent-adjuvant chemotherapy, 2) capecitabine/cisplatin (PX) in place of standard 5-FU/cisplatin (PF), and 3) accelerated versus conventional fractionation. Preliminary results at 3.3 years of follow-up suggest no significant benefit with switching from concurrent-adjuvant to induction-concurrent, more favorable toxicity with PX in place of PF, and no benefit but higher toxicities (mucositis and dehydration) with altered fractionation.

, Sun (Lancet Oncol 2016). 480 patients with Stages III–IVB (except T3-4N0) randomized to IMRT with concurrent 100 mg/m^2 cisplatin every 3 weeks × 3c vs. induction TPF (docetaxel 60 mg/m^2, cisplatin 60 mg/m^2, and continuous 5FU 600 mg/m^2 on day 1 to day 5, every 3 weeks × 3c) followed by the same IMRT-cisplatin concurrent regimen. Induction TPF chemo improved 3-year failure-free survival (80% vs. 72%). Induction TPF increased grade 3–4 neutropenia (42% vs. 7%), leucopenia (41% vs. 17%), and stomatitis (41% vs. 35%).

EBV DNA TITERS

- Lin (NEJM 2004): 99 patients with Stages III–IV (M0) received chemotherapy followed by radiotherapy. At one week after the completion of radiotherapy, patients with persistently detectable plasma EBV DNA had worse overall survival ($p < 0.001$) and relapse-free survival ($p < 0.001$) than patients with undetectable EBV DNA.
- Leung (JCO 2008): 376 patients. On multivariate analysis, high EBV DNA (>4000 copies/mL) and low EBV DNA (≤4000 copies/mL) were predictive of OS ($p = 0.005$). EBV DNA load was better prognostic than UICC staging especially for Stage II.
- Wang (Cancer 2013): 210 NPC patients, including 99 previously reported by Lin (NEJM 2004) with Stage III–IV disease, were treated with induction chemo and RT and were followed for at least 6 years. EBV titer <1500 copies/mL had increased OS and RFS. Persistently elevated EBV titer 1 week after completion of sequential chemo-RT had worse OS, RFS.
- NRG-HN001: Patients enter either phase II or phase III study based on post-chemoradiation EBV DNA plasma titers. If EBV is undetectable, phase III randomization to cisplatin/5FU adjuvant chemotherapy versus no further treatment. If EBV is detectable, phase II randomization to cisplatin/5FU versus gemcitabine/paclitaxel adjuvant chemotherapy.

IMRT

- UCSF (Lee IJROBP 2002, 2003): 67 patients treated with IMRT to 70 Gy. Excellent 4-year OS (88%) and LRC (97%).
- Lee (JCO 2009). RTOG 0225 phase II study for Stages I–IVB using IMRT (2.12/70 Gy) and (for T2b or N+)

concurrent cisplatin → cisplatin/5-FU × 3c. Two-year locoregional control 90.5%, PFS 73%, OS 79%.

- Kam (JCO 2007): 60 patients with T1-2bN01 NPC randomized to 2D vs. IMRT. IMRT reduced 1 year observer-rated severe xerostomia (82% vs. 39%) and improved salivary flow rate. Subjective feeling of recovery not significantly different between arms.

- Pow (IJROBP 2006): 51 patients with Stage II disease randomized to IMRT vs. 2DRT. The mean parotid dose was 68 Gy for 2DRT and 42 Gy for IMRT. At 1 year, IMRT patients had improved salivary flow and surveys indicated improved physical/emotional health.

ALTERED FRACTIONATION

- Lee (Radiother Oncol 2011): 189 patients with T3-4 N0-1M0 NPC randomized to one of four treatment arms (2x2 design: radiation alone versus radiation + concurrent cisplatin and adjuvant cisplatin/5FU; conventional versus altered fractionation). Chemo-RT with altered fractionation was the winning arm with highest 5-year failure free rate of 88%.

RADIATION TECHNIQUES

SIMULATION AND FIELD DESIGN

- Patient set-up supine and immobilized with head and neck thermoplastic mask or equivalent device.
- Planning CT scan obtained with IV contrast if available. A prechemo MRI is critical for definition of GTV. Use CT-MRI fusion if available.
- In every case, the entire GTV must be treated to the entire prescription dose. Except in the case of very early T1–T2 N0 tumors, it is not possible to accomplish this without exceeding normal tissue tolerances with conventional 2D planning. 3DCRT or IMRT is necessary for the final cone down.
- *IMRT volumes (Lee Radiother Oncol 2017):*
  - *High dose clinical target volume (CTVp1)*
    - Margin from GTVp
      - GTVp + 5 mm (+/– whole NP), can reduce to minimum 1 mm (if close proximity to critical OARS)

- *High dose clinical target volume (CTVn1)*
  - Margin from GTVn
    - GTVn + 5 mm (consider 10 mm if ECE)
- *Intermediate dose clinical target volume (CTVp2)*
  - Margin from GTV
    - GTVp + 10 mm + whole NP can reduce to minimum of 2 mm (if close proximity to critical OARS)
  - Nasal cavity – posterior part
    - At least 5 mm from choana
  - Maxillary sinuses – posterior part
    - At least 5 mm from posterior wall
  - Posterior ethmoid sinus
    - Include vomer
  - Skull base
    - Cover foramen ovale, rotundum, lacerum, and petrous tip
  - Cavernous sinus
    - If T3-4 (involved side only)
  - Pterygoid fossae and parapharyngeal spaces
    - Full coverage
  - Sphenoid sinus
    - Inferior ½ if T1-2; whole if T3-4
  - Clivus
    - 1/3 if no invasion; whole if invasion
- *Intermediate dose clinical target volume (CTVn2)*
  - CTVn1 + 5 mm
  - Lymph nodes – bilateral RP, level II, III, and Va
    - Include level VIIb plus at least ipsilateral one level below the involved levels
  - Level Ib
    - Cover if involvement of submandibular gland, structures that drain to level Ib as first echelon (oral cavity, anterior half of nasal cavity), level II with ECE
- *Low dose clinical target volume (CTVn3)*
  - Levels IV and Vb down to clavicle
    - Omit if N0 or N1 based solely on RPLN involvement
- IMRT plan can be matched isocentrically to a conventional low neck field.
- *Conventional set-up* (when IMRT not available) = 3 fields (lateral opposed fields covering the primary and upper neck, with isocentric match to a low neck field). Use a

central larynx block on the low neck field and then full cord block after 42 Gy.

˒ *Conventional borders*: superior = generously cover sphenoid sinus and base of skull. Inferior = match at plane above true vocal cords (to block larynx in AP field). Posterior = spinous processes. Anterior = 2–3 cm anterior to GTV (and include pterygoid plates and posterior 1/3 of maxillary sinuses).

˒ If supraclavicular nodes involved, historically used a mediastinal 8 cm wide T field with inferior border 5 cm below the head of the clavicle.

˒ Use wedges and compensators as needed.

DOSE PRESCRIPTIONS

˒ *IMRT per RTOG 0615*: CTV70 (GTV + 5 mm) = 2.12/70 Gy, CTV56-59.4 = 1.8/56–59.4 Gy, CTV54 1.64/54 Gy in 33 fractions.

˒ *Conventional*: 2/42 Gy → off cord boost to 50 Gy with a posterior neck electron field → cone down to GTV + 2 cm margin to 70 Gy. For the neck, N0 = 50 Gy, nodes <3 cm = 66 Gy, and nodes ≥3 cm = 70 Gy.

˒ *Rotterdam NPX applicator*: optional boost after 66–70 Gy to gross disease. Use 1 week after EBRT (T1–T3 60 Gy EBRT → HDR 3 Gy × 6; T4 70 Gy EBRT → HDR 3 Gy × 4).

DOSE LIMITATIONS

˒ Recommend careful contouring of organs at risk. See atlas by Sun and colleagues (Radiother Oncol 2014).

˒ *EBRT*: partial brain 60 Gy, brainstem 54 Gy (60 Gy point dose), cord 45 Gy, optic chiasm 54 Gy, retina 45 Gy, lens 10 Gy, lacrimal gland 30 Gy, ear (sensorineuronal hearing loss) 45 Gy, parotid mean dose 26 Gy, TMJ max dose 70 Gy.

˒ *SRS*: brainstem 12 Gy, optic nerves or chiasm 8 Gy.

COMPLICATIONS

˒ Acute: mucositis, dermatitis, xerostomia.

˒ Late: soft tissue fibrosis, trismus, xerostomia, hearing loss, vasculopathy, osteoradionecrosis, temporal lobe necrosis, hypothyroidism, hypopituitarism (if included).

FOLLOW-UP

꜌ H&P every 1–3 months for the first year, every 2–4 months second year, every 4–6 months years 3–5, and then every 6–12 months

꜌ MRI at 2 and 4 months post-RT and then every 6 months or as clinically indicated

꜌ TSH every 6–12 months

꜌ Dental cleaning every 3 months for lifetime

Acknowledgment We thank Gautam Prasad, MD, PhD; James Rembert, MD; and Eric K. Hansen, MD, for their work on the prior edition of this chapter.

REFERENCES

Al-Sarraf M, LeBlanc M, Giri PG, et al. Chemoradiotherapy versus radiotherapy in patients with advanced nasopharyngeal cancer: phase III randomized intergroup study 0099. J Clin Oncol. 1998;16:1310–7.

Blanchard P, et al. Chemotherapy and radiotherapy in nasopharyngeal carcinoma: an update of the MAC-NPC meta-analysis. Lancet Oncol. 2015;16(6):645–55.

Chan AT, Teo PM, Leung TW, Leung SF, Lee WY, Yeo W, Choi PH, Johnson PJ. A prospective randomized study of chemotherapy adjunctive to definitive radiotherapy in advanced nasopharyngeal carcinoma. International Journal of Radiation Oncology. Biology. Physics. 1995 Oct 15;33(3):569–77.

Chan AT, Leung SF, Ngan RK, et al. Overall survival after concurrent cisplatin-radiotherapy compared with radiotherapy alone in locoregionally advanced nasopharyngeal carcinoma. J Natl Cancer Inst. 2005b;97:536–9.

Chen L, et al. Concurrent chemoradiotherapy plus adjuvant chemotherapy versus concurrent chemoradiotherapy alone in patients with locoregionally advanced nasopharyngeal carcinoma: a phase 3 multicentre randomised controlled trial. Lancet Oncol. 2012; 13(2):163–71. Available at: https://doi.org/10.1016/S1470-2045(11)70320-5.

Chua DT, Sham JS, Choy D, et al. Preliminary report of the Asian-Oceanian clinical oncology association randomized trial comparing cisplatin and epirubicin followed by radiotherapy versus radiotherapy alone in the treatment of patients with locoregionally advanced nasopharyngeal carcinoma. Cancer. 1998;83:2270–83.

Garden AS. The nasopharynx. In: Cox JD, Ang KK, editors. Radiation oncology: rationale, technique, results. 8th ed. St. Louis: Mosby; 2003. p. 178–95.

International Nasopharynx Cancer Study Group. Preliminary results of a randomized trial comparing neoadjuvant chemotherapy (cisplatin, epirubicin, bleomycin) plus radiotherapy vs. radiotherapy alone in stage IV (≥ N2, M0) undifferentiated nasopharyngeal carcinoma: a positive effect on progression-free survival. Int J Radiat Oncol Phys. 1996;35:463–9.

Kam MK, Leung SF, Zee B, et al. Prospective randomized study of intensity-modulated radiotherapy on salivary gland function in early-stage nasopharyngeal carcinoma patients. J Clin Oncol. 2007;25:4873–9.

Lee N, Xia P, Quivey JM, et al. Intensity-modulated radiotherapy in the treatment of nasopharyngeal carcinoma: an update of the UCSF experience. Int J Radiat Oncol Biol Phys. 2002;53:12–22.

Lee N, Xia P, Fischbein NJ, et al. Intensity-modulated radiation therapy for head-and-neck cancer: the UCSF experience focusing on target volume delineation. Int J Radiat Oncol Biol Phys. 2003;57:49–60.

Lee N, Harris J, Garden AS, et al. Intensity-modulated radiation therapy with or without chemotherapy for nasopharyngeal carcinoma: radiation therapy oncology group phase II trial 0225. J Clin Oncol. 2009;27(22):3684–90.

Lee AWM, et al. A randomized trial on addition of concurrent-adjuvant chemotherapy and/or accelerated fractionation for locally-advanced nasopharyngeal carcinoma. Radiother Oncol. 2011;98(1):15–22.

Lee AWM, et al. Preliminary results of trial NPC-0501 evaluating the therapeutic gain by changing from concurrent-adjuvant to induction-concurrent chemoradiotherapy, changing from fluorouracil to capecitabine, and changing from conventional to accelerated radiotherapy fr. Cancer. 2015;121(8):1328–38.

Leung SF, Zee B, Ma BB, et al. Plasma Epstein-Barr viral deoxyribonucleic acid quantitation complements tumor-node-metastasis staging prognostication in nasopharyngeal carcinoma. J Clin Oncol. 2008;24:5414–8.

Lin JC, Wang WY, Chen KY, et al. Quantification of plasma Epstein-Barr virus DNA in patients with advanced nasopharyngeal carcinoma. N Engl J Med. 2004;350(24):2461–70.

Ma J, Mai HQ, Hong MH, et al. Results of a prospective randomized trial comparing neoadjuvant chemotherapy plus radiotherapy with radiotherapy alone in patients with locoregionally advanced nasopharyngeal carcinoma. J Clin Oncol. 2001;19:1350–7.

Pow EH, Kwong DL, McMillan AS, et al. Xerostomia and quality of life after intensity-modulated radiotherapy vs. conventional radiotherapy for early-stage nasopharyngeal carcinoma: initial report on a randomized controlled clinical trial. Int J Radiat Oncol Biol Phys. 2006;66:981–91.

Sun Y, Yu XL, Luo W, et al. Recommendation for a contouring method and atlas of organs at risk in nasopharyngealcarcinoma patients receiving intensity-modulated radiotherapy. Radiother Oncol. 2014;110(3):390–7.

Sun Y, et al. Induction chemotherapy plus concurrent chemoradiotherapy versus concurrent chemoradiotherapy alone in locoregionally advanced nasopharyngeal carcinoma: a phase 3, multicentre, randomised controlled trial. Lancet Oncol. 2016;17(11):1509–20.

Wang W-Y, et al. Long-term survival analysis of nasopharyngeal carcinoma by plasma Epstein-Barr virus DNA levels. Cancer. 2013;119(5):963–70.

Wee J, Tan EH, Tai BC, et al. Randomized trial of radiotherapy versus concurrent chemo-radiotherapy followed by adjuvant chemotherapy in patients with American Joint Committee on Cancer/International Union Against Cancer Stage III and IV nasopharyngeal cancer of the endemic variety. J Clin Oncol. 2005;23:6730–8.

III

Chapter 6
Nasal Cavity and Paranasal Sinus Cancer

III

Jason Chan and Sue S. Yom

PEARLS

- Epidemiology
  - 4500 cases per year in the USA.
  - Maxillary cancers are most common (70%).
  - Incidence higher in Japan and South Africa.
  - More common in males (2:1).
- Anatomy
  - Nasal cavity borders: base of skull (superior); hard palate (inferior); skin (anterior); choanae (posterior).
  - Nasal cavity subsites: vestibule, lateral walls, floor, septum.
  - Paranasal sinus borders: orbital floor (superior); hard palate (inferior); facial bone/zygomatic arch (anterior/anterior lateral); infratemporal fossa/pterygopalatine fossa (posterior/posterior lateral).
  - Paranasal sinus subsites: ethmoid, maxilla, sphenoid, frontal (named according to bones at the tumor location).
  - Ohngren's line runs from the medial canthus of the eye to the angle of the mandible.
    - Tumors superior-posterior to Ohngren's line historically had a poorer prognosis.
  - Lymphatic drainage of maxillary antrum to submandibular, parotid, jugulodigastric, retropharyngeal, and jugular nodes.
- Histology: most common is SCC (70%). Adenocarcinoma, adenoid cystic, mucoepidermoid carcinoma, neuroendocrine

(esthesioneuroblastoma/sinonasal undifferentiated carcinoma (SNUC)/sinonasal neuroendocrine carcinoma (SNEC)/small cell), plasmacytoma, lymphoma, melanoma, and sarcoma also seen.

, See Chap. 12 for more information on esthesioneuroblastoma.

WORKUP

, H&P, nasal endoscopy, CT/MRI, biopsy, CXR. Consider PET/CT for stage III/IV.

, Consider pretreatment baseline serum blood tests including IGF-1, free thyroxin, cortisol, and prolactin.

STAGING: NASAL CAVITY AND PARANASAL SINUS CANCER

Editors' note: All TNM stage and stage groups referred to elsewhere in this chapter reflect the 2010 AJCC staging nomenclature unless otherwise noted as the new system below was published after this chapter was written.

Table 6.1 (AJCC 7TH ED., 2010)

Primary tumor (T)
TX: Primary tumor cannot be assessed
T0: No evidence of primary tumor
Tis: Carcinoma in situ
Maxillary sinus
T1: Tumor limited to maxillary sinus mucosa with no erosion or destruction of bone
T2: Tumor causing bone erosion or destruction including extension into the hard palate and/or middle nasal meatus, except extension to posterior wall of maxillary sinus and pterygoid plates
T3: Tumor invades any of the following: bone of the posterior wall of maxillary sinus, subcutaneous tissues, floor or medial wall of orbit, pterygoid fossa, ethmoid sinuses
T4a: Moderately advanced local disease. Tumor invades anterior orbital contents, skin of cheek, pterygoid plates, infratemporal fossa, cribriform plate, sphenoid or frontal sinuses

Table 6.1 (continued)

Primary tumor (T)

T4b: Very advanced local disease. Tumor invades any of the following: orbital apex, dura, brain, middle cranial fossa, cranial nerves other than maxillary division of trigeminal nerve (V2), nasopharynx, or clivus

Nasal cavity and ethmoid sinus

T1: Tumor restricted to any one subsite, with or without bony invasion

T2: Tumor invading two subsites in a single region or extending to involve an adjacent region within the nasoethmoidal complex, with or without bony invasion

T3: Tumor extends to invade the medial wall or floor of the orbit, maxillary sinus, palate, or cribriform plate

T4a: Moderately advanced local disease. Tumor invades any of the following: anterior orbital contents, skin of nose or cheek, minimal extension to anterior cranial fossa, pterygoid plates, sphenoid or frontal sinuses

T4b: Very advanced local disease. Tumor invades any of the following: orbital apex, dura, brain, middle cranial fossa, cranial nerves other than (V2), nasopharynx, or clivus

Regional lymph nodes (N)

NX: Regional lymph nodes cannot be assessed

N0: No regional lymph node metastasis

N1: Metastasis in a single ipsilateral lymph node, 3 cm or less in greatest dimension

N2: Metastasis in a single ipsilateral lymph node, more than 3 cm, but not more than 6 cm in greatest dimension, or in multiple ipsilateral lymph nodes, not more than 6 cm in greatest dimension, or in bilateral or contralateral lymph nodes, not more than 6 cm in greatest dimension

N2a: Metastasis in a single ipsilateral lymph node, more than 3 cm, but not more than 6 cm in greatest dimension

N2b: Metastasis in multiple ipsilateral lymph nodes, not more than 6 cm in greatest dimension

N2c: Metastasis in bilateral or contralateral lymph nodes, not more than 6 cm in greatest dimension

N3: Metastasis in a lymph node, more than 6 cm in greatest dimension

Distant metastasis (M)

M0: No distant metastasis

M1: Distant metastasis

Anatomic stage/prognostic groups

Stage 0	Tis N0 M0
Stage I	T1 N0 M0
Stage II	T2 N0 M0
Stage III	T3 N0 M0
	T1–T3 N1 M0
Stage IVA	T4a N0 M0
	T4a N1 M0
	T1–T3 N2 M0
	T4a N2 M0
Stage IVB	T4b Any N M0
	Any T N3 M0
Stage IVC	Any T Any N M1

III

Table 6.2 (AJCC 8TH ED., 2017)

Definitions of AJCC TNM
Definition of Primary Tumor (T)
Maxillary sinus

T category	T criteria
TX	Primary tumor cannot be assessed
Tis	Carcinoma in situ
Tl	Tumor limited to the maxillary sinus mucosa with no erosion or destruction of the bone
T2	Tumor causing bone erosion or destruction including extension into the hard palate and/or middle nasal meatus, except extension to the posterior wall of the maxillary sinus and pterygoid plates
T3	Tumor invades any of the following: the bone of the posterior wall of the maxillary sinus, subcutaneous tissues, floor or medial wall of the orbit, pterygoid fossa, and ethmoid sinuses
T4	Moderately advanced or very advanced local disease
T4a	Moderately advanced local disease. Tumor invades anterior orbital contents, skin of the cheek, pterygoid plates, infratemporal fossa, cribriform plate, sphenoid, or frontal sinuses
T4b	Very advanced local disease. Tumor invades any of the following: orbital apex, dura, brain, middle cranial fossa, cranial nerves other than maxillary division of trigeminal nerve (V2), nasopharynx, or clivus

NASAL CAVITY AND ETHMOID SINUS

T category	T criteria
TX	Primary tumor cannot be assessed
Tis	Carcinoma in situ
T1	Tumor restricted to any one subsite, with or without bony invasion
T2	Tumor invading two subsites in a single region or extending to involve an adjacent region within the nasoethmoidal complex, with or without bony invasion
T3	Tumor extends to invade the medial wall or floor of the orbit, maxillary sinus, palate, or cribriform plate
T4	Moderately advanced or very advanced local disease
T4a	Moderately advanced local disease. Tumor invades any of the following: anterior orbital contents, skin of the nose or cheek, minimal extension to the anterior cranial fossa, pterygoid plates, sphenoid, or frontal sinuses
T4b	Very advanced local disease. Tumor invades any of the following: orbital apex, dura, brain, middle cranial fossa, cranial nerves other than (V2), nasopharynx, or clivus

DEFINITION OF REGIONAL LYMPH NODE (N)
Clinical N (CN)

N category	N criteria
NX	Regional lymph nodes cannot be assessed
N0	No regional lymph node metastasis
N1	Metastasis in a single ipsilateral lymph node, 3 cm or smaller in the greatest dimension and ENE(-)
N2	Metastasis in a single ipsilateral node larger than 3 cm but not larger than 6 cm in the greatest dimension and ENE(-) *or* metastases in multiple ipsilateral lymph nodes, not larger than 6 cm in the greatest dimension and ENE(-), *or* in bilateral or contralateral lymph nodes, not larger than 6 cm in the greatest dimension and ENE(-)
N2a	Metastasis in a single ipsilateral node larger than 3 cm but not larger than 6 cm in the greatest dimension and ENE(-)
N2b	Metastasis in multiple ipsilateral nodes, not larger than 6 cm in the greatest dimension and ENE(-)
N2c	Metastasis in bilateral or contralateral lymph nodes, not larger than 6 cm in the greatest dimension and ENE(-)
N3	Metastasis in a lymph node larger than 6 cm in the greatest dimension and ENE(-) *or* metastasis in any node(s) with clinically overt ENE(+)
N3a	Metastasis in a lymph node larger than 6 cm in the greatest dimension and ENE(-)
N3b	Metastasis in any node(s) with clinically overt ENE (ENE$_C$)

Note: A designation of "U" or "L" may be used for any N category to indicate metastasis above the lower border of the cricoid (U) or below the lower border of the cricoid (L) Similarly, clinical and pathological ENE should be recorded as ENE(-) or ENE(+)

PATHOLOGICAL N (PN)

N category	N criteria
NX	Regional lymph nodes cannot be assessed
N0	No regional lymph node metastasis
N1	Metastasis in a single ipsilateral lymph node, 3 cm or smaller in the greatest dimension and ENE(-)
N2	Metastasis in a single ipsilateral lymph node, 3 cm or smaller in the greatest dimension and ENE(+) *or* larger than 3 cm but not larger than 6 cm in the greatest dimension and ENE(-), *or* metastases in multiple ipsilateral lymph nodes, not larger than 6 cm in the greatest dimension and ENE(-), *or* in bilateral or contralateral lymph nodes, not larger than 6 cm in the greatest dimension and ENE(-)

continued

N category	N criteria
N2a	Metastasis in single ipsilateral or contralateral node 3 cm or less in the greatest dimension and ENE(+) *or* a single ipsilateral node larger than 3 cm but not larger than 6 cm in the greatest dimension and ENE(-)
N2b	Metastasis in multiple ipsilateral nodes, not larger than 6 cm in the greatest dimension and ENE(-)
N2c	Metastasis in bilateral or contralateral lymph nodes, not larger than 6 cm in the greatest dimension and ENE(-)
N3	Metastasis in a lymph node larger than 6 cm in the greatest dimension and ENE(-) *or* in a single ipsilateral node larger than 3 cm in the greatest dimension and ENE(+) *or* multiple ipsilateral, contralateral, or bilateral nodes, any with ENE(+)
N3a	Metastasis in a lymph node larger than 6 cm in the greatest dimension and ENE(-)
N3b	Metastasis in a single ipsilateral node larger than 3 cm in the greatest dimension and ENE(+) *or* multiple ipsilateral, contralateral, or bilateral nodes, any with ENE(+)

Note: A designation of "U" or "L" may be used for any N category to indicate metastasis above the lower border of the cricoid (U) or below the lower border of the cricoid (L) Similarly, clinical and pathological ENE should be recorded as ENE(-) or ENE(+)

DEFINITION OF DISTANT METASTASIS (M)

M category	M criteria
M0	No distant metastasis (no pathologic M0, use clinical M to complete stage group)
M1	Distant metastasis

AJCC PROGNOSTIC STAGE GROUPS

When T is...	And N is...	And M is...	Then the stage group is...
Tis	N0	M0	0
T1	N0	M0	I
T2	N0	M0	II
T3	N0	M0	III
T1, T2, T3	N1	M0	III
T4a	N0, N1	M0	IVA
T1, T2, T3, T4a	N2	M0	IVA
Any T	N3	M0	IVB
T4b	Any N	M0	IVB
Any T	Any N	M1	IVC

Used with permission of the American Joint Committee on Cancer (AJCC), Chicago, Illinois. The original and primary source for this information is the AJCC Cancer Staging Manual, Eighth Edition (2017) published by Springer International Publishing

TREATMENT RECOMMENDATIONS

Table 6.3 TREATMENT RECOMMENDATIONS

Stage	Recommended treatment
Nasal cavity and ethmoid sinus	T1-2N0: Resection → post-op RT for close/+ margins or PNI Alternatively, definitive RT. Choice depends on size, location, and expected cosmetic outcome T3-4N0: Resectable: resection → post-op RT Unresectable or inoperable: Definitive RT or chemo-RT N+: Resection + neck dissection → post-op RT or chemo-RT Alternatively, definitive chemo-RT
Maxillary sinus	T1-2N0: Resection → post-op RT for close margin, PNI, adenoid cystic. For + margin, re-resect (if possible) → post-op RT T3-4N0 resectable: Resection → post-op RT or chemo-RT Unresectable or inoperable: Definitive RT or chemo-RT N+: Resection + neck dissection → post-op RT or chemo-RT Alternatively, definitive chemo-RT
SNUC/SNEC/small cell	Include chemotherapy with treatment as above

STUDIES

NASAL CAVITY

ˌ Allen (IJROBP 2008): 68 patients with nasal cavity or nasal septum cancer. Forty-seven percent received definitive RT. Nineteen percent received neck RT. 5/10-yr LC 86/76%, DFS 86/78%, OS 82/62%.

PARANASAL SINUS

ˌ Le (IJROBP 2000): 97 patients with maxillary sinus tumors. Fifty-six had surgery first and 41 had pre-op or definitive RT. 12% LN relapse at 5 years. T3–4 SCC were associated with a high incidence of initial nodal involvement and nodal relapse. None of the patients presenting with SCC histology and N0 necks had nodal recurrence after elective neck radiation. Recommended elective ipsilateral neck RT for T3–4 SCC.

- Bristol (IJROBP 2007): 146 patients with maxillary sinus tumors treated with post-op radiotherapy. Group 1 included 90 patients treated before 1991. Group 2 included 56 patients treated after 1991, when radiotherapy technique incorporated coverage of the base of skull for patients with perineural invasion, elective neck RT in SCC or undifferentiated histology, and techniques to improve dose homogeneity to target. No difference in 5-yr OS (51% vs. 62%), RFS, LRC, DM between the two groups, but base of skull and nodal failures reduced in at-risk patients. Advanced age, need for enucleation, and positive margins were independent predictors of worse OS. Need for enucleation predicted worse LRC.

NASAL CAVITY AND PARANASAL SINUS

- Dulguerov (Cancer 2001): 220 patients with nasal cavity and paranasal sinus cancer. 5-yr OS 40%, LC 59%. Prognostic factors: histology, T stage, primary site, and treatment type. Local extension factors associated with worse survival: extension to pterygomaxillary fossa, extension to frontal and sphenoid sinuses, erosion of cribriform plate, and invasion of the dura. In the presence of an intraorbital invasion, enucleation was associated with better survival.
- Chen (IJROBP 2007): 127 patients with sinonasal carcinoma. 5-yr OS, LRC, and DFS were 52%, 62%, and 54%, respectively. No significant difference in 5-year OS rates for patients treated in the 1960s, 1970s, 1980s, 1990s, and 2000s. Significantly reduced incidence of severe (Grade 3 and 4) toxicity over the decades.
- Madani (IJROBP 2009): 73 primary and 11 locally recurrent sinonasal tumors definitively treated by IMRT. No chemo. 64% patients had adenocarcinoma histology. Median follow-up 40 mo with 5-year LRC, OS, and DFS were 71%, 58%, and 59%, respectively.
- Snyers (IJROBP 2009): 178 patients with sinonasal cancer. 62% of long-term survivors had hormonal disturbances and 24% had multiple hormonal deficiencies.
- Wiegner (IJROBP 2012): 52 patients with tumors of the nasal cavity and paranasal sinuses treated post-op or

definitively with IMRT. 2-year LRC, in-field LRC, FFDM, and OS were 64%, 74%, 71%, and 66%. Grade $\geq$ 3 mucositis 37%, dermatitis 15%, one late optic toxicity.

, Multiple other published series report that IMRT is safe and effective for sinonasal carcinomas (e.g., Askoxylakis, Radiat Oncol 2016) and that it is often the preferred radiotherapy technique in particular for normal tissue sparing (Chi, J Hematol Oncol 2013).

, Some physicians extrapolate from the Bernier and Cooper head and neck cancer studies (*NEJM* 2004, *Head and Neck* 2005) to support using post-op concurrent chemo and RT in patients with SCC of the paranasal sinuses having positive margins or extranodal extension.

INDUCTION CHEMOTHERAPY

, Hanna (Arch Otolaryngol Head Neck Surg 2011): 46 patients with T3–T4 squamous cell carcinoma of the paranasal sinuses or nasal cavity (maxillary sinus 67%). 26% had clinical evidence of nodal metastasis; 80% had stage IV. Induction chemotherapy was taxane-platinum in 80% or combined with ifosfamide or 5-fluorouracil, or taxane-5-fluorouracil. 67% of patients achieved at least partial response, 24% had progression, and 9% had stable disease. Surgery could be performed in 52% after induction. 2-year survival for stable or responding disease was 77% but was 36% for patients with progression on induction. The authors suggest that a lack of response to induction may indicate an inherently poor prognosis.

RADIATION TECHNIQUES

SIMULATION AND FIELD DESIGN

, Simulate supine with thermoplastic mask immobilization.
, Eyes open, straight ahead to keep posterior pole away from high dose region inferiorly.
, Consider tongue blade/cork to depress tongue out of fields.
, Consider filling surgical defects with tissue equivalent material.

‚ Recommend IMRT or 3DCRT planning to increase sparing of normal structures.

‚ GTV = clinical and/or radiographic gross disease.

‚ CTV1 = 1 cm margin on primary and/or nodal GTV.

‚ CTV2 = high-risk regions (depending on the presence or absence of anatomic boundaries to microscopic spread).

‚ CTV3 = elective neck.

‚ Individualized planning target volumes are used for the GTV, CTV1, CTV2, and CTV3 tailored to subsite and stage.

‚ Replanning may be considered during treatment if there is a potential for change in aeration of the sinuses in response to treatment, given the proximity to optic and central nervous system structures.

DOSE PRESCRIPTIONS

‚ EBRT 1.8–2 Gy/fx.

‚ Definitive RT or chemo-RT: CTV1 to 66–70 Gy, CTV2 to 60–63 Gy, CTV3 to 54–57 Gy.

‚ Post-op RT: CTV1 to 60 Gy with optional boost to 66 Gy to high-risk areas (close/+ margins, ECE, PNI). CTV2 to 50–54 Gy.

‚ For selected nasal septum tumors, brachytherapy may be appropriate.

DOSE LIMITATIONS

‚ Lens <10 Gy (cataracts).

‚ Retina <45 Gy (vision). May go higher if treating bid or partial volume.

‚ Optic chiasm and nerves <54 Gy at standard fractionation.

‚ Brain <60 Gy (necrosis).

‚ Mandible <60 Gy (osteoradionecrosis).

‚ Parotid mean dose <26 Gy (xerostomia).

‚ Lacrimal gland <30–40 Gy.

‚ Pituitary and hypothalamus mean dose <40 Gy.

COMPLICATIONS

‚ Acute = mucositis, skin erythema, nasal dryness, xerostomia

‚ Late = xerostomia, chronic keratitis and iritis, optic pathway injury, soft tissue or osteoradionecrosis, cataracts, radiation-induced hypopituitarism

FOLLOW-UP

, H&P, labs, and CXR every 3 months for the first year, every 4 months for second year, every 6 months for third year, and then annually. Imaging of the H&N at 3 months posttreatment and then as indicated.

III

Acknowledgment We thank Chien Peter Chen, MD, and Brian Missett, MD, for their work on the prior edition of this chapter.

REFERENCES

Allen MW, Schwartz DL, Rana V, et al. Long-term radiotherapy outcomes for nasal cavity and septal cancers. Int J Radiat Oncol Biol Phys. 2008;71:401–6.

Askoxylakis V, Hegenbarth P, Timke C, et al. Intensity modulated radiation therapy (IMRT) for sinonasal tumors: a single center long-term clinical analysis. Radiat Oncol. 2016;11:17.

Bernier J, Domenge C, Ozsahin M, et al. Postoperative irradiation with or without concomitant chemotherapy for locally advanced head and neck cancer. N Engl J Med. 2004;350:1945–52.

Bernier J, Cooper JS, Pajak TF, et al. Defining risk levels in locally advanced head and neck cancers: a comparative analysis of concurrent postoperative radiation plus chemotherapy trials of the EORTC (#22931) and RTOG (# 9501). Head Neck. 2005;27(10):843–50.

Bristol IJ, Ahamad A, Garden AS, et al. Postoperative radiotherapy for maxillary sinus cancer: long-term outcomes and toxicities of treatment. Int J Radiat Oncol Biol Phys. 2007;68:719–30.

Chen AM, Daly ME, Bucci MK, et al. Carcinomas of the paranasal sinuses and nasal cavity treated with radiotherapy at a single institution over five decades: are we making improvement? Int J Radiat Oncol Biol Phys. 2007;69:141–7.

Chi A, Nguyen NP, Tse W, et al. Intensity modulated radiotherapy for sinonasal malignancies with a focus on optic pathway preservation. J Hematol Oncol. 2013;6:4.

Dulguerov P, Jacobsen MS, Allal AS, et al. Nasal and paranasal sinus carcinoma: are we making progress? A series of 220 patients and a systematic review. Cancer. 2001;92:3012–29.

Hanna EY, et al. Induction chemotherapy for advanced squamous cell carcinoma of the paranasal sinuses. Arch Otolaryngol Head Neck Surg. 2011;137(1):78–81.

Le QT, Fu KK, Kaplan MJ, et al. Lymph node metastasis in maxillary sinus carcinoma. Int J Radiat Oncol Biol Phys. 2000;46:541–9.

Madani I, Bonte K, Vakaet L, et al. Intensity-modulated radiotherapy for sinonasal tumors: Ghent University Hospital update. Int J Radiat Oncol Biol Phys. 2009;73:424–32.

Snyers A, Janssens GO, Twickler MB, et al. Malignant tumors of the nasal cavity and paranasal sinuses: long-term outcome and morbidity with emphasis on hypothalamic-pituitary deficiency. Int J Radiat Oncol Biol Phys. 2009;73:1343–51.

Wiegner EA, et al. Intensity-modulated radiotherapy for tumors of the nasal cavity and paranasal sinuses: clinical outcomes and patterns of failure. Int J Radiat Oncol Biol Phy. 2012;83(1):243–51.

Chapter 7
Oropharyngeal Cancer

Christopher H. Chapman and Sue S. Yom

PEARLS

- Approximately 8500 cases/year in the USA with male predominance (3:1).
- Risk factors include use of tobacco, alcohol, and oncogenic human papilloma virus (HPV) infection.
- Recent decreases in the incidence of tobacco-related cancers and increases in HPV-associated cancers (now about 70–80% of oropharyngeal squamous cell carcinomas).
  - Attributed to decreased tobacco use and changing sexual practices.
  - HPV-associated cancers may occur at a younger age and have better survival rates across all stages compared to non-HPV-associated cancers.
- Historically second primary tumors in the upper aerodigestive tract and lung occur in ~25% of patients, but the rate is lower after HPV-associated cancer.
  - Risk of second primary cancers is doubled with continued smoking.
- Subsites: soft palate, palatine tonsils, tonsillar pillars, base of tongue (lingual tonsils, posterior to circumvallate papillae), and pharyngeal wall.
- Anatomic boundaries: superior = superior plane above soft palate; inferior = plane of superior hyoid bone (or floor of vallecula).

© Springer International Publishing AG, part of Springer Nature 2018   **171**
Eric K. Hansen and M. Roach III (eds.), *Handbook of Evidence-Based Radiation Oncology*, https://doi.org/10.1007/978-3-319-62642-0_7

- Deep (middle) ear pain may be referred from base of tongue via the tympanic nerve of Jacobson (CN IX) via the petrosal ganglion.
- Histology: 95% squamous cell carcinoma (SCC). Others: adenocarcinoma, mucoepidermoid, adenoid cystic, melanoma, small cell carcinoma of tonsil, non-Hodgkin's lymphoma of tonsil.
- Presentation: sore throat, dysphagia, otalgia, odynophagia, hot potato voice (with base of tongue invasion), hoarseness (with larynx invasion or edema).
- Major cervical lymph node levels (Fig. 7.1) (Grégoire *Radiother Oncol* 2014):
  - Ia: Midline, between anterior bellies of digastric muscles to hyoid bone.
  - Ib: Lateral to anterior belly of digastric muscle to posterior edge of submandibular gland.
  - II: Deep to sternocleidomastoid, extends to bottom of hyoid. Medial edge is medial border of internal carotid artery. Standard superior border is transverse process of C1 vertebral body; "high" superior border is jugular foramen (a.k.a. level VIIb). IIa is anterior to posterior edge of internal jugular vein; IIb is posterior.
  - Retropharyngeal (RPN): (a.k.a. level VIIa) from midline to medial edge of internal carotid arteries, same superior/inferior extent as level II. Posterior to pharyngeal constrictor muscles. "Medial RPN" are medial to plane at edge of longus capiti muscles.
  - III: Deep to sternocleidomastoid, including medial edge of internal carotid artery, inferior to hyoid, superior to cricoid cartilage.
  - IV: Deep to sternocleidomastoid, including medial edge of internal carotid artery, inferior to top of cricoid cartilage. IVa inferior border is 2 cm cranial to sternoclavicular joint; IVb extends to manubrium (a.k.a. medial supraclavicular).
  - V: Posterior to sternocleidomastoid, inferior to hyoid, anterior to plane at anterior edge of trapezius muscle, superior to transverse cervical vessels. Level Vc (a.k.a. lateral supraclavicular) extends to 2 cm cranial to sternoclavicular joint.
  - VI: Midline, between medial edges of sternocleidomastoid, inferior to hyoid, superior to manubrium.

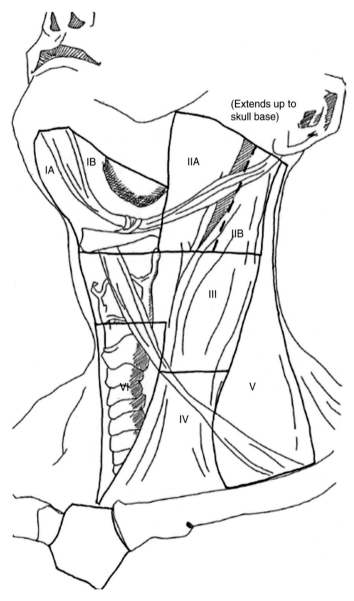

Fig. 7.1 Major cervical lymph node levels

WORKUP

- H&P with palpation, indirect mirror exam ± fiberoptic endoscopy.
- Panendoscopy (esophagoscopy, bronchoscopy, laryngoscopy) with biopsy.
- Labs: CBC, chemistries, BUN, Cr, and LFTs including alkaline phosphatase.
- HPV testing should be performed on primary tumor or nodal biopsy specimens. Immunohistochemistry of p16 protein is a surrogate marker for HPV infection with 80–90% concordance in the oropharynx (lower in other subsites).
- Imaging: MRI or CT scan with contrast of head and neck. Consider FDG-PET for stages III–IV. Otherwise CT chest to rule out metastatic disease.
  - Uninvolved tonsils, base of tongue, and salivary glands may show low levels of signal intensity on MRI or low SUV on FDG-PET.
- Preventive dental care with extractions at least 14 days before RT.
- Speech/swallow and nutrition consultations with follow-up during and after RT.

STAGING: OROPHARYNGEAL CANCER

Editors' note: All TNM stage and stage groups referred to elsewhere in this chapter reflect the 2010 AJCC staging nomenclature unless otherwise noted as the new system below was published after this chapter was written.

Table 7.1 (AJCC 7TH ED., 2010)

Primary tumor (T)	
TX:	Primary tumor cannot be assessed
T0:	No evidence of primary tumor
Tis:	Carcinoma in situ

Table 7.1 (continued)

T1:	Tumor 2 cm or less in greatest dimension
T2:	Tumor more than 2 cm but not more than 4 cm in greatest dimension
T3:	Tumor more than 4 cm in greatest dimension or extension to lingual surface of epiglottis
T4a:	Moderately advanced local disease. Tumor invades the larynx, extrinsic muscle of tongue, medial pterygoid, hard palate, or mandible*
T4b:	Very advanced local disease. Tumor invades lateral pterygoid muscle, pterygoid plates, lateral nasopharynx, or skull base or encases carotid artery

Note: Mucosal extension to lingual surface of epiglottis from primary tumors of the base of the tongue and vallecula does not constitute invasion of the larynx

Regional lymph nodes (N)

NX:	Regional lymph nodes cannot be assessed
N0:	No regional lymph node metastasis
N1:	Metastasis in a single ipsilateral lymph node, 3 cm or less in greatest dimension
N2:	Metastasis in a single ipsilateral lymph node, more than 3 cm, but not more than 6 cm in greatest dimension, or in multiple ipsilateral lymph nodes, not more than 6 cm in greatest dimension, or in bilateral or contralateral lymph nodes, not more than 6 cm in greatest dimension
N2a:	Metastasis in a single ipsilateral lymph node more than 3 cm but not more than 6 cm in greatest dimension
N2b:	Metastasis in multiple ipsilateral lymph nodes, not more than 6 cm in greatest dimension
N2c:	Metastasis in bilateral or contralateral lymph nodes, not more than 6 cm in greatest dimension
N3:	Metastasis in a lymph node more than 6 cm in greatest dimension

Note: Metastases at level VII (upper mediastinum) are considered regional lymph node metastases

Distant metastases (M)

MX:	Distant metastasis cannot be assessed
M0:	No distant metastasis

Stage grouping

0:	TisN0M0
I:	T1N0M0
II:	T2N0M0
III:	T3N0M0, T1-3N1M0
IVA:	T4aN0-1M0, T1-4aN2M0
IVB:	T4b, any N, M0; any T, N3M0
IVC:	Any T, any N, M1

Used with the permission from the American Joint Committee on Cancer (AJCC), Chicago, Illinois. The original source for this material is the AJCC Cancer Staging Manual, Seventh Edition (2010), published by Springer Science + Business Media

Table 7.2 (AJCC 8TH ED., 2017)

Definitions of AJCC TNM
Definition of Primary Tumor (T)
Oropharynx (p 16-)

T category	T criteria
TX	Primary tumor cannot be assessed
Tis	Carcinoma in situ
T1	Tumor 2 cm or smaller in greatest dimension
T2	Tumor larger than 2 cm but not larger than 4 cm in the greatest dimension
T3	Tumor larger than 4 cm in the greatest dimension or extension to the lingual surface of the epiglottis
T4	Moderately advanced or very advanced local disease
T4a	Moderately advanced local disease. Tumor invades the larynx, extrinsic muscle of tongue, medial pterygoid, hard palate, or mandible*
T4b	Very advanced local disease. Tumor invades the lateral pterygoid muscle, pterygoid plates, lateral nasopharynx, or skull base or encases the carotid artery

*Note: Mucosal extension to lingual surface of the epiglottis from primary tumors of the base of the tongue and vallecula does not constitute invasion of the larynx

DEFINITION OF REGIONAL LYMPH NODE (N)

CLINICAL N (cN): OROPHARYNX (P 16-) AND HYPOPHARYNX

N category	N criteria
NX	Regional lymph nodes cannot be assessed
N0	No regional lymph node metastasis
N1	Metastasis in a single ipsilateral lymph node, 3 cm or smaller in the greatest dimension and ENE(-)
N2	Metastasis in a single ipsilateral node larger than 3 cm but not larger than 6 cm in the greatest dimension and ENE(-) *or* metastases in multiple ipsilateral lymph nodes, not larger than 6 cm in the greatest dimension and ENE(-), *or* in bilateral or contralateral lymph nodes, not larger than 6 cm in the greatest dimension and ENE(-)
N2a	Metastasis in a single ipsilateral node larger than 3 cm but not larger than 6 cm in the greatest dimension and ENE(-)
N2b	Metastasis in multiple ipsilateral nodes, not larger than 6 cm in the greatest dimension and ENE(-)
N2c	Metastasis in bilateral or contralateral lymph nodes, not larger than 6 cm in the greatest dimension and ENE(-)
N3	Metastasis in a lymph node larger than 6 cm in the greatest dimension and ENE(-) *or* metastasis in any node(s) and clinically overt ENE(+)
N3a	Metastasis in a lymph node larger than 6 cm in the greatest dimension and ENE(-)
N3b	Metastasis in any node(s) and clinically overt ENE(+)

Note: A designation of "U" or "L" may be used for any N category to indicate metastasis above the lower border of the cricoid (U) or below the lower border of the cricoid (L)
Similarly, clinical and pathological ENE should be recorded as ENE(-) or ENE(+)

PATHOLOGICAL N (PN): OROPHARYNX (P 16-) AND HYPOPHARYNX

N category	N criteria
NX	Regional lymph nodes cannot be assessed
N0	No regional lymph node metastasis
N1	Metastasis in a single ipsilateral lymph node, 3 cm or smaller in the greatest dimension and ENE(-)
N2	Metastasis in a single ipsilateral lymph node, 3 cm or smaller in the greatest dimension and ENE(+) *or* larger than 3 cm but not larger than 6 cm in the greatest dimension and ENE(-), *or* metastases in multiple ipsilateral lymph nodes, not larger than 6 cm in the greatest dimension and ENE(-), *or* in bilateral or contralateral lymph nodes, not larger than 6 cm in the greatest dimension and ENE(-)
N2a	Metastasis in single ipsilateral or contralateral node 3 cm or smaller in the greatest dimension and ENE(+) *or* a single ipsilateral node larger than 3 cm but not larger than 6 cm in the greatest dimension and ENE(-)
N2b	Metastasis in multiple ipsilateral nodes, not larger than 6 cm in the greatest dimension and ENE(-)
N2c	Metastasis in bilateral or contralateral lymph nodes, not larger than 6 cm in the greatest dimension and ENE(-)
N3	Metastasis in a lymph node larger than 6 cm in the greatest dimension and ENE(-) *or* in a single ipsilateral node larger than 3 cm in greatest dimension and ENE(+) *or* multiple ipsilateral, contralateral, or bilateral nodes, any with ENE(+)
N3a	Metastasis in a lymph node larger than 6 cm in the greatest dimension and ENE(-)
N3b	Metastasis in a single ipsilateral node larger than 3 cm in the greatest dimension and ENE(+) *or* multiple ipsilateral, contralateral, or bilateral nodes, any with ENE(+)

Note: A designation of "U" or "L" may be used for any N category to indicate metastasis above the lower border of the cricoid (U) or below the lower border of the cricoid (L) Similarly, clinical and pathological ENE should be recorded as ENE(-) or ENE(+)

DEFINITION OF DISTANT METASTASIS (M) OROPHARYNX (PI6-) AND HYPOPHARYNX

M category	M criteria
M0	No distant metastasis
M1	Distant metastasis

AJCC PROGNOSTIC STAGE GROUPS

When T is...	And N is...	And M is...	Then the stage group is...
Tis	N0	M0	0
T1	N0	M0	I
T2	N0	M0	II
T3	N0	M0	III
T1, T2, T3	N1	M0	III
T4a	N0. 1	M0	IVA
T1, T2, T3, T4a	N2	M0	IVA
Any T	N3	M0	IVB
T4b	Any N	M0	IVB
Any T	Any N	M1	IVC

Used with permission of the American Joint Committee on Cancer (AJCC), Chicago, Illinois. The original and primary source for this information is the AJCC Cancer Staging Manual, Eighth Edition (2017) published by Springer International Publishing

OUTCOMES

- (O'Sullivan *Lancet Oncol* 2016): 1907 HPV+ pts, 696 HPV- pts 98% treated with primary RT, 2% with surgery. 5-yr OS:
  - HPV+ AJCC 8th Ed. Stages
    - I (T1-2N0-1): 85%
    - II (T1-2N2 or T3N02): 78%
    - III (T4 or N3): 53%
  - HPV- AJCC 7th Ed. Stages
    - I: 76%
    - II: 68%
    - III: 53%
    - IVA: 45%
    - IVB: 34%
- (O'Sullivan *JCO* 2013): AJCC 7th Ed stages. 899 pts treated with chemo-RT or RT. 3-yr LRC and DM:
  - HPV+
    - Low-risk (T1-3N0-2c): LRC 95%, DM 7%
    - High-risk (T4 or N3): LRC 82%, DM 24%
  - HPV-
    - Low-risk (T1-2N0-2c): LRC 76%, DM 7%
    - High-risk (T3-4 or N3): LRC 62%, DM 28%

TREATMENT RECOMMENDATIONS

Table 7.3 TREATMENT RECOMMENDATIONS

Clinical stage	Recommended treatment
T1-2N0	Definitive RT with consolidative surgery for < CR Alternative: surgical resection of primary ± ipsilateral or bilateral neck dissection. Post-op RT indicated for pT3–T4, close margin, multiple nodes, level IV–V nodes, PNI, or LVSI. Post-op chemo-RT indicated for positive margin or ECE
T3–4 or LN+	Preferred: concurrent chemo-RT with consolidative surgery for < CR Alternative: surgical resection of primary ± ipsilateral or bilateral neck dissection. Post-op RT indicated for pT3–T4, close margin, multiple nodes, level IV–V nodes, PNI, or LVSI. Post-op chemo-RT indicated for positive margin or ECE For patients not candidates for standard cisplatin chemo-RT, consider concurrent cetuximab If unable to tolerate concurrent chemo, altered fractionation RT may be used

SURGERY

- Transoral laser microsurgery (TLM) and/or transoral robotic surgery (TORS) is an emerging approach for resectable oropharynx cancers
  - T1–2 tumors arising within the tonsillar fossa, lateral pharyngeal wall, glossopharyngeal sulcus, or lateral tongue base may be amenable to TORS.
  - Recent meta-analyses report similar DSS and OS with primary transoral surgery or radiotherapy for early-stage tumors (de Almeida *Laryngoscope* 2014; Morisod *Head Neck* 2016). However, postoperative radiotherapy may be indicated in up to 90% of pts and about one third of patients receive postoperative chemoradiation.
  - Soft tissue necrosis reported in 23.5–28% of patients receiving adjuvant therapy after TORS; highest risk with fraction sizes >2 Gy/fraction (Lee 2016; Lukens 2014).

- Ongoing phase II and III trials are evaluating the role of TORS
  - ECOG 3311 observes low-risk HPV+ T1-2N0-1 patients with negative margins. High-risk pts with positive margins, >1 mm ECE, or >5 LN involved receive postoperative 66 Gy chemoradiation. Intermediate-risk patients with <1 mm ECE, 2–4 LN, PNI, or LVSI are randomized to 50 Gy vs 60 Gy post-op radiotherapy.
- For T3–4 primaries, tonsillar lesions may require radical tonsillectomy often with partial mandibulectomy; base of tongue lesions require partial or total glossectomy and myocutaneous flap reconstruction. Patients requiring removal of more than 1/2 of tongue or elderly patients with poor pulmonary function often experience subsequent aspiration. Therefore, for locally advanced oropharyngeal cancer, primary organ preservation approach with radiation or chemo-RT is often preferred.
- Types of neck dissection
  - Radical neck dissection (RND) removes levels I–V, sternocleidomastoid muscle, omohyoid muscle, internal and external jugular veins, CN XI, and the submandibular gland.
  - Modified RND leaves ≥1 of sternocleidomastoid muscle, internal jugular vein, or CN XI.
  - Selective neck dissection removes less than all of levels I–V:
    - Supraomohyoid neck dissection only removes levels I–III.
    - Lateral neck dissection only removes levels II–IV.

ALTERED FRACTIONATION

- Improved local control and survival with accelerated or hyperfractioned/dose escalated radiotherapy.
- *RTOG 90–03* (Fu *IJROBP* 2000; Beitler *IJROBP* 2014): 268 patients with locally advanced H&N SCC randomized to standard 2/70 Gy vs. hyperfractionated 1.2 BID/81.6 Gy vs. concomitant boost 72 Gy (1.8/54 Gy plus BID 1.5 Gy last 12 days) vs. split-course 1.6 BID/67.2 Gy (2 week break). At 5 years, reduction in LRF vs. standard was 6.5%, 6.6%, and 1.1%. Overall survival was

nonsignificantly improved for hyperfractionated and concomitant boost. All non-standard fractionation increased acute side effects, and accelerated fractionation increased late side effects.

, *DAHANCA 6 & 7* (Overgaard *Lancet* 2003): 1485 patients with H&N SCC of any stage all received 62–68 Gy definitive radiotherapy with radiosensitizer nimorazole. Randomized to 5 fractions per week vs. 6 fractions per week (weekend or one BID treatment). Accelerated fractionation significantly improved 5-year LRC (60 → 70%, entirely from primary site control) and DSS (68 → 74%). No difference in 5-year OS (44%). More/earlier grade 3 mucositis in accelerated arm (33 → 53%). No difference in late toxicity.

, *MARCH meta-analysis* (Bourhis *Lancet* 2006): 15 phase III trials of 6515 patients with H&N SCC. Significantly improved OS (3.4% benefit) and LRC (6.4% benefit) at 5 years for altered fractionation vs. conventional fractionation, with most benefit seen for hyperfractionation. Decreasing benefit with increasing age.

, For lower-risk pts unable to tolerate systemic therapy, primary RT offers good results:

, (Garden *Cancer* 2016): 324 pts with AJCC 7th T1-3N1-2b or T3N0 and <10 pack-years smoking with intact primary treated with RT without systemic therapy. 73% received standard fractionation (66 Gy at 2–2.2 Gy/fx), 27% altered fractionation. 5-yr PFS T1 90%, T2 83%, T3 70%. No significant difference in PFS compared to 439 pts given systemic therapy except trend for T3 pts (5-yr PFS 77%, $p = 0.07$). 5-yr LRC 95% with RT without systemic therapy.

CHEMO-RT ± ALTERED FRACTIONATION

, Improved local control and survival with concurrent chemotherapy, especially regimens including a platinum agent. Accelerated RT with 2 cycles cisplatin comparable to standard RT with 3 cycles cisplatin. Concurrent cetuximab superior to RT alone but no advantage when added to cisplatin-RT.

, *Intergroup* (Adelstein *JCO* 2003): 295 patients with stage III–IVB H&N SCC, randomized to 2/70 Gy vs.

2/70 Gy + 3 cycles cisplatin vs. split-course (2/30 Gy + 2 cycles cisplatin/5FU → resection if possible → 2/30–40 Gy + 1 cycle cisplatin/5FU). Continuous but not split-course chemo-RT significantly improved 3-year OS (23 → 37%) and DSS (33 → 51%) vs. RT alone. No difference in distant metastases. Chemo-RT increased acute toxicity.

- *GORTEC 94–01* (Denis *JCO* 2004): 226 patients with stage III–IVB oropharyngeal SCC randomized to 2/70 vs. 2/70 Gy + 3 cycles carboplatin/5-FU. Chemo-RT improved 5-year LC (25 → 48%), DFS (15 → 27%), and OS (16 → 23%), but increased acute toxicity. Trend for increased late toxicity.

- *MACH-NC Meta-analysis* (Pignon *Radiother Oncol* 2009): 93 phase III trials and 17,346 patients. 5-year OS benefit 4.5% with chemo-RT vs. RT alone. Greater OS benefit for concurrent (6.5%) vs. induction chemo (2.4%), no benefit from adjuvant chemo. Similar results with post-op RT, conventional, and altered fractionation. More benefit with regimens containing platinum. Decreasing chemo-RT benefit with age; none observed if age > 70 years.

- (Bonner *NEJM* 2006; *Lancet Oncol* 2010): 424 patients with stage III–IVB H&N SCC randomized to RT or RT + weekly cetuximab. RT not standardized; options included 2/70 Gy, 1.2 BID/72–76.8 Gy, or concomitant boost 72 Gy. Cetuximab improved 5-year OS (36 → 46%). Improved OS with concomitant boost vs. standard fractionation. Cetuximab patients with prominent acneiform rash had longer median survival (26 → 69 months). No difference by EGFR expression.

- *RTOG 01–29* (Ang *NEJM* 2010): 721 patients with stage III–IV H&N SCC randomized to concomitant boost 72 Gy + 2 cycles cisplatin vs. standard fractionation 2/70 Gy + 3 cycles cisplatin. No significant difference in 3-year OS, PFS, or relapse pattern. In 323 patients with HPV/p16 status available, 3-year OS 82% in HPV-positive vs. 57% in HPV-negative. RPA using HPV status, smoking history, and T/N stage: 3-year OS 93% for low-risk, 71% for intermediate-risk, and 46% for high-risk patients.

- *GORTEC 99–02* (Bourhis *Lancet Oncol* 2012): 840 patients with stage III–IVB H&N SCC randomized to conventional chemo-RT (70 Gy in 7 weeks +3 cycles carboplatin/5-FU) vs. accelerated chemo-RT (70 Gy in 6 weeks +2 cycles carboplatin/5-FU) vs. very accelerated RT alone (64.8 Gy in 3.5 weeks). Very accelerated RT had worse 3-year OS (43 → 37%), PFS (38 → 32%) and LRF (42 → 50%) vs. conventional chemo-RT, also worse mucositis and long-term PEG-tube dependence. No difference in accelerated vs. conventional chemo-RT.

, *RTOG 05-22* (Ang *JCO* 2014): 891 patients with stage III–IV H&N SCC randomized to accelerated chemo-RT with 2 cycles cisplatin ± neoadjuvant/concurrent cetuximab. No significant difference in 3-year OS, PFS, LRC, or DM. No interaction with p16 or EGFR status. More treatment-related deaths and interruption of radiation (15 → 27%) with cetuximab.

, Recently completed HPV-associated oropharyngeal cancer de-intensification trials:

, *RTOG 10–16*: Phase III equivalence trial of accelerated RT with concurrent cisplatin vs. cetuximab

, p16+, stratified by stage, KPS, smoking history.

, Arm 1 (control): 2/70 Gy IMRT (6 fx/week) + 2c cisplatin 100 mg/m2 q3 weeks.

, Arm 2: Same RT + cetuximab 400 mg/m2 loading pre-RT + 250 mg/m2 weekly during RT.

, *NRG-HN002*: Randomized phase II, dose-reduced RT ± cisplatin.

, p16+ with ≤10 pack-years smoking history, T1-3 N1-2b or T3 N0.

, Arm 1: 2/60 Gy IMRT (5 fx/week) + 6c cisplatin 40 mg/m2.

, Arm 2: 2/60 Gy IMRT (6 fx/week) with no chemotherapy.

POST-OPERATIVE CHEMO-RT

, Post-op RT alone indications (minor risk factors): close margin, multiple LN+, PNI, LVSI.

, Post-op chemo-RT indications (major risk factors): nodal extracapsular extension (ECE) and/or positive margin.

, *EORTC 22931* (Bernier *NEJM* 2004): 334 patients with operable H&N SCC stage pT3–4, pT1-2N2-3, oral cavity/oropharynx with levels IV–V involved, or T1-2N0-1 with ECE, +margin, LVSI, or PNI. Randomized to post-op RT 2/60–66 Gy or chemo-RT (+ cisplatin ×3 cycles). Chemo-RT improved 5-year DFS (36 → 47%), OS (40 → 53%), and LRC (69 → 82%). Chemo-RT increased acute grade ≥ 3 toxicity (21 → 41%).

ː *RTOG 95–01* (Cooper *NEJM* 2004, *IJROBP* 2012): 459 patients with operable H&N SCC who had ≥2 LN, ECE, or +margin randomized to post-op RT (2/60–66 Gy) vs. chemo-RT (2/60–66 + cisplatin ×3 cycles). Chemo-RT improved 2-year DFS (43 → 54%) and LRC (72 → 82%); only in ECE and/or +margin subset improved 10-year DFS (12 → 18%) and LRC (21 → 33%). Trend only for OS improvement. Chemo-RT increased acute toxicity, no significant increase in late toxicity.

ː *Combined analysis* (Bernier *Head Neck* 2005): In subset of ECE and/or +margin, post-op chemo-RT improves OS (30% ARR), DFS (23% ARR), and LRC (42% ARR) vs. RT alone. No significant benefit to concurrent chemo without these risk factors.

PRE-RT INDUCTION CHEMOTHERAPY

ː No survival advantage to induction chemotherapy before chemo-RT, in part due to toxicity and inability to complete chemo-RT. Slight advantage in distant metastasis in phase II setting. Three-agent regimens containing taxanes are superior.

ː Possible scenarios for induction chemotherapy: unavoidable delays in starting chemo-RT, markedly advanced disease, oligometastasis, or very high metastatic potential.

ː *TAX 324* (Posner *NEJM* 2007, Lorch *Lancet Oncol* 2011): Randomized 501 patients with stage III–IV H&N SCC to TPF (docetaxel, cisplatin, 5-FU) vs. PF induction chemotherapy followed by carboplatin chemo-RT (70–74 Gy). TPF improved median PFS (13 → 38 months) and OS (35 → 71 months). More acute hematologic toxicity with TPF, but more treatment delays with PF. No significant difference in late toxicity.

ː *PARADIGM* (Haddad *Lancet Oncol* 2013): Randomized 145 patients with T3–4 or N2–3 (except T1 N2) H&N SCC (55% oropharyngeal cancer) to cisplatin chemo-RT ± 3 cycles TPF induction. Induction arm received chemo-RT with weekly docetaxel if poor responder/incomplete induction or with weekly carboplatin if responded. RT given as 2/70 Gy in carboplatin group, as concomitant boost to 72 Gy in other groups. No difference in 3-year OS, PFS, or failure pattern between groups. More febrile neutropenia in induction arm.

˒ (Hitt *Ann Oncol* 2014): Randomized 439 patients with stage III–IV H&N SCC (98% stage IV, 43% oropharyngeal cancer) to 3 arms: induction with 3c TPF, induction with 3c PF, or no induction. All patients got concurrent chemo-RT with 3c cisplatin and 2/70 Gy. ~30% of induction patients did not proceed to chemo-RT. Median f/u ~ 24 months. No difference in LRC, PFS, or OS by intention to treat; however per protocol showed improved LRC and PFS with induction, particularly with TPF arm. More toxicity (neutropenia, odynophagia, stomatitis) with induction.

˒ *DeCIDE* (Cohen *JCO* 2014): Randomized 273 patients with N2 or N3 H&N SCC (58% with oropharyngeal cancer) to 2 cycles TPF vs. no induction. All patients got chemo-RT with DFHX (docetaxel/5-FU/hydroxyurea) and 1.5 Gy BID to 75 Gy. Median f/u 30 months, no difference in OS or PFS. More hematologic toxicity with induction chemo. More deaths from cancer without induction, but more deaths from other causes with induction. Higher rate of distant recurrence without local recurrence in no-induction arm (p = 0.043).

˒ Induction-based de-intensification trial for HPV-associated oropharyngeal cancer:

˒ ECOG 1308 (Marur *JCO* 2017): 80 pts with HPV/p16+ stages III–IV received 3c cisplatin, paclitaxel, and cetuximab. If CR at primary site on exam, then patients received 54 Gy with weekly cetuximab to primary site and received 69.3 Gy and cetuximab to primary or nodal regions not in CR on exam. 70% achieved primary site CR. 2-year progression-free survival 80%, 2-year overall survival 94%.

TECHNIQUES

SIMULATION AND FIELD DESIGN

˒ Simulate supine with neck gently extended, shoulders down. Immobilize with thermoplastic head and shoulder mask. Bolus if skin involved. Shield metal crowns or fillings with custom dental tray or dental putty mold.

- CT planning with fusion to MRI and/or PET/CT.
- IMRT provides improved normal tissue sparing to parotid and submandibular glands, mandible, larynx, thyroid, and pharyngeal constrictors.
  - *PARSPORT* (Nutting *Lancet Oncol* 2011): Reduction of grade ≥ 2 xerostomia at 24 months with parotid-sparing IMRT vs. conventional (83 → 29%). No difference in other late toxicities, LC, or OS.
- Conventional:
  - 3-field technique (opposed laterals superiorly, AP inferiorly).
  - Beam split at thyroid notch/arytenoids (not through gross disease).
  - Small anterior block to avoid double treatment of cord at the matchline
  - Superior: Include skull base and mastoid processes.
  - Anterior: Include faucial arch and 2 cm margin on tumor. If base of tongue, can exclude hard palate.
  - N0: Include levels II–IV and retropharyngeal nodes (RPN). For T1 N0 tonsil, may exclude levels IV–V.
  - N1: Include levels IB–IV and RPN.
  - N2-3: Include levels IB–V and RPN.
  - Spinal cord shielding after 42–45 Gy with posterior block on lateral fields. Boost blocked posterior neck with electrons.
- IMRT:
  - GTV = Clinical or radiographic gross disease (primary and nodes).
  - CTV1 = 5–10 mm margin on primary and 3–5 mm margin on nodes (depending on adjacent critical structures and anatomic boundaries to microscopic spread). Should include maxillary tuberosity and aryepiglottic fold for tonsil primary.
  - CTV2 = "High-risk" areas and nodal levels (e.g., pterygoid plates, next drainage site from involved nodes).
  - CTV3 = Elective nodal levels (same as conventional) and borders of high-risk areas.
  - PTV = CTV + 3–5 mm (depending on tumor motion and setup error).
  - Need for IMRT coverage of medial retropharyngeal LN is controversial.
  - Sparing contralateral IB (including submandibular gland) is recommended if contralateral II is uninvolved.

, Limited retrospective series suggest treating ipsilateral II–IV only for non-bulky ipsilateral nodes only (N1, no ECE).

, Typically 7–9 nonopposing beam angles or VMAT are used.

, Splitting fields at thyroid notch/arytenoids (IMRT superior, AP inferior) may reduce larynx dose.

, If primary or nodal disease is near or past the level of the larynx, extended-field whole neck IMRT or VMAT planning is indicated. Avoid purely lateral beam angles to avoid treating through shoulders.

, Unilateral RT:

, Multiple published series report that carefully selected well-lateralized T1-2N0-2a tonsil pts may be treated with unilateral RT with only 0–3% risk of failure in the contralateral neck, regardless of HPV status (Huang *IJROBP* 2017).

, Not recommended if ≥1 cm soft palate or base of tongue invasion or any posterior pharyngeal wall invasion.

, N2b or ECE is controversial (increased metastatic risk, potential for altered lymphatic flow).

DOSE PRESCRIPTIONS

, T1-2N0: definitive RT to 70 Gy at 2 Gy/fx (7 weeks) or 66 Gy at 2.2 Gy/fx (6 weeks).

, Select T1N1 and T2N0-1: definitive altered fractionation RT.

, Accelerated: Six fractions per week during weeks 2–6: 2/70 Gy (6 weeks) or 66 Gy at 2.2 Gy/fx (6 weeks).

, Concomitant boost: 72 Gy (1.8/54 Gy plus BID 1.5 Gy last 12 days).

, Hyperfractionation: 81.6 Gy as 1.2 Gy BID (7 weeks).

, T3–4 or LN+: concurrent chemo-RT.

, Standard fractionation RT (70 Gy at 2 Gy/fx) with cisplatin 100 mg/m^2 q3 weeks ×3c (alternatively, cisplatin 40 mg/m^2 weekly x6c or cetuximab).

, Definitive IMRT:

, UCSF 33 fractions simultaneous integrated boost technique:

, PTV1: 2.12 Gy/fx to 69.96 Gy.

, PTV2: 1.8 Gy/fx to 59.4 Gy.

, PTV3: 1.64 Gy/fx to 54.12 Gy.

- Alternative IMRT fractionation schemes:
  - Simultaneous integrated boost in 35 fractions:
    - PTV1: 2 Gy/fx to 70 Gy.
    - PTV2: 1.8 Gy/fx to 63 Gy.
    - PTV3: 1.6 Gy/fx to 56 Gy.
  - Sequential technique with two plans:
    - First 30 fractions: PTV3 54 Gy at 1.8 Gy/fx, PTV2 60 Gy at 2 Gy/fx.
    - Last 5 fractions: PTV1 boost to 70 Gy total at 2 Gy/fx.
  - Concomitant boost:
    - Subclinical targets daily, then boost as second daily treatment at end of course.
    - PTV1–3: 1.8 Gy/fx to 54 Gy.
    - PTV1: +1.5 Gy daily for last 12 days to 72 Gy total.
- Post-op RT:
  - 60–66 Gy at 2 Gy/fx to high-risk areas and the postoperative bed.
  - 54 Gy to elective nodal volumes (same as for definitive treatment).
  - Chemo-RT indicated for nodal ECE and/or +margin. Cisplatin 100 mg/m2 q3 weeks recommended (alternatively, cisplatin 40 mg/m2 weekly x6c or cetuximab).
  - RT alone for other risk features: pT3–4, pN2–3, PNI, LVSI.

DOSE LIMITATIONS

- Spinal cord max ≤45 Gy (≤ 35 Gy for BID), brainstem max ≤54 Gy (≤ 30 Gy to dorsal vagal complex), parotid gland mean ≤ 26 Gy and V20 Gy ≤ 50%, submandibular mean ≤ 39 Gy, mandible max ≤70 Gy, retina max ≤45 Gy, larynx mean ≤ 32 Gy and V50 Gy ≤ 66%, cochlea mean (max) ≤ 37 (45) Gy, thyroid mean (max) ≤ 35 (45) Gy.
- Minimizing dose to the larynx and pharyngeal constrictor muscles may reduce the risk of late swallowing dysfunction but not at the expense of covering at-risk RPN or primary tumor margins (Feng *JCO* 2010).

COMPLICATIONS

- Acute and chronic mucositis, xerostomia.
- Skin reaction treated with plain moisturizing emollients. Silver-impregnated dressings for moist desquamation.

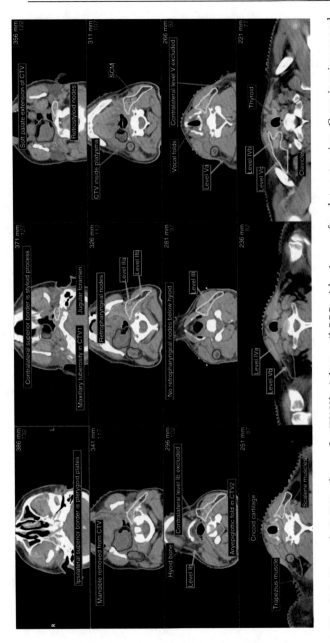

Fig. 7.2 Example IMRT volumes for T2N2b right tonsil SCC with >1 cm soft palate extension. *Green* is primary and nodal GTV, drawn with assistance of MRI fusion. *Red* is high-risk CTV. *Blue* is intermediate-risk CTV. *Yellow* is low-risk CTV. *Magenta* labels note anatomic landmarks. *Cyan* labels note nodal levels, and *Orange* labels note contouring boundaries. PTV expansion will be 3–5 mm from CTV, excluding 3–5 mm from skin surface

- Late toxicity includes skin/soft tissue fibrosis, hyperpigmentation, telangiectasias, swallowing dysfunction, voice alteration, alteration in taste, xerostomia, dental complications, chronic aspiration, acceleration of atherosclerosis, and thromboembolic disease.
- Preventive dental care with prophylactic extractions as needed at least 2 weeks before XRT, fluoride treatment, and mouth washing with antiseptics.
- Severe nutritional problems occur in 10% of patients. Proactive speech and swallowing support is mandatory. Need minimum 2000 cal/day diet. Use liquid nutritional supplements as needed. Prophylactic PEG-tube placement controversial.
- Risk of pharyngocutaneous fistula related to surgery, not RT. Flap reconstruction decreases complications.
- Mandibular necrosis uncommon with IMRT, carotid artery rupture <1%.
- Amifostine can be used to decrease acute and late xerostomia, but may be associated with significant hypotension and nausea/vomiting.

FOLLOW-UP

- 85–90% of locoregional recurrences occur within 3 years.
- H&P q 1–2 months for year 1, q 3 months for years 2–3, q 6 months for years 4–5, and then annually.
- Post-treatment PET/CT has high predictive value for long-term outcomes.
  - *PET-NECK* (Mehanna *NEJM* 2016): 564 patients with N2–3 H&N SCC randomized to PET-CT at 12 weeks post-treatment vs. planned neck dissection. Rate of neck dissection reduced 78 → 19%. Improved quality of life at 6 months. No difference in 5-year OS or LC.
- If recurrence suspected but biopsy is negative, follow up monthly until resolved.
- Speech, swallow, dental, and hearing evaluation/rehabilitation as indicated.
- Smoking cessation counseling if needed.

Acknowledgment We thank Siavash Jabbari MD, Kim Huang MD, and Jeanne Marie Quivey MD, FACR, for their work on the prior edition of this chapter.

REFERENCES

Adelstein DJ, Li Y, Adams GL, et al. An intergroup phase III comparison of standard radiation therapy and two schedules of concurrent chemoradiotherapy in patients with unresectable squamous cell head and neck cancer. J Clin Oncol. 2003;21:92–8.

de Almeida JR, Byrd JK, Wu R, et al. A systematic review of transoral robotic surgery and radiotherapy for early oropharynx cancer: a systematic review. Laryngoscope. 2014;124(9):2096–102.

Ang KK, Harris J, Wheeler R, et al. Human papillomavirus and survival of patients with oropharyngeal cancer. N Engl J Med. 2010;363(1):24–35.

Ang KK, Zhang Q, Rosenthal DI, et al. Randomized phase III trial of concurrent accelerated radiation plus cisplatin with or without cetuximab for stage III to IV head and neck carcinoma: RTOG 0522. J Clin Oncol. 2014;32(27):2940–50.

Beitler JJ, Zhang Q, Fu KK, et al. Final results of local-regional control and late toxicity of RTOG 9003: a randomized trial of altered fractionation radiation for locally advanced head and neck cancer. Int J Radiat Oncol Biol Phys. 2014;89(1):13–20.

Bernier J, Domenge C, Ozsahin M, et al. Postoperative irradiation with or without concomitant chemotherapy for locally advanced head and neck cancer. N Engl J Med. 2004;350:1945–52.

Bernier J, Cooper JS, Pajak TF, et al. Defining risk levels in locally advanced head and neck cancers: a comparative analysis of concurrent postoperative radiation plus chemotherapy trials of the EORTC (#22931) and RTOG (#9501). Head Neck. 2005;27(10):843–50.

Bonner JA, Harari PM, Giralt J, et al. Radiotherapy plus cetuximab for squamous-cell carcinoma of the head and neck. N Engl J Med. 2006;354:567–78.

Bonner JA, Harari PM, Giralt J, et al. Radiotherapy plus cetuximab for locoregionally advanced head and neck cancer: 5-year survival data from a phase 3 randomised trial, and relation between cetuximab-induced rash and survival. Lancet Oncol. 2010;11(1):21–8.

Bourhis J, Overgaard J, Audry H, et al. Hyperfractionated or accelerated radiotherapy in head and neck cancer: a meta-analysis. Lancet. 2006;368(9538):843–54.

Bourhis J, Sire C, Graff P, et al. Concomitant chemoradiotherapy versus acceleration of radiotherapy with or without concomitant chemotherapy in locally advanced head and neck carcinoma (GORTEC 99-02): an open-label phase 3 randomised trial. Lancet Oncol. 2012;13(2):145–53.

Cohen EEW, Karrison TG, Kocherginsky M, et al. Phase III randomized trial of induction chemotherapy in patients with N2 or N3 locally advanced head and neck cancer. J Clin Oncol. 2014;32(25):2735–43.

Cooper JS, Pajak TF, Forastiere AA, et al. Postoperative concurrent radiotherapy and chemotherapy for high-risk squamous-cell carcinoma of the head and neck. N Engl J Med. 2004;350:1937–44.

Cooper JS, Zhang Q, Pajak TF, et al. Long-term follow-up of the RTOG 9501/intergroup phase III trial: postoperative concurrent radiation therapy and chemotherapy in high-risk squamous cell carcinoma of the head and neck. Int J Radiat Oncol Biol Phys. 2012;84(5):1198–205.

Denis F, Garaud P, Bardet E, et al. Final results of the 94-01 French Head and Neck Oncology and Radiotherapy Group randomized trial comparing radiotherapy alone with concomitant radiochemotherapy in advanced-stage oropharynx carcinoma. J Clin Oncol. 2004;22:69–76.

Feng FY, Kim HM, Lyden TH, et al. Intensity-modulated chemoradiotherapy aiming to reduce dysphagia in patients with oropharyngeal cancer: clinical and functional results. J Clin Oncol. 2010;28(16):2732–8.

Fu KK, Pajak TF, Trotti A, et al. A Radiation Therapy Oncology Group (RTOG) phase III randomized study to compare hyperfractionation and two variants of accelerated fractionation to standard fractionation radiotherapy for head and neck squamous cell carcinomas: first report of RTOG 9003. Int J Radiat Oncol Biol Phys. 2000;48:7–16.

III

Garden AS, Fuller CD, Rosenthal DI, et al. Radiation therapy (with or without neck surgery) for phenotypic human papillomavirus-associated oropharyngeal cancer. Cancer. 2016;122:1702–7.

Grégoire V, Ang KK, Budach W, et al. Delineation of the neck node levels for head and neck tumors: a 2013 update. DAHANCA, EORTC, HKNPCSG, NCIC CTG, NCRI, RTOG, TROG consensus guidelines. Radiother Oncol. 2014;110(1):172–81.

Haddad R, O'Neill A, Rabinowits G, et al. Induction chemotherapy followed by concurrent chemoradiotherapy (sequential chemoradiotherapy) versus concurrent chemoradiotherapy alone in locally advanced head and neck cancer (PARADIGM): a randomised phase 3 trial. Lancet Oncol. 2013;14(3):257–64.

Hitt R, Grau JJ, López-Pousa A, et al. A randomized phase III trial comparing induction chemotherapy followed by chemoradiotherapy versus chemoradiotherapy alone as treatment of unresectable head and neck cancer. Ann Oncol. 2014;25:216–25.

Huang SH, Waldron J, Bratman SV, et al. Re-evaluation of ipsilateral radiation for T1-T2N0-N2b tonsil carcinoma at the Princess Margaret Hospital in the human papillomavirus era, 25 years later. Int J Radiat Oncol Biol Phys. 2017;98(1):159–69.

Lee YH, Kim YS, Chung MJ, et al. Soft tissue necrosis in head and neck cancer patients after transoral robotic surgery or wide excision with primary closure followed by radiation therapy. Medicine (Baltimore). 2016;95(9):e2852.

Lorch JH, Goloubeva O, Haddad RI, et al. Induction chemotherapy with cisplatin and fluorouracil alone or in combination with docetaxel in locally advanced squamous-cell cancer of the head and neck: long-term results of the TAX 324 randomised phase 3 trial. Lancet Oncol. 2011;12(2):153–9.

Lukens JN, Lin A, Gamerman V, et al. Late consequential surgical bed soft tissue necrosis in advanced oropharyngeal squamous cell carcinomas treated with transoral robotic surgery and postoperative radiation therapy. Int J Radiat Oncol Biol Phys. 2014;89(5):981–8.

Marur S, Li S, Cmelak AJ, et al. E1308: phase II trial of induction chemotherapy followed by reduced-dose radiation and weekly cetuximab in patients with HPV-associated resectable squamous cell carcinoma of the oropharynx–ECOG-ACRIN cancer research group. J Clin Oncol. 2017;35(5):490–7.

Mehanna H, Wong W-L, McConkey CC, et al. PET-CT surveillance versus neck dissection in advanced head and neck cancer. N Engl J Med. 2016;374(15):1444–54.

Morisod C, Simon C. Meta-analysis on survival of patients treated with transoral surgery versus radiotherapy for early-stage squamous cell carcinoma of the oropharynx. Head Neck. 2016;38(Suppl 1):E2143–50.

Nutting CM, Morden JP, Harrington KJ, et al. Parotid-sparing intensity modulated versus conventional radiotherapy in head and neck cancer (PARSPORT): a phase 3 multicentre randomised controlled trial. Lancet Oncol. 2011;12(2):127–36.

O'Sullivan B, Huang SH, Siu LL, et al. Deintensification candidate subgroups in human papillomavirus-related oropharyngeal cancer according to minimal risk of distant metastasis. J Clin Oncol. 2013;31(5):543–50.

O'Sullivan B, Huang SH, Su J, et al. Development and validation of a staging system for HPV-related oropharyngeal cancer by the International Collaboration on Oropharyngeal cancer Network for Staging (ICON-S): a multicentre cohort study. Lancet Oncol. 2016;17:440–51.

Overgaard J, Hansen HS, Specht L, et al. Five compared with six fractions per week of conventional radiotherapy of squamous-cell carcinoma of head and neck: DAHANCA 6&7 randomised controlled trial. Lancet. 2003;362(9388):933–40.

Pignon JP, le Maitre A, Maillard E, Bourhis J. Meta-analysis of chemotherapy in head and neck cancer (MACH-NC): an update on 93 randomised trials and 17,346 patients. Radiother Oncol. 2009;92(1):4–14.

Posner MR, Hershock DM, Blajman CR, et al. Cisplatin and fluorouracil alone or with docetaxel in head and neck cancer. N Engl J Med. 2007;357(17):1705–15.

Chapter 8
Cancer of the Lip and Oral Cavity

III

Christopher H. Chapman and Adam Garsa

PEARLS

- Oral cavity cancers are approximately 40% of head and neck cancers.
- The oral cavity consists of the upper and lower lips, gingivobuccal sulcus, buccal mucosa, upper and lower gingiva (including alveolar ridge), retromolar trigone, hard palate, floor of mouth, and anterior two-thirds of the tongue (anterior to circumvallate papillae).
- CN XII provides motor innervation of the tongue, and the lingual nerve (CN V) provides sensory innervation. Taste is mediated by the chorda tympani branch of CN VII for the anterior two-thirds of the tongue and CN IX for the posterior one-third.
- Extrinsic tongue muscles: hyoglossus, genioglossus, styloglossus, palatoglossus.
- Risk factors for oral cavity cancer include use of tobacco, alcohol, poor oral hygiene, and betel and areca nuts. Oral leukoplakia can proceed to cancer (4–18%) as can erythroplakia (30%). 1.5% will have synchronous cancers; 10–40% will develop second primaries.
- Presentation: pain, bleeding, poorly fitting dentures, speech alteration, neck lymphadenopathy.

- LN drainage (see Chapter 7 Fig. 7.1):
  - Upper lip: facial nodes and level IB.
  - Floor of mouth, lower lip, and lower gingiva: levels I, II, and III.
  - Anterior oral tongue: IA, IB, and II, and also directly to levels III–IV.
  - Bilateral node drainage is frequent, especially when the lesion approaches midline.
- Depth of invasion, increasing T size, and grade increase risk of involved LN.
- Approximate risk of LN involvement.
  - Lip: T1–2 = 5%, T3–4 = 33%
  - Floor of mouth: T1–2 = 10–20%, T3–4 = 33–67%
  - Oral tongue: T1–2 = 20%, T3–4 = 33–67%
  - Bucco-gingival mucosa: T1–2 = 10–20%, T3–4 = 33–67%
  - Retromolar trigone: 25–40%
- 90% of tumors are squamous cell carcinoma. Less common tumors include minor salivary gland cancers (common in the hard palate and include adenoid cystic carcinoma, mucoepidermoid carcinoma, and adenocarcinoma). Rare: lymphoma, melanoma, sarcoma, and ameloblastoma/ameloblastic carcinoma.

WORKUP

- H&P with palpation, indirect mirror exam ± fiberoptic endoscopy.
- Biopsy of tumor and/or lymph nodes.
- Labs: CBC, chemistries, BUN, Cr, and LFTs including alkaline phosphatase.
- Imaging:
  - CT and/or MRI with contrast of the head and neck (CT for cortical bone invasion, MRI for soft tissue delineation and perineural extension).
  - Consider FDG-PET for stages III–IV. Otherwise CT chest to rule out metastatic disease.
- Preventive dental care and extractions at least 14 days before RT.
- Speech/swallowing and nutrition consultations during and after RT.

STAGING: CANCER OF THE LIP AND ORAL CAVITY

Editors' note: All TNM stage and stage groups referred to elsewhere in this chapter reflect the 2010 AJCC staging nomenclature unless otherwise noted as the new system below was published after this chapter was written.

III

Table 8.1 (AJCC 7TH ED., 2010)

Primary tumor (T)

TX:	Primary tumor cannot be assessed
T0:	No evidence of primary tumor
Tis:	Carcinoma in situ
T1:	Tumor 2 cm or less in greatest dimension
T2:	Tumor more than 2 cm, but not more than 4 cm in greatest dimension
T3:	Tumor more than 4 cm in greatest dimension
T4a:	Moderately advanced local disease* (lip) Tumor invades through cortical bone, inferior alveolar nerve, floor of mouth, or skin of face, i.e., chin or nose (oral cavity). Tumor invades adjacent structures only (e.g., through cortical bone [mandible or maxilla] into deep [extrinsic] muscle of tongue [genioglossus, hyoglossus, palatoglossus, and styloglossus], maxillary sinus, skin of face)
T4b:	Very advanced local disease. Tumor invades masticator space, pterygoid plates, or skull base, and/or encases internal carotid artery*

Note: Superficial erosion alone of bone/tooth socket by gingival primary is not sufficient to classify a tumor as T4

Regional lymph nodes (N)

NX:	Regional lymph nodes cannot be assessed
N0:	No regional lymph node metastasis
N1:	Metastasis in a single ipsilateral lymph node, 3 cm or less in greatest dimension
N2a:	Metastasis in a single ipsilateral lymph node, more than 3 cm but not more than 6 cm in greatest dimension
N2b:	Metastasis in multiple ipsilateral lymph nodes, not more than 6 cm in greatest dimension
N2c:	Metastasis in bilateral or contralateral lymph nodes, not more than 6 cm in greatest dimension
N3:	Metastasis in a lymph node more than 6 cm in greatest dimension

Distant metastases (M)

M0:	No distant metastasis
M1:	Distant metastasis

continued

Table 8.1 (continued)

Anatomic stage/prognostic groups	
0:	Tis N0 M0
I:	T1 N0 M0
II:	T2 N0 M0
III:	T3 N0 M0
	T1–T3 N1 M0
IVA:	T4a N0 M0
	T4a N1 M0
	T1–T3 N2 M0
	T4a N2 M0
IVB:	Any T N3 M0
	T4b, any N M0
IVC:	Any T; any N M1

Used with permission from the American Joint Committee on Cancer (AJCC), Chicago, Illinois. The original source for this material is the AJCC Cancer Staging Manual, Seventh Edition (2010), published by Springer Science+Business Media

Table 8.2 (AJCC 8TH ED., 2017)

Definitions of AJCC TNM	
Definition of Primary Tumor (T)	
T category	**T criteria**
TX	Primary tumor cannot be assessed
Tis	Carcinoma in situ
T1	Tumor ≤ 2 cm, ≤ 5 mm depth of invasion (DOI) DOI is depth of invasion and not tumor thickness
T2	Tumor ≤ 2cm, DOI > 5 mm and ≤ 10 mm, *or* tumor>2 cm but ≤ 4cm, and< 10 mm DOI
T3	Tumor > 4 cm *or* any tumor > 10 mm DOI
T4	Moderately advanced or very advanced local disease
T4a	Moderately advanced local disease
	lip – tumor invades through the cortical bone or involves the inferior alveolar nerve, floor of mouth, or skin of the face (i.e., chin or nose)
	oral cavity – tumor invades adjacent structures only (e.g., through the cortical bone of the mandible or maxilla or involves the maxillary sinus or skin of the face)
	Note: Superficial erosion of the bone/tooth socket (alone) by a gingival primary is not sufficient to classify a tumor as T4
T4b	Very advanced local disease
	Tumor invades masticator space, pterygoid plates, or skull base and/ or encases the internal carotid artery

DEFINITION OF REGIONAL LYMPH NODE (N)
Clinical N (cN)

N category	N criteria
NX	Regional lymph nodes cannot be assessed
N0	No regional lymph node metastasis
N1	Metastasis in a single ipsilateral lymph node, 3 cm or smaller in the greatest dimension ENE(−)
N2	Metastasis in a single ipsilateral node larger than 3 cm but not larger than 6 cm in greatest dimension and ENE(−) *or* metastases in multiple ipsilateral lymph nodes, not larger than 6 cm in greatest dimension and ENE(−), *or* in bilateral or contralateral lymph nodes, not larger than 6 cm in the greatest dimension and ENE(−)
N2a	Metastasis in a single ipsilateral node larger than 3 cm but not larger than 6 cm in greatest dimension and ENE(−)
N2b	Metastasis in multiple ipsilateral nodes, not larger than 6 cm in the greatest dimension and ENE(−)
N2c	Metastasis in bilateral or contralateral lymph nodes, not larger than 6 cm in the greatest dimension and ENE(-)
N3	Metastasis in a lymph node larger than 6 cm in greatest dimension and ENE(−) *or* metastasis in any node(s) and clinically overt ENE(+)
N3a	Metastasis in a lymph node larger than 6 cm in the greatest dimension and ENE(−)
N3b	Metastasis in any node(s) and clinically overt ENE(+)

Note: A designation of "U" or "L" may be used for any N category to indicate metastasis above the lower border of the cricoid (U) or below the lower border of the cricoid (L) Similarly, clinical and pathological ENE should be recorded as ENE(−) or ENE(+)

Pathological N (pN)
AJCC Prognostic Stage Groups

N category	N criteria
NX	Regional lymph nodes cannot be assessed
NO0	No regional lymph node metastasis
N1	Metastasis in a single ipsilateral lymph node, 3 cm or smaller in the greatest dimension and ENE(−)
N2	Metastasis in a single ipsilateral lymph node, 3 cm or smaller in the greatest dimension and ENE(+) *or* larger than 3 cm but not larger than 6 cm in the greatest dimension and ENE(−), *or* metastases in multiple ipsilateral lymph nodes, not larger than 6 cm in the greatest dimension and ENE(−), *or* in bilateral or contracterai lymph nodes, not larger than 6 cm in the greatest dimension and ENE(−)
N2a	Metastasis in a single ipsilateral or contralateral node 3 cm or smaller in the greatest dimension and ENE(+) *or* a single ipsilateral node larger than 3 cm but not larger than 6 cm in greatest dimension and ENE(-)
N2b	Metastasis in multiple ipsilateral nodes, not larger than 6 cm in greatest dimension and ENE(−)
N2c	Metastasis in bilateral or contralateral lymph nodes, not larger than 6 cm in the greatest dimension and ENE(−)

continued

N3	Metastasis in a lymph node larger than 6 cm in the greatest dimension and ENE(−) *or* in a single ipsilateral node larger than 3 cm in the greatest dimension and ENE(+) *or* multiple ipsilateral, contralateral, or bilateral nodes any with ENE(+)
N3a	Metastasis in a lymph node larger than 6 cm in the greatest dimension and ENE(−)
N3b	Metastasis in a single ipsilateral node larger than 3 cm in the greatest dimension and ENE(+) *or* multiple ipsilateral, contralateral, or bilateral nodes any with ENE(+)

Note: A designation of "U" or "L" may be used for any N category to indicate metastasis above the lower border of the cricoid (U) or below the lower border of the cricoid (L) Similarly, clinical and pathological ENE should be recorded as ENE(−) or ENE(+)

DEFINITION OF DISTANT METASTASIS (M)

M category	M criteria
M0	No distant metastasis
M1	Distant metastasis

AJCC PROGNOSTIC STAGE GROUPS

When T is...	And N is...	And M is...	Then the stage group is...
T1	N0	M0	I
T2	N0	M0	II
T3	N0	M0	III
T1,2,3	N1	M0	III
T4a	N0,1	M0	IVA
T1,2,3,4a	N2	M0	IVA
Any T	N3	M0	IVB
T4b	Any N	M0	IVB
Any T	Any N	M1	IVC

Used with permission of the American Joint Committee on Cancer (AJCC), Chicago, Illinois. The original and primary source for this information is the AJCC Cancer Staging Manual, Eighth Edition (2017) published by Springer International Publishing

TREATMENT RECOMMENDATIONS

Table 8.3 TREATMENT RECOMMENDATIONS

Stage	Lip
T1-2N0	Preferred: surgical resection of primary. For positive margin only, re-excise if feasible. Post-op RT (including nodes if not dissected) indicated for close margin, PNI, or LVSI. Post-op chemo-RT indicated if positive margin Alternative: definitive EBRT ± brachytherapy. Salvage surgery for residual disease

Table 8.3 (continued)

T3–4a or N1–3	Preferred: surgical resection of primary and ipsilateral neck dissection (contralateral neck dissection if tumor approaches midline or N2c). Reconstruction as indicated. Consider post-op RT for all, post-op chemo-RT for positive margin or ECE. Alternatively: concurrent chemo-RT ± brachytherapy. If primary has < CR, consider salvage surgery and neck dissection. If residual neck involvement by imaging at 6–12 weeks, consider salvage neck dissection
Stage	**Oral cavity**
T1-2N0	Preferred: surgical resection of primary with ipsilateral or bilateral selective neck dissection (consider bilateral for midline, oral tongue, or floor of mouth). Neck treatment (dissection or RT) for lesions >2–3 mm thick. For positive margin only, re-excise if feasible. Post-op RT alone (including neck if not dissected) indicated for close margin (< 5 mm), PNI, or LVSI. Post-op chemo-RT for positive margin. Alternatively: definitive EBRT ± brachytherapy. Salvage surgery for residual disease
T3–4a or N1–3	Preferred: surgical resection of primary with ipsilateral or bilateral selective neck dissection (consider bilateral for tumors approaching midline, oral tongue, floor of mouth, N2c). Reconstruction as indicated. Consider post-op RT for all, post-op chemo-RT for positive margin or ECE
Unresectable	Preferred: concurrent chemo-RT with cisplatin based regimen. Alternative: induction chemotherapy followed by chemo-RT, or altered fractionation RT if unable to tolerate chemo. If primary has < CR, salvage surgery controversial. If residual neck involvement by imaging at 6–12 weeks, consider salvage neck dissection

SURGERY

- Surgery followed by adjuvant therapy as indicated is the standard of care for oral cavity cancers, due to high rates of complications and salvage with upfront RT ± chemo and better functional outcomes with oral cavity surgery versus other H&N subsites.
  - (Iyer *Cancer* 2015): 119 patients with stage III–IV H&N SCC (32 with oral cavity cancer) randomized to primary surgery and adjuvant radiation therapy vs. primary concurrent chemo-RT. No significant differences in survival between arms overall; however in subset of oral cavity primaries, surgery improved 5-year DSS 68% vs. 12% and DRFS 92% vs. 50% ($p \leq 0.05$).
- Surgical access technique: transoral, visor split, lip split, or mandibulotomy.

꜄ Surgical resection technique: en bloc; if mandibulectomy necessary, segmental mandibulectomy with free flap reconstruction or marginal mandibulectomy (no bone invasion/affixed tumor).

꜄ cN+: level I–V dissection. cN0: level I–III dissection. Consider level IV dissection for oral tongue (higher rate of skip metastasis to level IV).

꜄ (D'Cruz *NEJM* 2015): 500 patients with T1-2N0 oral cavity cancers randomized to neck dissection at time of initial surgery (elective) vs. at the time of nodal relapse (therapeutic). Elective neck dissection improved 3-year OS 80% vs. 68% and 3-year DFS 70% vs. 46%.

꜄ Sentinel lymph node biopsy as an alternative to neck dissection has been studied in T1–2 tumors with negative predictive values ≥90%, but is controversial due to high dependence on subsite and technical experience.

꜄ Preferred interval between resection and post-operative RT is ≤6 weeks.

STUDIES

POST-OP EBRT

꜄ Post-op RT superior to pre-op RT.

꜄ Indications for post-op RT: pT3–4, close margin, N2/3, level IV–V nodes, PNI, or LVSI. 60–66 Gy if no gross residual disease, otherwise 70 Gy.

꜄ *RTOG 73–03* (Kramer *Head Neck Surg* 1987, Tupchong *IJROBP* 1991): 354 patients with locally advanced H&N SCC randomized to 2/50 Gy pre-op vs. 2/50–60 Gy post-op. With median 7-year follow-up, post-op RT significantly improved LRC (58 → 70%) but not overall survival (20 → 29%). Similar rates of complications.

꜄ (Peters *IJROBP* 1993): 240 patients with H&N SCC, 90% stages III–IV, underwent surgery. Stratified by risk factors (T stage, margins, nerve invasion, N stage, number of nodes, number of nodal groups, size/ECE, direct invasion). Low risk randomized to post-op 1.8/52.2–54 Gy (later increased to 1.8/57.6 Gy) vs. 1.8/63 Gy. High risk randomized to post-op 1.8/63 Gy vs. 1.8/68.4 Gy. In low risk, worse 2-year LC with ≤54 Gy (63%) vs. ≥ 57.6 Gy (89–92%); no difference between 57.6 and 63 Gy. In high risk, no difference in 2-year LC between 63 and 68.4 Gy (81–89%). If ECE, significant increase in 2-year LC with ≥63 Gy (52 → 72–74%, p = 0.03). Needed four other risk factors to reach recurrence risk of ECE.

꞉ (Ang *IJROBP* 2001): 213 patients with locally advanced oral cavity, oropharynx, larynx, and hypopharynx cancers treated with surgery randomized by risk factors to post-op RT. Risk factors included >1 node group, ≥2 nodes, nodes >3 cm, microscopic +margins, PNI, oral cavity site, and ECE. No risk factors → no RT. One risk factor (not ECE) → 1.8/57.6 Gy. ECE or ≥2 risk factors → 1.8/63 Gy in 7 weeks or in 5 weeks with a concomitant boost. 5-year LRC/OS for low risk = 90/83%, intermediate risk = 94/66%, high risk = 68/42%. 5-year LRC improved with shorter total treatment time (<11 weeks: 76%, 11–13 weeks: 62%, >13 weeks: 38%). Trend for improved OS with concomitant boost in high risk group.

POST-OP CHEMO-RT

꞉ Indications for post-op chemo-RT: ECE and/or positive margins. See Chapter 7 for details of *EORTC 22931*, *RTOG 95-01*, and combined analysis. Concurrent cisplatin 100 mg/m^2 q3 weeks ×3c (alternatively, cisplatin 40 mg/m^2 weekly ×6c).

꞉ OCAT (Laskar, ASCO 2016): 900 postoperative oral cavity pts randomized to 56–60 Gy at 5 fx/week, same plus cisplatin 30 mg/m2 weekly, or 56–60 Gy at 6 fx/week. No difference in LRC or acute grade 3 toxicity overall, but pts with T3–4, N2–3, or ECE had improved LRC, DFS, and OS with chemo-RT vs. RT alone.

ALTERED FRACTIONATION

꞉ Improved local control and survival with accelerated or hyperfractioned/dose escalated in definitive RT ± chemo. See Chapter 7 for details of major trials and meta-analysis.

INDUCTION CHEMOTHERAPY

꞉ See Chapter 7 for details of major preradiation induction chemo randomized trials. Induction chemo before surgery is not currently the standard of care, but may have advantage in subsets of patient with high distant metastasis risk.

, (Zhong *JCO* 2013, *Oncotarget* 2015): Randomized 256 patients with resectable stage III–IV oral cavity SCC to docetaxel/cisplatin/5-FU induction chemo → surgery vs. upfront surgery. Acute grade 3 toxicity 7% with induction. No significant differences in 5-year OS, DFS, LRC, or DM with induction, except in subsets of cN2 (OS HR 0.47, $p = 0.044$; DM HR 0.47, $p = 0.046$) and female patients. All outcomes improved vs. controls in 28% of induction group with CR/near CR.

BRACHYTHERAPY

, May be useful as an adjunct to EBRT or as definitive therapy in early stage tumors, especially in cases of re-irradiation. Experience necessary due to risks of soft tissue and bone necrosis (Nag *IJROBP* 2001).

, (Wendt *IJROBP* 1990): retrospective of 103 patients with T1-2N0 oral tongue SCC treated with brachytherapy and/or EBRT. Combined RT given as 40–55 Gy brachytherapy and 16–32 Gy EBRT, or 20–40 Gy brachytherapy, and 40–50 Gy EBRT. Higher dose brachytherapy improved 5-year LC 92% vs. 65%. Higher dose EBRT improved 2-year neck control 73–93% vs. 56–63%. DFS and OS equivalent.

, (Grabenbauer *Strahlenther Onkol* 2001): 318 patients with primary (74%) and recurrent (26%) oral cavity (63%) or oropharynx (27%) SCC received post-op low dose rate (LDR) brachytherapy ± EBRT. Brachytherapy dose 45–55 Gy alone or 23–25 Gy after 50–60 Gy EBRT. 5-year LC 74% for primary and 57% for recurrent disease. With EBRT + brachytherapy, 5-year LC 92% for stages I–II and 65% for stages III–IV. 7.5% late necrosis.

, (Melzner *Radiother Oncol* 2007): 210 patients with oral cavity (77%) or oropharynx (23%) SCC received pulsed dose rate (PDR) brachytherapy either post-op or definitively. Median brachytherapy dose 24 Gy after median 50.4 Gy EBRT or 56.65 Gy alone. Median 2-year follow-up: OS 83%, LC 93%, soft tissue necrosis 11%, bone necrosis 8%.

, (Martinez-Monge *Brachytherapy* 2009): 40 patients with oral cavity (70%) or oropharynx (30%) SCC received perioperative high dose rate (HDR) brachytherapy (4 Gy BID × 4 for R0 resection or × 6 for R1 resection) and 45 Gy EBRT. 7-year LRC 82%, DFS 50%, OS 52%. Acute grade ≥ 3 toxicity 8%. Late grade ≥ 3 toxicity 20%, including 1 death.

₎ (Strnad *Strahlenther Onkol* 2015): 104 patients with H&N SCC in previously radiated site (59% oral cavity) received PDR brachytherapy (median 55 Gy) ± EBRT (32%, median 24 Gy) ± surgery (51%) ± chemotherapy (56%). 5-/10-year local control 82/59%. Improved 10-year LC with concurrent chemo (39 → 76%). Soft tissue necrosis 17%; bone necrosis 10%.

III

RADIATION TECHNIQUES

SIMULATION AND FIELD DESIGN

₎ Simulate supine with neck extended, shoulders down. Immobilize with thermoplastic head and shoulder mask. Wire scars. Cork and tongue blade to depress tongue from palate if appropriate. 2–5 mm bolus may be applied to scars.

₎ CT planning with fusion to MRI, contrast-enhanced CT, and/or PET-CT studies.

₎ Planning with IMRT alone (extended-field) if inferior disease or close to larynx, or split field at thyroid notch/arytenoids to reduce larynx dose (IMRT superior, AP or AP/PA inferior).

₎ With extended-field whole neck IMRT, use anterior obliques rather than lateral fields to avoid treating through shoulders.

IMRT

₎ UCSF IMRT volumes

  ₎ GTV = Clinical or radiographic gross disease, if present (primary and nodes).

  ₎ CTV1 = Entire postoperative bed, including ≥0.5–2 cm margin on GTV (depending on anatomic boundaries to microscopic spread), and areas of close/positive margins, ECE. Entire flap is covered if reconstructed.

  ₎ CTV2 = Elective neck (dissected neck, high risk cN0, contralateral neck).

  ₎ PTV = CTV + 3–5 mm (depending on tumor motion and setup error).

₎ IMRT (simultaneous integrated boost technique)

  ₎ GTV (if present) = 69.96 Gy in 2.12 Gy fractions

  ₎ CTV1 = 60–66 Gy in 2 Gy fractions

  ₎ CTV2 = 54 Gy in 1.8 Gy fractions

, For post-op chemo-RT recommend concurrent cisplatin 100 mg/m2 q3 weeks x3c (alternatively, cisplatin 40 mg/m2 weekly x6c).
, If using split-field technique, low anterior neck 50–50.4 Gy in 1.8–2 Gy fractions.

BRACHYTHERAPY
, Follow GEC-ESTRO recommendations for head and neck cancers (Mazeron, Radiother Oncol 2009; Kovács, Radiother Oncol 2016).

LIP
, T1–2 may be treated with EBRT (100–250 kV photons or 6–12 MeV electrons), with brachytherapy or both. Appositional field for EBRT. Borders determined clinically with 1–1.5 cm margin for orthovoltage or 2–2.5 cm margin for electrons. Bolus for superficial tumors. Wax-coated lead shield behind lip to reduce dose to mandible and oral cavity.
, T3–4 tumors typically treated with IMRT or opposed lateral 4–6 MV photons.
, Suggested nodal coverage: Levels I–II for T3, levels I–IV for T4 or LN+. May consider "moustache field" of elective RT to perifacial lymphatics for advanced upper lip lesions.
, HDR brachytherapy typically Ir-192 in catheters spaced 1 cm apart. A dental roll is placed between the lip and the gingiva to minimize dose to mandible and oral cavity.

ORAL TONGUE AND FLOOR OF MOUTH
, Low RT tolerance due to increased risk of soft tissue injury and osteoradionecrosis.
, Use cork and tongue blade to depress tongue from palate. Need secure setup due to tongue mobility.
, For superficial T1–2 lesions, brachytherapy or intraoral cone RT may be used in lieu of surgery.
  , LDR brachytherapy dose is 60–70 Gy. Intraoral cone dose is 3 Gy × 15–20 fractions.
, For definitive treatment of larger lesions, 3DCRT or IMRT techniques are generally recommended for advanced lesions in order to spare adjacent normal structures.

Brachytherapy (21–30 Gy) or intraoral cone (15–24 Gy) may be used for boost after EBRT (40–50 Gy).
, Suggested nodal coverage (all bilateral): Levels I–IV, include level V for +LN.

III

BUCCAL MUCOSA
, Wire ipsilateral commissure. The oral commissures and lips are excluded or shielded if possible. Consider intra-oral device to displace and shield tongue. May insert metal seeds into the periphery of the tumor for localization.
, Suggested nodal coverage:
  , T1-T4N0: Ipsilateral levels I–IV if well lateralized, otherwise consider covering contralateral neck.
  , LN+: Ipsilateral levels I–V, consider contralateral neck.

GINGIVA, HARD PALATE, AND RETROMOLAR TRIGONE
, Brachytherapy is generally avoided due to risk of osteoradionecrosis.
, EBRT superior border must include pterygoid plates (exception: inferior gingiva).
, For gingival tumors, if PNI is present the entire hemi-mandible from mental foramen to TMJ is included.
, MRI can help identify perineural spread along major nerves (e.g., inferior alveolar nerve). If radiographically or clinically involved, or extensive PNI present, cover nerve pathway at least to the base of skull foramina and consider covering to trigeminal ganglion.
, Suggested nodal coverage:
  , T1-4N0: ipsilateral levels I–IV if well lateralized, otherwise consider covering contralateral neck.
  , LN+: ipsilateral levels I–V, consider contralateral neck.

DOSE LIMITATIONS
, Same as oropharyngeal primary: see Chapter 7.

COMPLICATIONS
, Perioperative complications of surgery include bleeding, airway obstruction, infection, and wound complications.

Post-operative complications include wound breakdown, flap loss, aspiration, as well as functional speech and/or swallowing deficits.

, Osteoradionecrosis more common with brachytherapy. Other RT complications same as oropharyngeal primary: see Chapter 7.

FOLLOW-UP

, Same as oropharyngeal primary: see Chap. 7.

Acknowledgment We thank Eric K. Hansen MD, Sue S. Yom MD, Chien Peter Chen MD, and Naomi R. Schechter MD, for their work on the prior edition of this chapter.

REFERENCES

Ang KK, Trotti A, Brown BW, et al. Randomized trial addressing risk features and time factors of surgery plus radiotherapy in advanced head-and-neck cancer. Int J Radiat Oncol Biol Phys. 2001;51:571–8.

D'Cruz AK, Vaish R, Kapre N, et al. Elective versus therapeutic neck dissection in node-negative oral cancer. N Engl J Med. 2015;373(6):521–9.

Grabenbauer GG, Rodel C, Brunner T, et al. Interstitial brachytherapy with Ir-192 low-dose-rate in the treatment of primary and recurrent cancer of the oral cavity and oropharynx. Review of 318 patients treated between 1985 and 1997. Strahlenther Onkol. 2001;177:338–44.

Iyer NG, Tan DSW, Tan VK, et al. Randomized trial comparing surgery and adjuvant radiotherapy versus concurrent chemoradiotherapy in patients with advanced, non-metastatic squamous cell carcinoma of the head and neck: 10-year update and sub-set analysis. Cancer. 2015;121(10):1599–607.

Kovács G, Martinez-Monge R, Budrukka A, et al. GEC-ESTRO ACROP recommenda-tions for head & neck brachytherapy in squamous cell carcinomas: 1st update – improvement by cross sectional imaging based treatment planning and stepping source technology. Radiother Oncol. 2016;122(2):248–54.

Kramer S, Gelber RD, Snow JB, et al. Combined radiation therapy and surgery in the management of advanced head and neck cancer: final report of study 73-03 of the Radiation Therapy Oncology Group. Head Neck Surg. 1987;10:19–30.

Laskar SG, Chaukar D, Deshpande M, et al. Phase III randomized trial of surgery fol-lowed by conventional radiotherapy (5 fr/Wk) (Arm A) vs concurrent chemoradio-therapy (arm B) vs accelerated radiotherapy (6fr/Wk) (Arm C) in locally advanced, stage III and IV, resectable, squamous cell carcinoma of oral cavity- oral cavity adju-vant therapy (OCAT): final results (NCT00193843). J Clin Oncol. 2016;34(suppl; abstr 6004).

Martinez-Monge R, Gomez-Iturriaga A, Cambeiro M, et al. Phase I-II trial of periopera-tive high-dose-rate brachytherapy in oral cavity and oropharyngeal cancer. Brachytherapy. 2009;8:26–33.

Mazeron JJ, Ardiet JM, Haie-Méder C, et al. GEC-ESTRO recommendations for brachytherapy for head and neck squamous cell carcinomas. Radiother Oncol. 2009;91(2):150–6.

Melzner WJ, Lotter M, Sauer R, et al. Quality of interstitial PDR brachytherapy-implants of head-and-neck-cancers: predictive factors for local control and late toxicity? Radiother Oncol. 2007;82:167–73.

Nag S, Cano ER, Demanes DJ, et al. The American Brachytherapy Society recommendations for high-dose-rate brachytherapy for head-and-neck carcinoma. Int J Radiat Oncol Biol Phys. 2001;50(5):1190–8.

Peters LJ, Goepfert H, Ang KK, et al. Evaluation of the dose for postoperative radiation therapy of head and neck cancer: first report of a prospective randomized trial. Int J Radiat Oncol Biol Phys. 1993;26(1):3–11.

Strnad V, Lotter M, Kreppner S, Fietkau R. Reirradiation for recurrent head and neck cancer with salvage interstitial pulsed-dose-rate brachytherapy: long-term results. Strahlenther Onkol. 2015;191(6):495–500.

Tupchong L, Scott CB, Blitzer PH, et al. Randomized study of preoperative versus postoperative radiation therapy in advanced head and neck carcinoma: long-term follow-up of RTOG study 73-03. Int J Radiat Oncol Biol Phys. 1991;20:21–8.

Wendt CD, Peters LJ, Delclos L, et al. Primary radiotherapy in the treatment of stage I and II oral tongue cancers: importance of the proportion of therapy delivered with interstitial therapy. Int J Radiat Oncol Biol Phys. 1990;18(6):1287–92.

Zhong LP, Zhang CP, Ren GX, et al. Randomized phase III trial of induction chemotherapy with docetaxel, cisplatin, and fluorouracil followed by surgery versus upfront surgery in locally advanced resectable oral squamous cell carcinoma. J Clin Oncol. 2013;31:744–51.

Zhong LP, Zhang CP, Ren GX, et al. Long-term results of a randomized phase III trial of TPF induction chemotherapy followed by surgery and radiation in locally advanced oral squamous cell carcinoma. Oncotarget. 2015;6(21):18707–14.

III

Chapter 9
Larynx and Hypopharynx Cancer

III

Christopher H. Chapman and Adam Garsa

PEARLS

LARYNX

- Larynx cancer (including early-stage glottic tumors) is the most common cancer of the head and neck.
- Risk factors include use of tobacco, alcohol, and iron deficiency (Plummer-Vinson syndrome).
- Larynx subsites:
    - Supraglottis: suprahyoid and infrahyoid epiglottis, aryepiglottic folds, arytenoids, and vestibular folds (false cords).
    - Glottis: true vocal cords (TVCs) including the anterior and posterior commissures.
    - Subglottis: extends from the lower boundary of the glottis to the inferior aspect of the cricoid cartilage.
- TVCs attach to the thyroid cartilage at the center of the "figure of 8" on a lateral X-ray.
- LN drainage is common from the supraglottis (to levels II–V) and subglottis (to levels III–VI). Glottic tumors rarely spread to LN when T1–2 (<3%), but more commonly spread to LN when T3–4 (20–30%).
- Superior laryngeal nerves innervate the cricothyroid muscles that produce tension and elongation of the vocal cords. All other laryngeal muscles are innervated by the recurrent laryngeal nerves.

HYPOPHARYNX

- Portion of the pharynx extending from the plane of the superior border of the hyoid bone to the inferior border of the cricoid cartilage.
- Hypopharynx subsites: pyriform sinuses, postcricoid area, posterior and lateral hypopharyngeal walls.
- LN drainage from the hypopharynx is to levels II–V, the retropharyngeal LN, and to paratracheal and paraesophageal LN (when tumor involves the lowest portion of the hypopharynx and the postcricoid area).
- 95% of tumors of the larynx and hypopharynx are SCC.
- External auditory canal pain may be referred via the superior laryngeal nerve through the auricular nerve of Arnold (branch of CN X).
- A "hot potato" voice may be due to the involvement of the base of tongue.

WORKUP

- H&P, including hoarseness, pain, dysphagia, odynophagia, otalgia, trismus.
- All patients should have nasopharyngolaryngoscopy. Fixation of the true cord may be caused by invasion of the cricoarytenoid muscle or joint, or from recurrent laryngeal nerve injury.
- Esophagoscopy for hypopharynx tumors or if clinically indicated for laryngeal tumors.
- Bronchoscopy if clinically indicated.
- Biopsy tumor and/or lymph node(s).
- Labs include CBC, chemistries, BUN/Cr, LFTs, baseline TSH.
- Imaging includes thin-cut CT and/or MRI of the head and neck and chest imaging. Consider FDG-PET scan for stages III–IV.
- Preventive dental care and extractions should occur 10–14 days before RT.
- Baseline speech, swallowing, and nutrition evaluations. If locally advanced, consider baseline audiometry too.

STAGING: LARYNX AND HYPOPHARYNX CANCER

Editors' note: All TNM stage and stage groups referred to elsewhere in this chapter reflect the 2010 AJCC staging nomenclature unless otherwise noted as the new system below was published after this chapter was written.

III

Table 9.1 (AJCC 7TH ED., 2010)

Primary tumor (T)

Larynx

TX: Primary tumor cannot be assessed

T0: No evidence of primary tumor

Tis: Carcinoma in situ

Supraglottis

T1: Tumor limited to one subsite of supraglottis with normal vocal cord mobility

T2: Tumor invades mucosa of more than one adjacent subsite of supraglottis or glottis or region outside the supraglottis (e.g., mucosa of the base of tongue, vallecula, medial wall of pyriform sinus) without fixation of the larynx

T3: Tumor limited to larynx with vocal cord fixation and/or invades any of the following: postcricoid area, preepiglottic space, paraglottic space, and/or inner cortex of thyroid cartilage

T4a: Moderately advanced local disease. Tumor invades through the thyroid cartilage and/ or invades tissues beyond the larynx (e.g., trachea, soft tissues of neck including deep extrinsic muscle of the tongue, strap muscles, thyroid, or esophagus)

T4b: Very advanced local disease. Tumor invades prevertebral space, encases carotid artery, or invades mediastinal structures

Glottis

T1: Tumor limited to the vocal cord(s) (may involve anterior or posterior commissure) with normal mobility

T1a: Tumor limited to one vocal cord

T1b: Tumor involves both vocal cords

T2: Tumor extends to supraglottis and/or subglottis, and/or with impaired vocal cord mobility

T3: Tumor limited to the larynx with vocal cord fixation and/or invasion of paraglottic space, and/or inner cortex of the thyroid cartilage

T4a: Moderately advanced local disease. Tumor invades through the outer cortex of the thyroid cartilage and/or invades tissues beyond the larynx (e.g., trachea, soft tissues of neck including deep extrinsic muscle of the tongue, strap muscles, thyroid, or esophagus)

T4b: Very advanced local disease. Tumor invades prevertebral space, encases carotid artery, or invades mediastinal structures

continued

Subglottis

T1:   Tumor limited to the subglottis

T2:   Tumor extends to vocal cord(s) with normal or impaired mobility

T3:   Tumor limited to larynx with vocal cord fixation

T4a: Moderately advanced local disease. Tumor invades cricoid or thyroid cartilage and/ or invades tissues beyond the larynx (e.g., trachea, soft tissues of neck including deep extrinsic muscles of the tongue, strap muscles, thyroid, or esophagus)

T4b: Very advanced local disease. Tumor invades prevertebral space, encases carotid artery, or invades mediastinal structures

Hypopharynx

T1:   Tumor limited to one subsite of hypopharynx and/or 2 cm or less in greatest dimension

T2:   Tumor invades more than one subsite of hypopharynx or an adjacent site, or measures more than 2 cm, but not more than 4 cm in greatest dimension without fixation of hemilarynx

T3:   Tumor more than 4 cm in greatest dimension or with fixation of hemilarynx or extension to esophagus

T4a: Moderately advanced local disease. Tumor invades thyroid/cricoid cartilage, hyoid bone, thyroid gland, or central compartment soft tissue*

T4b: Very advanced local disease. Tumor invades prevertebral fascia, encases carotid artery, or involves mediastinal structures

Note: Central compartment soft tissue includes prelaryngeal strap muscles and subcutaneous fat

Regional lymph nodes (N)*

Larynx and hypopharynx

NX: Regional lymph nodes cannot be assessed N0; no regional lymph node metastasis

N1:   Metastasis in a single ipsilateral lymph node, 3 cm or less in greatest dimension

N2:   Metastasis in a single ipsilateral lymph node, more than 3 cm but not more than 6 cm in greatest dimension, or in multiple ipsilateral lymph nodes, not more than 6 cm in greatest dimension, or in bilateral or contralateral lymph nodes, not more than 6 cm in greatest dimension

N2a: Metastasis in a single ipsilateral lymph node, more than 3 cm but not more than 6 cm in greatest dimension

N2b: Metastasis in multiple ipsilateral lymph nodes, not more than 6 cm in greatest dimension

N2c: Metastasis in bilateral or contralateral lymph nodes, not more than 6 cm in greatest dimension

N3:   Metastasis in a lymph node, more than 6 cm in greatest dimension

Note: Metastases at level VII are considered regional lymph node metastases

Distant metastasis (M)

Larynx and hypopharynx

M0:   No distant metastasis

M1:   Distant metastasis

Anatomic stage/prognostic groups

Larynx and hypopharynx

0:	Tis N0 M0
I:	T1 N0 M0
II:	T2 N0 M0
III:	T3 N0 M0
	T1–T3 N1 M0
IVA:	T4a N0 M0
	T4a N1 M0
	T1–T3 N2 M0
	T4a N2 M0
IVB:	T4b Any N M0
	Any T N3 M0
IVC:	Any T Any N M1

Used with permission from the American Joint Committee on Cancer (AJCC), Chicago, Illinois. The original source for this material is the AJCC Cancer Staging Manual, Seventh Edition (2010), published by Springer Science + Business Media

Table 9.2 SUPRAGLOTTIS (AJCC 8TH ED., 2017)

Definitions of AJCC TNM

Definition of Primary Tumor (T)

Supraglottis

T category	T criteria
TX	Primary tumor cannot be assessed
Tis	Carcinoma in situ
T1	Tumor limited to one subsite of the supraglottis with normal vocal cord mobility
T2	Tumor invades the mucosa of more than one adjacent subsite of the supraglottis or glottis or region outside the supraglottis (e.g., mucosa of the base of the tongue, vallecula, medial wall of pyriform sinus) without fixation of the larynx
T3	Tumor limited to the larynx with vocal cord fixation and/or invades any of the following: postcricoid area, preepiglottic space, paraglottic space, and/or the inner cortex of the thyroid cartilage
T4	Moderately advanced or very advanced
T4a	Moderately advanced local disease. Tumor invades through the outer cortex of the thyroid cartilage and/or invades tissues beyond the larynx (e.g., trachea, soft tissues of the neck including the deep extrinsic muscle of the tongue, strap muscles, thyroid, or esophagus)
T4b	Very advanced local disease Tumor invades the prevertebral space, encases the carotid artery, or invades mediastinal structures

GLOTTIS

T category	T criteria
TX	Primary tumor cannot be assessed
Tis	Carcinoma in situ
T1	Tumor limited to the vocal cord(s) (may involve anterior or posterior commissure) with normal mobility
T1a	Tumor limited to one vocal cord
T1b	Tumor involves both vocal cords
T2	Tumor extends to the supraglottis and/or subglottis and/or with impaired vocal cord mobility
T3	Tumor limited to the larynx with vocal cord fixation and/or invasion of the paraglottic space and/or inner cortex of the thyroid cartilage
T4	Moderately advanced or very advanced
T4a	Moderately advanced local disease. Tumor invades through the outer cortex of the thyroid cartilage and/or invades tissues beyond the larynx (e.g., trachea, cricoid cartilage, soft tissues of the neck including the deep extrinsic muscle of the tongue, strap muscles, thyroid, or esophagus)
T4b	Very advanced local disease. Tumor invades the prevertebral space, encases the carotid artery, or invades mediastinal structures

SUBGLOTTIS

T category	T criteria
TX	Primary tumor cannot be assessed
Tis	Carcinoma in situ
Tl	Tumor limited to the subglottis
T2	Tumor extends to the vocal cord(s) with normal or impaired mobility
T3	Tumor limited to the larynx with vocal cord fixation and/or invasion of the paraglottic space and/or inner cortex of the thyroid cartilage
T4	Moderately advanced or very advanced
T4a	Moderately advanced local disease. Tumor invades the cricoid or thyroid cartilage and/or invades tissues beyond the larynx (e.g., trachea, soft tissues of the neck including deep extrinsic muscles of the tongue, strap muscles, thyroid, or esophagus)
T4b	Very advanced local disease. Tumor invades the prevertebral space, encases the carotid artery, or invades mediastinal structures

HYPOPHARYNX

T category	T criteria
TX	Primary tumor cannot be assessed
Tis	Carcinoma in situ
T1	Tumor limited to one subsite of the hypopharynx and/or 2 cm or smaller in the greatest dimension
T2	Tumor invades more than one subsite of the hypopharynx or an adjacent site or measures larger than 2 cm but not larger than 4 cm in the greatest dimension without fixation of hemilarynx
T3	Tumor larger than 4 cm in the greatest dimension or with fixation of hemilarynx or extension to the esophagus
T4	Moderately advanced and very advanced local disease
T4a	Moderately advanced local disease. Tumor invades the thyroid/cricoid cartilage, hyoid bone, thyroid gland, or central compartment soft tissue*
T4b	Very advanced local disease. Tumor invades the prevertebral fascia, encases the carotid artery, or involves mediastinal structures

Note: Central compartment soft tissue includes prelaryngeal strap muscles and subcutaneous fat

DEFINITION OF REGIONAL LYMPH NODES (N)
Clinical N (cN)

N category	N criteria
NX	Regional lymph nodes cannot be assessed
N0	No regional lymph node metastasis
N1	Metastasis in a single ipsilateral lymph node, 3 cm or smaller in the greatest dimension and ENE(−)
N2	Metastasis in a single ipsilateral node, larger than 3 cm but not larger than 6 cm in the greatest dimension and ENE(-), *or* métastases in multiple ipsilateral lymph nodes, not larger than 6 cm in the greatest dimension and ENE(−), *or* metastasis in bilateral or contralateral lymph nodes, not larger than 6 cm in greatest dimension and ENE(−)
N2a	Metastasis in a single ipsilateral node, larger than 3 cm but not larger than 6 cm in the greatest dimension and ENE(−)
N2b	Métastases in multiple ipsilateral nodes, not larger than 6 cm in the greatest dimension and ENE(−)
N2c	Metastasis in bilateral or contralateral lymph nodes, not larger than 6 cm in the greatest dimension and ENE(−)
N3	Metastasis in a lymph node, larger than 6 cm in the greatest dimension and ENE(−), or metastasis in any lymph node(s) with clinically overt ENE(+)

continued

| N3a | Metastasis in a lymph node, larger than 6 cm in the greatest dimension and ENE(−) |
| N3b | Metastasis in any lymph node(s) with clinically overt ENE(+) |

Note: A designation of "U" or "L" may be used for any N category to indicate metastasis above the lower border of the cricoid (U) or below the lower border of the cricoid (L) Similarly, clinical and pathological ENE should be recorded as ENE(−) or ENE(+)

Pathological N (pN)

N category	N criteria
NX	Regional lymph nodes cannot be assessed
N0	No regional lymph node metastasis
N1	Metastasis in a single ipsilateral lymph node, 3 cm or smaller in the greatest dimension and ENE(−)
N2	Metastasis in a single ipsilateral lymph node, 3 cm or smaller in the greatest dimension and ENE(+), *or* metastasis in a single ipsilateral lymph node, larger than 3 cm but not larger than 6 cm in the greatest dimension and ENE(−), *or* metastases in multiple ipsilateral lymph nodes, not larger than 6 cm in the greatest dimension and ENE(−), *or* metastasis in bilateral or contralateral lymph nodes, not larger than 6 cm in the greatest dimension and ENE(−)
N2a	Metastasis in a single ipsilateral or contralateral node, 3 cm or smaller in the greatest dimension and ENE(+), *or* metastasis in a single ipsilateral node, larger than 3 cm but not larger than 6 cm in the greatest dimension and ENE(−)
N2b	Metastasis in multiple ipsilateral nodes, not larger than 6 cm in the greatest dimension and ENE(-)
N2c	Metastasis in bilateral or contralateral lymph nodes, not larger than 6 cm in the greatest dimension and ENE(−)
N3	Metastasis in a lymph node, larger than 6 cm in the greatest dimension and ENE(−), *or* metastasis in a single ipsilateral node, larger than 3 cm in the greatest dimension and ENE(+), *or* metastases in multiple ipsilateral, contralateral, or bilateral lymph nodes and any with ENE(+)
N3a	Metastasis in a lymph node, larger than 6 cm in the greatest dimension and ENE(−)
N3b	Metastasis in a single ipsilateral node, larger than 3 cm in the greatest dimension and ENE(+), *or* metastases in multiple ipsilateral, contralateral, or bilateral lymph nodes and any with ENE(+)

Note: A designation of "U" or "L" may be used for any N category to indicate metastasis above the lower border of the cricoid (U) or below the lower border of the cricoid (L) Similarly, clinical and pathological ENE should be recorded as ENE(-) or ENE(+)

DEFINITION OF DISTANT METASTASIS (M)

M category	M criteria
M0	No distant metastasis
M1	Distant metastasis

III

AJCC PROGNOSTIC STAGE GROUPS

When T is...	And N is...	And M is...	Then the stage group is...
Tis	N0	M0	0
T1	N0	M0	I
T2	N0	M0	II
T3	N0	M0	III
T1, T2, T3	N1	M0	III
T4a	N0, N1	M0	IVA
T1, T2, T3, T4a	N2	M0	IVA
Any T	N3	M0	IVB
T4b	Any N	M0	IVB
Any T	Any N	M1	IVC

Used with permission of the American Joint Committee on Cancer (AJCC), Chicago, Illinois. The original and primary source for this information is the AJCC Cancer Staging Manual, Eighth Edition (2017) published by Springer International Publishing

TREATMENT RECOMMENDATIONS

Table 9.3 TREATMENT RECOMMENDATIONS

2010 stage	Larynx
Tis	Endoscopic resection (stripping/laser) Definitive RT
T1-2N0 glottic	Definitive RT Alternative: cordectomy or partial laryngectomy ± selective neck dissection. Post-op RT for close/+margin, PNI, LVSI
T1-2N0 supraglottic	Definitive RT Alternative: partial supraglottic laryngectomy ± selective neck dissection. Post-op chemo-RT for + margin; post-op RT for close margin, PNI, LVSI

continued

Table 9.3 (continued)

T1-2N+ or T3 requiring total laryngectomy	Concurrent chemo-RT. If < CR, salvage surgery ± neck dissection. If residual neck mass after RT or initial N2–3 post-RT, consider neck dissection Alternative: total laryngectomy and ipsilateral ± contralateral neck dissection. Post-op chemo-RT for +margin or nodal ECE. Post-op RT for pT3–4, pN2–3, close margin, PNI, LVSI, ≥1 cm subglottic extension, and/or cartilage invasion Induction chemo may be considered. If CR or PR, proceed with concurrent chemo-RT as above. If < PR or progression, proceed to surgery ± neck dissection as indicated
Resectable T4	Total laryngectomy and ipsilateral or bilateral neck dissection followed by post-op RT. Post-op chemo-RT for +margin or ECE Alternative (selected patients): Concurrent chemo-RT. Induction chemo may be considered. If CR or PR, proceed with concurrent chemo-RT as above. If < PR or progression, proceed to surgery ± neck dissection as indicated
Unresectable	Concurrent chemo-RT If unable to tolerate chemo, definitive RT with altered fractionation
2010 stage	**Hypopharynx**
Early T1–2	Definitive RT. If < complete response, salvage surgery and neck dissection as indicated. If complete response, neck dissection considered for N2–3 Alternative: partial laryngopharyngectomy and ipsilateral or bilateral selective neck dissection (N0) or comprehensive neck dissection (N+). Post-op chemo-RT for + margin or nodal ECE. Post-op RT (or chemo-RT if multiple factors) for pN2–3, close margin, PNI, LVSI, cartilage invasion
T2–4 requiring total laryngectomy	Concurrent chemo-RT as extrapolated from RTOG 91–11 Alternative: laryngopharyngectomy and selective (N0) or comprehensive neck dissection (N+ or T4). Post-op chemo-RT for + margin or nodal ECE. Post-op RT (or chemo-RT if multiple factors) for pT3–4, pN2–3, close margin, PNI, LVSI, cartilage invasion Consider induction chemo. If CR at primary site, proceed with definitive RT. If only PR at primary site, concurrent chemo-RT. Nonresponders to induction chemo should undergo surgery → post-op RT or chemo-RT as indicated. If residual neck mass after definitive RT or initial N2–3, post-RT neck dissection considered
Unresectable	Concurrent chemo-RT If unable to tolerate chemo, definitive RT with concomitant boost (CB) and consider concurrent cetuximab

Table 9.4 Surgical options

Operation	Indications	Removes	Contraindications/notes
Limited surgery (stripping or CO₂ laser)	Carcinoma in situ	Mucosa of cord	Can lead to thickened or harsh voice. Difficult to determine if invasive carcinoma present. Laser appropriate for lesions in middle 1/3 of cord
Cordectomy	Early T1a lesions of middle 1/3 of one TVC	Transoral laser excision of part of one cord	Afterward, pseudocord forms and patient has useful (but harsh) voice
Vertical partial (hemi-) laryngectomy	Voice preservation for TVC lesions involving 1 and <1/3 (<5 mm) of other TVC	Bisects larynx and removes 1/2 of thyroid cartilage, a portion or all of 1 TVC and up to 1/3 (5 mm) of other TVC	Contraindicated if TVC fixation, >5 mm posterior or >10 mm anterior subglottic extension (because it must preserve cricoid), or supraglottic extension to false cord or interarytenoid area
Supraglottic (horizontal partial) laryngectomy (SGL)	Early supraglottic lesions for voice preservation	Removes epiglottis, aryepiglottic folds, false cords, upper 1/3–1/2 of thyroid cartilage, ± hyoid bone (if epiglottic space involvement). Preserves one or both arytenoids and both TVCs	Contraindicated if exolaryngeal spread, vocal cord fixation, involvement of arytenoids, <3 mm between tumor and anterior commissure, thyroid/cricoid cartilage invasion, and/or inadequate pulmonary function (due to high aspiration risk)
Extended SGL	Supraglottic lesion with <1 cm base of tongue invasion	Same as SGL with removal of ipsilateral BOT up to circumvallate papillae	
Total laryngectomy (TL)	Indicated for advanced lesions with transglottic or extensive subglottic extension, most pyriform sinus lesions, and/or cartilage invasion	Removes hyoid, thyroid, and cricoid cartilages, epiglottis, strap muscles. Patient left with a permanent tracheostoma and pharynx reconstruction (by suturing to the base of tongue)	Most frequent sites of failure include tracheal stoma, base of tongue, and neck nodes. Rehabilitation options include tracheoesophageal speech, artificial electronic larynx, and esophageal speech
Partial laryngopharyngectomy	Used for small medial and anterior pyriform sinus lesions	Removes false cords, epiglottis, aryepiglottic fold, and pyriform sinus, but TVCs are preserved	Contraindicated if transglottic extension, cartilage invasion, vocal fold paralysis, pyriform apex invasion (b/c below level of TVCs), postcricoid invasion, exolaryngeal spread, or poor pulmonary reserve
Total laryngopharyngectomy	For more advanced hypopharyngeal lesions	TL plus removal of varying amount of pharyngeal wall	Requires flap or gut graft if total pharyngectomy

III

STUDIES

EARLY-STAGE (T1-2N0) GLOTTIC CANCER

⌄ Local control with primary RT: T1 85–95%, T2 65–85%.

⌄ Local control with primary RT including salvage surgery: T1 ~ 95%, T2 ~ 90%.

⌄ (Yamazaki *IJROBP* 2006): 180 patients with T1 N0 glottic carcinoma randomized to 2/60 Gy (if ≤2/3 TVC involved) or 66 Gy (if >2/3 TVC involved) vs. 2.25/56.25–63 Gy. Higher fraction size improved 5-year LC (77 → 92%), but not CSS (97 vs. 100%) or toxicity.

⌄ *RTOG 95–12* (Trotti *IJROBP* 2014): 250 patients with T2 N0 glottic cancer randomized to 70 Gy in 35 fx vs. 79.2 Gy at 1.2 Gy BID. Nonsignificant trend with BID for improved 5-year LC (70 → 79%, $p = 0.14$). Trial was underpowered. Higher acute toxicity with BID, no difference in late toxicity.

⌄ (Aaltonen *IJROBP* 2014): 60 patients with T1aN0 glottic cancer randomized to transoral laser surgery or RT 2/66 Gy. Voice quality rated at baseline and 6 and 24 months by experts blinded to voice recordings, patient self-rating, and videolaryngostroboscopy. With RT, less breathiness at 2 years (30% vs. 81%), less self-rated impact, and less irregular glottic closure.

ALTERED FRACTIONATION

⌄ *DAHANCA 6&7* (Overgaard *Lancet* 2003): 1485 patients with head and neck cancer, including 690 patients with glottic cancer and 218 with supraglottic larynx cancer. Patients received 2/62–68 Gy, randomized to 5 vs. 6 fractions per week (weekend or once weekly BID treatment). For larynx cancer, 6 fractions/week reduced 5-year LF (glottic 27 → 18%, supraglottic 48 → 33%) and improved 5-year voice preservation (68 → 80%, $p = 0.007$).

⌄ See Chapter 7 (Oropharynx) for other key trials of altered fractionation, most of which included patients with larynx/hypopharynx cancer.

LARYNX-PRESERVING CHEMO-RT FOR ADVANCED STAGE CANCER

, Estimated long-term (>2 years) larynx preservation rates:
  , RT alone: 60–70%.
  , Induction chemo → RT: 65–75%.
  , Concurrent chemo-RT: 80–85%.
  , Note: median overall survival 4–6 years; no difference by therapy.
, *VA Larynx Trial* (Wolf *NEJM* 1991): 332 patients with III–IV larynx (T1 N1 excluded), randomized to surgery and post-op RT (50–74 Gy) vs. induction cisplatin/5-FU × 2c (with a third cycle if PR/CR) → RT (66–76 Gy). If < PR/CR then surgery → RT. Larynx preservation at 2 years with induction chemo 64%. No difference in 2-year OS (68%). Induction chemo decreased DM, but had higher LF (12 vs. 2%). Salvage laryngectomy was required for 56% of T4 patients.
, *EORTC 24891* (Lefebvre *J Natl Cancer Inst* 1996, *Ann Oncol* 2012): 202 patients with T2–4 pyriform sinus or aryepiglottic tumors randomized to surgery → RT (50–64 Gy) vs. induction cisplatin/5-FU × 2c (with a third cycle if PR/CR) → RT (70 Gy). If < PR/CR then surgery → RT. 54% of patients had a CR after chemo. No significant difference in 5-/10-year LRF, PFS, or OS. In chemo arm, 5-/10-year survival with preserved larynx = 22%/9%.
, *RTOG 91–11* (Forastiere *NEJM* 2003, *JCO* 2013): 547 patients with stage III/IV larynx cancer (T2–3 or low-volume T4 [not invading through thyroid cartilage and <1 cm base of tongue invasion], or LN+) randomized to three arms: RT alone, chemo → RT, or concurrent chemo-RT (all 2/70 Gy). Induction chemo was cisplatin/5-FU × 2c (with a third cycle if PR/CR, otherwise surgery). Concurrent chemo was cisplatin × 3c. Over RT alone or induction chemo, concurrent chemo-RT improved 10-year larynx preservation (64 → 68 → 82%) and LRC (47 → 49 → 65%). Trend toward improved distant control with any chemo (76 → 83 → 84%). No significant difference in 10-year OS (32 → 39 → 28%), although more late deaths unrelated to disease with concurrent chemo-RT.
, *GORTEC 2000–01* (Pointreau *JNCI* 2009): 220 patients with locally advanced larynx/hypopharynx cancer randomized to

3c of TPF (docetaxel, cisplatin, 5-FU) vs. PF. If CR/PR and larynx mobility → RT. If no response → surgery and post-op RT. TPF improved overall response (59 → 80%) and 3-year larynx preservation (58 → 70%), but caused more neutropenia. No difference in 3-year OS or PFS.

, *TREMPLIN* (Lefebvre *JCO* 2013): 153 patients with stage III–IV larynx SCC received 3c induction TPF. < 50% response → salvage surgery. ≥ 50% response → randomized to RT (2/70 Gy) with concurrent cisplatin or cetuximab. 116 patients randomized after induction. No differences in 18-month larynx preservation or 3-year OS (albeit limited power). More protocol-modifying toxicity with cisplatin.

, *MD Anderson T4 retrospective* (Rosenthal *Cancer* 2015): 221 patients with T4 larynx SCC (46% ≥ full thickness thyroid cartilage invasion). 161 treated with total laryngectomy → RT; 60 treated with larynx-preserving RT (85% with chemo-RT). Improved 10-year LRC with laryngectomy (58 → 72%), however chemo-RT no different after salvage surgery (73%). Same median OS (64 months). 5-/10-year rate of disease free survival with fully functioning larynx in preservation group = 32/13%. LN+ biggest predictor of DM, DSS, and OS.

, See Chapter 7 (Oropharynx) for other major trials of induction chemotherapy and concurrent chemoradiotherapy, most of which included patients with larynx/hypopharynx cancer.

ADJUVANT THERAPY

, Indications for post-op RT: emergent tracheostomy, pT3–4, pN2–3, close margin (< 5 mm), PNI, or LVSI. Post-op chemo-RT for ECE and/or positive margin.

, See Chapter 7 (Oropharynx) for major trials of adjuvant therapy, most of which included patients with larynx/hypopharynx cancer.

RADIATION TECHNIQUES

SIMULATION AND FIELD DESIGN

, Simulate supine with neck extended, shoulders down. Immobilize with a thermoplastic head and shoulder mask. Wire neck scars. Bolus may be needed for anterior commissure tumors and over tracheostoma (if present).

, A 3D-conformal or IMRT plan should be used to spare normal tissues, except for simple opposed lateral fields for early-stage glottic cancer. Fluoroscopy may be useful to evaluate motion of larynx with swallowing to ensure appropriate superior border.

, Conventional plans for early-stage glottic cancer:

, T1 N0 glottic larynx: 5 × 5 cm opposed lateral fields. Superior border at the top of the thyroid cartilage, inferior border at the bottom of the cricoid, 1 cm skin flash anteriorly, and 2 cm margin posteriorly (or the anterior edge of the vertebral body) (Fig. 9.1). Use paired wedges (e.g., 15 degrees) for homogeneity, but avoid overwedging and underdosing anterior commissure. Consider 5 mm bolus if anterior ½ cord involved to ensure anterior commissure coverage.

, T2 N0 glottic larynx: increase field size to 6 × 6 cm with inferior border, one tracheal ring below the cricoid.

, IMRT:

, IMRT is not necessary for T1-2N0 glottic cancers, but recommended for advanced lesions for improved normal tissue sparing.

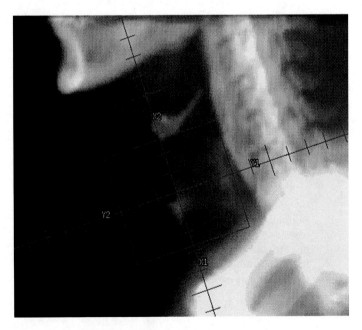

Fig. 9.1 Lateral DRR of a field used to treat a T1 glottic carcinoma

- GTV = clinical and/or radiographic gross disease (primary and nodes).
- CTV1 = 5 mm margin on primary and 3–5 mm margin on nodes (depending on adjacent critical structures and anatomic boundaries to microscopic spread).
- CTV2 = High-risk areas and nodal levels (entire larynx [for both larynx and hypopharynx cancers] involved and adjacent nodal levels).
- CTV3 = Elective nodal levels (same as conventional).
- PTV = CTV + 3–5 mm. For primary tumor, 5–10 mm PTV expansion (due to risk of intrafraction larynx/tumor motion).
- Extended-field whole neck IMRT preferred for larynx/hypopharynx. Use anterior obliques rather than lateral fields to avoid treating through shoulders.
- Nodal coverage:
  - Larynx
    - Levels II–IV. Include IB and V on the involved N+ neck, level VI if subglottic or soft tissue extension.
  - Hypopharynx
    - Levels II–IV, retropharyngeal nodes. Include IB and V on the involved N+ neck. Paratracheal nodal coverage in upper mediastinum if positive postcricoid involvement or nodal involvement in low neck.

DOSE PRESCRIPTIONS

- T1-2N0 glottic larynx
  - >2 Gy/fx preferred. If 2 Gy/fx is used, total dose >66 Gy.
  - UCSF uses 2.25 Gy/fx.
    - Tis: 56.25–60.75 Gy.
    - T1N0: 63 Gy.
    - T2N0: 65.25 Gy.
- T3–4 and LN+: concurrent chemo-RT
  - Standard-fractionation RT with cisplatin 100 mg/m^2 q3 weeks ×3c (alternatively, cisplatin 40 mg/m^2 weekly ×6c or cetuximab).
  - RT dose/fractionation for chemo-RT or definitive RT alone same as oropharyngeal cancer; see Chapter 7.

- Post-op RT: dose/fractionation same as oropharyngeal cancer, see Chapter 7.
  - High-risk volume includes tracheostoma if: emergent tracheostomy, subglottic extension, tumor invasion of soft tissues of neck, extranodal extension in level VI, close/positive margin. Otherwise cover tracheostoma in low-risk volume.
  - Post-op chemo-RT indicated for nodal ECE and/or +margin. Considered for other risk features, including pT3–4, pN2–3, PNI, LVSI. Concurrent single agent cisplatin 100 mg/m² q3 weeks x3c (alternatively, cisplatin 40 mg/m² weekly x6c or cetuximab).

DOSE LIMITATIONS
- Generally same as oropharyngeal primary; see Chapter 7.
- Thyroid should not be spared at the expense of target volume coverage: use TSH monitoring and levothyroxine supplementation for hypothyroidism.
- 70 Gy to larynx carries 5% risk of cartilage necrosis.

COMPLICATIONS
- Acute complications of RT include mucositis, dermatitis, xerostomia, laryngeal edema and dysgeusia. Long-term complications include soft tissue fibrosis, cartilage necrosis, dysphagia, swallowing dysfunction, xerostomia, dental complications, acceleration of atherosclerosis, osteoradionecrosis, secondary malignancy, and hypothyroidism.
- Perioperative complications of surgery include bleeding, airway obstruction, infection, and wound complications. Long-term post-op complications include webs, stenosis, chondritis, fistulas, and aspiration.
- Patients need ≥2000 calories/day to avoid malnutrition. Use liquid nutritional supplements as needed. Prophylactic PEG-tube placement controversial.

FOLLOW-UP

- Same as oropharyngeal primary; see Chapter 7.

Acknowledgment We thank Sunanda Pejavar MD, Eric K. Hansen MDb, Sue S. Yom MD, and Naomi R. Schechter MDa, for their work on the prior edition of this chapter.

REFERENCES

Aaltonen L-M, Rautiainen N, Sellman J, et al. Voice quality after treatment of early vocal cord cancer: a randomized trial comparing laser surgery with radiation therapy. Int J Radiat Oncol Biol Phys. 2014;90(2):255–60.

Forastiere AA, Goepfert H, Maor M, et al. Concurrent chemotherapy and radiotherapy for organ preservation in advanced laryngeal cancer. N Engl J Med. 2003;349:2091–8.

Forastiere AA, Zhang Q, Weber RS, et al. Long-term results of RTOG 91-11: a comparison of three nonsurgical treatment strategies to preserve the larynx in patients with locally advanced larynx cancer. J Clin Oncol. 2013;31(7):845–52.

Lefebvre JL, Chevalier D, Luboinski B, et al. Larynx preservation in pyriform sinus cancer: preliminary results of a European Organization for Research and Treatment of cancer phase III trial. EORTC head and neck cancer cooperative group. J Natl Cancer Inst. 1996;88:890–9.

Lefebvre JL, Andry G, Chevalier D, et al. Laryngeal preservation with induction chemotherapy for hypopharyngeal squamous cell carcinoma: 10-year results of EORTC trial 24891. Ann Oncol. 2012;23(10):2708–14.

Lefebvre JL, Pointreau Y, Rolland F, et al. Induction chemotherapy followed by either chemoradiotherapy or bioradiotherapy for larynx preservation: the TREMPLIN randomized phase II study. J Clin Oncol. 2013;31(7):853–9.

Overgaard J, Hansen HS, Specht L, et al. Five compared with six fractions per week of conventional radiotherapy of squamous-cell carcinoma of head and neck: DAHANCA 6&7 randomised controlled trial. Lancet. 2003;362(9388):933–40.

Pointreau Y, Garaud P, Chapet S, et al. Randomized trial of induction chemotherapy with cisplatin and 5-fluorouracil with or without docetaxel for larynx preservation. J Natl Cancer Inst. 2009;101(7):498–506.

Rosenthal DI, Mohamed ASR, Weber RS, et al. Long-term outcomes after surgical or non-surgical initial therapy for patients with T4 squamous cell carcinoma of the larynx: a 3-decade survey. Cancer. 2015;121(10):1608–19.

Trotti A, Zhang Q, Bentzen SM, et al. Randomized trial of hyperfractionation versus conventional fractionation in T2 squamous cell carcinoma of the vocal cord (RTOG 9512). Int J Radiat Oncol Biol Phys. 2014;89(5):958–63.

Wolf GT, Hong WK, Fisher SG, et al. Induction chemotherapy plus radiation compared with surgery plus radiation in patients with advanced laryngeal cancer. N Engl J Med. 1991;324(24):1685–90.

Yamazaki H, Nishiyama K, Tanaka E, et al. Radiotherapy for early glottic carcinoma (T1N0M0): results of prospective randomized study of radiation fraction size and overall treatment time. Int J Radiat Oncol Biol Phys. 2006;64(1):77–82.

Chapter 10
Salivary Gland Tumors

Christopher H. Chapman and Adam Garsa

PEARLS

- Salivary gland neoplasms account for ~3–5% of H&N cancers.
- Major salivary glands consist of the paired parotid, submandibular, and sublingual glands.
- Minor salivary glands are located throughout oral cavity, pharynx, and paranasal sinuses.
- Parotid glands located lateral to the mandibular ramus and masseter muscle.
  - Facial nerve divides parotid gland into superficial and deep lobes.
  - Parotid gland drains into oral cavity through Stensen's duct adjacent to upper second molar.
  - Lymphatic drainage from parotid gland is to intraparotid and periparotid nodes, followed by ipsilateral level I, II, and III nodes.
- Submandibular gland is located under the horizontal mandibular ramus.
  - Submandibular gland is lateral to lingual (V3) and hypoglossal nerves and is medial to mandibular and cervical branches of CN VII.
  - Submandibular glands drain into oral cavity through Wharton's duct.

© Springer International Publishing AG, part of Springer Nature 2018   **227**
Eric K. Hansen and M. Roach III (eds.), *Handbook of Evidence-Based Radiation Oncology*, https://doi.org/10.1007/978-3-319-62642-0_10

- ˒ Submandibular lymphatic drainage is to levels I, II, III.
- ˒ Drainage from parotid and submandibular glands to contralateral nodes is rare.
- ˒ Sublingual gland located superior to mylohyoid muscle and deep to mucous membrane. Sublingual glands drain into oral cavity through Rivinus ducts or Bartholin's duct.
- ˒ Incidence of LN involvement varies according to histology and site. Overall risk of lymph node involvement is less common than for SCC.
- ˒ LN metastases are most common with minor salivary gland tumors followed by submandibular gland tumors followed by parotid tumors.

HISTOLOGY

- ˒ Salivary gland neoplasms are notable for diversity of histology and behavior.
- ˒ Majority of salivary gland neoplasms are benign.
- ˒ Inverse relationship exists between size of gland and frequency of malignant vs. benign tumors.
  - ˒ Parotid: ~20% malignant.
  - ˒ Submandibular: ~50% malignant.
  - ˒ Sublingual and minor glands: 50–80% malignant.
- ˒ Pleomorphic adenoma is most common benign salivary gland neoplasm (5–10% risk of malignant transformation), followed by Warthin's tumor (papillary cystadenoma lymphomatosum; more common in smokers).
- ˒ Most common malignant histology of parotid gland is mucoepidermoid carcinoma.
- ˒ Most common malignant histology of submandibular and minor salivary glands is adenoid cystic carcinoma.
- ˒ Adenoid cystic carcinoma has the lowest frequency of cervical node metastasis (5–8%), but the highest propensity for perineural spread. High rate of distant metastases (primarily lung), which can occur years or decades later.
- ˒ Acinic cell carcinoma predominantly occurs in the parotid gland.
- ˒ Additional histologic subtypes include: polymorphic low-grade adenocarcinoma, salivary duct carcinoma,

carcinoma ex pleomorphic adenocarcinoma, mucinous adenocarcinoma, myoepithelial, others.

, Lymphoepithelial carcinoma is associated with Epstein-Barr virus (EBV) in Asian and Inuit populations.

, High-grade carcinoma associated with androgen receptor overexpression, especially salivary duct carcinoma.

, Squamous cell carcinoma is most often metastatic from skin cancer, not salivary primary.

PROGNOSIS AND FAILURE PATTERNS

, Prognostic variables include grade, postsurgical residual disease, and LN status.

, Larger tumor size and cranial nerve involvement associated with poor prognosis.

, Patterns of failure generally dominated by high rates of distant metastases.

, Most likely sites for DM are the lung and the bone and liver.

, Adenoid cystic, salivary duct carcinoma, and undifferentiated carcinoma have highest rates of DM.

WORKUP

, Most common presentation is painless mass. Malignant tumors more likely to be painful, affecting cranial nerves, and/or fixed deeply.

, H&P with bimanual palpation. Carefully examine cranial nerves and trismus.

, Fine-needle aspiration biopsy.

, CT and/or MRI of head and neck. Role for FDG-PET not clearly established for salivary gland tumors; may consider for distant staging in high grade or advanced primaries. Otherwise chest CT to rule out lung metastases.

, Dental evaluation prior to the start of RT.

, Note that minor salivary gland cancer is staged according to systems for the anatomic site of origin (e.g., oral cavity, sinuses, etc.).

STAGING: MAJOR SALIVARY GLAND

Editors' note: All TNM stage and stage groups referred to elsewhere in this chapter reflect the 2010 AJCC staging nomenclature unless otherwise noted as the new system below was published after this chapter was written.

Table 10.1 (AJCC 7th ed., 2010)

Primary tumor (T)	
TX:	Primary tumor cannot be assessed
T0:	No evidence of primary tumor
T1:	Tumor 2 cm or less in greatest dimension without extraparenchymal extension*
T2:	Tumor more than 2 cm but not more than 4 cm in greatest dimension without extraparenchymal extension*
T3:	Tumor more than 4 cm and/or tumor having extraparenchymal extension*
T4a:	Moderately advanced disease. Tumor invades skin, mandible, ear canal, and/or facial nerve
T4b:	Very advanced disease. Tumor invades skull base and/or pterygoid plates and/or encases carotid artery

Note: Extraparenchymal extension is clinical or macroscopic evidence of invasion of soft tissues. Microscopic evidence alone does not constitute extraparenchymal extension for classification purposes

Regional lymph nodes (N)	
NX:	Regional lymph nodes cannot be assessed
N0:	No regional lymph node metastasis
N1:	Metastasis in a single ipsilateral lymph node, 3 cm or less in greatest dimension
N2:	Metastasis in a single ipsilateral lymph node, more than 3 cm but not more than 6 cm in greatest dimension, or in multiple ipsilateral lymph nodes, not more than 6 cm in greatest dimension, or in bilateral or contralateral lymph nodes, not more than 6 cm in greatest dimension
N2a:	Metastasis in a single ipsilateral lymph node, more than 3 cm but not more than 6 cm in greatest dimension
N2b:	Metastasis in multiple ipsilateral lymph nodes, not more than 6 cm in greatest dimension
N2c:	Metastasis in bilateral or contralateral lymph nodes, not more than 6 cm in greatest dimension
N3:	Metastasis in a lymph node, more than 6 cm in greatest dimension

Distant metastasis (M)

M0: No distant metastasis

M1: Distant metastasis

Anatomic stage/prognostic groups

I:	T1 N0 M0
II:	T2 N0 M0
III:	T3 N0 M0
	T1–T3 N1 M0
IVA:	T4a N0 M0
	T4a N1 M0
	T1–T3 N2 M0
	T4a N2 M0
IVB:	T4b Any N M0
	Any T N3 M0
IVC:	Any T Any N M1

Used with the permission from the American Joint Committee on Cancer (AJCC), Chicago, Illinois. The original source for this material is the AJCC Cancer Staging Manual, Seventh Edition (2010), published by Springer Science + Business Media

Table 10.2 (AJCC 8th ed., 2017)

Definitions of AJCC TNM	
Definition of Primary Tumor (T)	
T category	**T criteria**
TX	Primary tumor cannot be assessed
T0	No evidence of primary tumor
Tis	Carcinoma in situ
T1	Tumor 2 cm or smaller in the greatest dimension without extraparenchymal extension*
T2	Tumor larger than 2 cm but not larger than 4 cm in the greatest dimension without extraparenchymal extension*
T3	Tumor larger than 4 cm and/or tumor having extraparenchymal extension*
T4	Moderately advanced or very advanced disease
T4a	Moderately advanced disease Tumor invades the skin, mandible, ear canal, and/or facial nerve
T4b	Very advanced disease Tumor invades the skull base and/or pterygoid plates and/or encases the carotid artery

*Extraparenchymal extension is a clinical or macroscopic evidence of invasion of soft tissues. Microscopic evidence alone does not constitute extraparenchymal extension for classification purposes

DEFINITION OF REGIONAL LYMPH NODE (N)
Clinical N (cN)

N category	N criteria
NX	Regional lymph nodes cannot be assessed
N0	No regional lymph node metastasis
N1	Metastasis in a single ipsilateral lymph node, 3 cm or smaller in the greatest dimension and ENE(–)
N2	Metastasis in a single ipsilateral node larger than 3 cm but not larger than 6 cm in the greatest dimension and ENE(–) *or* métastases in multiple ipsilateral lymph nodes, not larger than 6 cm in the greatest dimension and ENE(–), *or* in bilateral or contracterai lymph nodes, not larger than 6 cm in greatest dimension and ENE(–)
N2a	Metastasis in a single ipsilateral node larger than 3 cm but not larger than 6 cm in the greatest dimension and ENE(–)
N2b	Metastasis in multiple ipsilateral nodes, not larger than 6 cm in the greatest dimension and ENE(-)
N2c	Metastasis in bilateral or contralateral lymph nodes, not larger than 6 cm in the greatest dimension and ENE(–)
N3	Metastasis in a lymph node larger than 6 cm in the greatest dimension and ENE(-) *or* metastasis in any node(s) with clinically overt ENE(+)
N3a	Metastasis in a lymph node larger than 6 cm in the greatest dimension and ENE(–)
N3b	Metastasis in any node(s) with clinically overt ENE(+)

Note: A designation of "U" or "L" may be used for any N category to indicate metastasis above the lower border of the cricoid (U) or below the lower border of the cricoid (L). Similarly, clinical and pathological ENE should be recorded as ENEA(–) or ENE(+)

Pathological N (pN)

N category	N criteria
NX	Regional lymph nodes cannot be assessed
N0	No regional lymph node metastasis
N1	Metastasis in a single ipsilateral lymph node, 3 cm or smaller in the greatest dimension and ENE(–)
N2	Metastasis in a single ipsilateral lymph node, 3 cm or smaller in the greatest dimension and ENE(+) *or* larger than 3 cm but not larger than 6 cm in the greatest dimension and ENE(–), *or* métastases in multiple ipsilateral lymph nodes, not larger than 6 cm in the greatest dimension and ENE(–), *or* in bilateral or contralateral lymph nodes, not larger than 6 cm in the greatest dimension and ENE(–)

N2a	Metastasis in single ipsilateral or contralateral node 3 cm or smaller in the greatest dimension and ENE(+) *or* a single ipsilateral node larger than 3 cm but not larger than 6 cm in the greatest dimension and ENE(−)
N2b	Metastasis in multiple ipsilateral nodes, not larger than 6 cm in the greatest dimension and ENE(-)
N2c	Metastasis in bilateral or contralateral lymph nodes, not larger than 6 cm in the greatest dimension and ENE(-)
N3	Metastasis in a lymph node larger than 6 cm in the greatest dimension and ENE(-) *or* in a single ipsilateral node larger than 3 cm in the greatest dimension and ENE(+) *or* multiple ipsilateral, contralateral, or bilateral nodes any with ENE(+)
N3a	Metastasis in a lymph node larger than 6 cm in the greatest dimension and ENE(-)
N3b	Metastasis in a single ipsilateral node larger than 3 cm in the greatest dimension and ENE(+) *or* multiple ipsilateral, contralateral, or bilateral nodes any with ENE(+)

Note: A designation of "U" or "L" may be used for any N category to indicate metastasis above the lower border of the cricoid (U) or below the lower border of the cricoid (L). Similarly, clinical and pathological ENE should be recorded as ENE(-) or ENE(+)

DEFINITION OF DISTANT METASTASIS (M)

M category	M criteria
M0	No distant metastasis
M1	Distant metastasis

AJCC PROGNOSTIC STAGE GROUPS

When T is...	And N is...	And M is...	Then the stage group is...
Tis	N0	M0	0
T1	N0	M0	I
T2	N0	M0	II
T3	N0	M0	III
T0, T1, T2, T3	N1	M0	III
T4a	N0, NI	M0	IVA
T0, T1, T2, T3, T4a	N2	M0	IVA
Any T	N3	M0	IVB
T4b	Any N	M0	IVB
Any T	Any N	M1	IVC

Used with permission of the American Joint Committee on Cancer (AJCC), Chicago, Illinois. The original and primary source for this information is the AJCC Cancer Staging Manual, Eighth Edition (2017) published by Springer International Publishing

TREATMENT RECOMMENDATIONS

GENERAL POINTS

- Surgery is the mainstay of definitive treatment for salivary gland malignancies.
  - Neck dissection recommended for cN+ or high-grade histology.
  - Superficial parotidectomy can generally be performed for low-grade tumors.
  - Facial nerve sparing can often be performed to preserve function and cosmesis.
  - Complications of surgery include facial nerve dysfunction and Frey's syndrome (gustatory flushing and sweating).
- Adjuvant therapy indications are controversial as there are no randomized data.
  - Adjuvant RT recommended for residual gross disease or pathological LN involvement. Consider chemo-RT.
  - Consider adjuvant RT for close/+margins, adenoid cystic histology, intermediate/high grade, PNI, LVSI, T3–4 primary.
- RT alone indicated for medically inoperable and unresectable tumors.
  - LC rates with RT alone range from 20 to 80%.
  - Higher linear energy transfer (LET) radiation (e.g., neutrons) may achieve better LC for unresectable or inoperable tumors.
  - Brachytherapy or intraoperative RT can be considered for recurrent tumors.
  - IMRT reduces doses to normal structures and allows dose escalation to tumor.
- Despite high risk of distant metastases, so far there is no established role for chemotherapy.

Table 10.3 TREATMENT RECOMMENDATIONS

2010 stage	Recommended treatment
Resectable T1-2N0, superficial	Surgery followed by observation if low-grade Consider post-op RT if close/+margins, adenoid cystic histology, intermediate/high grade, PNI, LVSI
Resectable T3–4/N+	Surgery with neck dissection for N+ or high grade, followed by post-op RT
Unresectable	Definitive RT. LRC may be higher with neutrons than photons
Pleomorphic adenoma	Preferred: parotidectomy (vs. simple enucleation) Post-op RT controversial; consider if multifocal, recurrent, PNI, or residual disease

III

STUDIES

SURGERY ALONE

꜄ (Spiro *Head Neck Surg* 1986): retrospective of 2807 patients with salivary gland tumors (46% malignant). ~95% treated with surgery alone. 5-/10-/20-year DFS for malignant: parotid 55/40/33%, submandibular 31/22/14%, minor salivary glands 48/37/15%. 10-year OS highly related to grade (low ~90%, high ~25%) except for adenoid cystic (~50%).

꜄ (Chen *IJROBP* 2007a): retrospective of 207 patients with major salivary gland carcinoma, all treated with surgery alone. 5-/10-year LRC = 86/74%. Worse 10-year LRC with pN+ (37%), positive margins (59%), high-grade histology (62%), and T3–4 (63%). 5-/10-year OS = 83/62%. Worse 10-year OS with pN+ (24%).

SURGERY ± ADJUVANT RADIATION THERAPY
MAJOR SALIVARY GLANDS

꜄ (Armstrong *Arch Otolaryngol Head Neck Surg* 1990): matched pair analysis of 46 patients treated with surgery → RT (median 56.64 Gy) to 46 patients treated with surgery alone. For stages III–IV, post-op RT improved 5-year LC (17 → 51%) and DSS (10 → 51%). For pN+, post-op RT improved 5-year LC (40 → 69%) and DSS (19 → 49%).

, (Terhaard *IJROBP* 2005): retrospective of 538 patients. 72% had surgery → RT, 21% surgery alone, 7% RT alone. Post-op RT improved 10-year LC vs. surgery alone for patients with T3–4 tumors (18 → 84%), close (55 → 95%) and incomplete resection (44 → 82%), bone invasion (54 → 86%), and PNI (60 → 88%). For pN+, post-op RT improved 10-year neck control (57 → 83%).

, (Garden *IJROBP* 1997): retrospective of 166 patients with parotid gland malignancies treated with surgery → RT (median 60 Gy). 17% pN+, 34% PNI. 5-/10-/15-year LC: 92/90/90%. Worse LC with facial nerve sacrifice and pN+.

, (Al-Mamgani, IJROBP 2012): retrospective of 186 pts with parotid carcinoma treated with surgery and post-op RT. 5-yr LRC 89% overall. 5-yr EFS: acinic cell 89%, mucoepidermoid 78%, adenoid cystic 76%, adenocarcinoma 74%, squamous cell carcinoma 70%.

MINOR SALIVARY GLANDS

, (Garden *Cancer* 1994): retrospective of 160 patients treated with surgery → RT (median 60 Gy). 10-year LC 86%, DFS 62%, OS 65%. Distant metastasis was the predominant site of failure (27%). Higher local failure with paranasal primary, pN+, and increased interval between surgery and radiation (median 31 days).

, (Loh *Head Neck* 2009): retrospective of 171 patients treated with surgery alone (31%), surgery → RT (31%), or RT alone (38%). Post-op RT given for +margin or ECE. 5-year DFS/DSS/OS = 65/78/74%. 19% distant metastasis, most commonly lungs. Worse 5-year DSS with high-grade disease (45% vs. 95–100%). Worse DSS with radiation alone, although no significant difference after multivariate analysis.

ADENOID CYSTIC CARCINOMA

, (Garden *IJROBP* 1995): retrospective of 198 patients with adenoid cystic carcinoma treated with surgery → RT (median 60 Gy). 42% + margin, 28% major nerve invasion.

5-/10-year LC 95/86%. Worse 10-year LC with +margin (95 → 81%) or named nerve invasion (88 → 80%). Dose >56 Gy more effective with +margin.

- (Mendenhall *Head Neck* 2004): retrospective of 101 patients with adenoid cystic carcinoma. 10-year LC 43% with RT alone, 91% with surgery → RT. If cN0 (96%), 10-year neck control 90% with observation, 98% with elective RT. Clinical PNI associated with worse LRC, DM, OS, and CSS.

III

ELECTIVE NODAL IRRADIATION (ENI)

- (Armstrong *Cancer* 1992): retrospective of 474 previously untreated patients with major salivary gland cancers. Of all patients, 14% were cN+. Of cN0 patients, 12% were pN+. By multivariate analysis, higher risk of occult pN+ with size ≥4 cm (4 → 20%) and high-grade histology (7 → 49%).
- (Chen *IJROBP* 2007b): retrospective of 251 patients with cN0 salivary gland carcinomas treated with surgery (no neck dissection) → RT. 52% received ENI (median 50 Gy). 10-year nodal failure 13%; nodal was first site of failure in 4%. Median time to nodal failure 1.4 years. ENI reduced 10-year nodal failure 26 → 0%. Trend toward more nodal failure with T3-4 disease (13 vs. 6%). No nodal failures with adenoid cystic or acinic cell histology.

NEUTRONS AND CHARGED PARTICLES

- *RTOG/MRC* (Laramore *IJROBP* 1993): randomized 32 patients with inoperable salivary gland cancer to fast neutron RT vs. conventional RT with photons and/or electrons. Trial stopped early due to improved 10-year LRC with neutrons (17 → 56%). No difference in OS. Distant metastases accounted for most failures in neutron arm.
- *COSMIC* (Jensen *IJROBP* 2015): 53 patients with incompletely resected or inoperable adenoid cystic carcinoma (89%) or other malignant salivary gland tumors received carbon ion (C12) particle therapy 24 Gy(RBE) in 8 fractions, followed by 2/50 Gy IMRT. 3-year LC 90% (positive margin only), 87% (gross residual disease), and 75% (inoperable). Major site of failure is pulmonary metastasis.

CHEMOTHERAPY

ˌ (Tanvetyanon *Arch Otolaryngol Head Neck Surg* 2009): matched pair analysis of 24 patients with high-risk major salivary gland carcinoma treated with post-op RT or post-op concurrent chemo-RT (cisplatin or carboplatin). 3-year OS improved with chemo-RT (44 → 83%). Trend toward improved PFS. No difference in DM (25–33%). Chemo-RT increased Grade ≥ 3 toxicity (17 → 67%).

ˌ (Hsieh *Radiat Oncol* 2016): propensity score matched analysis of 93 patients with adenoid cystic salivary gland malignancies treated with surgery and post-op RT or post-op concurrent chemo-RT (94% cisplatin-based). Chemo-RT improved 8-year LRC (67 → 97%), but not DMFS, DFS, or OS. Greatest LRC benefit to chemo-RT in subgroups of +margins, PNI, and stage III–IV disease. More hematological toxicity with chemo-RT, otherwise no toxicity differences.

ˌ *RTOG 1008* (ongoing): Phase II/III study of post-op high-risk salivary pts with intermediate- to high-grade adenocarcinoma or mucoepidermoid carcinoma, high-grade acinic cell carcinoma or adenoid cystic carcinoma, and salivary duct carcinoma randomized to post-op RT (60–66 Gy) with or without cisplatin 40 mg/m^2 weekly × 7.

RADIATION TECHNIQUES

SIMULATION AND FIELD DESIGN

ˌ Simulate supine with neck gently extended, shoulders down. Immobilize with thermoplastic head and shoulder mask. Wire scar.

ˌ Place bolus for skin invasion, close or positive superficial margin, residual or unresectable tumor close to surface.

ˌ CT planning fusion to MRI and/or PET-CT. Contrast-enhanced MRI particularly useful for imaging perineural invasion.

ˌ GTV includes all gross residual disease and involved nodes.

- Post-op CTV includes entire surgical bed with 1–2 cm margin.
- For large or deep parotid tumors, include parapharyngeal space and retrostyloid nodes in high-risk CTV. For adenoid cystic histology or clinical/pathological perineural invasion, cover named nerves (e.g. CN V3, VII, XII) to base of skull foramina in high-risk CTV. If facial nerve is grossly involved, cover the facial nerve canal through the petrous temporal bone.
- Elective nodal RT should be considered for high-grade or T3-4 disease. Can be omitted for adenoid cystic and acinic cell cancers, due to low propensity for nodal metastasis.
- Elective nodal RT includes ipsilateral levels Ib-V for cN+, at least ipsilateral levels Ib-III for high-risk cN0. Consider covering contralateral neck for tumors approaching midline or high nodal disease burden.
- IMRT recommended for large operative beds or extended neck coverage.
- Conventional treatment can be performed with wedged-pair photon beams or mixed photon/electron beams. Neck field is angled obliquely to keep off the spinal cord and superior half-beam block with matching to primary field.
- PTV = CTV + 3–5 mm depending on expected motion.

DOSE PRESCRIPTIONS
- Postoperative and definitive dose/fractionation same as other head and neck sites; see prior chapters (e.g., "Oropharyngeal Cancer" Chapter 7, "Oral Cavity" Chapter 8).

DOSE LIMITATIONS
- Same as other head and neck sites; see prior chapters.
- Uninvolved salivary glands mean ≤ 24 Gy. Complete loss of salivary gland function after ≥35 Gy.

COMPLICATIONS
- Similar to other head and neck sites; see prior chapters.
- Late cranial nerve dysfunction can be seen after cranial nerve involvement.

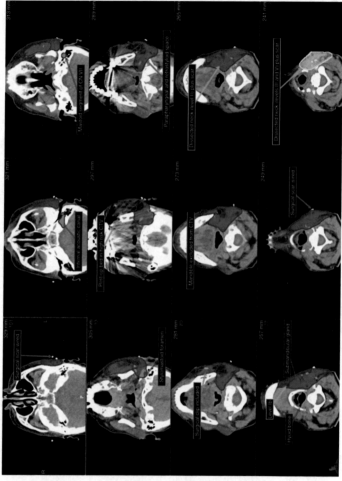

Fig. 10.1 Contours for pT3N0 high-grade salivary duct carcinoma of the left parotid gland, status-post parotidectomy and ipsilateral neck dissection.

Preoperative MRI demonstrated involvement of the tympanic portions of the left facial nerve. Superficial and deep margins were positive, and perineural invasion was present. *Red* contour is high-risk CTV covering the positive margins (66 Gy). *Blue* is intermediate-risk CTV (59.4 Gy). *Yellow* is low-risk CTV (54.12 Gy), treated in 33 fractions using IMRT

FOLLOW-UP

, Similar to other head and neck sites; see prior chapters.
, Consider posttreatment baseline MRI within 6 months and again as indicated.
, TSH every 6–12 months if neck irradiated.

III

Acknowledgment We thank Chien Peter Chen MD and Naomi R. Schechter MD for their work on the prior edition of this chapter.

REFERENCES

Al-Mamgani A, van Rooij P, Verduijn GM, et al. Long-term outcomes and quality of life of 186 patients with primary parotid carcinoma treated with surgery and radiotherapy at the Daniel den Hoed Cancer Center. Int J Radiat Oncol Biol Phys. 2012;84(1):189–95.

Armstrong JG, Harrison LB, Spiro RH, et al. Malignant tumors of major salivary gland origin. A matched-pair analysis of the role of combined surgery and postoperative radiotherapy. Arch Otolaryngol Head Neck Surg. 1990;116:290–3.

Armstrong JG, Harrison LB, Thaler HT, et al. The indications for elective treatment of the neck in cancer of the major salivary glands. Cancer. 1992;69:615–9.

Chen AM, Granchi PJ, Garcia J, et al. Local-regional recurrence after surgery without postoperative irradiation for carcinomas of the major salivary glands: implications for adjuvant therapy. Int J Radiat Oncol Biol Phys. 2007a;67:982–7.

Chen AM, Garcia J, Lee NY, Bucci MK, Eisele DW. Patters of nodal relapse after surgery and postoperative radiation therapy for carcinomas of the major and minor salivary glands: what is the role of elective neck irradiation? Int J Radiat Oncol Biol Phys. 2007b;67:988–94.

Garden AS, Weber RS, Ang KK, et al. Postoperative radiation therapy for malignant tumors of minor salivary glands. Cancer. 1994;73:2563–9.

Garden AS, Weber RS, Morrison WH, et al. The influence of positive margins and nerve invasion in adenoid cystic carcinoma of the head and neck treated with surgery and radiation. Int J Radiat Oncol Biol Phys. 1995;32:619–26.

Garden AS, El-Naggar AK, Morrison WH, et al. Postoperative radiotherapy for malignant tumors of the parotid gland. Int J Radiat Oncol Biol Phys. 1997;37:79–85.

Hsieh CE, Lin CY, Lee LY, et al. Adding concurrent chemotherapy to postoperative radiotherapy improves locoregional control but not overall survival in patients with salivary gland adenoid cystic carcinoma—a propensity score matched study. Radiat Oncol. 2016;11(47):1–10.

Jensen AD, Nikoghosyan AV, Lossner K, et al. COSMIC: a regimen of intensity modulated radiation therapy plus dose-escalated, raster-scanned carbon ion boost for malignant salivary gland tumors: results of the prospective phase 2 trial. Int J Radiat Oncol Biol Phys. 2015;93(1):37–46.

Laramore GE, Krall JM, Griffin TW, et al. Neutron versus photon irradiation for unresectable salivary gland tumors: final report of an RTOG-MRC randomized clinical trial. Radiation Therapy Oncology Group. Medical Research Council. Int J Radiat Oncol Biol Phys. 1993;27:235–40.

Loh KS, Barker E, Bruch G, et al. Prognostic factors in malignancy of the minor salivary glands. Head Neck. 2009;31:58–63.

Mendenhall WM, Morris CG, Amdur RJ, et al. Radiotherapy alone or combined with surgery for adenoid cystic carcinoma of the head and neck. Head Neck. 2004;26:154–62.

Spiro RH. Salivary neoplasms: overview of a 35-year experience with 2,807 patients. Head Neck Surg. 1986;68(3):177–84.

Tanvetyanon T, Qin D, Padhya T, et al. Outcomes of postoperative concurrent chemoradiotherapy for locally advanced major salivary gland carcinoma. Arch Otolaryngol Head Neck Surg. 2009;35(7):687–92.

Terhaard CH, Lubsen H, Rasch CR, et al. The role of radiotherapy in the treatment of malignant salivary gland tumors. Int J Radiat Oncol Biol Phys. 2005;61:103–11.

Chapter 11
Thyroid Cancer

Christopher H. Chapman and Adam Garsa

PEARLS

- Thyroid gland anatomy.
  - 10–20 g bilobed gland with isthmus.
  - Inferior to thyroid cartilage, anterior to cricoid cartilage.
  - 20–50% have third pyramidal lobe above isthmus.
  - Colloidal follicles surrounded by follicular cells and parafollicular C-cells.
  - Follicular cells take up iodide ions, including radioactive iodine (RAI).
  - Parafollicular C-cells produce calcitonin and other peptide hormones.
  - Lymphatic drainage is bilateral to central compartment (level VI): pretracheal, paratracheal, and prelaryngeal (a.k.a. Delphian node). Secondary drainage to cervical lymph nodes. Less commonly to the anterior mediastinal nodes and occasionally to the retropharyngeal nodes.
- Benign thyroid nodules are common.
  - Approximately 5% prevalence of clinically detected nodules for ages ≥50.
  - Up to 50% prevalence when examined by ultrasonography or surgery.
  - More common in women and after radiation exposure.

© Springer International Publishing AG, part of Springer Nature 2018   **243**
Eric K. Hansen and M. Roach III (eds.), *Handbook of Evidence-Based Radiation Oncology*, https://doi.org/10.1007/978-3-319-62642-0_11

- Lifetime risk of thyroid cancer is approximately 1%.
  - Female/male ratio 3:1.
  - Incidence increases starting in teenage years, peak at approximately age 50.
  - Incidence is increasing, likely due to increased detection with ultrasound, but mortality decreasing.
- Radiation exposure and iodine deficiency are the main environmental risk factors.
  - Risk with radiation exposure especially high if age < 10 years old.
  - Radiation exposure usually associated with well-differentiated thyroid cancers.
- Poor prognostic factors: older age, male sex, larger tumor size, extrathyroidal extension (ETE), histologic high grade, nodal metastasis, distant metastases, grossly incomplete resection.
- Large variation in behavior and prognosis by histologic subtype.
  - Differentiated thyroid cancers.
    - From follicular cells: produce thyroglobulin and take up iodine.
    - Papillary thyroid carcinoma (PTC).
      - 80–90% of thyroid cancers, ~95% 10-year survival.
      - Follicular variant PTC: *not* follicular carcinoma, good prognosis.
      - Poor prognosis variants: tall cell, columnar cell, diffuse sclerosing, solid, insular (poorly differentiated).
      - BRAF V600E and TERT promoter mutations may be associated with worse outcomes (Xing *JCO* 2014).
    - Follicular thyroid carcinoma (FTC).
      - 5–15% of thyroid cancers, ~85% 10-year survival.
      - Invasion distinguishes from benign adenoma: need preserved microarchitecture (core needle or surgical excision, not FNA).
    - Hürthle cell carcinoma (a.k.a. oncocytic or oxyphilic cell carcinoma).
      - 2–3% of thyroid cancers, ~75% 10-year survival.

- Classically a poor prognosis variant of FTC, PTC variants now recognized.
- Takes up iodine, but not as well as PTC/FTC.
- For all differentiated histologies, ~50% 5-year survival if metastatic. Longer survival if young, small metastases, lung only, and iodine uptake maintained.

- Medullary thyroid carcinoma (MTC)
  - From parafollicular C-cells: produce calcitonin, do not take up iodine.
  - ~2% of thyroid cancers, ~75% 5-year survival.
  - ~25% 5-year survival if metastatic: most often liver, lung, and bone.
  - ~50% cervical adenopathy at presentation.
  - Advanced disease associated with hormonal peptide syndromes and amyloidosis.
  - 20% are familial: multiple endocrine neoplasia (MEN) type 2.
    - Autosomal dominant mutations of *RET* proto-oncogene.
    - Codon 918 (exon 16) mutation associated with MEN 2B and worse outcomes.
    - MEN 2A: MTC, pheochromocytomas, parathyroid tumors.
    - MEN 2B: MTC, pheochromocytomas, Marfanoid habitus, mucosal neuromas.
    - Carriers have ~90% lifetime risk of MTC.
  - Anaplastic thyroid carcinoma (undifferentiated).
    - Develops from differentiated thyroid cancer, particularly with p53 loss.
    - Does not take up iodine or produce thyroglobulin.
    - ~1% of thyroid cancer, 1-year survival ~20%, median ~ 5 months.
    - Very locally aggressive, up to 50% of deaths due to airway obstruction.
    - 15–50% have distant metastases at presentation: lung > bone > others.

WORKUP

- The majority of thyroid malignancies present as asymptomatic nodules, either discovered by the patient or incidentally during physical exam, imaging, or surgical pathology. Most asymptomatic nodules are benign, especially if <1 cm.
- Risk of malignancy is greatly increased if symptomatic at presentation: rapidly growing mass, fixation, stridor, hoarseness, hemoptysis, dysphagia. Symptoms caused by recurrent laryngeal nerve paralysis or invasion of adjacent structures.
- Thyroid nodules may be initially evaluated with ultrasonography, serum TSH, and radioiodide imaging if TSH is suppressed. A hyperfunctioning nodule is unlikely to be malignant.
- Suspicious sonographic features include size >1 cm, solid, hypoechoic, microcalcifications, increased vascularity, infiltrative margins, taller than wide.
- FNA of suspicious thyroid nodules and cervical nodes is the most important diagnostic tool. Atypia of uncertain significance (AUS) or follicular lesion of uncertain significance (FLUS) can be evaluated with molecular testing and observation or proceed to lobectomy/thyroidectomy. FNA alone cannot diagnose follicular or Hürthle cell carcinoma.
- If FNA indicates medullary thyroid carcinoma:
  - Serum calcitonin, calcium, and CEA.
  - Pheochromocytoma screening with urine/serum metanephrines. If detected, remove before thyroid surgery to avoid hypertensive crisis.
  - Screen for germline *RET* proto-oncogene mutations and genetic counseling if positive. Therapy for family dependent on specific codon mutation.
- Obtain neck CT or MRI for symptomatic, fixed, bulky, or substernal lesions. For differentiated thyroid cancers, avoid iodinated contrast with CT as this may preclude treatment with RAI for up to 6 months. If the patient received iodinated contrast, can check urine iodine level prior to RAI administration.

‚ For high-risk medullary and anaplastic thyroid carcinoma, screen for metastatic disease with contrast-enhanced CT C/A/P or 18FDG-PET/CT.

‚ Laryngoscopy/bronchoscopy if concern for airway invasion.

III

STAGING: THYROID CANCER

Editors' note: All TNM stage and stage groups referred to elsewhere in this chapter reflect the 2010 AJCC staging nomenclature unless otherwise noted as the new system below was published after this chapter was written.

Table 11.1 (AJCC 7TH ED., 2010)

Primary tumor (T)

Note: All categories may be subdivided: (s) solitary tumor and (m) multifocal tumor (the largest determines the classification)

TX:	Primary tumor cannot be assessed
T0:	No evidence of primary tumor
T1:	Tumor 2 cm or less in greatest dimension limited to the thyroid
T1a:	Tumor 1 cm or less, limited to the thyroid
T1b:	Tumor more than 1 cm but not more than 2 cm in greatest dimension limited to the thyroid
T2:	Tumor more than 2 cm but not more than 4 cm in greatest dimension limited to the thyroid
T3:	Tumor more than 4 cm in greatest dimension limited to the thyroid or any tumor with minimal extrathyroid extension (e.g., extension to sternothyroid muscle or perithyroid soft tissues)
T4a:	Moderately advanced disease. Tumor of any size extending beyond the thyroid capsule to invade subcutaneous soft tissues, larynx, trachea, esophagus, or recurrent laryngeal nerve
T4b:	Very advanced disease. Tumor invades prevertebral fascia or encases carotid artery or mediastinal vessels

All anaplastic carcinomas are considered T4 tumors

T4a:	Intrathyroidal anaplastic carcinoma
T4b:	Anaplastic carcinoma with gross extrathyroid extension

Regional lymph nodes (N)

Regional lymph nodes are the central compartment, lateral cervical, and upper mediastinal lymph nodes

NX:	Regional lymph nodes cannot be assessed
N0:	No regional lymph node metastasis
N1:	Regional lymph node metastasis

continued

Table 11.1 (continued)

N1a:	Metastasis to Level VI (pretracheal, paratracheal, and prelaryngeal/Delphian lymph nodes)
N1b:	Metastasis to unilateral, bilateral, or contralateral cervical (Levels I, II, III, IV, and V) or retropharyngeal or superior mediastinal lymph nodes (Level VII)

Distant metastasis (M)

M0:	No distant metastasis
M1:	Distant metastasis

Anatomic stage/prognostic groups

Separate stage groupings are recommended for papillary or follicular (differentiated), medullary, and anaplastic (undifferentiated) carcinoma

Papillary or follicular (differentiated)

Under 45 years

I:	Any T Any N M0
II:	Any T Any N M1
	45 years and older
I:	T1 N0 M0
II:	T2 N0 M0
III:	T3 N0 M0
	T1-T3 N1a M0
IVA:	T4a N0 M0
	T4a N1a M0
	T1-T3 N1b M0
	T4a N1b M0
IVB:	T4b Any N M0
IVC:	Any T Any N M1

Medullary carcinoma (all age groups)

I:	T1 N0 M0
II:	T2–T3 N0 M0
III:	T1–T3 N1a M0
IVA:	T4a N0 M0
	T4a N1a M0
	T1–T3 N1b M0
	T4a N1b M0
IVB:	T4b Any N M0
IVC:	Any T Any N M1

Anaplastic carcinoma

All anaplastic carcinomas are considered Stage IV

IVA:	T4a Any N M0
IVB:	T4b Any N M0
IVC:	Any T Any N M1

Table 11.2 (AJCC 8TH ED., 2017)

Definitions of AJCC TNM

Definition of Primary Tumor (T)

Papillary, Follicular, Poorly Differentiated, Hurthle Cell and Anaplastic Thyroid Carcinoma

T category	T criteria
TX	Primary tumor cannot be assessed
T0	No evidence of primary tumor
T1	Tumor ≤2 cm in the greatest dimension limited to the thyroid
T1a	Tumor ≤1 cm in the greatest dimension limited to the thyroid
T1b	Tumor >1 cm but ≤2 cm in the greatest dimension limited to the thyroid
T2	Tumor >2 cm but ≤4 cm in the greatest dimension limited to the thyroid
T3	Tumor >4 cm limited to the thyroid or gross extrathyroidal extension invading only strap muscles
T3a	Tumor >4 cm limited to the thyroid
T3b	Gross extrathyroidal extension invading only strap muscles (sternohyoid, sternothyroid, thyrohyoid, or omohyoid muscles) from a tumor of any size
T4	Includes gross extrathyroidal extension
T4a	Gross extrathyroidal extension invading subcutaneous soft tissues, larynx, trachea, and esophagus or recurrent laryngeal nerve from a tumor of any size
T4b	Gross extrathyroidal extension invading prevertebral fascia or encasing the carotid artery or mediastinal vessels from a tumor of any size

Note: All categories may be subdivided: (s) solitary tumor and (m) multifocal tumor (the largest tumor determines the classification)

DEFINITION OF REGIONAL LYMPH NODE (N)

N category	N criteria
NX	Regional lymph nodes cannot be assessed
N0	No evidence of locoregional lymph node metastasis
N0a	One or more cytologically or histologically confirmed benign lymph nodes
N0b	No radiology or clinical evidence of locoregional lymph node metastasis
N1	Metastasis to regional nodes
N1a	Metastasis to level VI or level VII (pretracheal, paratracheal, or prelaryngeal/Delphian or upper mediastinal) lymph nodes. This can be unilateral or bilateral disease
N1b	Metastasis to unilateral, bilateral, or contralateral lateral neck lymph nodes (level I, II, III, IV, or V) or retropharyngeal lymph nodes

DEFINITION OF DISTANT METASTASIS (M)

M category	M criteria
M0	No distant metastasis
M1	Distant metastasis

AJCC PROGNOSTICS STAGE GROUPS
DIFFERENTIATED

When age at diagnosis is...	And T is...	And N is...	And M is...	Then the stage group is...
<55 years	Any T	Any N	M0	I
<55 years	Any T	Any N	M1	II
≥55 years	T1	N0/NX	M0	I
≥55 years	T1	N1	M0	II
≥55 years	T2	N0/NX	M0	I
≥55 years	T2	N1	M0	II
≥55 years	T3a/T3b	Any N	M0	II
≥55 years	T4a	Any N	M0	III
≥55 years	T4b	Any N	M0	IVA
≥55 years	Any T	Any N	M1	IVB

ANAPLASTIC

When T is...	And N is...	And M is...	Then the stage group is...
T1–T3a	N0/NX	M0	IVA
T1–T3a	N1	M0	IVB
T3b	Any N	M0	IVB
T4	Any N	M0	IVB
Any T	Any N	M1	IVC

Used with permission of the American Joint Committee on Cancer (AJCC), Chicago, Illinois. The original and primary source for this information is the AJCC Cancer Staging Manual, Eighth Edition (2017) published by Springer International Publishing

TREATMENT RECOMMENDATIONS

Table 11.3 TREATMENT RECOMMENDATIONS

Differentiated thyroid carcinoma	Treatment recommendations
High risk: history of radiation exposure, family history of thyroid cancer, high-grade histology, tumor > 4 cm, multifocal tumor, vascular invasion, ETE, +LN, or +DM	Total thyroidectomy with central neck dissection if cN+ Consider prophylactive central neck dissection if cN0 Lateral neck dissection for FNA-proven metastasis only Post-operative RAI Levothyroxine to TSH < 0.1 mU/L Consider EBRT for patients >45 years old with gross extrathyroid extension with high risk of having microscopic residual disease. Also consider for patients with gross ECE or non-iodine-avid disease
Low risk: None of the above	Preferred: total thyroidectomy ± RAI Alternative: lobectomy + isthmusectomy. Thyroglobin surveillance not possible. Completion thyroidectomy for positive margins, high-risk features on final pathology, or indication for RAI Levothyroxine to TSH 0.1—0.5 mU/L
Papillary microcarcinoma: PTC ≤ 1 cm without high-risk features	Lobectomy or observation alone (controversial). Completion surgery for high-risk features
Locoregional recurrence or residual disease	Cervical LN: neck dissection → RAI Superior mediastinum: dissection → RAI, or RAI alone Unresectable or no RAI uptake: EBRT Consider EBRT for persistent/recurrent disease following surgery and RAI, particularly if further surgery would be morbid
Metastatic	Total thyroidectomy if not done to allow for RAI treatment RAI treatment every 12–24 months until no longer amenable Continue TSH suppression with levothyroxine Local control/palliation: surgery, EBRT, ablative therapies Systemic: tyrosine kinase inhibitors, chemotherapy, bisphosphonates or denosumab
Medullary thyroid carcinoma	**Treatment recommendations**
Locoregional	Total thyroidectomy with central neck dissection ± ipsilateral or bilateral levels II–V if cN+. Consider prophylactic neck dissection for high-volume disease Consider adjuvant EBRT for incomplete resection, LN+, extensive ETE, or persistent calcitonin Levothyroxine to normalize TSH only. No role for RAI
Metastatic	Local control/palliation: surgery, EBRT, ablative therapies Systemic: vandetanib, cabozantinib, other kinase inhibitors, chemotherapy, octreotide for hormonal peptide syndromes

continued

Table 11.3 (continued)

Anaplastic thyroid carcinoma	Treatment recommendations
Locoregional	Gross total resection if possible (rare)
	If not possible, avoid morbid radical surgery but need airway management, consider tracheostomy
	Post-op chemo-RT for local control and palliation. Consider accelerated fractionation schedules
	Levothyroxine to normalize TSH only. No role for RAI
	Clinical trials and early palliative care involvement recommended for all patients
Metastatic	Local control/palliation: surgery, EBRT, ablative therapies
	Systemic: chemotherapy, targeted agents on clinical trial

STUDIES

SURGERY AND RAI FOR DIFFERENTIATED THYROID CANCER (DTC)

- Although most DTC cases can be resected completely, there is an increased risk of microscopic residual disease when the tumor is shaved off the recurrent laryngeal nerve, trachea, or larynx or if a limited resection of the esophageal muscularis or jugular vein sacrifice is required.
- The American Thyroid Association guidelines (Haugen, Thyroid 2016) describe the use of adjuvant RAI for DTC. The details of treatment with RAI are beyond the scope of this book; readers are referred to nuclear medicine literature.
- After surgery, RAI (I-131) is considered for DTC with T2–4, N1, or M1, high-risk features, post-operative unstimulated thyroglobulin >5–10 ng/mL, unresectable, and recurrent disease.
- Pretreatment thyroxine withdrawal and/or recombinant TSH with low iodine diet to maximize iodine uptake.
- Depending on volume of iodine-avid disease, dose ranges from 30 to 200 mCi.
- Rescan 7–10 days after treatment to identify additional foci of uptake undetected on the diagnostic scan and to document sites of disease treated.

˒ Repeat diagnostic RAI scan ~4–6 months later. Can retreat approximately every 6 months. Continue until RAI imaging negative. Once negative, repeat in 1–2 years. If negative then, follow clinically and with thyroglobulin.

˒ Avoid use of iodinated contrast in a patient who will need RAI within 3–6 months.

˒ RAI success is lower for pts with poorly differentiated, tall cell, columnar, insular, and Hürthle cell carcinomas, older age, recurrent disease (especially after prior RAI) and pts with low RAI uptake on whole body scan with known residual disease.

EBRT FOR DTC

˒ No prospective randomized trials of EBRT for thyroid cancer have successfully enrolled adequate patient numbers. Most data are from retrospective reviews.

˒ The Endocrine Surgery Committee of the American Head and Neck Society has published recommendations regarding EBRT for DTC (Kiess, Head Neck 2016).

˒ EBRT is recommended for pts with gross residual or unresectable locoregional disease, except for pts <45 years old with limited gross disease that is RAI-avid.

˒ Multiple retrospective studies report good long-term locoregional control with EBRT for pts with gross residual or unresectable DTC:

  ˒ *Hong Kong* (Chow *Endocrine-Related Cancer* 2006): retrospective of 1297 patients with PTC treated with surgery ± RAI ± EBRT (2/60 Gy). Mean follow-up 9.9 years. Among 217 pts with gross residual disease, EBRT improved 10-year LC (24 → 64%) and CSS (50 → 74%). If pT4, EBRT and RAI together improved 10-year LC (41 → 88%).

  ˒ MSKCC (Romesser, J Surg Oncol 2014). 66 pts with gross residual/unresectable non-anaplastic thyroid cancer treated with EBRT +/− concurrent chemotherapy. 3-yr LRC overall 77%; adding chemo improved LRC for poorly differentiated (89% vs. 66%).

˒ After complete resection, EBRT may be considered in select pts >45 years old with high likelihood of microscopic residual disease and low likelihood of responding to RAI:

- *Princess Margaret* (Brierley *Clin Endocrinol* 2005): retrospective of 729 patients treated with surgery and/or RAI and/or EBRT. Median follow-up 11 years. EBRT significantly improved LRC (66% → 86%) and CSS (65% → 81%) among patients age > 60 with extrathyroid extension and no gross residual disease (n = 70).
- *Keum* (2006). 68 pts with DTC shaved off trachea. EBRT improved 10 yr local PFS (89% vs. 38%).
- Cervical lymph node involvement alone should not be an indication for adjuvant EBRT. RAI is usually effective at clearing microscopic residual nodal disease, and nodal recurrences are more easily salvaged with neck dissection.
- There is no consensus on timing of adjuvant RAI and EBRT, but EBRT may be preferred first for bulky gross disease and/or low likelihood of responding to RAI.

MEDULLARY THYROID CANCER (MTC)

- The role of EBRT for MTC is less clear than for DTC. It may benefit microscopic residual, extrathyroid extension, and/or node-positive pts.
- *SEER analysis* (Martinez *J Surg Oncol* 2010): 534 pts had surgery, 12% received post-op EBRT. 10-year OS 87% with EBRT vs. 70% without (not significant). EBRT had survival benefit in node-positive patients on univariate, but not multivariate analysis. Increased age and tumor size predicted mortality.
- *Princess Margaret* (Brierley *Thyroid* 1996): retrospective of 73 patients with thyroidectomy ± EBRT (median 40 Gy). Among 40 high-risk pts (microscopic residual, +LN, or extrathyroid extension), EBRT improved 10-year LRC (86% vs. 52%)

ANAPLASTIC THYROID CARCINOMA

- *NCDB* (Haymart, Cancer 2013). 2742 pts with anaplastic thyroid cancer. Omission of treatment increased mortality: thyroidectomy or chemotherapy increased MS from 2 to 6 months, radiotherapy increased MS from 2 to 5. MS with surgery, RT, and chemotherapy was 11 mo for intrathyroidal resectable (stage IVA), 9 mo for extrathyroidal unresectable (stage IVB), and 5 mo if distant mets (stage IVC).
- *SEER analysis* (Kebebew *Cancer* 2005): 516 patients treated with surgery and/or EBRT. 6-/12-month CSS 32/19%. On multivariate analysis, age < 60 years, no ETE, and combined surgery + EBRT predicted improved CSS.

RADIATION TECHNIQUES

SIMULATION AND FIELD DESIGN

- Simulate patient supine with neck gently extended, shoulders down. Immobilize with thermoplastic head and shoulders mask.
- Preoperative imaging may be useful for planning EBRT. Simulation CT with fusion to MRI and/or diagnostic CT.
- Target volumes:
  - Customized for each patient according to risk of local and regional recurrence.
  - Advanced differentiated or medullary thyroid cancer: thyroid bed from hyoid bone to aortic arch, tracheoesophageal groove, bilateral nodal levels II to VI, and upper mediastinal nodes to the aortic arch. Consider extending mediastinal coverage inferiorly to the carina if +LN in low neck or upper mediastinum. May include retropharyngeal nodes and/or level I if adjacent level II nodes involved.

       ˶   If primary indication for RT is ETE or +margins, may consider treating thyroid bed alone. This extends from the bottom of the hyoid to just below the suprasternal notch.

       ˶   Anaplastic thyroid cancer: gross disease and post-surgical bed, trachea-esophageal groove, bilateral nodal levels II to VI, upper mediastinum, tracheostomy site if present. May include level I and/or retropharyngeal nodes if at risk.

   ˶   IMRT is often recommended to achieve dose levels below and to improve sparing of larynx, spinal cord, salivary glands, esophagus, pharyngeal constrictors, and lungs, brachial plexus.

   ˶   Image guidance (e.g., conebeam CT) is recommended when available to improve setup accuracy.

DOSE PRESCRIPTIONS

   ˶   CTV 66–70 Gy: Unresectable, gross residual, or +margin(s).

   ˶   CTV 59.4–66 Gy: High-risk areas, such as thyroid bed, tracheoesophageal groove, level VI, or involved nodal levels.

   ˶   CTV 54 Gy: Lower risk elective coverage, such as uninvolved levels II–V and VII, tracheostomy site if present.

   ˶   Fraction size: ≤2 Gy for DTC.

   ˶   Anaplastic: In pts with good PS without metastasis, either standard fractionation (1.8–2 Gy/fx, 5 days/wk) or accelerated hyperfractionated (1.5–1.6 Gy BID, 5 days/wk) schedules may be used.

   ˶   For palliation, shorter courses may be considered (e.g., 3 Gy × 10 fractions over 2 weeks or 20 Gy in 5 fractions with option of 2nd course 2–4 weeks later).

DOSE LIMITATIONS

   ˶   From EBRT: Parotid gland mean ≤ 26 Gy, V30 Gy ≤ 50% (consider RAI also affects salivary function). Otherwise similar to other head and neck sites (see Chapter 7 Oropharyngeal Cancer).

ˌ From RAI: Recommended ≤2 Gy to blood and bone marrow; however dosimetry requires serial serum measurements.

COMPLICATIONS
ˌ From EBRT
  ˌ Acute: dermatitis, esophagitis, mucositis, dysphagia, changes in taste, xerostomia, laryngitis.
  ˌ Late: neck fibrosis and lymphedema, xerostomia, dental caries, esophageal stenosis, chronic feeding tube dependence (~5% with IMRT).
ˌ From RAI:
  ˌ Acute: sialadenitis, xerostomia, cystitis, gastritis, diarrhea, pain, transient leucopenia/thrombocytopenia, transient oligospermia. Rarely, thyrotoxicosis due to tumor lysis. Radiation pneumonitis if extensive pulmonary metastases are present.
  ˌ Late: increased risk of leukemia with cumulative doses >800 mCi, increased risk of breast and bladder cancer with doses >1000 mCi. Pulmonary fibrosis if extensive pulmonary metastases. No increased incidence of chronic infertility or birth defects, although most advise that patients wait 6 months before attempting pregnancy.

FOLLOW-UP

ˌ H&P every 6–12 months.
ˌ Differentiated thyroid cancer: TSH, thyroglobulin, and antithyroglobulin antibodies at 6 and 12 months and then annually if negative. Periodic neck ultrasound, can be deferred if low risk. If thyroglobulin is rising, consider RAI imaging and/or ultrasound. If RAI imaging negative, consider neck/chest CT and/or PET-CT.

> Medullary thyroid cancer: calcitonin and CEA at 2–3 months and annually. If elevated, neck imaging with ultrasound. If calcitonin ≥150 pg/mL, include cross-section imaging of neck, chest, and abdomen.
> Anaplastic thyroid cancer: No established guidelines, consider PET-CT 3–6 months after initial therapy if clinically NED.

Acknowledgment We thank Jennifer S. Yu MD, PhD, Joy Coleman MD, and Jeanne Marie Quivey MD, FACR, for their work on the prior edition of this chapter.

REFERENCES

Brierley J, Tsang R, Simpson WJ, et al. Medullary thyroid cancer: analyses of survival and prognostic factors and the role of radiation therapy in local control. Thyroid. 1996;6(4):305–10.

Brierley J, Tsang R, Panzarella T, et al. Prognostic factors and the effect of treatment with radioactive iodine and external beam radiation on patients with differentiated thyroid cancer seen at a single institution over 40 years. Clin Endocrinol. 2005;63(4):418–27.

Chow SM, Yau S, Kwan CK, et al. Local and regional control in patients with papillary thyroid carcinoma: specific indications of external radiotherapy and radioactive iodine according to T and N categories in AJCC 6th edition. Endocr Relat Cancer. 2006;13(4):1159–72.

Haugen BR, Alexander EK, Bible KC, et al. 2015 American Thyroid Association management guidelines for adult patients with thyroid nodules and differentiated thyroid cancer: the American Thyroid Association guidelines task force on thyroid nodules and differentiated thyroid cancer. Thyroid. 2016;26(1):1–133.

Haymart MR, Banerjee M, Yin H, et al. Marginal treatment benefit in anaplastic thyroid cancer. Cancer. 2013;119:3133–9.

Kebebew E, Greenspan FS, Clark OH, et al. Anaplastic thyroid carcinoma. Treatment outcome and prognostic factors. Cancer. 2005;103(7):1330–5.

Keum KC, Suh YG, Koom WS, et al. The role of postoperative external-beam radiotherapy in the management of patients with papillary thyroid cancer invading the trachea. Int J Radiat Oncol Biol Phys. 2006;65(2):474–80.

Kiess AP, Agrawal N, Brierley JD, et al. External-beam radiotherapy for differentiated thyroid cancer locoregional control: a statement of the American Head and Neck Society. Head Neck. 2016;38(4):493–8.

Martinez SR, Beal SH, Chen A, et al. Adjuvant external beam radiation for medullary thyroid carcinoma. J Surg Oncol. 2010;102(2):175–8.

Romesser PB, Sherman EJ, Shaha AR, et al. External beam radiotherapy with or without concurrent chemotherapy in advanced or recurrent non-anaplastic non-medullary thyroid cancer. J Surg Oncol. 2014;110(4):375–82.

Xing M, Liu R, Liu X, et al. BRAF V600E and TERT promoter mutations cooperatively identify the most aggressive papillary thyroid cancer with highest recurrence. J Clin Oncol. 2014;32(25):2718–25.

Chapter 12
Unusual Neoplasms of the Head and Neck

Jason Chan and Adam Garsa

PEARLS

- **Chloromas** (also called *granulocytic sarcomas* or *myeloid sarcomas*) are solid extramedullary tumors consisting of early myeloid precursors associated with AML. The name derives from the green color of affected tissues. They are more frequent with AML M4 and M5 subtypes, and are associated with t(8;21). They may herald AML relapse after remission. They present in the CNS with increased intracerebral pressure, or in the orbit with exophthalmos.
- **Chordomas** originate from the primitive notochord. 50% occur in the sacrococcygeal area, 35% in the base of skull, and 15% in cervical vertebrae. The most common age is in the range of 50–60. They are more common in men (2–3:1). They are locally invasive with slow growth. Metastases occur in up to 25% of patients, but lymph node spread is uncommon. Gross total resection is accomplished in only 10–20% of patients. Protons offer improved local control.
- **Chondrosarcomas** are malignant primary bone tumors that arise in cartilaginous elements. They frequently arise in the base of skull, commonly in the sphenoid bone. They can be either high or low grade, with the majority being low grade.
- **Esthesioneuroblastomas** arise in the olfactory receptors of the nasal mucosa or cribriform plate. They present most commonly at ages 11–20 or 40–60 years, and the most

© Springer International Publishing AG, part of Springer Nature 2018   **259**
Eric K. Hansen and M. Roach III (eds.), *Handbook of Evidence-Based Radiation Oncology*, https://doi.org/10.1007/978-3-319-62642-0_12

common symptoms are epistaxis and nasal blockage. LN spread is ≤10% for early-stage disease, but is as high as 50% for Kadish stage C disease.

- **Glomus tumors** are also called *paragangliomas, chemo-dectomas* (when nonchromaffin producing), or *carotid body tumors* (when chromaffin producing). They arise from the carotid body, jugular bulb, or middle ear from the tympanic nerve (of Jacobson) or auricular nerve (of Arnold). They rarely spread to nodes or metastasize (<5%). The mean age is in the 40s. They are more common in women (3:1). They present with ear pain, pulsations, tinnitus, cranial nerve palsies, or a painless mass. Biopsies may cause severe bleeding. They are associated with neurofibromatosis, MEN syndromes, and thyroid CA.

- **Hemangioblastomas** are benign vascular tumors. The most common age is in the 20–30s. Most are found in the cerebellum. It is the most common cerebellar tumor in adults. It is associated with von-Hippel Lindau disease (cerebellar and retinal hemangioblastomas, pancreatic and renal cysts, renal cell carcinoma).

- **Hemangiopericytomas** are sarcomatous lesions arising from the smooth muscle around vessels. They most commonly present in the base of the skull. They grow slowly and are locally invasive and hypervascular. They may be confused for meningioma. In the nose, they present with epistaxis. In the orbit, they present as painless proptosis. Meningeal hemangiopericytomas have >80% LR. Late metastases occur in 50–80% of patients.

- **Juvenile nasopharyngeal angiofibromas** arise most frequently in pubertal boys, but age ranges from 9 to 30 years. They present with nasal obstruction or epistaxis. They have a pronounced tendency for hemorrhage, so biopsy is contraindicated. They often contain androgen receptors and may regress with estrogen therapy. Less than 4% of patients are female.

- **Nasal NK/T cell lymphoma** (called also *lethal midline granuloma* or midline polymorphic reticulosis) presents with progressive ulceration and necrosis of midline facial tissues, and is associated with EBV. The differential diagnosis includes Wegener's granulomatosis, polymorphic reticulosis, cocaine abuse, sarcoidosis, and infection. The cause is idiopathic. It is more common in men, and presents most commonly in the nasal cavity and paranasal sinuses. The most common age is in the 50s. Must rule out Wegener's because it responds to steroids.

, *NUT midline carcinoma (NMC)* is a lethal tumor defined by translocation involving the *NUT* gene on chromosome 15q14, resulting in the BRD4-NUT fusion oncogene. NMC does not have a clear age predilection and does not arise from a specific tissue type or organ. It presents as a poorly differentiated carcinoma from midline locations such as the head and neck or mediastinum. These tumors are refractory to conventional treatments, and the median survival is only about 7 months (Bauer et al. 2012).

WORKUP

, H&P, CT, MRI, angiogram (optional), CBC, chemistries, audiogram (to establish baseline hearing), visual testing (optional), neurosurgical consultation with biopsy only as indicated (radiographic appearance may be pathognomonic).

, For hemangioblastoma, MRI brain ± CT angiography ± MRI spine (if VHL+).

, For hemangiopericytoma, consider CT chest abdomen pelvis to rule out metastases.

, For NK/T cell lymphoma, CT of abdomen and pelvis and/ or whole body PET/CT, and bone marrow biopsy.

STAGING

, AML has three stages: untreated, in remission, or recurrent.

, Chordomas and chondrosarcomas are staged like sarcomas.

, *Esthesioneuroblastoma* is staged according to the *Kadish System* (A = confined to nasal cavity; B = extends to ≥1 of the paranasal sinuses; C = extends beyond nasal cavity or paranasal sinuses; D = distant metastasis).

, *Glomus tumors* are staged according to the Glassock-Jackson classification or the McCabe-Fletcher classification based on anatomic location, extension, and tumor volume.

, *Hemangiopericytomas* are staged as localized or metastatic.

، ***Nasopharyngeal angiofibromas*** are staged according to one of two systems: *Chandler* (I = confined to nasopharynx; II = extends to nasal cavity or sphenoid sinus; III = extends to antrum, ethmoid, pterygomaxillary and infratemporal fossa, orbit, and/or cheek; IV = intracranial extension) or *Sessions* (Ia = limited to nasopharynx and posterior nares; Ib = extends to paranasal sinuses; IIa/b/c = extends to other extracranial locations; III = intracranial extension).

، ***NK/T cell lymphomas*** are currently staged in the Ann Arbor lymphoma staging system.

TREATMENT RECOMMENDATIONS

Table 12.1 TREATMENT RECOMMENDATIONS

Stage	Recommended treatment	Results
Chloroma	Often respond to systemic therapy for AML Definitive RT (24–30 Gy)	>80–90% LC
Chordoma and chondrosarcoma	Maximal safe resection. If gross total resection, post-op RT (50–60 Gy). If subtotal resection, post-op RT (66 Gy) For small tumors, may use SRS Protons may be preferred due to sharp dose gradient and ability to dose escalate (up to 70.2 CGE to microscopic disease; 77.4 CGE to gross disease)	LC dependent on extent of resection and RT dose Chordoma: LC ~ 70% Chondrosarcoma: LC 50–100%
Esthesioneuroblastoma	Surgery or RT alone (65–70 Gy) for small, low-grade tumors confined to ethmoids Usually, combine surgery, with pre-op RT (50 Gy) or post-op RT (60 Gy), and chemo	LC: Stage A 70%, Stage B 50–65%, Stage C 30–50%
Glomus tumor	Pre-op embolization → maximal safe resection → post-op RT (50 Gy) Alternative SRS 12–14 Gy or EBRT (IMRT) 45–54 Gy	LC > 90%
Hemangioblastoma	Maximal safe resection. If GTR, observe. If STR/unresectable, SRS or EBRT (50–60 Gy) with 1–2 cm margin	LC 60–90%

Table 12.1 (continued)

Hemangiopericytoma	Pre-op embolization → maximal safe resection + post-op RT (60–65 Gy) with wide margins up to 5 cm. SRS may be used (12–20 Gy). Need long-term follow-up due to DM	LC ~70–90%
Nasopharyngeal angiofibroma	If extracranial and resectable, surgery ± embolization. Residual disease may be observed, or treated with RT if symptoms develop. If intracranial, orbital, or pterygopalatine extension, treat with RT (30–50 Gy in 2–3 Gy fractions)	RT LC ~80%, but tumors regress slowly (up to 2 years)
NK/T cell lymphoma	Definitive RT (54 Gy) usually with chemotherapy	OS 50–60%
NUT midline carcinoma	No clearly superior treatment paradigm. Generally multimodality treatment with surgical resection, chemotherapy, and RT	OS ~ 20% at 2 years

RADIATION TECHNIQUES

, Depend on histology and location. Refer to primary literature for details.

COMPLICATIONS

, Depend on the location, and they are in common with other head and neck sites described in this Handbook.

FOLLOW-UP

, Regular H&P, and follow-up imaging. Long-term follow-up may be needed due to late recurrences.

Acknowledgment We thank Sunanda Pejavar MD, Eric K. Hansen MD, and Sue Yom MD PhD MAS for their work on the prior edition of this chapter. And we thank Dr. M. Kara Bucci for her contribution to this chapter in the first edition.

REFERENCES

Bauer DE, et al. Clinicopathologic features and long-term outcomes of NUT midline carcinoma. Clin Cancer Res. 2012;18(20):5773–9.

Carew JF, Singh B, Kraus DH. Hemangiopericytoma of the head and neck. Laryngoscope. 1999;109:1409–11.

Chao KS, Kaplan C, Simpson JR, et al. Esthesioneuroblastoma: the impact of treatment modality. Head Neck. 2001;23:749–57.

Chen HH, Fong L, Su IJ, et al. Experience of radiotherapy in lethal midline granuloma with special emphasis on centrofacial T-cell lymphoma: a retrospective analysis covering a 34-year period. Radiother Oncol. 1996;38:1–6.

Hinerman RW, Mendenhall WM, Amdur RJ. Definitive radiotherapy in the management of chemodectomas arising in the temporal bone, carotid body, and glomus vagale. Head Neck. 2001;23:363–71.

Ivan ME, Sughrue ME, Clark AJ, et al. A meta-analysis of tumor control rates and treatment related morbidity for patients with glomus jugulare tumors. J Neurosurg. 2011;114:1299–305.

Khairi S, Ewend MG. Chordoma. Curr Treat Options Neurol. 2002;4:167–73.

Lee JT, Chen P, Safa A, et al. The role of radiation in the treatment of advanced juvenile angiofibroma. Laryngoscope. 2002;112:1213–20.

Pellitteri PK, Rinaldo A, Myssiorek D, et al. Paragangliomas of the head and neck. Oral Oncol. 2004;40:563–75.

Perez CA, Thorstad WL. Unusual Nonepithelial tumors of the head and neck. In: Halperin EC, Perez CA, Brady LW, editors. Principles and practice of radiation oncology. 6th ed. Philadelphia: Lippincott Williams & Wilkins; 2013. p. 868–902.

Sasaki R, Yasuda K, Abe E, et al. Multi-institutional analysis of solitary extramedullary plasmacytoma of the head and neck treated with curative radiotherapy. Int J Radiat Oncol Biol Phys. 2012;82(2):626–34.

Sohrabi S, Drabick JJ, Crist H, et al. Neoadjuvant concurrent chemoradiation for advanced esthesioneuroblastoma: a case series and review of the literature. J Clin Oncol. 2011;29(13):e358–61.

Tsao MN, Wara WM, Larson DA. Radiation therapy for benign central nervous system disease. Semin Radiat Oncol. 1999;9:120–33.

Chapter 13
Management of the Neck and Unknown Primary of the Head and Neck

III

Jason Chan and Sue S. Yom

CONSENSUS LEVELS OF THE NECK (FIG. 13.1)

- Ia: Submental
  - Bounded anteriorly by mandible, posteriorly by body of hyoid bone, superiorly by inferior edge of mandible, inferiorly by midhyoid bone, and laterally by medial edge of anterior belly of digastric
  - Drains skin of chin, mid lower lip, tip of tongue, and anterior floor of mouth
- Ib: Submandibular
  - Bounded anteriorly by mandible, posteriorly by posterior edge of the submandibular gland, superiorly by superior edge of submandibular gland, inferiorly by midhyoid bone, laterally by inner side of mandible, and medially by lateral edge of anterior belly of digastric muscle
  - Drains lower nasal cavity, hard and soft palate, maxillary and mandibular alveolar ridges, cheek, upper and lower lips, and most of anterior tongue

© Springer International Publishing AG, part of Springer Nature 2018   **265**
Eric K. Hansen and M. Roach III (eds.), *Handbook of Evidence-Based Radiation Oncology*, https://doi.org/10.1007/978-3-319-62642-0_13

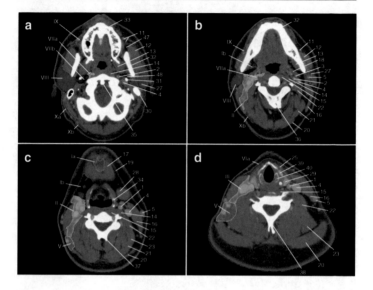

Fig. 13.1 Neck node levels using the radiological boundaries detailed above. Each node level corresponds to node groups and thus does not include any security margin for organ motion or setup inaccuracy. CT sections were taken at the level of the top edge of C1 (panel **a**), the bottom edge of C2 (panel **b**), mid C4 (panel **c**), the bottom edge of C6 (panel **d**), mid Th1 (panel **e**), and top edge of Th2 (panel **f**). (*1*) Common carotid artery; (*2*) internal carotid artery; (*3*) external carotid artery; (*4*) internal jugular vein; (*5*) external jugular vein; (*6*) anterior jugular vein; (*7*) right brachiocephalic trunk; (*8*) right brachiocephalic vein; (*9*) left subclavian artery; (*10*) left subclavian vein; (*11*) facial vessels; (*12*) masseter m.; (*13*) pterygoid m.; (*14*) longus capitis m.; (*15*) longus colli m.; (*16*) sternocleidomastoid m.; (*17*) digastric (ant. Belly) m.; (*18*) digastric (post. Belly) m.; (*19*) platysma m. (*20*) trapezius m.; (*21*) splenius capitis m.; (*22*) scalenus m.; (*23*) levator scapulae m.; (*24*) serratus anterior m.; (*25*) thyrohyoid m.; (*26*) sternohyoid m.; (*27*) parotid gland; (*28*) sub-mandibular gland; (*29*) thyroid gland; (*30*) mastoid; (*31*) styloid process; (*32*) mandible; (*33*) maxilla; (*34*) hyoid bone; (*35*) odontoid process; (*36*) 2nd cervical vertebra; (*37*) 4th cervical vertebra; (*38*) 6th cervical vertebra; (*39*) thyroid cartilage; (*40*) cricoid cartilage; (*41*) clavicle; (*42*) 1st thoracic vertebra; (*43*) 2nd thoracic vertebra; (*44*) rib; (*45*) lung apex; (*46*) esophagus; (*47*) Bichat's fat pad; (*48*) prestyloid parapharyngeal space (Reprinted from Grégoire et al. (2014), with permission from Elsevier)

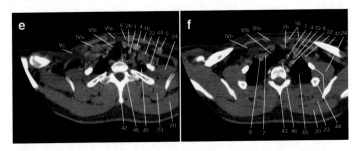

Fig. 13.1 (continued)

- II: Upper jugular
  - Bounded superiorly by the inferior edge of lateral process of C1, inferiorly by inferior edge of hyoid, laterally by medial edge of sternocleidomastoid muscle (SCM), and medially by medial edge of carotid and paraspinal muscles
  - IIa/IIb: subdivide level II by drawing an artificial line at the posterior edge of the internal jugular vein
  - Drains face, parotid, submandibular, submental, and retropharyngeal nodes, nasal cavity, pharynx, larynx, external auditory canal, middle ear, and sublingual and submandibular glands
- III: Midjugular
  - Bounded superiorly by inferior edge of hyoid, inferiorly by inferior edge of cricoid, anteriorly by anterior edge of SCM, posteriorly by posterior edge of SCM, laterally by medial edge of SCM, and medially by medial edge of carotid and paraspinal muscles
  - Drains level II and IV, retropharyngeal, pretracheal, and recurrent laryngeal nodes, base of tongue, tonsils, larynx, hypopharynx, and thyroid gland
- IVa: Lower jugular
  - Bounded superiorly by inferior edge of cricoid, inferiorly at a plane 2 cm above the sternoclavicular joint, anteriorly by anteromedial edge of SCM, posteriorly by posterior edge of SCM, laterally by medial edge of SCM, and medially by medial edge of carotid and paraspinal muscles

- Drains levels III and V, retropharyngeal, pretracheal, and recurrent laryngeal nodes, hypopharynx, larynx, thyroid gland, cervical esophagus, and rarely anterior oral cavity
- IVb: Medial supraclavicular nodes
  - Bounded superiorly by the plane 2 cm above the sterno-clavicular joint (inferior level IVa); inferiorly by the superior edge of the sternal manubrium; anteriorly by the SCM and clavicle; posteriorly by the anterior edge of the posterior scalene muscle and apex of the lung, the brachiocephalic vein and artery (right side), and common carotid artery and subclavian artery (left side); medially by level VI and medial edge of common carotid artery; and laterally by the lateral edge of the scalene muscle
  - Drains IVa, Vc, pretracheal, and recurrent laryngeal nodes, hypopharynx, esophagus, larynx, trachea, and thyroid gland
- V: Posterior triangle
  - Bounded superiorly by superior edge of hyoid, inferiorly by plane crossing cervical transverse vessels, anteriorly by posterior edge of SCM, posteriorly by anterior border of trapezius, laterally by platysma muscle and skin, and medially by levator scapulae (superiorly) and posterior scalene muscles (inferiorly)
  - Drains occipital and retroauricular nodes, occipital and parietal scalp, lateral and posterior neck and shoulder skin, nasopharynx, oropharynx, and thyroid gland
- Vc: Lateral supraclavicular
  - Bounded superiorly by plane just below transverse cervical vessels (inferior level V), inferiorly to 2 cm above sternal manubrium (similar to inferior IVa border), laterally by trapezius muscle (superiorly) and clavicle (inferiorly), medially by scalenus muscle and lateral edge of sternocleidomastoid muscle and lateral edge of IVa, anteriorly by skin, and posteriorly by anterior border of trapezius (superiorly) and serratus anterior (inferiorly)
  - Drains Va and Vb and nasopharynx
- VIa: Anterior jugular nodes
  - Bounded superiorly by inferior edge of hyoid or submandibular gland (whichever is more inferior), inferi-

orly by manubrium, anteriorly by skin and platysma muscle, posteriorly by anterior aspect of infrahyoid (strap) muscles, and laterally by the anterior edge of the sternocleidomastoids

- VIb: Prelaryngeal, pretracheal, paratracheal/recurrent laryngeal nerve nodes
  - Bounded superiorly by inferior edge of thyroid cartilage; inferiorly by manubrium; anteriorly by posterior edge of infrahyoid (strap) muscles; posteriorly by anterior aspect of larynx, thyroid, trachea, prevertebral muscles (right) and esophagus (left); laterally by the common carotid artery; and medially by lateral aspect of trachea and esophagus
  - Drain anterior floor of mouth, tip of tongue, lower lip, thyroid, glottic and supraglottic larynx, hypopharynx, and cervical esophagus
- VIIa: Retropharyngeal nodes
  - Bounded superiorly by the superior edge of C1 body/hard palate, inferiorly by superior edge of hyoid bone, anteriorly by posterior edge of superior or middle pharyngeal constrictor muscles, posteriorly by the prevertebral muscles, medially by line parallel to lateral edge of longus capitis muscle, and laterally by the medial edge of the internal carotid
  - Drain nasopharynx, Eustachian tube, soft palate, posterior pharyngeal wall, and tonsillar fossa
- VIIb: Retrostyloid nodes
  - Bounded superiorly by base of skull (jugular foramen), inferiorly by inferior edge of lateral process of C1, anteriorly by posterior edge of prestyloid parapharyngeal space, posteriorly by the C1 vertebral body and base of skull, laterally by the styloid process and deep parotid lobe, and medially by the medial edge of the internal carotid
  - Drain nasopharynx, any head and neck primary with upper level II involvement due to retrograde lymph flow
- VIII: Parotid nodes
  - Bounded superiorly by zygomatic arch and external auditory canal, inferiorly by angle of mandible, anteriorly by posterior edge of mandibular ramus and masseter muscle (laterally) and medial pterygoid muscle (medially), posteriorly by anterior edge of sternocleido-

mastoid (laterally) and posterior belly of digastric muscle (medially), laterally by subcutaneous tissue, and medially by styloid process and styloid muscle

- Drain parotid gland, frontal and temporal skin, eyelids, conjunctiva, auricle, external acoustic meatus, tympanum, nasal cavities, root of nose, nasopharynx, and Eustachian tube

- IX: Bucco-facial nodes
  - Bounded superiorly by inferior edge of orbit, inferiorly by inferior edge of mandible, anteriorly by subcutaneous tissue, posteriorly by anterior edge of masseter muscle and Bichat's fat pad, laterally by subcutaneous tissue, and medially by buccinators muscle
  - Drain nose, eyelids, cheek, buccal mucosa, and maxillary sinus

- Xa: Retroauricular nodes
  - Bounded superiorly by superior edge of external auditory canal, inferiorly by mastoid tip, anteriorly by anterior edge of mastoid and posterior edge of external auditory canal, posteriorly by anterior border of occipital nodes to posterior edge of sternocleidomastoid, laterally by subcutaneous tissue, and medially by splenius capitis muscle and temporal bone
  - Drain nose, eyelids, cheek, buccal mucosa, and maxillary sinus

- Xb: Occipital nodes
  - Bounded superiorly by external occipital protuberance, inferiorly by level V, anteriorly by posterior edge of sternocleidomastoid, posteriorly by anterior lateral edge of trapezius muscle, laterally by subcutaneous tissue, and medially by splenius capitis muscle

- Comment
  - The above nodal levels include the node-negative, node-positive, and post-operative situations
  - For larger nodes abutting or infiltrating adjacent structures, such as sternocleidomastoid, an expansion of the nodal level into these structures is recommended by 1–2 cm

NECK STAGING

- Most subsites of the head and neck use the same AJCC neck staging system, including the lip, oral cavity, p16-oropharynx, hypopharynx, larynx, and major salivary glands.
- p16+ oropharyngeal carcinoma has its own neck staging system.
- Nasopharyngeal cancer has a different neck staging system.
- Please refer to these other chapters for details of neck staging.

GENERAL TREATMENT RECOMMENDATIONS FOR NECK MANAGEMENT

- These are general; specific guidelines for primary site, histology, and stage should be followed.
- Clinically negative neck:
  - If risk of occult metastasis exists
    - Surgery for primary with elective neck dissection
      - (a) If N0, follow.
      - (b) If N1 with no extracapsular extension (ECE), follow.
      - (c) If >pN1 and/or ECE, postoperative RT or chemo-RT.
    - Alternatively, RT or chemo-RT for primary and RT for elective neck; surgery for persistent disease.
- Clinically positive neck:
  - N1
    - Surgery for primary with modified radical neck dissection
      - (a) If pN0, follow.
      - (b) If pN1 with no ECE, follow.

      - (c) If >pN1 and/or ECE, postoperative RT or chemo-RT.

III

, Alternatively, RT or chemo-RT for primary and involved neck and RT for elective neck; surgery and/ or neck dissection for persistent disease.

, N2–3

, Surgery for primary with modified radical, radical, or extended radical neck dissection

(a) If pN1 with no ECE, follow.

(b) If >pN1 and/or ECE, postoperative RT or chemo-RT.

, Alternatively, RT or chemo-RT for primary and involved neck with comprehensive RT for neck; surgery and/or neck dissection for persistent disease and/ or node >3 cm.

STUDIES OF POSTRADIOTHERAPY NECK DISSECTION

PLANNED SURGERY VS. SURVEILLANCE

, Observation is recommended in patients with radiographic complete response to definitive RT ± chemotherapy due to morbidity of routine neck dissection.

, Narayan (Head Neck 1999): 52 patients with ≥1 node, ≥3 cm (94% stage N2–3). Most common primary tumor was oropharyngeal carcinoma (56%), 60% had T2 or T3 primaries, and all patients were AJCC stage IV. Patients were treated with high-dose RT (various fractionation schemes) followed by radical or modified radical neck dissection after confirmation of CR at primary site. Five-year actuarial overall neck control rate was 83% and in-field control rate was 88%. Only 1/28 with pathologically negative neck specimens had an in-field failure vs. 5/24 patients with pathologic evidence of residual disease. Five-year actuarial DFS was 57% and OS was 38%. Seventeen percent had significant postoperative complications.

, Liauw (JCO 2006): 550 patients with LN+ head and neck cancer treated with RT ± chemotherapy (24%). 341 pts underwent planned post-RT neck dissection. Thirty-day post-RT CT in 211 was correlated with neck dissection pathology to determine criteria associated with a low likelihood of having residual disease. Radiographic CR (rCR) defined as absence of large (>1.5 cm) or focally abnormal lymph node. NPV of 77% for clinical exam CR vs. 94% for rCR. There was no significant difference in the 5-year neck control rate (100%) and CSS (72%) in 32 rCR patients who did not undergo neck dissection vs. patients with negative post-RT neck dissection.

Surveillance PET/CT at 12 weeks after chemo-RT may be safely considered instead of planned neck dissection for N2 disease.

Mehanna (NEJM 2016): Non-inferiority study that randomized 564 patients with N2–N3 disease to planned dissection versus neck dissection only if PET/CT performed 12 weeks after the end of chemo-RT showed an incomplete or equivocal response. 84% were oropharynx, 78% N2a–b, 18% N2c, 3% N3. No significant difference in p16 expression between the two groups. Median follow-up was 36 months. 221 dissections were performed in the planned surgery group versus 54 in the surveillance group. Two-year overall survival was 81.5% in the planned surgery group and 84.9% in the surveillance group.

UNKNOWN PRIMARY OF THE HEAD AND NECK

PEARLS

Definition = metastatic carcinoma in one or more lymph nodes within the head and neck region that are not solely in the supraclavicular region, with no primary site evident after history, physical exam, and initial imaging.

Unknown primary of the head and neck is staged as T0 (not Tx).

- Most unknown primary cancers in the body = adenocarcinoma originating below the clavicles; SCC arising in the cervical nodes <10% of all unknown primary.
- Most likely head and neck primary site: tonsil 45% > base of tongue 40% > pyriform sinus 10%.
  - Most cases especially with level II adenopathy are p16-positive/HPV-associated oropharyngeal cancer (Motz, JAMA Otolaryngol Head Neck Surg 2016; Keller, Head Neck 2014), but p16 positivity in a level II node does not rule out cutaneous primary (McDowell, Cancer 2016).
  - If the adenopathy is centered in level III or IV, the larynx and hypopharynx should be considered as potential primary sites.
  - If the adenopathy is centered in level I, the oral cavity (including lip) should be considered as a potential primary site.
  - Adenopathy in level V may be associated with cutaneous or nasopharyngeal primary origin.
- Patients with upper neck lymphadenopathy have much better prognosis than those with low cervical or supraclavicular lymphadenopathy.
- Lymphadenopathy in low internal jugular chain or supraclavicular fossa may be associated with primary lesions below the clavicles, with much worse prognosis, so workup should proceed accordingly.
  - Isolated supraclavicular lymphadenopathy, even if SCC, almost always originates from cancer in the skin or a primary site beneath the clavicles.
- Pathology
  - Most are squamous cell carcinoma or poorly differentiated (undifferentiated) carcinoma.
  - Adenocarcinoma in the neck is almost always associated with a primary lesion below the clavicles but must rule out salivary gland, thyroid, or parathyroid primary tumors.
  - Others = lymphoma, sarcoma.

WORKUP

- Specialist examination, imaging, and panendoscopy identify primary site >50% of the time.
- H&P including in-office nasopharyngolaryngoscopy with examination of oral cavity, pharynx, and larynx.
- Imaging:
  - Chest X-ray
  - CT and/or MRI of head and neck
  - PET/CT useful in prebiopsy setting as it increases primary site detection rate by approximately 25% (Rudmik, Head Neck 2011; Johansen, Head Neck 2008)
  - Chest CT for N stage ≥N2b, or low neck or bulky lymphadenopathy to evaluate for pulmonary metastases
- Labs:
  - CBC
  - Chemistries including electrolytes, BUN/Cr, LFTs
  - EBV and HPV testing
- EUA with panendoscopy (sometimes called "triple endoscopy") and biopsies of nasopharynx, both tonsils, base of tongue, both pyriform sinuses, and any other suspicious areas seen during examination.
  - Identifies 40% of primaries (but only 25% if no CT or MRI)
- Ipsilateral or bilateral tonsillectomy may also be performed in those with adequate lymphoid tissue in tonsillar fossae.
  - Evaluate tumor samples for EBV DNA in patients who have ethnicity from regions where nasopharyngeal carcinoma is endemic.
  - Detects 30% of primaries.
  - Bilateral tonsillectomy identifies contralateral tonsillar primary in 10%; may make surveillance exam easier.
  - Transoral robotic surgery (TORS) to perform a lingual tonsillectomy improves identification of primary site (Nagel, Head Neck 2014; Patel, JAMA Otolaryngol Head Neck Surg 2013).
- If lymphoma is suspected: core needle or excisional biopsy of node preferred; staging and treatment per lymphoma guidelines.
- Dental examination and cleaning; extractions done before any RT.

Table 13.1 TREATMENT RECOMMENDATIONS

, Two main goals for treatment: control disease in the neck and prevent posttreatment primary tumor emergence.

, Typically irradiate nasopharynx, oropharynx, and both sides of neck

  , Hypopharynx and larynx were irradiated historically; eliminated more recently because they are rarely the primary site and including these sites greatly increases morbidity of treatment.

  , Consider hypopharyngeal and laryngeal irradiation for adenopathy centered in level III/IV.

  , Oral cavity is not irradiated unless submandibular lymphadenopathy is present.

    If submandibular lymphadenopathy: perform neck dissection and observe or irradiate oral cavity and oropharynx but not nasopharynx.

, If only 1 cN+

  , Selective or modified radical neck dissection first (benefit = directs pathology and post-op RT dose is lower, but disadvantage is more surgical morbidity)

    If no additional lymphadenopathy or extracapsular extension (ECE), may observe

    If ≥2 LN or ECE on pathology: post-op RT or chemo-RT

, If ≥2 cN+

  , Selective or modified radical neck dissection first

    N2A: RT

    N2–N3 or ECE: RT or chemo-RT

  , Alternative: Definitive RT or chemo-RT with surveillance PET/CT in 12 weeks with salvage surgery reserved for persistence/recurrence

, Neck control rates with primary RT

  , N1–N2a: 90–100%

  , N2b–N2c: 80%

  , N3: 50–60%

, Rate of DM

  , N1–N2a: <10%

  , N2b–N2c: 15%

  , N3: 25%

, Five-year OS: 40–60% depending on the extent of disease.

, 10% of pts have emergence of a head and neck SCC primary after treatment. Most common location for mucosal site failure is oropharynx, particularly the base of the tongue.

STUDIES
SURGERY +/– PORT

, Several series report that with surgery alone the mucosal emergence rate is about 10–25% and that the risk of ipsilateral neck failure is about 10–15% for N1 disease vs. 25–35% for N2–3 disease, so surgery alone is generally limited to patients with N1 disease without ECE (Galloway, JCO 2015).

, Nieder (IJROBP 2001): systemic review of published studies up to 2000. A combined analysis of four studies with surgery alone estimated mucosal primary emergence rate of 25% without radiation. This is one of the highest estimated rates in the literature.

, Patel (Arch Otolaryngol Head Neck Surg 2007): 70 patients treated with neck dissection. Post-op RT given only for ≥pN2 or ECE. 65 with pN2 or greater disease, 26 with ECE. Median follow-up 42 months. 5-year ipsilateral and contralateral neck controls were 84% and 93%. 5-year DFS was 62%. Crude risk of neck failure with pN2 and ECE or pN3 disease was 35%. Primary tumor site emergence in 8 patients (11%).

DEFINITIVE RT

, Balaker (Laryngoscope 2012). Literature review of 17 studies with 1726 pts. Survival outcomes are most influenced by N stage at diagnosis. No difference in 5-year survival was noted between pts treated with RT or chemo-RT vs. those who also received surgery.

, Grau (Radiother Oncol 2000): 277 pts treated with RT to the bilateral neck, nasopharynx, oropharynx larynx, hypopharynx, and larynx (81%) or only ipsilateral neck (10%). Surgery alone was used in 8% of pts. Emergence of primary occurred in 15% of RT cohort vs. 54% of surgery alone cohort. Pts treated with ipsilateral RT had nonsignificantly lower neck control (43% vs. 52%) and mucosal control (77% vs. 87%) than pts treated with bilateral neck and mucosal RT. Contralateral neck failure was 4% with ipsilateral RT vs. 2% with bilateral RT.

, Wallace (Am J Otolaryngol 2011). 179 pts treated with definitive RT, 39% without neck dissection and 58% with unilateral neck dissection. RT covered potential mucosal primary sites and was bilateral for 97% of pts. 5-yr neck control N1 94%, N2a 98%, N2b 86%, N2c 71%, N3 48%. Eliminating larynx and hypopharynx from RT portals did not compromise outcome.

, Several series have reported low rates of mucosal emergence (~5–15%) and contralateral neck failure (≤5%) for selected patients treated with unilateral RT (Galloway, JCO 2015), but an EORTC randomized trial of bilateral neck and mucosal RT vs. ipsilateral neck RT alone was closed due to poor accrual and no results have been reported.

, Mourad (Anticancer Res 2014): single institution series of 68 non-Asian patients. RT delivered to the bilateral retropharyngeal and neck nodes and oropharynx as only potential primary site; 56% received concurrent chemo. At median follow-up 3.5 years, 3-year LRC 95.5%. Emergence of primary in one patient (1.5%). Suggests that nasopharynx, hypopharynx, and larynx can be spared in select cases. To date there is no data directly comparing different radiation field designs.

RADIATION TECHNIQUES
SIMULATION AND FIELD DESIGN

- Patient setup: supine, hyperextend head, wire neck scars, may need bolus, consider wiring oral commissures, shoulders pulled down with straps, immobilization with thermoplastic mask or bite block.
- Volumes
  - Nasopharynx, oropharynx, bilateral retropharyngeal nodes and levels IB-IV, ipsilateral ± contralateral supraclavicular nodes
  - Include oral cavity only if submandibular adenopathy present, and may eliminate nasopharynx in that case
- IMRT: Recommended to spare contralateral parotid gland in patients with ipsilateral neck lymphadenopathy; low neck may be treated with a separate anterior field using isocentric match to upper IMRT fields.
- Conventional treatment borders (when IMRT not available)
  - Parallel-opposed lateral fields at 1.8–2 Gy/fraction
    - Superior = covers nasopharynx and level Ib and V to base of tongue
    - Posterior = behind spinous processes to C2
    - Anterior = 2 cm margin on nasopharynx and the base of tongue; shield skin and subcutaneous tissue of submentum as much as possible
    - Inferior = thyroid notch
  - Reduction of spinal cord at 42–45 Gy; supplement posterior neck with 9–12 MeV electron fields.
  - Advanced lymphadenopathy receives additional boost with anteroposterior or oblique beams to 66–70 Gy.
  - Anterior supraclavicular field
    - Larynx block is tapered inferiorly to stop at cricoid.
    - Cover ipsilateral ± contralateral supraclavicular fossa (generally very low risk of recurrence).

DOSE PRESCRIPTIONS
- UCSF definitive IMRT doses
  - GTV 2.12/69.96 Gy, high-risk CTV 2/66 Gy, intermediate-risk CTV 1.8/59.4 Gy, low-risk CTV 1.64/54 Gy in 33 fractions
- Conventional definitive = 42–45 Gy followed by off-cord boost to 70 Gy, or if using concomitant boost, 72 Gy
- Postoperative
  - With no adverse features = 50–54 Gy to potential primary mucosal sites and bilateral neck
  - Boost high-risk areas to 60–66 Gy (e.g., for perineural invasion, ECE, close/+ margin)

DOSE LIMITATIONS
- IMRT limits
  - Mandible <70 Gy, spinal cord <45 Gy, brainstem <54 Gy, mean parotid dose <26 Gy, optic nerves and chiasm 54 Gy, retina 45 Gy

COMPLICATIONS
- Surgical
  - Operative mortality 2–3%
  - Morbidity = infection; hematoma/seroma; lymphedema; wound dehiscence; chyle fistula; pharyngocutaneous fistula; cranial nerve VII, X, XI, XII injury; carotid exposure; or rupture
  - Incidence of complications greater with RT doses >60 Gy
- Radiation therapy
  - Acute and chronic mucositis, xerostomia
  - Skin reaction
  - Subcutaneous fibrosis
  - Lymphedema of larynx and submentum
  - Mandibular necrosis uncommon
  - Carotid artery rupture <1%

FOLLOW-UP
- Every 1–2 months for first year, every 3 months for years 2–3, every 6 months for years 4–5, then every year.
- If recurrence suspected but biopsy negative, follow-up every 1 month until resolved.
- 85–90% of recurrences occur within 3 years.

Acknowledgment We thank Tania Kaprealian MD for her work on the prior edition of this chapter.

REFERENCES

Balaker AE, Abemayor E, Elashoff D, et al. Cancer of unknown primary: does treatment modality make a difference? Laryngoscope. 2012;122:1279–82.

Galloway TJ, Ridge JA. Management of squamous cancer metastatic to cervical nodes with an unknown primary site. J Clin Oncol. 2015;33(29):3328–37.

Grau C, et al. Cervical lymph node metastases from unknown primary tumours. Results from a national survey by the Danish Society for Head and Neck Oncology. Radiother Oncol. 2000;55(2):121–9.

Grégoire V, Ang K, Budach W, et al. Delineation of the neck node levels for head and neck tumors: a 2013 update. DAHANCA, EORTC, HKNPCSG, NCIC CTG, NCRI, RTOG, TROG consensus guidelines. Radiother Oncol. 2014;110(1):172–81.

Johansen J, et al. Prospective study of 18FDG-PET in the detection and management of patients with lymph node metastases to the neck from an unknown primary tumor. Results from the DAHANCA-13 study. Head Neck. 2008;30(4):471–8.

Keller LM, et al. p16 status, pathologic and clinical characteristics, biomolecular signature, and long-term outcomes in head and neck squamous cell carcinomas of unknown primary. Head Neck. 2014;36(12):1677–84.

Liauw SL, Mancuso AA, Amdur RJ, et al. Postradiotherapy neck dissection for lymph node-positive head and neck cancer: the use of computed tomography to manage the neck. J Clin Oncol. 2006;24(9):1421–7.

McDowell LJ, et al. p16-positive lymph node metastases from cutaneous head and neck squamous cell carcinoma: no association with high-risk human papillomavirus or prognosis and implications for the workup of the unknown primary. Cancer. 2016;122(8):1201–8.

Mehanna H, et al. PET-CT surveillance versus neck dissection in advanced head and neck cancer. N Engl J Med. 2016;374:1–11.

Mendenhall WM, Mancuso AA, Parsons JT, Stringer SP, Cassisi NJ. Diagnostic evaluation of squamous cell carcinoma metastatic to cervical lymph nodes from an unknown head and neck primary site. Head Neck. 1998;20(8):739–44.

Motz K, et al. Changes in unknown primary squamous cell carcinoma of the head and neck at initial presentation in the era of human papillomavirus. JAMA Otolaryngol Head Neck Surg. 2016;142(3):223–8.

Mourad WF, et al. Initial experience with oropharynx-targeted radiation therapy for metastatic squamous cell carcinoma of unknown primary of the head and neck. Anticancer Res. 2014;34(1):243–8.

Nagel TH, et al. Transoral laser microsurgery for the unknown primary: role for lingual tonsillectomy. Head Neck. 2014;36(7):942–6.

Narayan K, Crane CH, Kleid S, Hughes PG, Peters LJ. Planned neck dissection as an adjunct to the management of patients with advanced neck disease treated with definitive radiotherapy: for some or for all? Head Neck. 1999;21(7):606–13.

Nieder C, Gregoire V, Ang KK. Cervical lymph node metastases from occult squamous cell carcinoma: cut down a tree to get an apple? Int J Radiat Oncol Biol Phys. 2001;50(3):727–33.

Patel RS, et al. Squamous cell carcinoma from an unknown head and neck primary site: a "selective treatment" approach. Arch Otolaryngol Head Neck Surg. 2007;133(12):1282–7.

Patel SA, et al. Robotic surgery for primary head and neck squamous cell carcinoma of unknown site. JAMA Otolaryngol Head Neck Surg. 2013;139(11):1203–11.

Rudmik L, et al. Clinical utility of PET/CT in the evaluation of head and neck squamous cell carcinoma with an unknown primary: a prospective clinical trial. Head Neck. 2011;33(7):935–40.

Wallace A, Richards GM, Harari PM, et al. Head and neck squamous cell carcinoma from an unknown primary site. Am J Otolaryngol. 2011;32(4):286–90.

III

PART IV
Thorax

Chapter 14
Small Cell Lung Cancer

Michael Wahl and Adam Garsa

IV

PEARLS

- SCLC accounts for 15–20% of lung cancer cases with decreasing incidence.
- Approximately 1/3 of patients present with limited stage disease and the remainder present with extensive stage disease.
- More than 95% of cases are associated with a history of tobacco exposure.
- Ten to 15% of patients present with brain metastases and 2-year incidence after chemo-RT is 50–80%.
- SCLC is the most common solid tumor associated with paraneoplastic syndromes: SIADH, ACTH production syndrome, and Eaton–Lambert syndrome.
- Histopathologic hallmarks include dense sheets of small, round to fusiform cells with scant cytoplasm, extensive necrosis, and a high mitotic rate.
- Pathologic subtypes (pure or classic, variant, and mixed) carry the same prognosis.
- Most important prognostic factors are stage and performance status.

© Springer International Publishing AG, part of Springer Nature 2018   **285**
Eric K. Hansen and M. Roach III (eds.), *Handbook of Evidence-Based Radiation Oncology*, https://doi.org/10.1007/978-3-319-62642-0_14

WORKUP

- H&P.
- Labs: CBC, chemistries, BUN/Cr, LFTs, LDH.
- Diagnosis: sputum, FNA, bronchoscopic biopsy, or CT-guided biopsy.
- Pathologic mediastinal staging only if T1-2N0 and patient is surgical candidate.
- Imaging: CT chest and abdomen, MRI brain, PET/CT.
- Additional: PFTs, pathology review, smoking cessation intervention.

STAGING

- See Chap. 15 for details of the AJCC Staging for Lung Cancer.
- In practice, SCLC has been divided into limited stage and extensive stage disease.
  - Limited Stage (LS): classically defined as disease fitting into a single radiation port, typically confined to one hemithorax and regional nodes.
  - With modern conformal radiotherapy techniques, LS now effectively characterized as stage I-III disease that can safely be treated with definitive radiotherapy.
  - Extensive Stage (ES): Any disease not meeting limited stage criteria.

TREATMENT RECOMMENDATIONS

Stage	Recommended treatment	Outcome
Limited	Concurrent cisplatin and etoposide (4c every 3 weeks) with early RT during cycle 1 or 2 (45 Gy/1.5 Gy b.i.d. or 6070 Gy QD). If CR or near-CR, prophylactic cranial RT (25 Gy in 10 fx)	MS 20 months, 5-year OS 20–26%
	For <5% of patients with cT1-2 N0 disease with negative mediastinoscopy (or endoscopic biopsy), lobectomy and mediastinal node dissection/sampling may be performed initially. If pN0, chemotherapy alone. If pN+, concurrent chemoradiation as above. PCI (25 Gy in 10 fx) for all patients post-operatively	

Extensive	Combination platinum-based chemotherapy ± palliative RT to symptomatic sites. For patients with PR or CR to chemotherapy, prophylactic cranial RT (25 Gy in 10 fx), consider consolidative thoracic RT (ex. 30 Gy in 10 fx (Slotman *Lancet* 2015)). If brain metastases present, WBRT (30–37.5 Gy in 10–15 fx)	MS 12 months, 5-year OS <5–10%

STUDIES

IV

LIMITED STAGE (LS-SCLC)
ROLE OF SURGERY

- Multiple older studies did not show benefit to surgical resection over chemoradiation, but recent data suggests it may play a role in patients with node negative disease after full staging with pathologic mediastinal evaluation, PET/CT and MRI.
- JCOG9101 (*J Thorac Cardiovasc Surg* 2005): Phase II study of 61 patients with stage I-IIIA SCLC (90% stage I/II) who underwent complete surgical resection followed by adjuvant chemotherapy (cisplatin/etoposide x 4c). 3y OS 61% (I: 68%, II: 56%, III: 13%).

THORACIC RADIATION

- Pignon (*NEJM* 1992): metaanalysis of 13 trials and 2140 patients with LS-SCLC treated with chemo ± thoracic RT. Thoracic RT improved 3-year OS by 5.4% vs. chemo alone (14.3 vs. 8.9%).
- Metaanalyses of randomized controlled trials performed on LS-SCLC patients receiving chemo and early vs. late timing of thoracic RT demonstrate improved survival for early concurrent integration of RT with platinum-based chemo (De Ruysscher *JCO* 2006a,b, Pijls-Johannesma *Cancer Treat Rev* 2007).
- *INT 0096* (Turrisi *NEJM* 1999): 417 patients with LS-SCLC randomized to concurrent cisplatin/etoposide with either 45 Gy/1.8 Gy QD or 45 Gy/1.5 Gy BID. Twice daily arm decreased local failure (36 vs. 52%) and increased 5-year OS (26 vs. 16%) compared to QD arm. Grade 3 esophagitis more frequent with b.i.d. regimen (27 vs. 11%). Criticism: hyperfractionation arm had higher BED than standard fractionation, so positive

result may be a consequence of dose escalation and not hyperfractionation per se.

- *RTOG 0239* (Komaki *JCO* 2009): phase II trial using accelerated high-dose thoracic RT (AHTRT) with concurrent etoposide/cisplatin. RT was given to large field to 28.8 Gy /1.8 Gy QD, then 14.4 Gy/1.8 Gy b.i.d. (1.8 Gy AP/PA in am; 1.8 Gy boost in pm). Total RT dose 61.2 Gy in 5 weeks. Two-year OS 37%, 2-year LC 80%, and 18% acute severe esophagitis, improved compared to INT 0096.

- CALGB 30610/RTOG 0538 (ongoing): Patients with LS-SCLC randomized to 3 RT regimens: standard fractionation (70 Gy/2 Gy daily), Turrisi regimen (45 Gy/1.5 Gy BID) or RTOG 0239 dose escalation (61.2 Gy in 5 weeks). RTOG 0239 based arm dropped at planned interim analysis to facilitate accrual.

- CONVERT (Faivre-Finn, ASCO 2016). 547 patients randomized to 45 Gy (1.5 Gy BID over 3 weeks) vs. 66 Gy (2 Gy daily over 6.5 weeks) on day 22 cycle 1 chemotherapy (4–6 cycles cisplatin etoposide), followed by PCI as indicated (received by ~87% of patients). No significant difference in 2-yr OS (BID 56%, QD 51%), MS (BID 30 mo, QD 25 mo), or toxicities (grade 2 esophagitis 55–63%, grade 3/4 esophagitis 19%, grade 3/4 pneumonitis 2.2–2.5%).

PROPHYLACTIC CRANIAL IRRADIATION

- Auperin (*NEJM* 1999): metaanalysis of seven trials of SCLC patients in CR comparing prophylactic cranial irradiation (PCI) vs. no PCI. PCI reduced the 3-year incidence of brain metastases (59 vs.33%) and increased 3-year OS (15.3 vs. 20.7). Neurocognitive function not assessed.

- RTOG 0212/Intergroup (Le Pechoux *Lancet* 2009): 720 LS-SCLC patients in CR to chemo-RT randomized to standard dose (25 Gy/2.5 Gy QD) vs. higher dose (36 Gy/2 Gy QD or 36 Gy/1.5 Gy b.i.d.) PCI. No significant difference in 2-year incidence of brains metastases. Reduced 2-year OS in higher dose group (37 vs. 42%) probably due to increased cancer-related mortality.

EXTENSIVE STAGE (ES-SCLC)

, Jeremic (*JCO* 1999): 210 ES-SCLC patients treated with three cycles cisplatin/etoposide with local PR or CR and distant CR randomized to accelerated hyperfractionated RT (54 Gy/1.5 Gy b.i.d.) and chemo vs. four cycles chemo alone. Patients receiving chemo-RT had improved 5-year OS (9.1 vs. 3.7%) and MS (17 vs. 11 months) vs. those treated with chemo alone.

, *EORTC* (Slotman *NEJM* 2007): 286 patients with ES-SCLC with response to chemotherapy randomized to PCI vs. no further treatment. PCI reduced 1-year incidence of symptomatic brain mets (14.6 vs. 40.4%) and improved OS (27.1 vs. 13.3%) compared to the control group.

, CREST (Slotman *Lancet* 2015): 498 patients with ES-SCLC without brain metastases with CR or PR to chemo randomized to PCI (25 Gy/10 fractions) and thoracic RT (30 Gy/10 fractions) vs. PCI alone. RT targeted post-chemo tumor volume plus any initially involved nodal stations. Trend towards improved 1y OS (33 vs. 28%), with improved 2y OS (13 vs. 3%), and improved PFS at 6 months (24 vs. 7%). Rate of isolated introthoracic progression was cut in half (46 vs. 20%).

RADIATION TECHNIQUES

SIMULATION AND FIELD DESIGN

, Supine, arms up with wingboard or alpha cradle.

, 4DCT to account for respiratory motion.

, GTV = Gross primary and nodal disease.

, CTV = GTV + 0.5–1 cm + pre-chemo involved nodal stations.

, Traditional mediastinal fields covered ipsilateral hilum and bilateral mediastinum from thoracic inlet to subcarinal region, but recent evidence suggests limited risk of isolated nodal failure away from clinically node positive disease.

, Van Loon (*IJROBP* 2010): 60 patients with LS-SCLC prospectively treated chemo-RT to primary and pre-

IV

chemo involved nodes on PET/CT only. 3% isolated nodal failure rate.

- MDACC (Shirvani *IJROBP* 2012): Retrospective analysis of 60 patients with LS-SCLC underwent chemo-RT to primary and pre-chemo involved nodes on PET/CT. 2% isolated nodal failure rate.
- If RT is preceded by chemotherapy, target volumes should be defined on the RT planning CT scan. However, the pre-chemotherapy originally involved lymph node regions should be included.

DOSE PRESCRIPTIONS

- LS-SCLC: 45 Gy in 1.5 b.i.d. fx (6 hour interval) or 60–70 Gy at 1.8–2.0 Gy QD.
- PCI: 25 Gy in 10 fx.
- Brain metastases: 30–37.5 Gy in 10–15 fx.

DOSE LIMITATIONS

- Spinal cord: limit maximum dose to ≤36 Gy with 1.5 Gy b.i.d. RT or ≤46 Gy at 1.8–2 Gy/fx QD.
- See Chapter 15 for additional dose limitations for thoracic RT.

COMPLICATIONS

- Acute: esophagitis, dermatitis, cough, fatigue.
- Subacute/late: radiation pneumonitis, pulmonary fibrosis, esophageal stricture or perforation, pericarditis, coronary artery disease, brachial plexopathy, rib fracture.

FOLLOW-UP

- Clinic visits every 2–4 months initially (H&P, CT chest/abdomen, and blood work at each visit), then decrease frequency to every 3–6 months, then annually.

Acknowledgment We thank R. Scott Bermudez MD, Brian Missett MD, and Daphne A. Haas-Kogan MD for their work on the prior edition of this chapter.

REFERENCES

Auperin A, Arriagada R, Pignon JP, et al. Prophylactic cranial irradiation for patients with small-cell lung cancer in complete remission. Prophylactic cranial irradiation overview collaborative group. N Engl J Med. 1999;341:476–84.

De Ruysscher D, Pijls-Johannesma M, Vansteenkiste J, et al. Systematic review and meta-analysis of randomised, controlled trials of the timing of chest radiotherapy in patients with limited-stage, small-cell lung cancer. Ann Oncol. 2006a;17:543–52.

De Ruysscher D, Pijls-Johannesma M, Bentzen S, et al. Time between the first day of chemotherapy and the last day of chest radiation is the most important predictor of survival in limited-disease small cell lung cancer. J Clin Oncol. 2006b;24:1057–63.

Faivre-Finn C, Snee M, Ashcroft L, et al. CONVERT: an international randomised trial of concurrent chemo-radiotherapy (cCTRT) comparing twice-daily (BD) and once-daily (OD) radiotherapy schedules in patients with limited stage small cell lung cancer (LS-SCLC) and good performance status (PS). J Clin Oncol. 2016;34. (suppl; abstr 8504).

Jeremic B, Shibamoto Y, Nikolic N. Role of radiation therapy in the combined-modality treatment of patients with extensive disease small-cell lung cancer: a randomized study. J Clin Oncol. 1999;17:2092–9.

Komaki R, Paulus R, Ettinger DS, Videtic GM, Bradley JD, Glisson BS, Choy H. A phase II study of accelerated high-dose thoracic radiation therapy (AHTRT) with concurrent chemotherapy for limited small cell lung cancer: RTOG 0239. J Clin Oncol. 2009;27:7s (suppl; abstr 7527).

Le Pechoux C, Dunant A, Senan S, et al. Standard-dose versus higher-dose prophylactic cranial irradiation (PCI) in patients with limited-stage small-cell lung cancer in complete remission after chemotherapy and thoracic radiotherapy (PCI 99-01, EORTC 2203-08004, RTOG 0212, and IFCT 99-01): a randomised clinical trial. Lancet Oncol. 2009;10:467–74.

National comprehensive cancer network clinical practice guidelines in oncology: small cell lung cancer. Available at: http://www.nccn.org/professionals/physician_gls/PDF/sclc.pdf. Accessed 31 Aug 2016.

Pignon JP, Arriagada A, Ihde DC, et al. A meta-analysis of thoracic radiotherapy for small-cell lung cancer. N Engl J Med. 1992;3:1618–24.

Pijls-Johannesma M, De Ruysscher D, Vansteenkiste J, et al. Timing of chest radiotherapy in patients with limited stage small cell lung cancer: a systematic review and meta-analysis of randomized controlled trials. Cancer Treat Rev. 2007;33(5):461–73.

Shirvani SM, Komaki R, Heymach JV, et al. Positron emission tomography/computed tomography-guided intensity-modulated radiotherapy for limited-stage small-cell lung cancer. Int J Radiat Oncol Biol Phys. 2012;82(1):e91–7.

Slotman B, Faivre-Finn C, Kramer G, et al. Prophylactic cranial irradiation in extensive small-cell lung cancer. N Engl J Med. 2007;357:664–72.

Slotman B, van Tinteren H, Praag JO, et al. Use of thoracic radiotherapy for extensive stage small-cell lung cancer. Lancet. 2015;385:36–42.

Tsuchiya R, Suzuki K, Ichinose Y, et al. Phase II trial of postoperative adjuvant cisplatin and etoposide in patients with completely resected stage I-IIIa small cell lung cancer: the Japan Clinical Oncology Lung Cancer Study Group Trial (JCOG9101). J Thorac Cardiovasc Surg. 2005;129(5):977–833.

Turrisi AT III, Kim K, Blum R, et al. Twice-daily compared with once-daily thoracic radiotherapy in limited small-cell lung cancer treated concurrently with cisplatin and etoposide. N Engl J Med. 1999;340:265–71.

Van Loon J, De Ruysscher D, Wanders R, et al. Selective nodal irradiation on basis of (18)FDG-PET scans in limited-disease small-cell lung cancer: a prospective study. Int J Radiat Oncol Biol Phys. 2010;77(2):329–36.

IV

Chapter 15
Non-small Cell Lung Cancer

Michael Wahl, Matthew A. Gubens, and Sue S. Yom

PEARLS

- #1 non-cutaneous cancer in the world.
- #2 most common cancer in the United States, behind prostate in men and breast in women.
- #1 cause of cancer death in the United States and worldwide.
- >90% of cases are associated with active or passive smoking. Second most common cause in the United States is radon. Asbestos exposure is associated with 3–4% of cases.
- Screening with low-dose CT is standard of care for strong smoking history.
- After initial cancer, risk of tobacco-induced second primary is ~2–3% per year.
- Surgical lymph node levels 1–9 correspond to N2 nodes, and levels 10–14 correspond to N1 nodes. International Association for the Study of Lung Cancer lymph node definition contouring atlas has been published (Lynch, PRO 2013) (Fig. 15.1).

© Springer International Publishing AG, part of Springer Nature 2018   **293**
Eric K. Hansen and M. Roach III (eds.), *Handbook of Evidence-Based Radiation Oncology*, https://doi.org/10.1007/978-3-319-62642-0_15

- Pathology
  - Adenocarcinoma comprises 40–50% of cases. It tends to be peripherally located; squamous cell carcinoma tends to be centrally located.
  - TTF-1 is positive only in adenocarcinomas of primary lung and thyroid origin (not metastases); napsin is differentiating as it is positive in 80% of lung and only 10% of thyroid adenocarcinomas.
  - Large cell carcinoma behaves similarly to small cell lung cancer, with high propensity to metastasize, especially to brain.
  - Adenocarcinoma in situ (AIS) or minimally invasive adenocarcinoma (MIS), formerly referred to as bronchoalveolar carcinoma, is a subtype of adenocarcinoma with weak association with smoking. Frequently harbor EGFR or ALK mutations (sensitive to gefitinib, erlotinib, crizotinib, etc.).
- Pancoast tumor = apical (superior sulcus) tumor + either chest wall (rib) invasion or Pancoast syndrome [shoulder pain or brachial plexus palsy, ±Horner's syndrome (ptosis, meiosis, and ipsilateral anhidrosis)].
- Carcinoid tumors are rare. Tend to be endobronchial. Most common site is GI tract, but 25% in lung. 70–90% are typical carcinoids, which rarely metastasize and are not associated with smoking. 10–30% are atypical carcinoids, which more frequently metastasize and are associated with smoking, and have poorer prognosis. Only 10–15% of patients with carcinoid tumors present with carcinoid syndrome (flushing, diarrhea, and wheezing), but up to 2/3 eventually develop symptoms.
- Presentation: stage I 10%, II 20%, III 30%, IV 40%.
- Prognostic factors: stage, weight loss (>10% body weight over 6 months), KPS, pleural effusion.
  - RTOG RPA analysis (Werner-Wasik IJROBP 2000): KPS <90, use of chemo, age > 70 years, pleural effusion, N stage. Worst survival in patients with malignant pleural effusion (5 months).
  - For N2, single station disease has more favorable outcomes than multi-station (5-year OS 34% vs 11%, Andre JCO 2000).

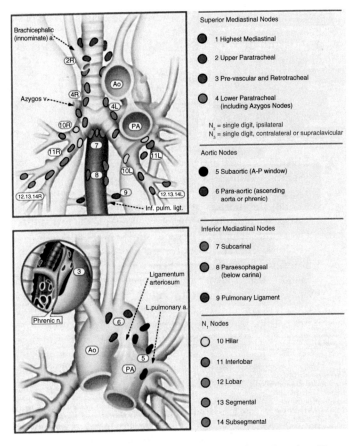

Fig. 15.1 Pulmonary and mediastinal lymph node atlas (From Rusch et al. (2009). Reprinted with permission from Elsevier)

WORKUP

, H&P, including performance status, weight loss, and smoking status.

, Cough, dyspnea, hemoptysis, postobstructive pneumonia, pleural effusion, pain, hoarseness (left recurrent

laryngeal nerve), SVC syndrome, clubbing, Pancoast syndrome.
- Labs: CBC, BUN, Cr, LFTs, alkaline phosphatase, LDH.
- Imaging:
  - CT chest and abdomen (to rule out adrenal or liver metastasis).
    - Mediastinal LN sensitivity ~60%, specificity ~80% (Gould 2003).
    - Approximately 10–20% false negative rate for CT depending on T stage and size.
  - PET/CT: Mediastinal LN sensitivity 77%, specificity 90% (Schmidt-Hansen 2014).
  - Brain MRI for stage II–IV, or for neurologic symptoms.
  - MRI of the thoracic inlet for superior sulcus tumors to assess vertebral body and/or brachial plexus invasion.
  - Octreotide scan for carcinoid tumor.
- Pathology: Thoracentesis for pleural effusions. For central lesions, bronchoscopy because sputum cytology has ~65–80% sensitivity. For peripheral lesions, CT-guided biopsy. Endobronchial ultrasound (EBUS)-guided biopsy to reach peripheral lesions less invasively. Thoracoscopic (surgical) biopsy can be diagnostic and therapeutic.
  - Molecular testing for Kras activation, EGFR mutation, ROS/ALK rearrangements.
- Many prescribe SBRT without pathologic confirmation for FDG-avid nodules that are new or growing (<6% false positive rate).
- Pathologic mediastinal staging recommended for all patients per NCCN, but not universally performed for cN0 patients. Mediastinoscopy or bronchoscopic biopsy to confirm any CT+ or PET+ nodes, and for all superior sulcus tumors. If T3 or central T1–2, perform mediastinoscopy to evaluate superior mediastinal nodes.
  - Cervical mediastinoscopy assesses nodal levels 1–4R.
  - Anterior (Chamberlain) mediastinoscopy assesses levels 4 L (left lower paratracheal), 5, 6, and 7.
  - Endobronchial Ultrasound (EBUS): Levels 2, 3, 4, 7, 10.
  - Esophageal Ultrasound (EUS): Levels 4 L, 7, 8, 9.
- Pulmonary function testing for presurgical and/or preradiotherapy evaluation:

- Desire FEV1 $\geq$ 1.2–2 L (if pneumonectomy >2.5 L, if lobectomy >1.2 L) or >75% predicted or predicted post-op FEV1 > 0.8 L; also DLCO >60%.
- Medically inoperable is generally FEV1 < 40% or <1.2 L, DLCO <60%, FVC <70% but less restrictive if wedge/segmentectomy is planned.

- Paraneoplastic syndromes.
  - Hypercalcemia (SqCC).
  - Hypertrophic pulmonary osteoarthropathy (adenocarcinoma).
  - Hypercoagulable (adenocarcinoma).
  - Gynecomastia (large cell).
  - VIP-induced diarrhea (carcinoid).

IV

STAGING: NON-SMALL CELL LUNG CANCER

Editors' note: All TNM stage and stage groups referred to elsewhere in this chapter reflect the 2010 AJCC staging nomenclature unless otherwise noted.

STAGING (AJCC 7TH ED., 2010)

Primary tumor (T)

TX: Primary tumor cannot be assessed, or tumor proven by the presence of malignant cells in sputum or bronchial washings, but not visualized by imaging or bronchoscopy

T0: No evidence of primary tumor

Tis: Carcinoma in situ

T1: Tumor 3 cm or less in greatest dimension, surrounded by lung or visceral pleura, without bronchoscopic evidence of invasion, more proximal than the lobar bronchus (i.e., not in the main bronchus)*

T1a: Tumor 2 cm or less in greatest dimension

T1b: Tumor more than 2 cm but 3 cm or less in greatest dimension

T2: Tumor more than 3 cm but 7 cm or less or tumor with any of the following features (T2 tumors with these features are classified T2a if 5 cm or less); involves main bronchus, 2 cm or more distal to the carina; invades visceral pleura (pl1 or pl2); associated with atelectasis or obstructive pneumonitis that extends to the hilar region but does not involve the entire lung

continued

T2a:	Tumor more than 3 cm but 5 cm or less in greatest dimension
T2b:	Tumor more than 5 cm but 7 cm or less in greatest dimension
T3:	Tumor more than 7 cm or one that directly invades any of the following: parietal pleural (PL3) chest wall (including superior sulcus tumors), diaphragm, phrenic nerve, mediastinal pleura, and parietal pericardium; or tumor in the main bronchus (less than 2 cm distal to the carina*) but without involvement of the carina; or associated atelectasis or obstructive pneumonitis of the entire lung or separate tumor nodule(s) in the same lobe
T4:	Tumor of any size that invades any of the following: mediastinum, heart, great vessels, trachea, recurrent laryngeal nerve, esophagus, vertebral body, carina, separate tumor nodule(s) in a different ipsilateral lobe

*The uncommon superficial spreading tumor of any size with its invasive component limited to the bronchial wall, which may extend proximally to the main bronchus, is also classified as T1a

Regional lymph nodes (N)

NX:	Regional lymph nodes cannot be assessed
N0:	No regional lymph node metastases
N1:	Metastasis in ipsilateral peribronchial and/or ipsilateral hilar lymph nodes and intrapulmonary nodes, including involvement by direct extension
N2:	Metastasis in ipsilateral mediastinal and/or subcarinal lymph node(s)
N3:	Metastasis in contralateral mediastinal, contralateral hilar, ipsilateral or contralateral scalene, or supraclavicular lymph node(s)

Distant metastasis (M)

M0:	No distant metastasis
M1:	Distant metastasis
M1a:	Separate tumor nodule(s) in a contralateral lobe tumor with pleural nodules or malignant pleural (or pericardial) effusion
M1b:	Distant metastasis

Anatomic stage/prognostic groups

Occult carcinoma: TX N0 M0

0:	Tis N0 M0
IA:	T1a N0 M0
	T1b N0 M0
IB:	T2a N0 M0
IIA:	T2b N0 M0
	T1a N1 M0
	T1b N1 M0
	T2a N1 M0
IIB:	T2b N1 M0
	T3 N0 M0
IIIA:	T1a N2 M0
	T1b N2 M0
	T2a N2 M0
	T2b N2 M0
	T3 N1 M0
	T3 N2 M0
	T4 N0 M0
	T4 N1 M0

IIIB:	T1a N3 M0
	T1b N3 M0
	T2a N3 M0
	T2b N3 M0
	T3 N3 M0
	T4 N2 M0
	T4 N3 M0
IV:	Any T Any N M1a
	Any T Any N M1b

Used with the permission from the American Joint Committee on Cancer (AJCC) (2010) Chicago, Illinois. The original source for this material is the AJCC cancer staging manual, 7th edn, Springer + Business Media

IV

~5-year survival	~Median survival
IA:50–70%	IA:5–10 years
IB:40–60%	IB:3–7 years
IIA:34–55%	IIA:3–4 years
IIB:20–40%	IIB:1.5–3 years
IIIA:10–25%	IIIA:14–23 months
IIIB:7–9%	IIIB:10–16 months
IV:2–13%	IV:6–18 months (best supportive care 3–6 months; better with chemo; even better with targetable mutations)
Superior sulcus: 3 years 50%	

*Range represents clinical vs pathologic staging

STAGING (AJCC 8TH ED., 2017)

Definitions of AJCC TNM

Definition of primary tumor (T)

T category	T criteria
TX	Primary tumor that cannot be assessed or tumor proven by the presence of malignant cells in sputum or bronchial washings but not visualized by imaging or bronchoscopy
T0	No evidence of primary tumor
Tis	Carcinoma in situ Squamous cell carcinoma in situ (SCIS) Adenocarcinoma in situ (AIS): adenocarcinoma with pure lepidic pattern, ≤3 cm in the greatest dimension
T1	Tumor ≤3 cm in the greatest dimension, surrounded by the lung or visceral pleura, without bronchoscopic evidence of invasion more proximal than the lobar bronchus (i.e., not in the main bronchus)
T1mi	Minimally invasive adenocarcinoma: adenocarcinoma (<3 cm in the greatest dimension) with a predominantly lepidic pattern and ≤5 mm invasion in the greatest dimension

continued

T1a	Tumor ≤1 cm in the greatest dimension. A superficial, spreading tumor of any size whose invasive component is limited to the bronchial wall and may also extend proximal to the main bronchus is classified as T1a, but this tumor is uncommon
T1b	Tumor >1 cm but ≤2 cm in the greatest dimension
T1	Tumor >2 cm but ≤3 cm in the greatest dimension
T2	Tumor >3 cm but ≤5 cm or having any of the following features: Involves the main bronchus regardless of the distance to the carina but without involvement of the carina Invades the visceral pleura (PL1 or PL2) Associated with atelectasis or obstructive pneumonitis that extends to the hilar region, involving part or all of the lung T2 tumors with these features are classified as T2a if ≤4 cm or if the size cannot be determined and T2b if >4 cm but ≤5 cm
T2a	Tumor >3 cm but ≤4 cm in the greatest dimension
T2b	Tumor >4 cm but ≤5 cm in the greatest dimension
T3	Tumor >5 cm but ≤7 cm in the greatest dimension or directly invading any of the following—parietal pleura (PL3), chest wall (including superior sulcus tumors), phrenic nerve, and parietal pericardium—or separate tumor nodule(s) in the same lobe as the primary
T4	Tumor >7 cm or tumor of any size invading one or more of the following—diaphragm, mediastinum, heart, great vessels, trachea, recurrent laryngeal nerve, esophagus, vertebral body, or carina— separate tumor nodule(s) in an ipsilateral lobe different from that of the primary

DEFINITION OF REGIONAL LYMPH NODE (N)

N category	N criteria
NX	Regional lymph nodes cannot be assessed
N0	No regional lymph node metastasis
N1	Metastasis in ipsilateral peribronchial and/or ipsilateral hilar lymph nodes and intrapulmonary nodes, including involvement by direct extension
N2	Metastasis in ipsilateral mediastinal and/or subcarinal lymph node(s)
N3	Metastasis in contralateral mediastinal, contralateral hilar, ipsilateral or contralateral scalene, or supraclavicular lymph node(s)

DEFINITION OF DISTANT METASTASIS (M)

M category	M criteria
M0	No distant metastasis
M1	Distant metastasis
M1a	Separate tumor nodule(s) in a contralateral lobe; tumor with pleural or pericardial nodules or malignant pleural or pericardial effusion. Most pleural (pericardial) effusions with lung cancer are a result of the tumor. In a few patients, however, multiple microscopic examinations of pleural (pericardial) fluid are negative for tumor, and the fluid is nonbloody and not an exudate. If these elements and clinical judgment dictate that the effusion is not related to the tumor, the effusion should be excluded as a staging descriptor
M1b	Single extrathoracic metastasis in a single organ (including involvement of a single nonregional node)
M1c	Multiple extrathoracic metastases in a single organ or in multiple organs

IV

AJCC PROGNOSTIC STAGE GROUPS

When T is...	And N is...	And M is...	Then the stage group is...
TX	N0	M0	Occult carcinoma
Tis	N0	M0	0
T1mi	N0	M0	IA1
T1a	N0	M0	IA1
T1a	N1	M0	IIB
T1a	N2	M0	IIIA
T1a	N3	M0	IIIB
T1b	N0	M0	IA2
T1b	N1	M0	IIB
T1b	N2	M0	IIIA
T1b	N3	M0	IIIB
T1c	N0	M0	IA3
T1c	N1	M0	IIB
T1c	N2	M0	IIIA
T1c	N3	M0	IIIB
T2a	N0	M0	IB
T2a	N1	M0	IIB
T2a	N2	M0	IIIA
T2a	N3	M0	IIIB
T2b	N0	M0	IIA
T2b	N1	M0	IIB
T2b	N2	M0	IIIA
T2b	N3	M0	IIIB
T3	N0	M0	IIB
T3	N1	M0	IIIA
T3	N2	M0	IIIB
T3	N3	M0	IIIC

continued

T4	N0	M0	IIIA
T4	N1	M0	IIIA
T4	N2	M0	IIIB
T4	N3	M0	IIIC
Any T	Any N	M1a	IVA
Any T	Any N	M1b	IVA
Any T	Any N	M1c	IVB

Used with permission of the American Joint Committee on Cancer (AJCC), Chicago, Illinois. The original and primary source for this information is the AJCC Cancer Staging Manual, Eighth Edition (2017) published by Springer International Publishing

TREATMENT RECOMMENDATIONS

Stage	Recommended treatment	Outcome
I–II operable	Lobectomy (~2–3% mortality) preferred over pneumonectomy (~5–7% mortality) if anatomically feasible Wedge resection only if physiologically compromised LN sampling or dissection generally indicated because ~15% of cT1–2N0 found to have +LN For resected T1–2N1, adjuvant chemo For resected T2N0, consider adjuvant chemo esp if >4 cm For resected T3N0, give adjuvant chemo For close/+ margin, re-resect or consider post-op RT	LRF: lobectomy 6%, wedge 18% 5-year OS stage I: 70–80%
I–II inoperable	T1-2N0: Definitive SBRT not 3D Consider adjuvant chemo for T2N0 > 4 cm T3N0: Definitive chemo-RT or hypofractionated RT or SBRT T1-2N1: Definitive chemo-RT to 60–66 Gy	SBRT: 2–3-year LC 85–95%, OS 55%
IIIA operable or marginally operable	If candidate for lobectomy and non-bulky N2 disease: Concurrent chemo-RT (45 Gy) → restage → if no progression → surgery → chemo Alternatively, chemo alone → restage → if no progression → surgery → chemo and post-op RT for +margin or N2 disease Otherwise, definitive concurrent chemo-RT (60–66 Gy)	5-year OS 20–25%, MS 16–17 months Induction chemo-RT pCR 15–30% and mediastinal clearance rate ~ 50% Induction chemo pCR 5–10% and mediastinal clearance rate ~ 30–35%
IIIA inoperable	Concurrent chemo-RT (60–66 Gy) If unacceptable risk of pneumonitis with upfront RT, may consider mid-course replanning or alternatively induction chemo for downstaging → concurrent chemo-RT (to postchemo volume) if no progression	~5-year OS and MS Concurrent chemo-RT: 20–25%, 16–17 mo Sequential chemo-RT: 20%, 13–15 mo RT alone: <10%, 10–12 mo

Stage	Recommended treatment	Outcome
IIIB	Concurrent chemo-RT (60–66 Gy) If unacceptable risk of pneumonitis with upfront RT, consider mid-course replanning or alternatively induction chemo for downstaging → concurrent chemo-RT (to postchemo volume) if no progression If T4N0-1, may treat with surgery → chemo ± RT (if +margin or N2), or chemo ± RT → surgery → chemo	
Typical chemo	*Postsurgery* Cisplatin 100 mg/m² d1 and etoposide 100 mg/m² d1–3 every 4 weeks × 4 cycles Other cisplatin combinations with vinorelbine, vinblastine, gemcitabine, pemetrexed, and docetaxel may be considered Alternative if not able to tolerate cisplatin: carboplatin, paclitaxel every 3 weeks for 4 cycles *Concurrent with RT* Cisplatin 50 mg/m² d1, 8, 29, and 36 and etoposide 50 mg/m² d1–5 and 29–33 Carboplatin AUC 2 and paclitaxel 45 mg/m2 weekly then after RT completion, carboplatin AUC 6 and paclitaxel 200 mg/m2 every 3 weeks × 2 cycles Alternatives: cisplatin week 1 and 4, vinblastine weekly; or carboplatin and paclitaxel weekly; or for nonsquamous, cisplatin and pemetrexed *Sequential chemo → RT* Cisplatin 100 mg/m² d1, 29 and vinblastine 5 mg/m² weekly × 5 weeks Alternative: carboplatin and paclitaxel every 3 weeks × 2 cycles *Consolidation chemo after chemo-RT* Carboplatin and paclitaxel every 3 weeks × 2 cycles	
IV	If EGFR mutation or ALK/ROS1 translocation detected, initial therapy with appropriate targeted agent. If PD-L1 tumor expression >50%, pembrolizumab Otherwise: ECOG PS 0–2: platinum-based chemo ± palliative RT ECOG PS 3–4: best supportive care Immune checkpoint inhibitors (anti-PD1, anti-PDL1) for disease progression after a platinum doublet Phase 3 data on combination regimens containing immunotherapy in 1st and subsequent lines are forthcoming	

continued

Stage	Recommended treatment	Outcome
Superior sulcus	If operable or marginally resectable, concurrent chemo-RT (45 Gy) → restage → if no progression → surgery → chemo. If unresectable (initially or after restaging), complete definitive concurrent chemo-RT (60–66 Gy)	50% achieve pCR or minimal microscopic residual after initial chemo-RT. 5-year OS 45%. Most common site failure in brain (40%)
Pulmonary carcinoid	For stage I–III, surgery preferred (lobectomy or other anatomic resection +/– mediastinal LN dissection or sampling). Adjuvant RT considered for atypical histology, involved LN, +margin, subtotal resection. No definite role for chemo since response rate is only 20–30%, but many institutions consider cisplatin/etoposide with RT. For stage III, if surgery is not feasible, definitive RT (for typical) or chemo-RT (for atypical). For stage IV, systemic therapy is used. Octreotide considered if octreotide scan positive or symptoms of carcinoid syndrome	5-year OS: Resected typical carcinoid >70–90% Resected atypical carcinoid: 25–70% Metastatic carcinoid: 20–40%

STUDIES
SCREENING

˒ National Lung Screening Trial (Aberle NEJM 2011): 53,454 patients aged 55–74, current or former smokers with >30 pack-year history randomized to annual CXR vs low-dose CT × 3 years. CT-based screening reduced mortality from lung cancer and from any cause (20% and 6.7% relative improvement, respectively).

SURGERY

˒ For T1–2 N0, surgery has 80–90% LRC and 50–70% CSS. 25–35% percent pathologic upstaging from clinical stage.

˒ Video-assisted thoracoscopic surgery (VATS) + lymphadenectomy may have equivalent oncologic results as open thoracotomy in properly selected cases.

˒ LCSG 821 (Ginsberg, Ann Thorac Surg 1995): 247 patients with peripheral T1 N0 randomized to lobectomy vs wedge resection with a 2 cm margin of normal lung. Wedge resection tripled LRF (6 → 18%).

SBRT

- Indiana (Timmerman JCO 2006; Fakiris, IJROBP 2009): 70 patients with T1–3N0 (≤7 cm) treated with 60–66 Gy in 3 fx over 1–2 weeks. Three-year LC 88%, CSS 82%, OS 43%, regional failure 9%, and distant failure 13%. Patients with central tumors had increased risk of grade 3–5 toxicity (27% vs 10%). Established "no-fly-zone" of 2 cm surrounding proximal bronchial tree for 3-fraction treatment.

- Onishi (Cancer, 2004): 245 patients with T1–2N0 treated with 18–75 Gy in 1–22 fx. LF was 8% for BED ≥100 Gy vs 26% for BED <100 Gy. Three-year OS was 88% for BED ≥100 Gy vs 69% for BED <100 Gy.

- RTOG 0236 (Timmerman 2010): Phase II study of patients with T1–3N0 (≤5 cm) medically inoperable tumors >2 cm from proximal bronchial tree treated with SBRT 20 Gy × 3 over 1.5–2 weeks (54 Gy applying heterogeneity correction). GTV = CTV. PTV = 0.5 cm axial margin and 1 cm superior/inferior margin. 5-year LC 93%, LRC 62%, 31% DM, DFS 26%, OS 40%.

- RTOG 0915 (Videtic IJROBP 2015): Phase II randomized study of 34 Gy in 1 fraction vs 48 Gy in 4 fractions for medically inoperable T1-3N0 (≤5 cm) NSCLC. Single fraction arm had lower risk of serious adverse events (10.3 vs 13.3%). 2-year primary control, OS, and DFS were 97% vs 93%, 61% vs 77%, and 56% vs 71%, respectively.

- RTOG 0618 (Timmerman ASCO 2013): Patients with medically operable T1-T3N0 (≤5 cm) NSCLC >2 cm from proximal bronchial tree treated with 60 Gy in 3 fractions (54 Gy with heterogeneity correction). 2-year primary failure rate 7.8%, local failure (including ipsilateral lobe) 19.2%, OS 84%. 16% grade 3 toxicity.

- RTOG 0813 (Bezjak ASTRO 2016) Phase I/II dose escalation trial for medically inoperable early-stage NSCLC with centrally located lesions (<2 cm from the bronchial tree). Dose escalated from 50 Gy in 5 fractions to 60 Gy in 5 fractions. 38 pts 57.5 Gy, 33 pts 60 Gy. 2 yr LC 88–89%, PFS 52–55%, OS 70–73%, grade 3 toxicity 6–7%.

- VUMC (Senthi, Lancet Oncol 2012). 676 pts with PET+ clinical stage T1–2 N0 NSCLC. 65% no histology attained. 2/5-yr LF 5/11%, regional failure 8/13%, DM 15/20%. Earlier report from same institution (Verstegen, Radiother Oncol 2011) compared 209 pts with pathologic

IV

confirmation vs 382 with clinical diagnosis only treated with SBRT and reported no difference in LC, regional control, DM, or OS, suggesting that SBRT results are unlikely to be biased substantially by inclusion of benign lesions.

SBRT VS SURGERY

- Two randomized trials of surgery vs SBRT for operable early-stage NSCLC failed to accrue (STARS and ROSEL).
- Combined ROSEL/STARS analysis (Chang Lancet Oncol 2015): 58 patients from two trials with T1-T2 (<4 cm) N0 medically operable NSCLC. Randomized to SBRT (54 Gy in 3 fractions, 50 Gy in 4 fractions if central) vs lobectomy and mediastinal lymph node dissection. 3-year OS improved for SBRT (95%) vs surgery (79%). Grade 3–4 toxicity 10% for SBRT vs 44% for surgery.
- New randomized trials: JoLT-Ca STABLE-MATES trial (NCT02468024), VALOR (Veterans Affairs Lung cancer surgery Or stereotactic Radiotherapy trial, NCT02984761) in the United States, SABRTOOTH (NCT02629458) in the United Kingdom.

PERIOPERATIVE CHEMOTHERAPY

- Multiple trials report that adjuvant chemotherapy after surgery improves survival for LN+ (stage II–III disease) and high-risk IB tumors >4 cm.
  - LACE (Pignon JCO 2008): Meta-analysis of 5 largest adjuvant chemotherapy trials (>4000 patients). 5.4% absolute overall survival benefit at 5 years with the addition of chemotherapy. Benefit most pronounced in stage II/III disease.
- Several trials also report that preoperative chemo is beneficial for stage II–III disease.
  - Meta-analysis (Song, J Thorac Oncol 2010) of 13 randomized trials reported that preoperative chemo improved survival vs surgery alone.
- Some studies suggest that preoperative chemo is as effective and better tolerated than adjuvant chemo, but a randomized trial for early-stage disease found no survival or quality of life difference (Westeel, Eur J Cancer 2013).

PRE-OP RT

, There is no improvement in survival with pre-op RT alone (without chemo) as noted in two collaborative studies from 1970s (VA and NCI).

, ASTRO guideline (Rodrigues, PRO 2015):

, There is no level 1 evidence for pre-op chemo-RT (≥45 Gy) for operable pts, but it may be considered for pts with minimal N2 disease, treatable with lobectomy, with good PS, and no/minimal weight loss.

, Pre-op chemo-RT is recommended for resectable superior sulcus tumors.

, German trial (Thomas, Lancet Oncol 2008): 524 patients with IIIA/IIIB (69% IIIB) treated with neoadjuvant cisplatin/etoposide × 3c, then randomized to pre-op hyperfractionated chemo-RT vs immediate surgery → post-op RT. Pre-op chemo-RT was 1.5 b.i.d./45 Gy with carboplatin/vindesine × 3c → surgery if possible → RT boost (1.5 b.i.d./24 Gy) if inoperable or R1/R2 resection. Post-op RT was 1.8/54 Gy or 1.8/68.4 Gy if inoperable or R1/R2 resection.

, No difference in 5-year OS or PFS (16% vs 14%).

, Pre-op chemo-RT increased complete resection rates (37% vs 32%), and in those with complete resection, increased mediastinal downstaging (46% vs 29%).

, Pre-op chemo-RT increased G3-4 hematologic toxicity and esophagitis, and was associated with 14% treatment-related mortality in pts undergoing pneumonectomy.

POST-OP RT

, Historically, post-op RT (PORT) utilized large fields covering comprehensive nodal fields. Multiple older studies showed no survival benefit to PORT, and PORT meta-analysis (Lancet 1998, 2005) showed a survival detriment, leading to PORT falling out of favor. Analysis criticized because 25% of patients were N0, many pts were treated with Co-60, older studies used inadequate staging, and unpublished data were included.

IV

- PORT is detrimental for pN0-1 pts with negative margins.
- Recent data suggest benefit of modern linear accelerator PORT for pN2 pts:
  - *SEER* (Lally JCO 2006): 7465 patients with stage II–III resected NSCLC, 48% received PORT. PORT used most often for patients <50 years, T3–4, larger T size, increased N stage. PORT improved 5-year OS for N2 patients (20 → 27%, HR 0.85), but reduced OS for N0 (41 → 31%, HR 1.2), and N1 (34 → 30%, HR 1.1) patients.
  - ANITA subgroup analysis (Douillard IJROBP 2008): Retrospective analysis of data from ANITA adjuvant chemotherapy trial. 232 of 840 patients on the trial received PORT. Median survival detriment to PORT seen in pN1 patients receiving chemo (94 → 47 months), but improved MS in pN1 not receiving chemo (26 → 50 months) and for pN2 regardless of chemo (24 → 47 months for if chemo, 12 → 13 months if no chemo). PORT reduced local/regional failure (first site) for both N1 and N2 patients.
  - National Cancer Database – N2 (Robinson JCO 2015): 4483 pts with pN2 disease, 48% underwent PORT, all received adjuvant chemo. PORT improved 5-year OS (35% → 39%) and remained prognostic of OS on multivariate analysis.
  - Patel (Lung Cancer 2014). Review of 3 prospective and 8 retrospective studies of 2728 N2 pts treated with linear accelerator PORT or not. PORT improved OS and locoregional recurrence free survival.
  - Lung ART (EORTC 22055–08053, ongoing): Randomizes patients with resected N2 disease to post-op conformal RT 54 Gy vs observation. Pre-op or post-op chemo allowed before RT, but not concurrent with RT.
- ASTRO guideline (Rodrigues, PRO 2015):
  - PORT (50–54 Gy) after R0 resection for pN2 pts should be delivered sequentially after adjuvant chemo.
  - PORT (54–60 Gy) may be considered after R1 resection or for extracapsular nodal extension, with either concurrent or sequential chemo.

, National Cancer Database – Positive Margins (Wang JCO 2015): 3395 pts with positive margins after surgery, 36% underwent PORT, all received adjuvant chemo. PORT improved 5-year OS (24% → 32%) and remained prognostic of OS on MVA.

, PORT (at least 60 Gy) is indicated after R2 resection, with concurrent or sequential chemo.

ROLE OF SURGERY FOR N2 PTS

IV

, The role of surgery for N2 disease is controversial, but this population is heterogeneous and there could be a benefit for selected pts [e.g., single station N2 nodes <3 cm, planned lobectomy (vs pneumonectomy), good PS, no/minimal weight loss, or other subsets].

, Intergroup/RTOG 0139 (Albain, Lancet 2009): 396 patients with T1–3pN2M0 treated with concurrent chemo × 2c + 45 Gy → restaging → randomized to [surgery (if no progression) → chemo × 2c] vs [concurrent chemo-RT to 61 Gy (no surgery)) → chemo × 2c]. Chemo was cisplatinum and etoposide. Surgery improved 5-year PFS (11% → 22%) and median PFS (10.5 → 12.8 months) with fewer local-only relapses (10% vs 22%). There was no significant difference in MS (23.6 vs 22.2 months, $p = 0.24$), although there was a 5-year OS trend in favor of surgery (20% vs 27%, $p = 0.1$). Increased treatment-related deaths with surgery (8% vs 2%), particularly when pneumonectomy required. 14% pCR rate, with 42% 5-year OS if pCR. In unplanned exploratory subgroup analysis, MS was improved for pts undergoing lobectomy compared to matched cohort undergoing nonoperative treatment (MS 22 → 33 months).

, EORTC 08941 (Van Meerbeeck, JNCI 2007): 579 patients with initially unresectable pIIIA(N2) disease treated with induction cisplatin-based chemo. 332 patients (61%) showing response randomized to surgery or definitive RT. Post-op RT (56 Gy) given to 40% of pts with an incomplete resection. pCR was 5%, and 47% had pneumonectomy. 4% surgical mortality. Definitive RT was to tumor and involved mediastinum to 60–62 Gy with 46 Gy to uninvolved mediastinum. One RT patient died of RT pneumonitis. No difference in MS (16–17 months) or PFS

(9–11 months). Fewer local/regional failures (32% vs 55%), but more DM (61% vs 39%) with surgery. Patients with pneumonectomy, incomplete resection, or persistent pN2 disease fared worst.

, ESPATUE (Eberhardt JCO 2015): 246 patients with resectable IIIA(N2) or IIIB disease (70% IIIB) received induction chemo (cisplatin/paclitaxel x 3c) → chemo-RT (45 Gy/1.5 Gy BID with cisplatin/vinorelbine). Patients then randomized to surgery (2/3 received lobectomy) vs chemo-RT boost (20 Gy in 10 fractions with cisplatin/vinorelbine). Trial closed early due to non-accrual. No significant difference in 5-year PFS (32–35%) or OS (40–44%). 33% pCR rate in surgery arm.

DEFINITIVE RT AND CHEMO FOR LOCALLY ADVANCED NSCLC

, ASTRO has published a practice guideline for locally advanced NSCLC (Rodrigues PRO 2015).
, *RT alone*: MS 10–12 months, 5-year OS 7%.
 , RT alone is superior to observation or chemo alone at the cost of side effects (e.g., esophagitis, pneumonitis).
 , Consider for pts not eligible for chemo (e.g., poor PS, comorbidities, extensive weight loss, or pt preference).
 , Dose options: 60 Gy/30 fx, 45 Gy/15 fx (hypofractionation), 54 Gy/36 fx TID (CHART), 60 Gy/40 fx TID (CHARTWEL).
, *Sequential chemo → RT*: MS 13–15 months, 5-year OS 20%
 , For pts who cannot tolerate concurrent chemo-RT, sequential chemo-RT improves survival vs RT alone [e.g., CALGB 8433 (Dillman, NEJM 1990) and RTOG 8808 (Sause, Chest 2000)].
 , With sequential chemo and RT, optimal RT dose is unknown, although accelerated hyperfractionated RT (CHARTWEL 60 Gy/40 fx TID over 18 days) may improve LC vs standard RT (66 Gy/33 fx over 6.5 wks) at cost of toxicity.
, *Concurrent chemo-RT*: MS 16–17 months, 5-year OS 20–30%.
 , Multiple randomized studies report improved survival, local control, and response rate with concurrent over sequential treatment. For example:

RTOG 9410 (Curran, JNCI 2011). 610 pts with unresectable or inoperable II/III (98% III) treated with sequential cisplatin/vinblastine then 63 Gy vs concurrent cisplatin/vinblastine +63 Gy QD vs concurrent cisplatin/etoposide +69.6 Gy / 1.2 Gy BID. Concurrent chemo-RT improved MS: 14.6 mo vs 17 mo vs 15.2 mo, respectively.

Auperin (JCO 2010): Meta-analysis of 1205 patients from six trials undergoing sequential vs concurrent chemo-RT. Sequential treatment improved 5-year OS (15% vs 10%) and 5-year PFS (16% vs 13%) at the cost of increased esophageal toxicity (grade 3+ esophagitis 18% vs 4%). No difference in pulmonary toxicity.

IV

- There is no proven role for induction chemo before chemo-RT, although it may be considered for bulky tumors to allow for RT planning after chemo response

  CALGB 39801 (Vokes, JCO 2007): 366 patients with unresectable IIIA/IIIB randomized to concurrent weekly carbo-Taxol chemo + RT (66 Gy) vs induction carbo-Taxol q3 weeks × 2c → same concurrent chemo-RT. No difference in MS (12–14 months) or OS. Induction chemo increased toxicity (20% grade 3–4 neutropenia).

- There is no proven role for consolidation chemo after chemo-RT, but it is routinely given for potential micrometastatic disease if full systemic chemo doses were not delivered during RT.

- Dose escalation beyond 60 Gy with conventional fractionation has not demonstrated any clinical benefit with concurrent chemo.

  RTOG 0617 (Bradley, Lancet Oncol 2015): 544 patients with inoperable IIIA/IIIB treated with concurrent chemo-RT carboplatin/Taxol underwent 2x2 randomization to 60 vs 74 Gy, and +/− weekly cetuximab. All patients received 2 cycles consolidation carboplatin/Taxol. Trial closed early due to interim analysis showing futility for survival endpoint. 74 Gy arm had decreased MS (20 mo vs 28 mo), nonsignificantly higher local failure (39% vs 31%), and worse grade 3+ esophagitis (43% vs 16%). Cetuximab did not improve OS but had increased toxicity. Reason for survival detriment hotly debated; possible explanations include decreased tumor coverage in 74 Gy arm, low volume centers' lack of expertise (Eaton JNCI 2016), increased acute or late toxicity, decreased quality of life in 74 Gy arm. IMRT produced similar local control and 2-year survival but lower rates of severe pneumonitis and cardiac dose (Chun JCO 2017).

, RTOG 1106 (ongoing): Randomized phase III trial comparing standard concurrent chemo-RT to 60 Gy vs concurrent chemo with adaptive dose escalation to 66–80.4 Gy, with doses constrained by mean lung dose <20 Gy.

SUPERIOR SULCUS

, SWOG 9416/Int 0160 (Rusch 2001): phase II trial of 111 patients with T3–4N0–1 superior sulcus tumors treated with concurrent chemo-RT (45 Gy) → restaging → surgery (if no progression) → chemo × 2c. Chemo was platinum/etoposide. If progression on restaging, complete definitive chemo-RT to 63 Gy without surgery. 86% of patients had surgery. 56% had pCR or minimal microscopic residual disease. The most common site of relapse was in the brain.

PROPHYLACTIC CRANIAL RT (PCI)

, Brain is the site of failure for ~15% of early-stage patients and >15% for advanced stage patients. Three older randomized trials have investigated PCI in advanced NSCLC. PCI delayed and reduced the incidence of brain failure, but had no impact on OS. Extracranial disease was the cause of death for most patients, and may be a source of CNS re-seeding after PCI.

, RTOG 0214 (Gore JCO 2011): 356 patients with definitively treated stage IIIA/B disease randomized to prophylactic cranial RT (30 Gy/15 fractions) or observation. No difference in 1-year OS or DFS, but PCI reduced rate of brain metastasis at 1 year (8% vs 18%).

RADIATION TECHNIQUES

SIMULATION AND FIELD DESIGN

- Simulate patient supine with arms up.
- Immobilize with a wingboard, body cradle, or SBRT immobilization device (with arms up).
- 4DCT to account for respiratory motion.
- Use a 3D conformal or IMRT plan.
  - IMRT associated with decreased pneumonitis risk (Yom IJROBP 2007, Chun JCO 2017).
- Favor 6–10 MV photons over higher energies, which can cause underdosing in regions of electronic disequilibrium such as the tumor/lung interface.
- GTV: gross primary and nodal disease, including LN(s) ≥1 cm or hypermetabolic on PET scan or harboring tumor cells per mediastinoscopy.
- CTV: typically includes the GTV plus 5–10 mm margin.
  - Giraud (IJROBP 2000): 6–8 mm margin required to cover 95% of microscopic disease.
- PTV: add 5–10 mm margin to CTV depending on respiratory motion management.
- Respiratory tracking or gating systems or 4D CT planning to generate ITV may allow for decreased PTV margins.
- Comprehensive elective nodal RT generally not recommended due to low observed rates of failure in uninvolved nodes without elective treatment:
  - MSKCC (Rosenzweig JCO 2007): 524 patients with NSCLC treated with 3DCRT to only tumor and histologically or radiographically involved LN regions. No elective nodal RT. Only 6% of patients developed failure in an initially uninvolved LN region in the absence of local failure. Many patients experienced treatment failure in multiple LN regions simultaneously.
  - Yuan (AJCO 2007): 200 patients with inoperable stage III disease. Randomized to elective nodal RT to 60–64 Gy vs IFRT to 68–74%. IFRT improved 5-year local control (51% vs 36%) and decreased rate of pneumonitis (17% vs 29%).
  - At UCSF, we commonly treat involved nodal station + immediately adjacent nodal stations felt to be at highest risk for subclinical disease.

IV

, Post-op RT:
  , If N2 and margins are negative:
    , CTV = Involved LN region ± paratracheal ± ipsilateral hilum ± subcarinal LN regions to 50.4 Gy depending on the extent of node dissection, number, bulk, and location of mediastinal disease and primary tumor; wide variations seen in Lung ART contouring study (Spoelstra IJROBP 2010).
  , If + margin: favor initial post-op chemo-RT or RT → adjuvant chemo. Limit field to area of +margin if N0–1 disease (i.e., no elective mediastinal nodal coverage).
  , If gross residual disease: recommend concurrent chemo-RT to 60–66 Gy.

DEFINITIVE RT DOSE PRESCRIPTIONS

, Stage I SBRT: Several dose/fractionation regimens have been published. At UCSF we typically give 50 Gy in 5 fractions for central/chest wall lesions, or 54 Gy in 3 fractions for peripheral lesions not abutting chest wall, with heterogeneity corrections. See NCCN guidelines for other 1–5 fraction SBRT schemes and dose constraints:
  , To account for or reduce internal motion, respiratory gating, active breath holding techniques, and/or abdominal compression may be used.
  , For planning, the GTV = CTV. ITV generated from 4DCT if real-time tumor tracking not performed. PTV = ITV + 5 mm.
  , Generally treat every other day, particularly if central lesion or abutting chest wall.
, Stage II–III
  , Primary and involved LN: 60–66 Gy at 1.8–2 Gy per fraction with chemo.
  , May consider treating up to 77.4 Gy without concurrent chemo (keep $V20 \leq 35\%$).
  , When chemo will not be tolerated, consider hypofractionated (e.g., 45 Gy at 3 Gy/fx) (Fig. 15.2).

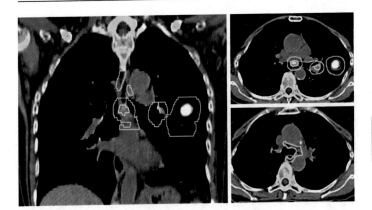

Fig. 15.2 Example contours for preoperative RT for patient with cT1N2 NSCLC with single subcarinal lymph node on PET. GTV shown in *pink* (primary) and *yellow* (nodal disease), with CTV in *blue* (primary) and *green* (nodal disease). CTVs encompass 7 mm margin on gross disease, with elective coverage of adjacent nodal regions (8: Paraesophageal, 4: Pretracheal). Prescriptions was 45 Gy in 25 fractions

NEOADJUVANT AND ADJUVANT RT DOSE PRESCRIPTIONS

- Preoperative: 45 Gy
- Postoperative:
  - If N2: 50.4 Gy
  - If ECE or +margin, boost to 54–60 Gy
  - If gross residual tumor, boost to 60–66 Gy (Fig. 15.3)

PALLIATIVE RT DOSE PRESCRIPTION

- ASTRO guideline (Rodrigues, PRO 2011): 30 Gy/10 fx or greater equivalent preferred over shorter courses (e.g., 20 Gy/5 fx, 17 Gy/2 weekly fx, 10 Gy/1 fx) for pts with good PS

DOSE LIMITATIONS
Standard Fractionation

- Spinal cord:
  - RT alone: maximum dose <50 Gy.
  - Chemo-RT: maximum dose <46 Gy at 1.8–2 Gy/fx QD or <36 Gy with bid RT.

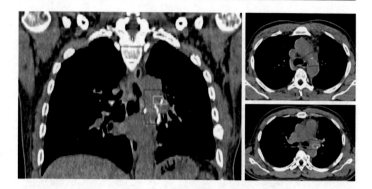

Fig. 15.3 Example contours for postoperative RT for patient with cT2aN1 NSCLC found to have single level 5 node at surgery (pT2aN2). Location of involved node shown in *blue*, with CTV shown in *purple* encompassing level 5 (AP window) and adjacent levels (4: Pretracheal, 6: Para-aortic). Prescription was 50 Gy in 25 fractions

- Lung:
  - Combined volume of both normal lungs receiving ≥20 Gy (V20): <35%.
  - Mean lung dose: <20 Gy.
  - Utility of V5 controversial, with data from RTOG 0617 suggesting a lack of prognostic value. V5 < 65% if used
  - Pneumonitis grading
    - Grade 1: asymptomatic radiographic changes.
    - Grade 2: changes requiring steroids or diuretics; dyspnea on exertion.
    - Grade 3: requires oxygen; shortness of breath at rest.
    - Grade 4: requires assisted ventilation.
    - Grade 5: death.
- Esophagus:
  - Maximum dose <105% of prescription dose
  - Mean < 34 Gy.
- Heart: V40 < 80%, V45 < 60%, V60 < 30%, Mean < 35 Gy.
- Pacemakers/internal cardiac defibrillators (ICD):
  - Increased risk of pacemaker malfunction at ~2 Gy, depending on manufacturer and model. Assess level of patient's dependence on device. Attempt to get RT tolerance specifications from manufacturer. Contour device and exclude it from radiation field. Determine actual dose with radiation dosimeter. If total dose >2 Gy, move out of field.

, Use energy <10 MV based on increased rates of malfunction with neutron-producing RT (Grant JAMA Oncol 2015).
, ICDs can be more sensitive to radiation than pacemakers. Consider deactivating ICD during RT and replace as needed with ECD (external cardiac defibrillator, temporary).
, Cardiology (electrophysiology) should evaluate and interrogate pacemaker/ICD before, weekly during RT, and immediately after RT.
, Have CPR equipment available. Monitoring of vital signs advisable during RT.
, Netherlands has published a guideline for pacemaker/ICD pts (Hurkmans, Radiation Oncology 2012)
, Brachial plexus: maximum dose <66 Gy.

SBRT
, See TG-101(Benedict Med Phys 2010) and NCCN guidelines for full constraints for 1, 3 and 5 fractions.
, Spinal cord: Dmax <18 Gy (3 fx) or <30 Gy (5 fx).
, Trachea/proximal bronchial tree: Dmax <30 Gy (3 fx) or <105% of PTV prescription (5 fx).
, Brachial Plexus: Dmax <24 Gy (3 fx) or <32 Gy (5 fx).
, Heart/pericardium: Dmax <30 Gy (3 fx) or <105% of PTV prescription (5 fx).
, Great vessels: <105% of PTV prescription (5 fx).
, Esophagus: <27 Gy (3 fx) or <105% of PTV prescription (5 fx).
, Rib: <30 Gy (3 fx).
, Skin: <24 Gy (3 fx) or 32 Gy (5 fx).

COMPLICATIONS
, Acute RT complications include fatigue, esophagitis, dermatitis, and/or cough.
, Subacute and late complications include pneumonitis, pericarditis, pulmonary fibrosis, bronchial or esophageal stricture, brachial plexopathy, rib fracture or intercostal nerve pain.
, Radiation pneumonitis occurs ~6 weeks after RT. It presents with cough, dyspnea, hypoxia, and fever. Treat symptomatic radiation pneumonitis with prednisone (1 mg/kg/d) or 60 mg/day and trimethoprim/sulfamethoxazole for PCP

prophylaxis. Often produces dramatic and quick response in symptoms, but very gradual and prolonged taper (>12 weeks) is critical for durable symptom resolution.

FOLLOW-UP

- H&P and chest CT every 3–6 months for 3 years, then annually.
- For patients after peripheral SBRT, low-dose non-contrast CT sufficient.
  - Solid mass-like component commonly seen 6–12 months after SBRT due to inflammation/scarring, easily confused for recurrence. Follow with short interval CT to assess for resolution.

Acknowledgment We thank Siavash Jabbari MD, Eric K. Hansen MD, and Daphne A. Haas-Kogan MD for their work on the prior edition of this chapter.

REFERENCES

Albain KS, Swann RS, Rusch VW, Turrisi AT, Shepherd FA, Smith C, et al. Radiotherapy plus chemotherapy with or without surgical resection for stage III non-small-cell lung cancer: a phase III randomised controlled trial. Lancet. 2009;374(9687):379–86.

Andre F, Grunenwald D, Pignon JP, Dujon A, Pujol JL, Brichon PY, et al. Survival of patients with resected N2 non-small-cell lung cancer: evidence for a subclassification and implications. J Clin Oncol. 2000;18(16):2981–9.

Aupérin A, Le Péchoux C, Rolland E, Curran WJ, Furuse K, Fournel P, et al. Meta-analysis of concomitant versus sequential radiochemotherapy in locally advanced non-small-cell lung cancer. J Clin Oncol. 2010;28(13):2181–90.

Benedict SH, Yenice KM, Followill D, Galvin JM, Hinson W, Kavanagh B, et al. Stereotactic body radiation therapy: the report of AAPM task group 101. Med Phys. 2010;37(8):4078–101.

Bezjak A, Paulus R, Gaspar LE, Timmerman RD, Straube WL, Ryan WF, et al. Primary study endpoint analysis for NRG Oncology/RTOG 0813 trial of stereotactic body radiation therapy (SBRT) for centrally located non-small cell lung cancer (NSCLC). Int J Radiat Oncol Biol Phys. 2016;94(1):5–6.

Bradley JD, Paulus R, Komaki R, Masters G, Blumenschein G, Schild S, et al. Standard-dose versus high-dose conformal radiotherapy with concurrent and consolidation carboplatin plus paclitaxel with or without cetuximab for patients with stage IIIA or IIIB non-small-cell lung cancer (RTOG 0617): a randomised, two-by-two factorial phase 3 study. Lancet Oncol. 2015;16(2):187–99.

Chang JY, Senan S, Paul MA, Mehran RJ, Louie AV, Balter P, et al. Stereotactic ablative radiotherapy versus lobectomy for operable stage I non-small-cell lung cancer: a pooled analysis of two randomised trials. Lancet Oncol. 2015;16:630–7.

Chun SG, Hu C, Choy H, et al. Impact of Intensity-Modulated Radiation Therapy Technique for Locally Advanced Non-Small-Cell Lung Cancer: A Secondary Analysis of the NRG Oncology RTOG 0617 Randomized Clinical Trial. Journal of Clinical Oncology. 2017;35(1):56–62.

Curran WJ, Paulus R, Langer CJ, Komaki R, Lee JS, Hauser S, et al. Sequential vs concurrent chemoradiation for stage III non-small cell lung cancer: randomized phase III trial RTOG 9410. J Natl Cancer Inst. 2011;103(19):1452–7.

Dillman RO, Seagren SL, Propert KJ, Guerra J, Eaton WL, Perry MC, et al. A randomized trial of induction chemotherapy plus high-dose radiation versus radiation alone in stage III non-small-cell lung cancer. N Engl J Med. 1990;323(14):940–5.

Douillard J-Y, Rosell R, De Lena M, Riggi M, Hurteloup P, Mahe M-A, Adjuvant Navelbine International Trialist Association. Impact of postoperative radiation therapy on survival in patients with complete resection and stage I, II, or IIIA non-small-cell lung cancer treated with adjuvant chemotherapy: the adjuvant Navelbine International Trialist Association (ANITA) randomized trial. Int J Radiat Oncol Biol Phys. 2008;72(3):695–701.

Eaton BR, Pugh SL, Bradley JD, et al. Institutional Enrollment and Survival Among NSCLC Patients Receiving Chemoradiation: NRG Oncology Radiation Therapy Oncology Group (RTOG) 0617. J Natl Cancer Inst. 2016;108(9).

Eberhardt WEE, Pöttgen C, Gauler TC, Friedel G, Veit S, Heinrich V, et al. Phase III study of surgery versus definitive concurrent chemoradiotherapy boost in patients with resectable stage IIIA(N2) and selected IIIB non-small-cell lung cancer after induction chemotherapy and concurrent chemoradiotherapy (ESPATUE). J Clin Oncol. 2015;33(35):4194–201.

Fakiris AJ, McGarry RC, Yiannoutsos CT, Papiez L, Williams M, Henderson MA, Timmerman R. Stereotactic body radiation therapy for early-stage non-small-cell lung carcinoma: four-year results of a prospective phase II study. Int J Radiat Oncol Biol Phys. 2009;75(3):677–82.

Ginsberg RJ, Rubinstein LV. Randomized trial of lobectomy versus limited resection for T1 N0 non-small cell lung cancer. Ann Thorac Surg. 1995;60(3):615–23.

Giraud P, Antoine M, Larrouy A, Milleron B, Callard P, De Rycke Y, et al. Evaluation of microscopic tumor extension in non-small-cell lung cancer for three-dimensional conformal radiotherapy planning. Int J Radiat Oncol Biol Phys. 2000;48(4):1015–24.

Gore EM, Bae K, Wong SJ, Sun A, Bonner JA, Schild SE, et al. Phase III comparison of prophylactic cranial irradiation versus observation in patients with locally advanced non-small-cell lung cancer: primary analysis of radiation therapy oncology group study RTOG 0214. J Clin Oncol. 2011;29(3):272–8.

Gould MK, Kuschner WG, Rydzak CE, Maclean CC, Demas AN, Shigemitsu H, et al. Test performance of positron emission tomography and computed tomography for mediastinal staging in patients with non-small-cell lung cancer: a meta-analysis. Ann Intern Med. 2003;139(11):879–92.

Grant JD, Jensen GL, Tang C, et al. Radiotherapy-Induced Malfunction in Contemporary Cardiovascular Implantable Electronic Devices: Clinical Incidence and Predictors. JAMA Oncol. 2015;1(5):624–32.

Hurkmans CW, Knegjens JL, Oei BS, Maas AJJ, Uiterwaal GJ, van der Borden AJ, et al. Management of radiation oncology patients with a pacemaker or ICD: a new comprehensive practical guideline in The Netherlands. Dutch Society of Radiotherapy and Oncology (NVRO). Radiat Oncol. 2012;7:198.

Lally BE. Postoperative radiotherapy for stage II or III non-small-cell lung cancer using the surveillance, epidemiology, and end results database. J Clin Oncol. 2006;24(19):2998–3006.

Lynch R, Pitson G, Ball D, Claude L, Sarrut D. Computed tomographic atlas for the new international lymph node map for lung cancer: a radiation oncologist perspective. Pract Radiat Oncol. 2013;3(1):54–66.

IV

National Lung Screening Trial Research Team, Aberle DR, Adams AM, Berg CD, Black WC, Clapp JD, et al. Reduced lung-cancer mortality with low-dose computed tomographic screening. N Engl J Med. 2011;365(5):395–409.

Onishi H, Araki T, Shirato H, Nagata Y, Hiraoka M, Gomi K, et al. Stereotactic hypofractionated high-dose irradiation for stage I nonsmall cell lung carcinoma: clinical outcomes in 245 subjects in a Japanese multiinstitutional study. Cancer. 2004;101(7):1623–31.

Patel SH, Ma Y, Wernicke AG, Nori D, Chao KSC, Parashar B. Evidence supporting contemporary post-operative radiation therapy (PORT) using linear accelerators in N2 lung cancer. Lung Cancer. 2014;84(2):156–60.

Pignon J-P, Tribodet H, Scagliotti GV, Douillard J-Y, Shepherd FA, Stephens RJ, et al. Lung adjuvant cisplatin evaluation: a pooled analysis by the LACE collaborative group. J Clin Oncol. 2008;26(21):3552–9.

PORT Meta-analysis Trialists Group. Postoperative radiotherapy in non-small-cell lung cancer: systematic review and meta-analysis of individual patient data from nine randomised controlled trials. PORT Meta-analysis Trialists Group. Lancet. 1998;352(9124):257–63.

PORT Meta-analysis Trialists Group. Postoperative radiotherapy for non-small cell lung cancer. Cochrane Database Syst Rev. 2005;2:CD002142.

Robinson CG, Patel AP, Bradley JD, DeWees T, Waqar SN, Morgensztern D, et al. Postoperative radiotherapy for pathologic N2 non-small-cell lung cancer treated with adjuvant chemotherapy: a review of the National Cancer Data Base. J Clin Oncol. 2015;33(8):870–6.

Rodrigues G, Videtic GMM, Sur R, Bezjak A, Bradley J, Hahn CA, et al. Palliative thoracic radiotherapy in lung cancer: an American Society for Radiation Oncology evidence-based clinical practice guideline. Pract Radiat Oncol. 2011;1(2):60–71.

Rodrigues G, Choy H, Bradley J, Rosenzweig KE, Bogart J, Curran WJ Jr, et al. Definitive radiation therapy in locally advanced non-small cell lung cancer: executive summary of an American Society for Radiation Oncology (ASTRO) evidence-based clinical practice guideline. Pract Radiat Oncol. 2015;5(3):141–8.

Rosenzweig KE, Sura S, Jackson A, Yorke E. Involved-field radiation therapy for inoperable non small-cell lung cancer. J Clin Oncol. 2007;25(35):5557–61.

Rusch VW, Giroux DJ, Kraut MJ, Crowley J, Hazuka M, Johnson D, et al. Induction chemoradiation and surgical resection for non-small cell lung carcinomas of the superior sulcus: initial results of Southwest Oncology Group Trial 9416 (Intergroup Trial 0160). J Thorac Cardiovasc Surg. 2001;121(3):472–83.

Rusch VW, Asamura H, Watanabe H, Giroux DJ, Rami-Porta R, Goldstraw P, Members of IASLC Staging Committee. The IASLC lung cancer staging project: a proposal for a new international lymph node map in the forthcoming seventh edition of the TNM classification of lung cancer. J Thorac Oncol. 2009;4(5):568–77.

Sause W, Kolesar P, Taylor SIV, Johnson D, Livingston R, Komaki R, et al. Final results of phase III trial in regionally advanced unresectable non-small cell lung cancer: radiation therapy oncology group, eastern cooperative oncology group, and southwest oncology group. Chest. 2000;117(2):358–64.

Schmidt-Hansen M, Baldwin DR, Hasler E, Zamora J, Abraira V, Roqué I, Figuls M. PET-CT for assessing mediastinal lymph node involvement in patients with suspected resectable non-small cell lung cancer. Cochrane Database Syst Rev. 2014;11:CD009519.

Senthi S, Lagerwaard FJ, Haasbeek CJA, Slotman BJ, Senan S. Patterns of disease recurrence after stereotactic ablative radiotherapy for early stage non-small-cell lung cancer: a retrospective analysis. Lancet Oncol. 2012;13(8):802–9.

Song W-A, Zhou N-K, Wang W, Chu X-Y, Liang C-Y, Tian X-D, et al. Survival benefit of neoadjuvant chemotherapy in non-small cell lung cancer: an updated meta-analysis of 13 randomized control trials. J Thorac Oncol. 2010;5(4):510–6.

Thomas M, Rübe C, Hoffknecht P, Macha HN, Freitag L, Linder A, et al. Effect of preoperative chemoradiation in addition to preoperative chemotherapy: a randomised trial in stage III non-small-cell lung cancer. Lancet Oncol. 2008;9(7):636–48.

Timmerman R, McGarry R, Yiannoutsos C, Papiez L, Tudor K, DeLuca J, et al. Excessive toxicity when treating central tumors in a phase II study of stereotactic body radiation therapy for medically inoperable early-stage lung cancer. J Clin Oncol. 2006;24(30):4833–9.

Timmerman R, Paulus R, Galvin J, Michalski J, Straube W, Bradley J, et al. Stereotactic body radiation therapy for inoperable early stage lung cancer. JAMA. 2010;303(11):1070–6.

Timmerman R, Paulus R, Pass H, Gore E, Edelman M, Galvin J, et al. Stereotactic body radiation therapy (SBRT) to treat operable early-stage lung cancer patients. J Clin Oncol. 2013;31:(suppl; abstr 7523).

van Meerbeeck JP, Kramer GWPM, Van Schil PEY, Legrand C, Smit EF, Schramel F, et al. Randomized controlled trial of resection versus radiotherapy after induction chemotherapy in stage IIIA-N2 non-small-cell lung cancer. J Natl Cancer Inst. 2007;99(6):442–50.

Verstegen NE, Lagerwaard FJ, Haasbeek CJA, Slotman BJ, Senan S. Outcomes of stereotactic ablative radiotherapy following a clinical diagnosis of stage I NSCLC: comparison with a contemporaneous cohort with pathologically proven disease. Radiother Oncol. 2011;101(2):250–4.

Videtic GMM, Hu C, Singh AK, Chang JY, Parker W, Olivier KR, et al. A randomized phase 2 study comparing 2 stereotactic body radiation therapy schedules for medically inoperable patients with stage I peripheral non-small cell lung cancer: NRG oncology RTOG 0915 (NCCTG N0927). Int J Radiat Oncol Biol Phys. 2015;93(4):757–64.

Vokes EE, Herndon JE, Kelley MJ, Cicchetti MG, Ramnath N, Neill H, et al. Induction chemotherapy followed by chemoradiotherapy compared with chemoradiotherapy alone for regionally advanced unresectable stage III non-small-cell lung cancer: cancer and leukemia group B. J Clin Oncol. 2007;25(13):1698–704.

Wang EH, Corso CD, Rutter CE, Park HS, Chen AB, Kim AW, et al. Postoperative radiation therapy is associated with improved overall survival in incompletely resected stage II and III non-small-cell lung cancer. J Clin Oncol. 2015;33:2727–34.

Werner-Wasik M, Scott C, Cox JD, Sause WT, Byhardt RW, Asbell S, et al. Recursive partitioning analysis of 1999 radiation therapy oncology group (RTOG) patients with locally-advanced non-small-cell lung cancer (LA-NSCLC): identification of five groups with different survival. Int J Radiat Oncol Biol Phys. 2000;48(5):1475–82.

Westeel V, Quoix E, Puyraveau M, Lavolé A, Braun D, Laporte S, et al. A randomised trial comparing preoperative to perioperative chemotherapy in early-stage non-small-cell lung cancer (IFCT 0002 trial). Eur J Cancer. 2013;49(12):2654–64.

Yom SS, Liao Z, Liu HH, Tucker SL, Hu C-S, Wei X, et al. Initial evaluation of treatment-related pneumonitis in advanced-stage non-small-cell lung cancer patients treated with concurrent chemotherapy and intensity-modulated radiotherapy. Int J Radiat Oncol Biol Phys. 2007;68(1):94–102. https://doi.org/10.1016/j.ijrobp.2006.12.031.

Yuan S, Sun X, Li M, Yu J, Ren R, Yu Y, et al. A randomized study of involved-field irradiation versus elective nodal irradiation in combination with concurrent chemotherapy for inoperable stage III nonsmall cell lung cancer. Am J Clin Oncol. 2007;30(3):239–44.

IV

Chapter 16
Mesothelioma and Thymic Tumors

Michael Wahl and Adam Garsa

MESOTHELIOMA

PEARLS

- Rare: only 2000–3000 cases per year in the United States.
- Eighty percent cases involve asbestos exposure; smoking history increases risk.
- Can affect visceral pleura, parietal pleura, peritoneum, pericardium, and tunica vaginalis.
- Cytology from pleural effusions generally low yield for diagnosis (~20%).
- May mimic adenocarcinoma on pathologic examination; immunohistochemical staining required for definitive diagnosis.
- Pathologic subtypes: Epithelioid (favorable, 40%), mixed (35%), sarcomatoid (unfavorable, 25%).
- <5% are surgically resectable at diagnosis.
- Surgical options include:
  - Pleurectomy/decortication (P/D): complete removal of pleura and all gross tumor. Perioperative mortality: 2–5%.
  - Extrapleural pneumonectomy (EPP): En bloc resection of pleura, ipsilateral lung, mediastinal lymph nodes, ipsilateral diaphragm, +/− pericardium. Perioperative mortality: 4–30%.

© Springer International Publishing AG, part of Springer Nature 2018   **323**
Eric K. Hansen and M. Roach III (eds.), *Handbook of Evidence-Based Radiation Oncology*, https://doi.org/10.1007/978-3-319-62642-0_16

 ͵ Adjuvant RT controversial after P/D due to high rates of pulmonary toxicity.
 ͵ Local progression leading to respiratory compromise is the most common cause of death.

WORKUP

 ͵ H&P, including occupational history for asbestos.
 ͵ Imaging: CXR, CT/MRI chest, PET/CT.
 ͵ On CT, look for pleural thickening, effusions, contraction of ipsilateral hemithorax.
 ͵ Functional imaging important because prior talc pleurodesis results in pleural thickening, which may be indistinguishable from disease-related plaques.
 ͵ Circumferential pleural thickening, mediastinal/chest wall/diaphragm involvement, and/or irregular pleural contour are most likely malignant.
 ͵ PFTs.
 ͵ Stage I-III: Pathologic mediastinal evaluation (mediastinoscopy or EBUS) to rule out N2 disease if potential surgical candidate.

Table 16.1 STAGING (AJCC 7TH ED., 2010) MESOTHELIOMA

Primary tumor (T)

TX:	Primary tumor cannot be assessed
T0:	No evidence of primary tumor
T1:	Tumor limited to the ipsilateral parietal pleura with or without mediastinal pleura and with or without diaphragmatic pleural involvement
T1a:	No involvement of the visceral pleura
T1b:	Tumor also involving the visceral pleura
T2:	Tumor involving each of the ipsilateral pleural surfaces (parietal, mediastinal, diaphragmatic, and visceral pleura) with at least one of the following:
	Involvement of diaphragmatic muscle
	Extension of tumor from visceral pleura into the underlying pulmonary parenchyma
T3:	Locally advanced but potentially resectable tumor. Tumor involving all of the ipsilateral pleural surfaces (parietal, mediastinal, diaphragmatic, and visceral pleura) with at least one of the following:
	Involvement of the endothoracic fascia

Table 16.1 (continued)

Primary tumor (T)

    Extension into the mediastinal fat

    Solitary, completely resectable focus of tumor

    Extending into the soft tissues of the chest wall

    Nontransmural involvement of the pericardium

T4: Locally advanced technically unresectable tumor. Tumor involving all of the ipsilateral pleural surfaces (parietal, mediastinal, diaphragmatic, and visceral pleura) with at least one of the following:

    Diffuse extension or multifocal masses of tumor in the chest wall, with or without associated rib destruction

    Direct transdiaphragmatic extension of tumor to the peritoneum

    Direct extension of tumor to the contralateral pleura

    Direct extension of tumor to mediastinal organs

    Direct extension of tumor into the spine

    Tumor extending through to the internal surface of the pericardium with or without a pericardial effusion or tumor involving the myocardium

Regional lymph nodes (N)

NX: Regional lymph nodes cannot be assessed

N0: No regional lymph node metastases

N1: Metastases in the ipsilateral bronchopulmonary or hilar lymph nodes

N2: Metastases in the subcarinal or the ipsilateral mediastinal lymph nodes including the ipsilateral internal mammary and peridiaphragmatic nodes

N3: Metastases in the contralateral mediastinal, contralateral internal mammary, ipsilateral or contralateral supraclavicular lymph nodes

Distant metastasis (M)

M0: No distant metastasis

M1: Distant metastasis present

Anatomic stage/prognostic groups

I: T1 N0 M0

IA: T1a N0 M0

IB: T1b N0 M0

II: T2 N0 M0

III: T1, T2 N1 M0

    T1, T2 N2 M0

    T3 N0, N1, N2 M0

IV: T4 Any N M0

    Any T N3 M0

    Any T Any N M1

IV

Table 16.2 STAGING (AJCC 8TH ED., 2017)

Definitions of AJCC TNM

Definition of primary tumor (T)

T category	T criteria
TX	Primary tumor cannot be assessed
T0	No evidence of primary tumor
T1	Tumor limited to the ipsilateral parietal with or without involvement of: Visceral pleura Mediastinal pleura Diaphragmatic pleura
T2	Tumor involving each of the ipsilateral pleural surfaces (parietal, mediastinal, diaphragmatic, and visceral pleura) with at least one of the following features: Involvement of diaphragmatic muscle Extension of tumor from visceral pleura into the underlying pulmonary parenchyma
T3	Describes locally advanced but *potentially resectable* tumor Tumor involving all the ipsilateral pleural surfaces (parietal, mediastinal, diaphragmatic, and visceral pleura) with at least one of the following features: Involvement of the endothoracic fascia Extension into the mediastinal fat Solitary, completely resectable focus of tumor extending into the soft tissues of the chest wall Nontransmural involvement of the pericardium
T4	Describes locally advanced *technically unresectable* tumor. Tumor involving all the ipsilateral pleural surfaces (parietal, mediastinal, diaphragmatic, and visceral pleura) with at least one of the following features: Diffuse extension or multifocal masses of tumor in the chest wall, with or without associated rib destruction Direct transdiaphragmatic extension of tumor to the peritoneum Direct extension of tumor to the contralateral pleura Direct extension of tumor to the mediastinal organs Direct extension of tumor into the spine Tumor extending through the internal surface of the pericardium with or without a pericardial effusion or tumor involving the myocardium

DEFINITION OF REGIONAL LYMPH NODE (N)

N category	N criteria
NX	Regional lymph nodes cannot be assessed
N0	No regional lymph node metastases
N1	Metastases in the ipsilateral bronchopulmonary, hilar, or mediastinal (including the internal mammary, peridiaphragmatic, pericardial fat pad, or intercostal) lymph nodes
N2	Metastases in the contralateral mediastinal, ipsilateral, or contralateral supraclavicular lymph nodes

IV

DEFINITION OF DISTANT METASTASIS (M)

M category	M criteria
M0	No distant metastasis
M1	Distant metastasis present

AJCC PROGNOSTIC STAGE GROUPS

When T is...	And N is...	And M is...	Then the stage group is...
T1	N0	M0	IA
T2 or T3	N0	M0	IB
T1	N1	M0	II
T2	N1	M0	II
T3	N1	M0	IIIA
T1–3	N2	M0	IIIB
T4	Any N	M0	IIIB
Any T	Any N	M1	IV

Used with permission of the American Joint Committee on Cancer (AJCC), Chicago, Illinois. The original and primary source for this information is the AJCC Cancer Staging Manual, Eighth Edition (2017) published by Springer International Publishing

TREATMENT RECOMMENDATIONS

Table 16.3 TREATMENT RECOMMENDATIONS

Stage	Recommended treatment	~MS

I–III, epithelial or mixed histology	Resectable/N0-1: Surgical resection (P/D or EPP) with combined neoadjuvant or adjuvant cisplatin/pemetrexed chemotherapy
	    Adjuvant hemithoracic RT (54 Gy in 30 fractions) if EPP resection
	    Consider hemithoracic RT after P/D (50.4 Gy in 28 fractions) if appropriate institutional experience
	Potentially resectable/N0-1: Neoadjuvant chemo → restaging, P/D or EPP as above if resectable
	N2, or medical or surgically inoperable: Primary chemotherapy
		Stage I: 38 months
		Stage II: 17 months
		Stage III: 11 months

IV or sarcomatoid histology	PS 0-2: Primary chemotherapy vs observation and treatment at progression PS 3-4: Best supportive care RT may be used for palliation	Stage IV: 7 months

STUDIES
SURGICAL MANAGEMENT

- EPP vs P/D controversial. P/D associated with less perioperative mortality.
- MSKCC (Flores et al. J Thorac Cardiovasc Surg 2008): Retrospective review of 663 patients treated with EPP or P/D. P/D had lower perioperative mortality (4% vs 7%) and was associated with improved survival (MS 16 vs 12 months).
- Cao et al. (Lung Cancer 2014): Meta-analysis of series comparing EPP with extended P/D. P/D had lower perioperative mortality (3% vs 7%) and morbidity (28% vs 62%), with comparable median survival.
- MARS (Treasure et al. Lancet Oncol 2011): 50 patients randomized after induction chemotherapy to EPP and hemithoracic RT vs no EPP. Survival was worse in EPP group (MS 19.5 vs 14.4 months), with 3 perioperative deaths. Study criticized since primary outcome was feasibility and was not powered to detect survival difference.

RESECTABLE DISEASE

- No randomized data supporting adjuvant RT, but several retrospective and phase II studies established favorable outcomes with trimodality therapy.

, Adjuvant radiotherapy after P/D more controversial, with high reported toxicity in some studies, but with recent study using IMRT showing promising results.

, Rusch (J Thorac Cardiovasc Surg 2001): phase II trial of 88 patients treated with EPP and adjuvant hemithoracic RT (54 Gy). MS 34 months for Stage I–II and 10 months for advanced stage. Toxicity included fatigue and esophagitis.

, Flores (J Thorac Oncol 2006): phase II trial of stage III or IV patients treated with induction chemo (gemcitabine/cisplatin), EPP, and adjuvant radiotherapy (54 Gy). MS: resectable patients 33.5 months, unresectable patients 9 months, all patients 19 months.

, Allen (IJROBP 2007a): retrospective review of outcomes associated with moderate dose hemithoracic RT (MDRT) vs. high dose hemithoracic RT (HDRT) in 39 patients after EPP. (MDRT = 30 Gy to hemithorax, 40 Gy to mediastinum, and boost to positive margins or nodes to 54 Gy with concurrent CT; HDRT = 54 Gy with sequential CT). Median OS 19 months. HDRT yield lower LF rate (27%) vs. MDRT (50%; p = ns). RT technique was not predictive of local failure, distant failure, or OS.

, EORTC 08031 (Van Schil, European Respiratory Journal 2010). Phase II study, 57 patients underwent 3 cycles induction cisplatin/pemetrexed - > EPP - > hemithoracic RT (54 Gy in 30 fractions). LR of 16% for patients completing treatment, but only 65% completed treatment. Median OS: 18.4 months.

, MSKCC (Gupta IJROBP 2005): Retrospective study of 125 patients receiving RT after P/D. High rate of toxicity, with 2 deaths within 1 month of treatment. LC only 40%.

, IMRT: Harvard (Allen, IJROBP 2006). 13 patients treated with IMRT, contralateral lung limited to V20 < 20% and mean lung dose <15 Gy. 6 of 13 patients developed fatal radiation pneumonitis.

, Rimmer (JCO 2016): Phase II study, 26 patients underwent induction chemo, P/D followed by IMRT to hemithorax (50.4 Gy in 28 fractions). 7% Grade 3 pneumonitis. Median OS: 24 months.

UNRESECTABLE DISEASE

, Generally treated with systemic therapy alone.

, No benefit to routine prophylactic radiotherapy to drain/biopsy tract based on multiple larger studies.

⸎ Vogelzang (JCO 2003): phase III study of pemetrexed and cisplatin vs. cisplatin alone in chemo naïve patients with malignant pleural mesothelioma. Addition of pemetrexed improved response rate (17 → 41%) and MS (9 → 12 months).

⸎ MAPS (Zalcman et al., Lancet 2016): Phase III study randomizing 448 patients with unresectable disease to cisplatin/pemetrexed ± bevacizumab. Survival improved with bevacizumab (MS 16 → 19 months).

⸎ Boutin (Chest 1995): randomized study of 40 patients treated with 21 Gy in 3 fx with electrons to drain sites vs. observation. RT to drain sites decreased LF 40–0%.

⸎ O'Rourke (Radiother Oncol 2007). Randomized study of 61 patients after chest drain or pleural biopsy treated with 21 Gy in 3 fx to drain site vs. best supportive care. No difference in the risk of tract metastases between arms (<10%).

⸎ UK (Clive Lancet Oncol 2016): Phase III study randomized 203 patients to prophylactic radiotherapy to procedure tracts (21 Gy in 3 fx) vs deferred radiotherapy after development of procedure tract metastasis (PTM). Prophylactic RT marginally reduced incidence of PTM from 16% to 9% (p = ns) without difference in QoL or survival. Subgroup analysis suggested that prophylactic RT may reduce the risk for PTM in patients with epithelioid histology or patients who did not receive chemotherapy.

RADIATION TECHNIQUES

SIMULATION AND FIELD DESIGN

⸎ Hemithoracic RT 4–8 weeks post resection.

⸎ Simulate and CT pt supine, arms overhead, immobilization.

⸎ Conventional AP/PA borders: superior = top of T1; inferior = bottom L2; medial = contralateral edge of vertebral body (if mediastinum negative) or 1.5 cm beyond contralateral edge of vertebral body (if mediastinum involved), lateral = flash.

⸎ Blocks: liver and stomach (covers diaphragm/abdomen interface), kidney, humerus, heart (after 19.8 Gy), spinal cord (after 41.4 Gy, shift medial border to ipsilateral edge of vertebral body).

- Scar: include in field, bolus, or boost to scar may be needed.
- Electron boost to areas of chest wall blocked for abdominal or cardiac protection.
- Cover surgical scars with bolus.
- Initial studies suggested IMRT associated with increased complications and/or deaths (Allen et al. 2006). However, studies by the same group (Allen et al. 2007a, b) and others (Krayenbuhl 2007; Rice 2007; Miles 2008) have shown decreased toxicity with careful planning.
- Helical tomotherapy may yield improved dosimetry (Sterzing, Radiother Oncol 2008).
- If using conformal technique, CTV = Entire pleural surface and surgical clips.
- Elective nodal radiation not recommended.

IV

DOSE PRESCRIPTIONS

- Postoperative RT: 54 Gy in 30 fractions, boost gross disease to 60 Gy.
- If AP/PA technique, give electrons concurrent with photon treatment, 1.53 Gy/fx (15% scatter under blocks from photon fields). Choose energy so that chest wall is covered by 90% IDL.

DOSE LIMITATIONS

- Spinal cord: ≤45 Gy
- Lung
  - Mean contralateral lung dose ≤8–10 Gy; V20 ≤ 7%; V5 ≤ 75%
  - If RT after P/D, mean total lung V20% < 37%
- Heart: limit 50% <25–40 Gy
- Esophagus: limit 1/3 to <60 Gy; 2/3 to <55 Gy; 3/3 to <45 Gy

COMPLICATIONS

- Acute: may include skin reactions, fatigue, nausea, vomiting, dysphagia, odynophagia, cough, dyspnea, acute pneumonitis, pneumonia
- Late: may include pericarditis, restrictive cardiomyopathy, myocardial infarction, CHF, pulmonary fibrosis

THYMIC TUMORS

PEARLS

- Thymoma has an indolent, predominantly locally invasive growth pattern, but can metastasize.
- Thymoma accounts for 20% of mediastinal tumors and 50% of anterior mediastinal masses in adults; most common age at diagnosis = 40–60 years.
- Most common presentation is as an anterior mediastinal mass on CXR performed for other reasons; 40–50% are asymptomatic.
- DDx for anterior mediastinal mass: Lymphoma, thymoma, carcinoid, germ cell tumor.
- Thymomas are often associated with immune and nonimmune mediated paraneoplastic syndromes: myasthenia gravis (MG; 30%), pure red cell aplasia (PRCA; 5–10%), and hypogammaglobulinemia (Good's syndrome; 3–6%).
- Only 10–15% of patients with MG have a thymoma; 50% of patients with PRCA have a thymoma.
- Common presenting symptoms include fatigue, chest pain, cough, dyspnea, hoarseness, symptoms of superior vena cava syndrome, and/or paraneoplastic symptoms (i.e., MG: muscle weakness, dysphagia, blurred vision).
- Prognosis is related to stage and completeness of resection; on multivariate analysis, treatment dose ≥50 Gy is a prognostic factor (Zhu et al. 2004).
- Thymomas are chemosensitive tumors; complete and partial response rates = 1/3 and 2/3, respectively.
- Thymoma histologic classification (WHO):
  - Type A,AB,B1: Long-term survival ~90%
  - Type B2-B3: Long-term survival 40–60%
  - Type C: Thymic Carcinoma, 30% rate of DM, long-term survival ~25%
  - Thymic carcinoid: more locally aggressive with 30% LN and 30–40% DM, associated with MEN, Cushing's, Eaton–Lambert, SIADH, and hypercalcemia paraneoplastic syndromes

WORKUP

- H&P, CXR, and preoperative chest imaging, mainly CT chest with contrast; MRI and PET–CT have been used.

> Be careful to note entire pre-op tumor volume including anterior extension to sternum or anterior chest wall or posterior extension into the mediastinum.
> Serum studies to rule out germ cell tumor (β-HCG, LDH, AFP).
> Serum antiacetylcholine receptor antibody levels. If patient has MG, treat prior to surgery to avoid risk of respiratory failure.
> No biopsy required if resectable and thymoma is strongly suspected based on clinical and radiographic findings. Otherwise, core needle biopsy or open biopsy to establish diagnosis.

IV

Table 16.4 STAGING

Stage grouping (Masaoka system)		~5-year survival
I:	Macroscopically completely encapsulated and microscopically no capsular invasion	I: 93–100%
II:	(a) microscopic invasion into capsule, or (b) macroscopic invasion into surrounding fatty tissue or mediastinal pleura	II: 86%
III:	Macroscopic invasion into neighboring structures, i.e., mediastinum, pericardium, great vessels, or lung. (a) without invasion of great vessels, (b) with invasion of great vessels	III: 70%
IVa:	Pleural or pericardial dissemination	IV: 50%
IVb:	Lymphatic or hematogenous metastasis	

From Masaoka A, Monden Y, Nakahara K, et al. Follow-up study of thymomas with special reference to their clinical stages. Cancer 1981;48:2485. Reprinted with permission from John Wiley & Sons

Table 16.5 (AJCC 8TH ED., 2017) THYMOMA

Definitions OF AJCC TNM

Definition of primary tumor (T)*, **

T category	T description
TX	Primary tumor cannot be assessed
T0	No evidence of primary tumor
T1	Tumor encapsulated or extending into the mediastinal fat; may involve the mediastinal pleura
T1a	Tumor with no mediastinal pleura involvement
T1b	Tumor with direct invasion of mediastinal pleura
T2	Tumor with direct invasion of the pericardium (either partial or full thickness)
T3	Tumor with direct invasion into any of the following: lung, brachiocephalic vein, superior vena cava, phrenic nerve, chest wall, or extrapericardial pulmonary artery or veins

(continued)

Table 16.5 (continued)

T4	Tumor with invasion into any of the following: aorta (ascending, arch, or descending), arch vessels, intrapericardial pulmonary artery, myocardium, trachea, esophagus

*Involvement must be microscopically confirmed in pathological staging, if possible
**T categories are defined by "levels" of invasion; they reflect the highest degree of invasion regardless of how many other (lower level) structures are invaded. T1, level 1 structures, thymus, anterior mediastinal fat, and mediastinal pleura; T2, level 2 structures, pericardium; T3, level 3 structures, lung, brachiocephalic vein, superior vena cava, phrenic nerve, chest wall, and hilar pulmonary vessels; T4, level 4 structures, aorta (ascending, arch, or descending), arch vessels, intrapericardial pulmonary artery, myocardium, trachea, and esophagus

Table 16.6 Definition of Regional Lymph Node (N)*

N category	N description
NX	Regional lymph nodes cannot be assessed
N0	No regional lymph node metastasis
N1	Metastasis in anterior (perithymic) lymph nodes
N2	Metastasis in deep intrathoracic or cervical lymph nodes

*Involvement must be microscopically confirmed in pathological staging, if possible

Table 16.7 Definition of Distant Metastasis (M)

M category	M description
M0	No pleural, pericardial, or distant metastasis
M1	Pleural, pericardial, or distant metastasis
M1a	Separate pleural or pericardial nodule(s)
M1b	Pulmonary intraparenchymal nodule or distant organ metastasis

When T is...	And N is...	And M is...	Then the stage group is...
T1a,b	N0	M0	I
T2	N0	M0	II
T3	N0	M0	IIIA
T4	N0	M0	IIIB
Any T	N1	M0	IVA
Any T	N0,1	M1a	IVA
Any T	N2	M0,M1a	IVB
Any T	Any N	M1b	IVB

Used with permission of the American Joint Committee on Cancer (AJCC), Chicago, Illinois. The original and primary source for this information is the AJCC Cancer Staging Manual, Eighth Edition (2017) published by Springer International Publishing

Table 16.8 TREATMENT RECOMMENDATIONS

˒ Complete surgical resection (R0) is the mainstay of treatment.
˒ The role for radiotherapy in the management of thymoma remains somewhat controversial; no randomized studies exist comparing treatment; retrospective data suffer from heterogeneity in treatment techniques.
˒ Forty percent of completely resected thymomas recur; median time to local recurrence (LR) ~4 years, but late recurrences (>10 years) possible.

IV

Treatment recommendations

Stage	Recommended treatment	5 year OS
Stage I–III resectable	R0 resection: post-op RT if stage III, consider for stage II R1 resection: post-op RT R2 resection: post-op RT +/– chemo	70–100%
Initially unresectable	Induction chemotherapy (cisplatin based) – surgery. Consider post-op RT based on pathologic findings Definitive RT if unresectable after induction chemotherapy	50–80%
Thymic carcinoma	R0 resection: post-op RT for stage II and above R1 resection: post RT +/– chemo R2 resection or unresectable: Chemo + RT	20–30%
Metastatic	Chemo with site-directed RT as needed	10–50%

STUDIES
ADJUVANT RADIOTHERAPY

˒ No prospective data evaluating adjuvant radiotherapy.
˒ Multiple retrospective reviews suggest that RT reduces recurrence rates and improves outcomes for incompletely resected stage II–IV thymoma. The role of post-op RT for completely resected stage II–III thymoma is controversial.
˒ Adjuvant chemotherapy generally not indicated for localized disease, but recommended after any R2 resection or R1 resection of thymic carcinoma.

- Curran (JCO 1988): retrospective study of 103 patients with thymoma. No recurrences among stage I patients after total resection without RT. Fifty-three percent with stage II/III thymoma had mediastinal recurrence without RT vs. 0% after total resection with RT, and 21% after subtotal resection or biopsy with RT.

- Kondo (Ann Thorac Surg 2003): review of 1320 patients with thymic epithelial tumors. Stage I treated with surgery alone. Stage II–III thymoma and thymic carcinoid treated with surgery and RT. Stage IV thymoma and thymic carcinoma treated with RT and chemo. Masaoka clinical stage is an excellent predictor of prognosis for thymoma and thymic carcinoma, but not thymic carcinoid. Complete resection is the most important prognostic factor. Post-op RT did not significantly reduce recurrence rate for patients with completely resected stage II–III thymoma.

- Utsumi (Cancer 2009): Retrospective review of 324 patients with thymoma after complete resection. Post-op RT did not improve CSS for all patients (93 vs 94%) or for patients with stage III thymoma (85 vs 87%). Pleural dissemination most common failure pattern.

- Korst (Ann Thorac Surg 2009): Meta-analysis of 22 retrospective studies, no reduction in local recurrence after RT for completely resected thymoma.

- Forquer (IJROBP 2010): review of 901 patients with surgically resected thymoma or thymic carcinoma in SEER database. Post-op RT improved 5-year OS for patients with Stage II–III disease (66 → 76%), but not CSS (91 vs. 86%). No benefit of post-op RT Stage I patients.

- Lim (J Thorac Oncol 2015): SEER analysis of 529 patients using propensity matching. PORT improved OS in patients with stage III and IV thymoma.

- Omasa (Cancer 2015): Retrospective study of 1265 patients with stage II and III thymoma and thymic carcinoma after surgery. PORT improved RFS but not OS in patients with thymic carcinoma; no improvement in RFS or OS for patients with thymoma and no benefit in stage III subgroup.

COMBINED MODALITY

- Mornex (IJROBP 1995): retrospective review of 90 patients treated with surgery and RT (30–70 Gy) ± chemo (cisplatin based). Five out of ten year OS was 51/39%. Extent of surgery impacted 10-year OS (43% for partial resection vs. 31% for biopsy only). Stage, histology, and chemo were not prognostic.
- Kim (Lung Cancer 2004): phase II study of a multidisciplinary approach with induction chemotherapy, followed by surgical resection, radiation therapy, and consolidation chemotherapy for unresectable malignant thymomas. Induction chemo 77% response rate. OS rates 95% (5-year) and 79% (7-year). PFS rates 77% (5-year) and 77% (7-year).
- Wright (Ann Thorac Surg 2008): 10 patients with stage III–IVA thymoma treated with 2 cycles of cisplatin and etoposide with concurrent RT followed by surgery. Four patients had >90% necrosis in resected specimen. Eight patients had R0 resection. Seven patients received 2 more cycles of chemo. Five-year OS 69%.
- Loehrer (JCO 1997): 26 patients with unresectable unresectable thymoma, treated with induction platinum-based chemotherapy followed by RT to 54 Gy. 5-year OS 53%.

RADIATION TECHNIQUES
SIMULATION AND FIELD DESIGN

- Simulate patient supine with arms overhead and adequate immobilization.
- Conformal, image-based planning techniques are preferred (IMRT, 3D–CRT, tomotherapy) to minimize dose to surrounding normal structures.
- Surgical clips denoting the extent of surgical resection and/or regions of residual disease are important for design of post-op fields.
- Volumes
  - CTV = GTV + tumor bed + surgical clips.
  - PTV = CTV + 0.5–1 cm margin.
- Elective nodal radiation generally not performed given low propensity for LN spread.

IV

DOSE PRESCRIPTIONS
- Pre-op RT: 1.8 Gy/fx to 45 Gy
- Post-op RT (1.8–2 Gy/fx)
  - R0: 45–50 Gy
  - R1: 54 Gy
  - R2: 60–70 Gy
- Unresectable: 60–70 Gy

DOSE LIMITATIONS
- Spinal cord: ≤45 Gy
- Lung: limit the volume receiving >20 Gy (V20) to <20–30%
- Heart: V40 < 50%
- Esophagus: Mean < 34 Gy, V33 < 60 Gy; V66 < 55 Gy

COMPLICATIONS
- Acute: may include skin reactions, fatigue, dysphagia, odynophagia, cough, dyspnea, acute pneumonitis, pneumonia
- Late: may include pericarditis, restrictive cardiomyopathy, myocardial infarction, CHF, radiation myelopathy, esophageal stricture, radiation pneumonitis, pulmonary fibrosis

FOLLOW-UP
- Late recurrences are not uncommon; long-term follow-up is indicated.
- Post-op RT has no impact on the incidence of subsequent pleural spread (outside of RT field).

Acknowledgment We thank Fred Y. Wu MD, PhD, Brian Lee MD, PhD, and Joycelyn L. Speight MD, PhD for their work on the prior edition of this chapter.

REFERENCES
Allen AM, Czerminska M, Janne PA, et al. Fatal pneumonitis associated with intensity-modulated radiation therapy for mesothelioma. Int J Radiat Oncol Biol Phys. 2006;65(3):640–5.

Allen AM, Schoenfield MS, Hacker F, et al. Restricted field IMRT dramatically enhances IMRT planning for mesothelioma. Int J Radiat Oncol Biol Phys. 2007a;69(5): 1587–92.

Allen AM, Den R, Wong JS, et al. Influence of radiotherapy technique and dose on patterns of failure for mesothelioma patients after extrapleural pneumonectomy. Int J Radiat Oncol Biol Phys. 2007b;68(5):1366–74.

Boutin C, Rey F, Viallat R, et al. Prevention of malignant seeding after invasive diagnostic procedures in patients with pleural mesothelioma. A randomized trial of local radiotherapy. Chest. 1995;108(3):754–8.

Cao C, Tian D, Park J, et al. A systematic review and meta-analysis of surgical treatments for malignant pleural mesothelioma. Lung Cancer. 2014;83(2):240–5.

Clive A, Taylor H, Dobson L, et al. Prophylactic radiotherapy for the prevention of procedure-tract metastases after surgical and large-bore pleural procedures in malignant pleural mesothelioma (SMART): a multicenter, open-label, phase 3, randomized controlled trial. Lancet Oncol. 2016;17(8):1094–104.

Curran WJ Jr, Kornstein MJ, Brooks JJ, et al. Invasive thymoma: the role of mediastinal irradiation following complete or incomplete surgical resection. J Clin Oncol. 1988;6:1722–7.

Flores R, Krug L, Rosenzweig K, et al. Induction chemotherapy, extrapleural pneumonectomy, and postoperative high-dose radiotherapy for locally advanced malignant pleural mesothelioma: a phase II trial. J Thorac Oncol. 2006;1:289–95.

Flores R, Pass H, Seshan V, et al. Extrapleural pneumonectomy versus pleurectomy/decortication in the surgical management of malignant pleural mesothelioma: results in 663 patients. J Thorac Cardiovasc Surg. 2008;135(3):620–6.

Forquer JA, Rong N, Fakiris AJ, et al. Postoperative radiotherapy after surgical resection of thymoma: differing roles in localized and regional disease. Int J Radiat Oncol Biol Phys. 2010;76(2):440–5.

Gupta V, Mychalczak B, Krug L, et al. Hemithoracic radiation therapy after pleurectomy/decortication for malignant pleural mesothelioma. Int J Radiat Oncol Biol Phys. 2005;63(4):1045–52.

Kim E, Putnam J, Komaki R, et al. Phase II study of a multidisciplinary approach with induction chemotherapy, followed by surgical resection, radiation therapy, and consolidation chemotherapy for unresectable malignant thymomas: final report. Lung Cancer. 2004;44:369–79.

Komaki R, Travis EL, Cox JD. The lung and thymus. In: Cox JD, Ang KK, editors. Radiation oncology: rationale, technique, results. 8th ed. St. Louis: Mosby; 2003. p. 399–427.

Kondo K, Monden Y. Therapy for thymic epithelial tumors: a clinical study of 1,320 patients from Japan. Ann Thorac Surg. 2003;76(3):878–84.

Korst R, Kansler A, Christos P, et al. Adjuvant radiotherapy for thymic epithelial tumors: a systematic review and meta-analysis. Ann Thorac Surg. 2009;87(5):1641–7.

Krayenbuhl J, OErtel S, Davis JB, et al. Combined photon and electron three-dimensional conformal versus intensity-modulated radiotherapy with integrated boost for adjuvant treatment of malignant pleural mesothelioma after pleuropneumectomy. Int J Radiat Oncol Biol Phys. 2007;69(5):1593–9.

Lim Y, Kim H, Wu HG. Role of postoperative radiotherapy in nonlocalized thymoma: propensity-matched analysis of surveillance, epidemiology and end results database. J Thorac Oncol. 2015;10(9):1357–63.

Loehrer PJ, Chen M, Kim K, et al. Cisplatin, doxorubicin, and cyclophosphamide plus thoracic radiation therapy for limited-stage unresectable thymoma: an intergroup trial. J ClinOncol. 1997;15(9):3093–9.

Masaoka A, Monden Y, Nakahara K, et al. Follow-up study of thymomas with special reference to their clinical stages. Cancer. 1981;48:2485.

Miles EF, Larrier NA, Kelsey CR, et al. Intensity modulated radiotherapy for restricted mesothelioma: the Duke experience. Int J Radiat Oncol Biol Phys. 2008;71(4):1143–50.

Mornex F. Radiotherapy and chemotherapy for invasive thymomas: a multicentric retrospective review of 90 cases. Int J Radiat Oncol Biol Phys. 1995;2:651–9.

IV

O'Rourke N, Garcia JC, Paul J, et al. A randomized controlled trial of intervention site radiotherapy in malignant pleural mesothelioma. Radiother Oncol. 2007;84(1):18–22.

Omasa M, Date H, Sozu T, et al. Postoperative radiotherapy is effective for thymic carcinoma but not for thymoma in stage II and III thymic epithelial tumors: the Japanese Association for Research on the Thymus Database Study. Cancer. 2015;121(7):1008–16.

Rice DC, Stevens CW, Correa AM, et al. Outcomes after extrapleural pneumonectomy and intensity-modulated radiation therapy for malignant pleural mesothelioma. Ann Thorac Surg. 2007;84(5):1685–92.

Rimmer A, Zauderer M, Gomez D, et al. Phase II study of hemithoracic intensity-modulated pleural radiation (IMPRINT) as part of lung-sparing multimodality therapy in patients with malignant pleural mesothelioma. J Clin Oncol. 2016;34(23):2761–8.

Rusch VW, Rosenzweig K, Venkatraman E, et al. A phase II trial of surgical resection and adjuvant high-dose hemithoracic radiation for malignant pleural mesothelioma. J Thorac Cardiovasc Surg. 2001;122:788–95.

Sterzing F, Sroka-Perez G, Schubert K, et al. Evaluating target coverage and normal tissue sparing in the adjuvant radiotherapy of malignant pleural mesothelioma: helical tomotherapy compared with step and shoot IMRT. Radiother Oncol. 2008;86(2):251–7.

Treasure T, Lang-Lazdunski L, Waller D, et al. Extra-pleural pneumonectomy vs no extra-pleural pneumonectomy for patients with malignant pleural mesothelioma: clinical outcomes of the mesothelioma and radical surgery (MARS) randomized feasibility study. Lancet Oncol. 2011;12(8):763–72.

Utsumi T, Shiono H, Kadota Y, et al. Postoperative radiation therapy after complete resection of thymoma has little impact on survival. Cancer. 2009;115(23):5413–20.

Van Schil P, Baas P, Gaafar R, et al. Trimodality therapy for malignant pleural mesothelioma: results from an EORTC phase II multicenter trial. Eur Respir J. 2010;36(6):1362–9.

Vogelzang NJ, Rusthoven JJ, Symanowski J, et al. Phase III study of pemetrexed in combination with cisplatin versus cisplatin alone in patients with malignant pleural mesothelioma. J Clin Oncol. 2003;21:2636–44.

Wright CD, Choi NC. Wain JC, et al induction chemoradiotherapy followed by resection for locally advanced Masaoka stage III and IVA thymic tumors. Ann Thorac Surg. 2008;85(2):385–9.

Zalcman G, Mazieres J, Margery J, et al. Bevacizumab for newly diagnosed pleural mesothelioma in the Mesothelioma Avastin Cisplatin Pemetrexed Study (MAPS): a randomized, controlled, open-label, phase 3 trial. Lancet. 2016;387(10026):1405–14.

Zhu G, He S, Fu X, Jiang G, Liu T. Radiotherapy and prognostic factors for thymoma: a retrospective study of 175 patients. Int J Radiat Oncol Biol Phys. 2004;60(4):1113–9. doi:10.1016/j.ijrobp.2004.05.013.

PART V

Breast

Chapter 17
Breast Cancer

Anna K. Paulsson, Tracy Sherertz, and Catherine C. Park

EPIDEMIOLOGY

- The most common cancer (excluding skin) among women in the United States, with a lifetime risk of <12%.
- Approximately 231,840 invasive and 60,290 in situ cases/year in the United States.
- Second leading cause of cancer deaths in women (40,290 deaths/year in the United States).
- The most important risk factor for breast cancer development is age.
- Risk also affected by age at menarche, first pregnancy, menopause, family history, obesity, and mammographic breast density.
- The use of exogenous estrogen increases risk for breast cancer.

GENETICS

- Approximately 10% of breast cancer cases are associated with germline mutation, including p53 (Li-Fraumeni), Cowden syndrome, BRCA1, BRCA2, and PALB2.
  - BRCA1 mutation carriers have 40–85% lifetime risk of breast and 25–65% lifetime risk of ovarian cancer. BRCA2 mutation carriers have similar risk of breast cancer but lower 10–15% lifetime risk of ovarian cancer.

The original version of this chapter was revised. An erratum to this chapter can be found at https://doi.org/10.1007/978-3-319-62642-0_44

© Springer International Publishing AG, part of Springer Nature 2018   **343**
Eric K. Hansen and M. Roach III (eds.), *Handbook of Evidence-Based Radiation Oncology*, https://doi.org/10.1007/978-3-319-62642-0_17

- PALB2 appears to have a risk profile similar to BRCA2.
- Prophylactic bilateral salpingo-oophorectomy decreases ovarian/fallopian tube cancers by 80% and breast cancers by 50% (Rebbeck, JNCI 2009).
- Prophylactic mastectomy nearly eliminates the risk of breast cancers, but does not alter the risk of ovarian/fallopian tube cancer.
- Chemoprevention with a selective estrogen receptor modulator (SERM) is an alternative strategy.
- MRI may have an increasing role in the screening and diagnosis of breast cancer in BRCA mutation carriers.
- Germline mutation panels are an expanding and actively evolving area. Check with your institutional genetic counselor regarding available panels at your institution

CHEMOPREVENTION

- SERMs, e.g., tamoxifen or raloxifene, can be considered in high-risk cohorts, including strong immediate family history, history of LCIS, confirmed adverse gene carrier, or deemed high risk by various risk assessment tools (Gail model).
- *Meta-analysis of Chemoprevention with SERMs* (Lancet 2013): 9 trials including 83,399 patients with median f/u of 65 months. SERMs reduced breast cancer (including DCIS) by 38%: cumulative incidence 6.3% vs. 4.2% with SERM. The overall frequency of ER-positive cancer was reduced from 4.0% to 2.1%. Rates of endometrial cancer were higher with SERM, particularly tamoxifen, and rates of thromboembolic events were increased overall.

ANATOMY

- Medial and lateral borders of breast tissue: typically the sternum and midaxillary line.
- Cranial and caudal borders: typically the second anterior rib and sixth anterior rib.
- Primary lymphatic drainage is to axillary, internal mammary, and SCV nodes.

- Axillary lymph nodes divided into three levels by relation to pectoralis minor muscle.
- Level I (low axillary) = nodes inferior/lateral to pectoralis minor muscle.
- Level II (midaxillary) = nodes directly beneath the pectoralis minor muscle.
  - Rotter's (interpectoral) nodes considered level II and are located between pectoralis major and minor muscles.
- Level III (apical or infraclavicular) = nodes superior/medial to pectoralis minor muscle.
- Internal mammary LN (IMLN) located in first to fifth intercostal spaces (first to third most commonly involved), 3–3.5 cm from midline.

IMAGING

SCREENING

- Screening yields 20–35% decrease in breast cancer mortality between the ages of 50–69, with slightly less impact for ages 40–49.
- Approximately 10% of all breast cancers are mammographically occult.
- Clinical breast exam every 1–3 years and periodic self-exam is generally recommended beginning in young adulthood.
- Annual clinical breast exam and screening mammography are generally recommended to begin at age 40–50 in the United States.
- Screening mammography (± adjunct MRI) should begin earlier in high-risk populations, such as prior thoracic RT (e.g., mantle-field RT), genetic predisposition or strong family history, or prior history of LCIS/atypical hyperplasia.
- For specific guidelines, please see National Comprehensive Cancer Network (www.nccn.org) and/or American College of Radiology (www.acr.org).
- The Breast Imaging Reporting and Data System (BI-RADS) provides a standardized classification for mammographic studies and demonstrates good correlation with the likelihood of malignancy.

Table 17.1 BREAST IMAGING REPORTING AND DATA SYSTEM (BI-RADS)

BI-RADS category	Assessment	Clinical management recommendation(s)
0	Assessment incomplete	Need additional imaging evaluation and/or prior mammograms for comparison
1	Negative	Continue routine screening
2	Benign finding	Continue routine screening
3	Probably benign finding (up to 2% likelihood)	Short-term follow-up mammogram at 6 months, then every 6–12 months for 1–2 years
4	Suspicious 4A: Low suspicion for malignancy (2–10% likelihood) 4B: Moderate suspicion for malignancy (10–50% likelihood) 4C: High suspicion for malignancy (50–95% likelihood)	Perform biopsy, preferably needle biopsy
5	Highly suggestive of malignancy (>95% chance of malignancy)	Biopsy and treatment, as necessary
6	Known biopsy-proven malignancy	Surgical excision when clinically appropriate

Adapted from American College of Radiology (ACR) BI-RADS 5th edition; visit www.acr.org/birads for more information

- Annual screening using MRI (in addition to mammography) is recommended by the American Cancer Society for women who:
  - Have a BRCA 1 or 2 mutation
  - Have a first-degree relative with a BRCA 1 or 2 mutation and are untested
  - Have a lifetime risk of breast cancer of 20–25% or more using standard risk assessment models (BRCAPRO, Claus, Tyrer-Cuzick)
  - Received radiation treatment to the chest between ages 10 and 30, such as for Hodgkin's disease
  - Carry or have a first-degree relative who carries a genetic mutation in the TP53 or PTEN genes (Li-Fraumeni syndrome and Cowden and Bannayan-Riley-Ruvalcaba syndromes)

DIAGNOSTIC STUDIES
- Bilateral diagnostic mammography (including magnification and compression views as indicated):
  - Sensitivity and specificity ≥90%.

- Note masses, areas of architectural distortion, suspicious calcifications (present in 85–90% of DCIS).
- Post lumpectomy mammogram should be routinely obtained to rule out residual microcalcifications if mammographic presentation associated with malignant-appearing calcifications (for both invasive and in situ disease).
- Ultrasound of breast (especially in young and/or dense breasts) and axilla.
- Optimal use of breast MRI continues to evolve. Associated with high false-positive rates, but may have utility in select patients (i.e., invasive lobular cancers, axillary adenopathy with occult breast primary, Paget's disease without evidence of underlying tumor, assessing response to neoadjuvant chemotherapy, young women with dense breasts, and BRCA 1/2 mutation careers).

PATHOLOGY

- Ductal carcinoma in situ (DCIS) comprises about 20% of all breast cancer:
  - DCIS represents confinement of malignant cells within basement membrane.
  - One-third of patients with DCIS develop invasive disease within 10 years.
  - Mortality risk from DCIS ≈10% of recurrence risk after breast-conserving surgery.
  - Prognostic variables for DCIS include tumor size, margins, nuclear grade, necrosis, multifocality, and age.
  - High-grade DCIS: tends to be continuous, 25% ER+.
  - Low-grade DCIS: increased multifocality and multicentricity, 90% ER+.
- Lobular carcinoma in situ (LCIS) is the marker for bilateral breast cancer:
  - Approximately 12% of in situ disease.
  - Approximately 20–25% lifetime risk for developing ipsilateral or contralateral cancer; risk dependent on age of diagnosis of LCIS.
  - Often mammographically silent.
  - Usually ER/PR+ Her2neu–.
  - About 25% associated with DCIS or invasive disease, treat according to DCIS or invasive disease indications.

- Invasive (infiltrating) ductal carcinoma (IDCA) is the most common type of breast cancer (85% of invasive cases).
- Invasive lobular carcinoma (ILCA) has prognosis similar to that of ductal carcinoma:
  - Associated with increased risk of bilateral, multifocal breast cancer.
- E-cadherin distinguishes DCIS/IDCA (E-cadherin +) from LCIS/ILCA (E-cadherin−).
- Tubular, medullary, and mucinous carcinomas generally have better prognosis:
  - Medullary carcinoma is typically high grade and associated with BRCA1/2.
- Paget's disease is nipple involvement associated with an underlying cancer:
  - Pathologically, tumor cells can be seen involving the epidermis.
  - Treat per underlying tumor characteristics; not a contraindication to breast-conserving therapy (BCT), but the nipple–areolar complex must be excised.
- Multicentricity is disease in multiple quadrants and is a contraindication to BCT.
- Multifocality is multiple foci within same quadrant and is not a contraindication to BCT.
- Pathological status of axillary lymph nodes is among the most important prognostic variables:
  - T1–2: 10–40% pLN+.
  - Predictors for pLN+ status: size >1 cm, G2–3, high S-phase ratio, +LVSI.
- Risk of internal mammary node (IMLN) involvement ranges from 1–10% if axilla pLN0 vs. 20–50% if axilla pLN+, based on older radical mastectomy series of locoregionally advanced disease:
  - Risk of clinical IMLN failure in modern series is ≤1%.
  - Approximately 5% of sentinel lymph node biopsy (SLNB) procedures localize to IMLN as first echelon drainage.
- Extensive intraductal component: 25% or more of primary invasive tumor is comprised of DCIS, and DCIS is present in surrounding normal breast tissue.
- Inflammatory carcinoma is a clinical diagnosis:
  - Confirmed by pathological findings of cancer cells in dermal lymphatics.

- Pathologic findings in the absence of clinical signs/symptoms are not diagnostic of inflammatory carcinoma.
- Presents with rapid onset of erythema, warmth, and edema of breast; localized inflammatory changes do not qualify.
- Underlying mass often cannot be appreciated for inflammatory carcinoma.

GENE EXPRESSION PROFILING AND MOLECULAR SUBTYPES

- Molecular subtypes approximated by receptor status include:
- *Luminal A:* ER/PR+ Her2neu–.
- *Luminal B:* ER/PR+ Her2neu + basal-like: ER/PR – Her2neu – (triple negative).
- *Her2neu+:* ER/PR – Her2neu+.
  - Her2neu + amplification is a negative prognosticator in both mastectomy and BCT cohorts.
- Commercially available gene expression profiling assays include OncotypeDx® and MammaPrint®:
- MammaPrint® predicts prognostic category (low vs. high risk) in terms of DMFS and OS in treated and untreated, ER-positive and ER-negative, and LN-positive and LN-negative patients. Requires fresh–frozen tissue (and on-site) processing.
- OncotypeDx® predicts prognostic category (low vs. intermediate vs. high risk) in terms of DMFS and OS and magnitude of chemotherapy benefit in tamoxifen-treated, ER+, LN-negative patients and can assay a fixed specimen (obviating need for on-site testing).
- PAM50 predicts residual risk of distant recurrence after endocrine therapy in post-menopausal women with ER+ breast cancer. This assay can be performed in a hospital laboratory, rather than a central referral laboratory.

WORKUP

- Breast cancer-specific history including risk factors, gynecologic history, menopausal status, and general physical exam.
- Breast exam (tumor size, satellites, skin/chest wall, nipple changes, symmetry).

V

- Lymph node exam (axillary, supraclavicular/infraclavicular).
- Biopsy with estrogen and progesterone receptor studies; Her-2-neu status, ki-67.
- CBC, blood chemistries, liver function labs.
- CXR.
- Breast imaging as above.
- Bone scan, head imaging (MRI preferred to CT), PET–CT when clinically indicated.
- Careful histologic assessment of breast specimens.
- Consider ultrasound-guided FNA of suspicious nodes (especially if neoadjuvant chemo considered):
  - cN0 axilla: 30% pN+.
  - cN+ axilla: 20–40% pN0.

STAGING: BREAST CANCER

Editors' note: All TNM stage and stage groups referred to elsewhere in this chapter reflect the 2010 AJCC staging nomenclature unless otherwise noted as the new system below was published after this chapter was written.

Table 17.2 AJCC 7TH ED., 2010

Primary tumor (T)
The T classification of the primary tumor is the same regardless of whether it is based on clinical or pathologic criteria, or both. Size should be measured to the nearest millimeter. If the tumor size is slightly less than or greater than a cut-off for a given T classification, it is recommended that the size be rounded to the millimeter reading that is closest to the cut-off. For example, a reported size of 1.1 mm is reported as 1 mm, or a size of 2.01 cm is reported as 2.0 cm. Designation should be made with the subscript "c" or "p" modifier to indicate whether the T classification was determined by clinical (physical examination or radiologic) or pathologic measurements, respectively. In general, pathologic determination should take precedence over clinical determination of T size

TX:	Primary tumor cannot be assessed
T0:	No evidence of primary tumor
Tis:	Carcinoma in situ
Tis (DCIS):	Ductal carcinoma in situ
Tis (LCIS):	Lobular carcinoma in situ

continued

Tis (Paget's): Paget's disease of the nipple not associated with invasive carcinoma and/or carcinoma in situ (DCIS and/or LCIS) in the underlying breast parenchyma. Carcinomas in the breast parenchyma associated with Paget's disease are categorized based on the size and characteristics of the parenchymal disease, although the presence of Paget's disease should still be noted

T1:   Tumor ≤20 mm in greatest dimension

T1mi: Tumor ≤1 mm in greatest dimension

T1a: Tumor >1 mm, but ≤5 mm in greatest dimension

T1b: Tumor >5 mm, but ≤10 mm in greatest dimension

T1c: Tumor >10 mm, but ≤20 mm in greatest dimension

T2:   Tumor >20 mm, but ≤50 mm in greatest dimension

T3:   Tumor >50 mm in greatest dimension

T4:   Tumor of any size with direct extension to the chest wall and/or to the skin (ulceration or skin nodules). Note: Invasion of the dermis alone does not qualify as T4

T4a: Extension to the chest wall, not including only pectoralis muscle adherence/invasion

T4b: Ulceration and/or ipsilateral satellite nodules and/or edema (including peau d'orange) of the skin, which do not meet the criteria for inflammatory carcinoma

T4c: Both T4a and T4b

T4d: Inflammatory carcinoma (see "Rules for Classification")

Posttreatment ypT. Clinical (pretreatment) T will be defined by clinical and radiographic findings, while y pathologic (posttreatment) T will be determined by pathologic size and extension

The ypT will be measured as the largest single focus of invasive tumor, with the modifier "m" indicating multiple foci. The measurement of the largest tumor focus should not include areas of fibrosis within the tumor bed. The inclusion of additional information in the pathology report, such as the distance over which tumor foci extend, the number of tumor foci present, or the number of slides/blocks in which tumor appears, may assist the clinician in estimating the extent of disease. A comparison of the cellularity in the initial biopsy to that in the posttreatment specimen may also aid in the assessment of response

Note: If a cancer was designated as inflammatory before neoadjuvant chemotherapy, the patient will be designated to have inflammatory breast cancer throughout, even if the patient has complete resolution of inflammatory findings

Regional lymph nodes (N)

Clinical

NX: Regional lymph nodes cannot be assessed (e.g., previously removed)

N0:   No regional lymph node metastases

N1:   Metastases to movable ipsilateral level I, II axillary lymph node(s)

N2:   Metastases in ipsilateral level I, II axillary lymph nodes that are clinically fixed or matted; or in clinically detected* ipsilateral internal mammary nodes in the *absence* of clinically evident axillary lymph node metastases

N2a: Metastases in ipsilateral level I, II axillary lymph nodes fixed to one another (matted) or to other structures

N2b: Metastases only in clinically detected* ipsilateral internal mammary nodes and in the *absence* of clinically evident level I, II axillary lymph node metastases

continued

N3:	Metastases in ipsilateral infraclavicular (level III axillary) lymph node(s) with or without level I, II axillary lymph node involvement; or in clinically detected* ipsilateral internal mammary lymph node(s) with clinically evident level I, II axillary lymph node metastases; or metastases in ipsilateral supraclavicular lymph node(s) with or without axillary or internal mammary lymph node involvement
N3a:	Metastases in ipsilateral infraclavicular lymph node(s)
N3b:	Metastases in ipsilateral internal mammary lymph node(s) and axillary lymph node(s)
N3c:	Metastases in ipsilateral supraclavicular lymph node(s)

Note: *Clinically detected* is defined as detected by imaging studies (excluding lymphoscintigraphy) or by clinical examination and having characteristics highly suspicious for malignancy or a presumed pathologic macrometastasis based on fine needle aspiration biopsy with cytologic examination. Confirmation of clinically detected metastatic disease by fine needle aspiration without excision biopsy is designated with an (f) suffix, for example, cN3a(f). Excisional biopsy of a lymph node or biopsy of a sentinel node, in the absence of assignment of a pT, is classified as a clinical N, for example, cN1. Information regarding the confirmation of the nodal status will be designated in site-specific factors as clinical, fine needle aspiration, core biopsy, or sentinel lymph node biopsy. Pathologic classification (pN) is used for excision or sentinel lymph node biopsy only in conjunction with a pathologic T assignment

Pathologic (pN)*

pNX:	Regional lymph nodes cannot be assessed (e.g., previously removed, or not removed for pathologic study)
pN0:	No regional lymph node metastasis identified histologically
Note:	Isolated tumor cell clusters (ITC) are defined as small clusters of cells not greater than 0.2 mm, or single tumor cells, or a cluster of fewer than 200 cells in a single histologic cross section. ITCs may be detected by routine histology or by immunohistochemical (IHC) methods. Nodes containing only ITCs are excluded from the total positive node count for purposes of N classification but should be included in the total number of nodes evaluated
pN0(i−):	No regional lymph node metastases histologically, negative IHC
pN0(i+):	Malignant cells in regional lymph node(s) no greater than 0.2 mm (detected by H&E or IHC including ITC)
pN0(mol−):	No regional lymph node metastases histologically, negative molecular findings (RT-PCR)
pN0(mol+):	Positive molecular findings (RT-PCR), **but no regional lymph node metastases detected by histology or IHC
pN1:	Micrometastases; or metastases in 1–3 axillary lymph nodes; and/or in internal mammary nodes with metastases detected by sentinel lymph node biopsy, but not clinically detected***
pN1mi:	Micrometastases (greater than 0.2 mm and/or more than 200 cells, but none greater than 2.0 mm)
pN1a:	Metastases in 1–3 axillary lymph nodes, at least one metastasis greater than 2.0 mm
pN1b:	Metastases in internal mammary nodes with micrometastases or macrometastases detected by sentinel lymph node biopsy, but not clinically detected***
pN1c:	Metastases in 1–3 axillary lymph nodes and in internal mammary lymph nodes with micrometastases or macrometastases detected by sentinel lymph node biopsy, but not clinically detected

continued

pN2:	Metastases in 4–9 axillary lymph nodes; or in clinically detected[d] internal mammary lymph nodes in the *absence* of axillary lymph node metastases
pN2a:	Metastases in 4–9 axillary lymph nodes (at least one tumor deposit greater than 2.0 mm)
pN2b:	Metastases in clinically detected**** internal mammary lymph nodes in the *absence* of axillary lymph node metastases
pN3:	Metastases in ten or more axillary lymph nodes; or in infraclavicular (level III axillary) lymph nodes; or in clinically detected**** ipsilateral internal mammary lymph nodes in the *presence* of one or more positive level I, II axillary lymph nodes; or in more than three axillary lymph nodes and in internal mammary lymph nodes with micrometastases or macrometastases detected by sentinel lymph node biopsy, but not clinically detected****; or in ipsilateral supraclavicular lymph nodes
pN3a:	Metastases in ten or more axillary lymph nodes (at least one tumor deposit greater than 2.0 mm); or metastases to the infraclavicular (level III axillary lymph) nodes
pN3b:	Metastases in clinically detected**** ipsilateral internal mammary lymph nodes in the *presence* of one or more positive axillary lymph nodes; or in more than three axillary lymph nodes and in internal mammary lymph nodes with micrometastases or macrometastases detected by sentinel lymph node biopsy, but not clinically detected[c]
pN3c:	Metastases in ipsilateral supraclavicular lymph nodes

Notes: *Classification is based on axillary lymph node dissection with or without sentinel lymph node biopsy. Classification based solely on sentinel lymph node biopsy without subsequent axillary lymph node dissection is designated (sn) for "sentinel node," for example, pN0(sn)

**RT-PCR: reverse transcriptase/polymerase chain reaction

***"Not clinically detected" is defined as not detected by imaging studies (excluding lymphoscintigraphy) or not detected by clinical examination

****"Clinically detected" is defined as detected by imaging studies (excluding lymphoscintigraphy) or by clinical examination and having characteristics highly suspicious for malignancy or a presumed pathologic macrometastasis based on fine needle aspiration biopsy with cytologic examination

Posttreatment ypN

Posttreatment yp "N" should be evaluated as for clinical (pretreatment) "N" methods above. The modifier "sn" is used only if a sentinel node evaluation was performed after treatment. If no subscript is attached, it is assumed that the axillary nodal evaluation was by axillary node dissection (AND)

The X classification will be used (ypNX) if no yp posttreatment SN or AND was performed

N categories are the same as those used for pN

Distant metastases (M)

M0:	No clinical or radiographic evidence of distant metastases
cM0(i+):	No clinical or radiographic evidence of distant metastases, but deposits of molecularly or microscopically detected tumor cells in circulating blood, bone marrow, or other nonregional nodal tissue that are no larger than 0.2 mm in a patient without symptoms or signs of metastases
M1:	Distant detectable metastases as determined by classic clinical and radiographic means and/or histologically proven larger than 0.2 mm

continued

Posttreatment yp M classification. The M category for patients treated with neoadjuvant therapy is the category assigned in the clinical stage, prior to the initiation of neoadjuvant therapy

Identification of distant metastases after the start of therapy in cases where pretherapy evaluation showed no metastases is considered progression of disease. If a patient was designated to have detectable distant metastases (M1) before chemotherapy, the patient will be designated as M1 throughout

Anatomic stage/prognostic groups	
0:	Tis N0 M0
IA:	T1* N0 M0
IB:	T0 N1mi M0
	T1* N1mi M0
IIA:	T0 N1** M0
	T1* N1** M0
	T2 N0 M0
IIB:	T2 N1 M0
	T3 N0 M0
IIIA:	T0 N2 M0
	T1* N2 M0
	T2 N2 M0
	T3 N1 M0
	T3 N2 M0
IIIB:	T4 N0 M0
	T4 N1 M0
	T4 N2 M0
IIIC:	Any T N3 M0
IV:	Any T Any N M1

Notes: *T1 includes T1mi

**T0 and T1 tumors with nodal micrometastases only are excluded from stage IIA and are classified stage IB

M0 includes M0(i+)

The designation pM0 is not valid; any M0 should be clinical

If a patient presents with M1 prior to neoadjuvant systemic therapy, the stage is considered stage IV and remains stage IV regardless of response to neoadjuvant therapy

Stage designation may be changed if postsurgical imaging studies reveal the presence of distant metastases, provided that the studies are carried out within 4 months of diagnosis in the absence of disease progression and provided that the patient has not received neoadjuvant therapy

Postneoadjuvant therapy is designated with "yc" or "yp" prefix. Of note, no stage group is assigned if there is a complete pathologic response (CR) to neoadjuvant therapy, for example, ypT0ypN0cM0

Table 17.3 (AJCC 8TH ED., 2017)

Definition OF AJCC TNM
Definition of primary tumor (T) – clinical and pathological

T category	T criteria
TX	Primary tumor cannot be assessed
T0	No evidence of primary tumor
Tis (DCIS)*	Ductal carcinoma in situ
Tis (Paget)	Paget disease of the nipple NOT associated with invasive carcinoma and/or ductal carcinoma in situ (DCIS) in the underlying breast parenchyma. Carcinomas in the breast parenchyma associated with Paget disease are categorized based on the size and characteristics of the parenchymal disease, although the presence of Paget disease should still be noted
T1	Tumor ≤ 20 mm in greatest dimension
T1mi	Tumor ≤ 1 mm in greatest dimension
T1a	Tumor > 1 mm but ≤ 5 mm in greatest dimension (round any measurement 1.0-1.9 mm to 2 mm)
T1b	Tumor > 5 mm but ≤ 10 mm in greatest dimension
T1c	Tumor > 10 mm but ≤ 20 mm in greatest dimension
T2	Tumor > 20 mm but ≤ 50 mm in greatest dimension
T3	Tumor > 50 mm in greatest dimension
T4	Tumor of any size with direct extension to the chest wall and/or to the skin (ulceration or macroscopic nodules); invasion of the dermis alone does not qualify as T4
T4a	Extension to the chest wall; invasion or adherence to pectoralis muscle in the absence of invasion of chest wall structures does not qualify as T4
T4b	Ulceration and/or ipsilateral macroscopic satellite nodules and/or edema (including peau d'orange) of the skin that does not meet the criteria for inflammatory carcinoma
T4c	Both T4a and T4b are present
T4d	Inflammatory carcinoma (see "Rules for Classification")

Note: Lobular carcinoma in situ (LCIS) is a benign entity and is removed from TNM staging in the AJCC Cancer Staging Manual, Eighth Edition

DEFINITION OF REGIONAL LYMPH NODES – CLINICAL (CN)

cN category	cN criteria
cNX*	Regional lymph nodes cannot be assessed (e.g., previously removed)
cN0	No regional lymph node metastases (by imaging or clinical examination)
cN1	Metastases to movable ipsilateral Levels I and II axillary lymph node(s)
cN1mi**	Micrometastases (approximately 200 cells, larger than 0.2 mm, but not larger than 2.0 mm)

continued

cN category	cN criteria
cN2	Metastases in ipsilateral Levels I and II axillary lymph nodes that are clinically fixed or matted *or* in ipsilateral internal mammary nodes in the absence of axillary lymph node metastases
cN2a	Metastases in ipsilateral Levels I and II axillary lymph nodes fixed to one another (matted) or to other structures
cN2b	Metastases only in ipsilateral internal mammary nodes in the absence of axillary lymph node metastases
cN3	Metastases in ipsilateral infraclavicular (Level III axillary) lymph node(s) with or without Levels I and II axillary lymph node involvement, in ipsilateral internal mammary lymph node(s) with Levels I and II axillary lymph node metastases, *or* in ipsilateral supraclavicular lymph node(s) with or without axillary or internal mammary lymph node involvement
cN3a	Metastases in ipsilateral infraclavicular lymph node(s)
cN3b	Metastases in ipsilateral internal mammary lymph node(s) and axillary lymph node(s)
cN3c	Metastases in ipsilateral supraclavicular lymph node(s)

Note: (sn) and (f) suffixes should be added to the N category to denote confirmation of metastasis by sentinel node biopsy and fine-needle aspiration/core needle biopsy, respectively

*The cNX category is used sparingly in cases where regional lymph nodes have previously been surgically removed or where there is no documentation of physical examination of the axilla

**cN1mi is rarely used but may be appropriate in cases where sentinel node biopsy is performed before tumor resection, most likely to occur in cases treated with neoadjuvant therapy

DEFINITION OF REGIONAL LYMPH NODES – PATHOLOGICAL (PN)

pN category	pN criteria
pNX	Regional lymph nodes cannot be assessed (e.g., not removed for pathological study or previously removed)
pN0	No regional lymph node metastasis identified or ITCs only
pN0(i+)	ITCs only (malignant cell clusters not larger than 0.2 mm) in regional lymph node(s)
pN0(mol+)	Positive molecular findings by reverse transcriptase polymerase chain reaction (RT-PCR); no ITCs detected
pN1	Micrometastases or metastases in 1–3 axillary lymph nodes and/or clinically negative internal mammary nodes with micrometastases or macrometastases by sentinel lymph node biopsy
pN1mi	Micrometastases (approximately 200 cells, larger than 0.2 mm, but not larger than 2.0 mm)

continued

pN category	pN criteria
pN1a	Metastases in 1–3 axillary lymph nodes, at least one metastasis larger than 2.0 mm
pN1b	Metastases in ipsilateral internal mammary sentinel nodes, excluding ITCs
pN1c	pN1a and pN1b combined
pN2	Metastases in 4–9 axillary lymph nodes or positive ipsilateral internal mammary lymph nodes by imaging in the absence of axillary lymph node metastases
pN2a	Metastases in 4–9 axillary lymph nodes (at least one tumor deposit larger than 2.0 mm)
pN2b	Metastases in clinically detected internal mammary lymph nodes with or without microscopic confirmation; with pathologically negative axillary nodes
pN3	Metastases in 10 or more axillary lymph nodes, in infraclavicular (Level III axillary) lymph nodes, positive ipsilateral internal mammary lymph nodes by imaging in the presence of one or more positive Levels I and II axillary lymph nodes, in more than three axillary lymph nodes and micrometastases or macrometastases by sentinel lymph node biopsy in clinically negative ipsilateral internal mammary lymph nodes, *or* in ipsilateral supraclavicular lymph nodes
pN3a	Metastases in 10 or more axillary lymph nodes (at least one tumor deposit larger than 2.0 mm) *or* metastases to the infraclavicular (Level III axillary) lymph nodes
pN3b	pN1a or pN2a in the presence of cN2b (positive internal mammary nodes by imaging) *or* pN2a in the presence of pN1b
pN3c	Metastases in ipsilateral supraclavicular lymph nodes

Note: (sn) and (f) suffixes should be added to the N category to denote confirmation of metastasis by sentinel node biopsy or FNA/core needle biopsy, respectively, with N0 further resection of nodes

DEFINITION OF DISTANT METASTASIS (M)

M category	M criteria
M0	No clinical or radiographic evidence of distant metastases*
cM0(i+)	No clinical or radiographic evidence of distant metastases in the presence of tumor cells or deposits not larger than 0.2 mm detected microscopically or by molecular techniques in circulating blood, bone marrow, or other nonregional nodal tissues in a patient without symptoms or signs of metastases
M1	Distant metastases detected by clinical and radiographic means (cM) and/or histologically proven metastases larger than 0.2 mm (pM)

*Note that imaging studies are not required to assign the cM0 category

AJCC ANATOMIC AND PROGNOSTIC STAGE GROUPS
AJCC ANATOMIC STAGE GROUPS

When T is...	And N is...	And M is...	Then the stage group is...
Tis	N0	M0	0
T1	N0	M0	IA
T0	N1mi	M0	IB
T1	N1mi	M0	IB
T0	N1	M0	IIA
T1	N1	M0	IIA
T2	N0	M0	IIA
T2	N1	M0	IIB
T3	N0	M0	IIB
T0	N2	M0	IIIA
T1	N2	M0	IIIA
T2	N2	M0	IIIA
T3	N1	M0	IIIA
T3	N2	M0	IIIA
T4	N0	M0	IIIB
T4	N1	M0	IIIB
T4	N2	M0	IIIB
Any T	N3	M0	IIIC
Any T	Any N	M1	IV

CLINICAL PROGNOSTIC STAGE

When TNM is...	And Grade is...	And HER2 Status is...	And ER Status is...	And PR Status is...	Then the Clinical Prognostic Stage Group is...
Tis N0 M0	Any	Any	Any	Any	0
T1* N0 M0	G1	Positive	Positive	Positive	IA
T0 N1mi M0				Negative	IA
T1* N1mi M0			Negative	Positive	IA
				Negative	IA
		Negative	Positive	Positive	IA
				Negative	IA
			Negative	Positive	IA
				Negative	IB
	G2	Positive	Positive	Positive	IA
				Negative	IA
			Negative	Positive	IA
				Negative	IA
		Negative	Positive	Positive	IA
				Negative	IA
			Negative	Positive	IA
				Negative	IB
	G3	Positive	Positive	Positive	IA
				Negative	IA
			Negative	Positive	IA
				Negative	IA
		Negative	Positive	Positive	IA
				Negative	IB
			Negative	Positive	IB
				Negative	IB

When TNM is...	And Grade is...	And HER2 Status is...	And ER Status is...	And PR Status is...	Then the Clinical Prognostic Stage Group is...
T0 N1** M0 T1* N1** M0 T2 N0 M0	G1	Positive	Positive	Positive	IB
				Negative	IIA
			Negative	Positive	IIA
				Negative	IIA
		Negative	Positive	Positive	IB
				Negative	IIA
			Negative	Positive	IIA
				Negative	IIA
	G2	Positive	Positive	Positive	IB
				Negative	IIA
			Negative	Positive	IIA
				Negative	IIA
		Negative	Positive	Positive	IB
				Negative	IIA
			Negative	Positive	IIA
				Negative	IIB
	G3	Positive	Positive	Positive	IB
				Negative	IIA
			Negative	Positive	IIA
				Negative	IIA
		Negative	Positive	Positive	IIA
				Negative	IIB
			Negative	Positive	IIB
				Negative	IIB

When TNM is...	And Grade is...	And HER2 Status is...	And ER Status is...	And PR Status is...	Then the Clinical Prognostic Stage Group is...
T2 N1*** M0 T3 N0 M0	G1	Positive	Positive	Positive	IB
				Negative	IIA
			Negative	Positive	IIA
				Negative	IIB
		Negative	Positive	Positive	IIA
				Negative	IIB
			Negative	Positive	IIB
				Negative	IIB
	G2	Positive	Positive	Positive	IB
				Negative	IIA
			Negative	Positive	IIA
				Negative	IIB
		Negative	Positive	Positive	IIA
				Negative	IIB
			Negative	Positive	IIB
				Negative	IIIB
	G3	Positive	Positive	Positive	IB
				Negative	IIB
			Negative	Positive	IIB
				Negative	IIB
		Negative	Positive	Positive	IIB
				Negative	IIIA
			Negative	Positive	IIIA
				Negative	IIIB

V

When TNM is...	And Grade is...	And HER2 Status is...	And ER Status is...	And PR Status is...	Then the Clinical Prognostic Stage Group is...
T0 N2 M0	G1	Positive	Positive	Positive	IIA
T1* N2 M0				Negative	IIIA
T2 N2 M0			Negative	Positive	IIIA
T3 N1*** M0				Negative	IIIA
T3 N2 M0		Negative	Positive	Positive	IIA
				Negative	IIIA
			Negative	Positive	IIIA
				Negative	IIIB
	G2	Positive	Positive	Positive	IIA
				Negative	IIIA
			Negative	Positive	IIIA
				Negative	IIIA
		Negative	Positive	Positive	IIA
				Negative	IIIA
			Negative	Positive	IIIA
				Negative	IIIB
	G3	Positive	Positive	Positive	IIB
				Negative	IIIA
			Negative	Positive	IIIA
				Negative	IIIA
		Negative	Positive	Positive	IIIA
				Negative	IIIB
			Negative	Positive	IIIB
				Negative	IIIC

When TNM is...	And Grade is...	And HER2 Status is...	And ER Status is...	And PR Status is...	Then the Clinical Prognostic Stage Group is...
T4 N0 M0	G1	Positive	Positive	Positive	IIIA
T4 N1*** M0				Negative	IIIB
T4 N2 M0			Negative	Positive	IIIB
Any T N3 M0				Negative	IIIB
		Negative	Positive	Positive	IIIB
				Negative	IIIB
			Negative	Positive	IIIB
				Negative	IIIC
	G2	Positive	Positive	Positive	IIIA
				Negative	IIIB
			Negative	Positive	IIIB
				Negative	IIIB
		Negative	Positive	Positive	IIIB
				Negative	IIIB
			Negative	Positive	IIIB
				Negative	IIIC
	G3	Positive	Positive	Positive	IIIB
				Negative	IIIB
			Negative	Positive	IIIB
				Negative	IIIB
		Negative	Positive	Positive	IIIB
				Negative	IIIC
			Negative	Positive	IIIC
				Negative	IIIC

V

When TNM is...	And Grade is...	And HER2 Status is...	And ER Status is...	And PR Status is...	Then the Clinical Prognostic Stage Group is...
Any T Any N M1	Any	Any	Any	Any	IV

*T1 includes T1mi

**N1 does not include N1mi. T1 N1mi M0 and T0 N1mi M0 cancers are included for prognostic staging with T1 N0 M0 cancers of the same prognostic factor status

***N1 includes N1mi. T2, T3, and T4 cancers and N1mi are included for prognostic staging with T2 N1, T3 N1 and T4 N1, respectively

Notes:

1. Because N1mi categorization requires evaluation of the entire node, and cannot be assigned on the basis of an FNA or core biopsy, N1mi can only be used with Clinical Prognostic Staging when clinical staging is based on a resected lymph node in the absence of resection of the primary cancer, such as the situation where sentinel node biopsy is performed prior to receipt of neoadjuvant chemotherapy or endocrine therapy

2. For cases with lymph node involvement with no evidence of primary tumor (e.g. T0 N1, etc.) or with breast ductal carcinoma *in situ* (e.g. Tis N1, etc.), the grade, HER2, ER, and PR information from the tumor in the lymph node should be used for assigning stage group

3. For cases where HER2 is determined to be "equivocal" by ISH (FISH or CISH) testing under the 2013 ASCO/CAP HER2 testing guidelines, the HER2 "negative" category should be used for staging in the Clinical Prognostic Stage Group table.[81, 82]

4. The prognostic value of these Prognostic Stage Groups is based on populations of persons with breast cancer that have been offered and mostly treated with appropriate endocrine and/or systemic chemotherapy (including anti-HER2 therapy)

PATHOLOGIC PROGNOSTIC STAGE

When TNM is...	And Grade is...	And HER2 Status is...	And ER Status is...	And PR Status is...	Then the Pathological Prognostic Stage Group is...
Tis N0 M0	Any	Any	Any	Any	0
T1* N0 M0	G1	Positive	Positive	Positive	IA
T0 N1mi M0				Negative	IA
T1* N1mi M0			Negative	Positive	IA
				Negative	IA
		Negative	Positive	Positive	IA
				Negative	IA
			Negative	Positive	IA
				Negative	IA
	G2	Positive	Positive	Positive	IA
				Negative	IA
			Negative	Positive	IA
				Negative	IA
		Negative	Positive	Positive	IA
				Negative	IA
			Negative	Positive	IA
				Negative	IB
	G3	Positive	Positive	Positive	IA
				Negative	IA
			Negative	Positive	IA
				Negative	IA
		Negative	Positive	Positive	IA
				Negative	IA
			Negative	Positive	IA
				Negative	IB

V

When TNM is...	And Grade is...	And HER2 Status is...	And ER Status is...	And PR Status is...	Then the Pathological Prognostic Stage Group is...
T0 N1** M0 T1* N1** M0 T2 N0 M0	G1	Positive	Positive	Positive	IA
				Negative	IB
			Negative	Positive	IB
				Negative	IIA
		Negative	Positive	Positive	IA
				Negative	IB
			Negative	Positive	IB
				Negative	IIA
	G2	Positive	Positive	Positive	IA
				Negative	IB
			Negative	Positive	IB
				Negative	IIA
		Negative	Positive	Positive	IA
				Negative	IIA
			Negative	Positive	IIA
				Negative	IIA
	G3	Positive	Positive	Positive	IA
				Negative	IIA
			Negative	Positive	IIA
				Negative	IIA
		Negative	Positive	Positive	IB
				Negative	IIA
			Negative	Positive	IIA
				Negative	IIA

When TNM is...	And Grade is...	And HER2 Status is...	And ER Status is...	And PR Status is...	Then the Pathological Prognostic Stage Group is...
T2 N1*** M0 T3 N0 M0	G1	Positive	Positive	Positive	IA
				Negative	IIB
			Negative	Positive	IIB
				Negative	IIB
		Negative	Positive	Positive	IA
				Negative	IIB
			Negative	Positive	IIB
				Negative	IIB
	G2	Positive	Positive	Positive	IB
				Negative	IIB
			Negative	Positive	IIB
				Negative	IIB
		Negative	Positive	Positive	IB
				Negative	IIB
			Negative	Positive	IIB
				Negative	IIB
	G3	Positive	Positive	Positive	IB
				Negative	IIB
			Negative	Positive	IIB
				Negative	IIB
		Negative	Positive	Positive	IIA
				Negative	IIB
			Negative	Positive	IIB
				Negative	IIIA

When TNM is...	And Grade is...	And HER2 Status is...	And ER Status is...	And PR Status is...	Then the Pathological Prognostic Stage Group is...
T0 N2 M0	G1	Positive	Positive	Positive	IB
T1* N2 M0				Negative	IIIA
T2 N2 M0			Negative	Positive	IIIA
T3 N1*** M0				Negative	IIIA
T3 N2 M0		Negative	Positive	Positive	IB
				Negative	IIIA
			Negative	Positive	IIIA
				Negative	IIIA
	G2	Positive	Positive	Positive	IB
				Negative	IIIA
			Negative	Positive	IIIA
				Negative	IIIA
		Negative	Positive	Positive	IB
				Negative	IIIA
			Negative	Positive	IIIA
				Negative	IIIB
	G3	Positive	Positive	Positive	IIA
				Negative	IIIA
			Negative	Positive	IIIA
				Negative	IIIA
		Negative	Positive	Positive	IIB
				Negative	IIIA
			Negative	Positive	IIIA
				Negative	IIIC

When TNM is...	And Grade is...	And HER2 Status is...	And ER Status is...	And PR Status is...	Then the Pathological Prognostic Stage Group is...
T4 N0 M0	G1	Positive	Positive	Positive	IIIA
T4 N1*** M0				Negative	IIIB
T4 N2 M0			Negative	Positive	IIIB
Any T N3 M0				Negative	IIIB
		Negative	Positive	Positive	IIIA
				Negative	IIIB
			Negative	Positive	IIIB
				Negative	IIIB
	G2	Positive	Positive	Positive	IIIA
				Negative	IIIB
			Negative	Positive	IIIB
				Negative	IIIB
		Negative	Positive	Positive	IIIA
				Negative	IIIB
			Negative	Positive	IIIB
				Negative	IIIC
	G3	Positive	Positive	Positive	IIIB
				Negative	IIIB
			Negative	Positive	IIIB
				Negative	IIIB
		Negative	Positive	Positive	IIIB
				Negative	IIIC
			Negative	Positive	IIIC
				Negative	IIIC

When TNM is...	And Grade is...	And HER2 Status is...	And ER Status is...	And PR Status is...	Then the Pathological Prognostic Stage Group is...
Any T Any N M1	Any	Any	Any	Any	IV

*T1 includes T1mi

**N1 does not include N1mi. T1 N1mi M0 and T0 N1mi M0 cancers are included for prognostic staging with T1 N0 M0 cancers of the same prognostic factor status

***N1 includes N1mi. T2, T3, and T4 cancers and N1mi are included for prognostic staging with T2 N1, T3 N1 and T4 N1, respectively

Notes:

1. For cases with lymph node involvement with no evidence of primary tumor (e.g. T0 N1, etc.) or with breast ductal carcinoma *in situ* (e.g. Tis N1, etc.), the grade, HER2, ER, and PR information from the tumor in the lymph node should be used for assigning stage group

2. For cases where HER2 is determined to be "equivocal" by ISH (FISH or CISH) testing under the 2013 ASCO/CAP HER2 testing guidelines, HER2 "negative" category should be used for staging in the Clinical Pathological Prognostic Stage Group Table.[81, 82]

3. The prognostic value of these Prognostic Stage Groups is based on populations of persons with breast cancer that have been offered and mostly treated with appropriate endocrine and/or systemic chemotherapy (including anti-HER2 therapy)

GENOMIC PROFILE FOR PATHOLOGIC PROGNOSTIC STAGING

When OncotypeDx Score is Less than 11

And TNM is...	And Grade is...	And HER2 Status is...	And ER Status is...	And PR Status is...	Then the Pathological Prognostic Stage Group is...
T1 N0 M0 T2 N0 M0	Any	Negative	Positive	Any	IA

Notes:

1. Obtaining genomic profiles is NOT required for assigning Pathological Prognostic Stage. However genomic profiles may be performed for use in determining appropriate treatment. If the OncotypeDx® test is performed in cases with a T1N0M0 or T2N0M0 cancer that is HER2-negative and ER-positive, and the recurrence score is less than 11, the case should be assigned Pathological Prognostic Stage Group IA

2. If OncotypeDx® is not performed, or if it is performed and the OncotypeDx® score is not available, or is 11 or greater for patients with T1–2 N0 M0 HER2–negative, ER-positive cancer, then the Prognostic Stage Group is assigned based on the anatomic and biomarker categories shown above

3. OncotypeDx® is the only multigene panel included to classify Pathological Prognostic Stage because prospective Level I data supports this use for patients with a score less than 11. Future updates to the staging system may include results form other multigene panels to assign cohorts of patients to Prognostic Stage Groups based on the then available evidence. Inclusion or exclusion in this staging table of a genomic profile assay is not an endorsement of any specific assay and should not limit appropriate clinical use of any genomic profile assay based on evidence available at the time of treatment

TREATMENT RECOMMENDATIONS

SURGERY

- Breast conservation surgery (BCS) may consist of (in order of decreasing tissue removed) quadrantectomy, wide excision, and lumpectomy (local excision).
- Variations of mastectomy:
  - Radical mastectomy: removal of breast, pectoralis minor and major muscles, axillary LN dissection (ALND) (levels I–III).
  - Modified radical mastectomy: removal of breast to the level of pectoralis minor muscle, ALND (levels I–II), and pectoralis major is spared.
  - Total (simple) mastectomy: removal of breast to the level of pectoralis minor muscle with no lymph node dissection.
  - Skin sparing mastectomy preserves skin of breast for enhanced reconstructive cosmetic outcomes.
  - Total skin sparing mastectomy preserves skin and nipple/areolar complex for enhanced reconstructive outcome.
- Reconstructive options postmastectomy include delayed vs. immediate and autologous tissue vs. expander/implant.

MANAGEMENT OF REGIONAL LYMPH NODES

- Surgical evaluation/treatment of axilla:
  - Axillary LN dissection (ALND)
  - Level I/II axillary node dissection performed with modified radical mastectomy
- Sentinel lymph node biopsy (SLNbx) has replaced ALND for the clinically negative axilla:
  - Performed with injection of radiotracer and/or methylene blue dye into breast skin and/or tumor.
  - False-negative rate is similar to ALND (~2–12%) and likely not increased with neoadjuvant chemotherapy.
  - Completion of ALND or radiotherapy coverage is indicated in the case of involved SLNB. Nomograms may be used to assess risk for non-sentinel node positivity (http://nomograms.mskcc.org/breast/BreastAdditional NonSLNMetastasesPage.aspx).

- *NSABP B-04* (NEJM 2002b, c): 1079 patients with clinically negative axillary LN randomized to 1 of 3 arms: radical mastectomy vs. total mastectomy (TM) without axillary dissection but with post-op RT vs. total mastectomy plus axillary dissection if LN pathologically positive. Also 586 patients with clinically + axillary LN randomized to 1 of 2 arms (radical mastectomy vs. total mastectomy without axillary dissection but with post-op RT). No systemic therapy. At 25-year follow-up, no significant differences in DFS or OS among the three groups of patients with clinically negative LN or the two groups of patients with clinically + LN. The use of systemic therapy in modern cohorts likely alters patterns of distant vs. LR recurrence, increasing the need for LR control. Approximately 40% of cN0 patients were found to be pLN+ after ALND. Among cN0 patients, axillary failure was <4% if addressed surgically or with RT vs. 19% in TM alone arm.

- Louis-Sylvestre (JCO 2004): 658 cN0 patients with <3 cm primary randomized to ALND or axillary RT. All had wide excision of primary and breast RT, and <10% had systemic therapy. Twenty-one percent of the patients in the axillary dissection group were pN+. Five-year survival benefit in ALND group, but identical OS at 15 years (73.8 vs. 75.5%). Decreased isolated axillary recurrences in ALND group at 15 years (1 vs. 3%; $p = 0.04$). No difference in breast, supraclavicular, and distant recurrence.

- *NSABP B-32* (Krag, Lancet Oncol 2010): Randomized trial of SLNbx (with ALND if +) vs. upfront ALND. SLNbx had an overall accuracy of 97.1%, false-negative rate of 9.8%, and negative predictive value of 96.1%. Only 1.4% of SLN specimens were outside of axillary levels I and II. No difference in 8-year OS, DFS, or sites of first treatment failure for upfront ALND vs. SLNBx.

- *ACOSOG Z-11* (Ann Surg 2010, JAMA 2011, San Antonio Breast Conference 2012 abstract): 856 pts with positive SLN randomized to lumpectomy + SLND with or without completion ALND. 97% received systemic therapy and 89% received whole breast RT. In ALND arm, 27% of pts had additional involved LNs. No significant difference in LR (2.8% SLND vs. 4.1% completion ALND). Regional recurrences (axilla, SCV) were 0.5% and 0.9%, respectively:

- About 1/3 of pts who received RT had detailed RT records (n = 228), and most patients were treated with tangents alone (n = 540), some with high tangents. 89 patients (15%) received radiation directed at the SCV, which were more likely to be patients with higher numbers of involved LN.
- *AMAROS* (Lancet Oncol 2014): Randomized non-inferiority trial of 1425 patients with +SLN to receive either ALND or axillary RT. 5-year rate of axillary recurrence was not significantly different (0.43% for ALND vs. 1.19% for axillary RT). Patients with ALND had higher rates of clinical lymphedema and increase in arm circumference > 10%, though the latter was only significant at 5 years.
- *MA-20* (NEJM 2015): 1832 patients with T1-3, N0-1 invasive breast cancer randomized to whole breast irradiation (WBI) +/− regional nodal irradiation (RNI). With a median follow-up of 9.5 years, isolated regional recurrence was 6.8% with WBI vs. 4.3% for WBI + RNI and regional recurrence alone was 2.5% vs. 0.5%, respectively. RNI improved 10-yr DFS (82% vs. 77%). On subgroup analysis, the N0 pts had greatest benefit of RNI. Adding RNI increased radiation pneumonitis by 1% and lymphedema by 4%.
- *EORTC Internal Mammary and SCV Nodal Irradiation* (NEJM 2015): 4004 patients treated with mastectomy (N = 955) or BCS (N = 3049) and either ALND or SNB followed by ALND if node positive, randomized to either +/− RNI. With median f/u 10.9 years, local recurrence was 5.5% across arms. RNI reduced regional recurrence from 4.2% to 2.7% (IMN recurrence 0.8% to 0.2%). RNI improved 10-yr DFS (72% vs. 69%) and breast cancer mortality (12.5% vs. 14.4%).

SYSTEMIC THERAPY

ADJUVANT ENDOCRINE THERAPY

- Generally recommended for all ER-positive tumors, regardless of age, menopausal status, node status, or whether chemotherapy is administered.
- The need for complete ovarian suppression/ablation in premenopausal women is currently under investigation.

- SERMs (e.g., tamoxifen, raloxifene) indicated for both pre- and postmenopausal women:
  - For ER+ disease, adjuvant tamoxifen reduces annual recurrence risk by 39%. 5 years of tamoxifen is more effective than 1–2 years of tamoxifen, and extending tamoxifen for up to 10 years further reduces absolute recurrence risk by 3.7% (ATLAS trial).
  - Side effects include hot flashes, night sweats, vaginal dryness, increased risk of thromboembolic disease, and endometrial proliferation or uterine cancer (1.5–3% absolute risk over 5–10 years).
- Aromatase inhibitors (AIs: anastrozole, letrozole, exemestane) are indicated for postmenopausal patients (they are not active in premenopausal patients):
  - AIs may be given as initial adjuvant endocrine therapy, after 2–3 years of tamoxifen, or as extended therapy following 5 years of tamoxifen. The optimal sequence is not clear.
  - Two randomized trials report fewer recurrences, but no survival difference with initial adjuvant AIs vs. tamoxifen (ATAC, BIG 1-98).
  - A meta-analysis of randomized trials reports fewer recurrences, but no clear OS benefit by adding AIs after initial tamoxifen vs. tamoxifen alone.
  - Side effects include hot flashes, night sweats, vaginal dryness, musculoskeletal symptoms/arthralgia, and osteoporosis.

CYTOTOXIC CHEMOTHERAPY

- Generally recommended for >1 cm tumors or node-positive disease.
- Consider for all triple negative tumors, given high rates of recurrence and lack of options for targeted or endocrine therapies.
- The EBCTCG meta-analysis (Lancet 2005a, b) reported that chemotherapy reduces annual breast cancer death rate by about 38% for women younger than 50 years and

by about 20% for women 50–69 years. For women over 70 years, there are insufficient data to make definitive chemotherapy recommendations.
- There are many gene-based assays to predict prognosis:
  - Patients with high recurrence score on 21-gene assay clearly benefit from chemotherapy, whereas low-score patients do not appear to benefit from chemotherapy as supported by the TAILORx study.
  - Long-term follow-up of the TAILORx study will clarify the use of chemotherapy for ER+, HER2-negative, LN-negative patients with intermediate score between 11–25.
- Several combination chemotherapy regimens are appropriate to consider when indicated. NCCN guidelines provide a detailed description for providers.
- Anthracycline (doxorubicin)-based regiments (± taxanes for high-risk disease) have been associated with superior outcomes as compared to non-anthracycline-containing regimens.
- Recent evidence suggests increased DFS and OS with taxane-based therapy as compared to anthracycline-based therapy.
- Dose-dense regimens may have increased efficacy in high-risk patients.
- Common regimens:
  - AC = adriamycin and cyclophosphamide.
  - AC-Taxol = AC followed by paclitaxel.
  - TC = Taxotere and cyclophosphamide.
  - CMF (lowest incidence of alopecia) = cyclophosphamide, methotrexate, and 5-fluorouracil.
  - FAC = 5-fluorouracil, adriamycin, and cyclophosphamide.
  - TAC = Taxotere (docetaxel), adriamycin, and cyclophosphamide.
  - FEC = 5-fluorouracil, epirubicin, and cyclophosphamide.
- Randomized trials have demonstrated that neoadjuvant chemotherapy is equivalent to adjuvant chemotherapy, including both patients with operable and inoperable disease. Neoadjuvant treatment can include cytotoxic

chemotherapy, endocrine therapy, or HER2 targeted therapy:

- Typically, indications are similar as adjuvant therapy.
- Advantages of neoadjuvant chemotherapy: assessment of disease response, increased rate of breast conserving therapy (BCT), can render inoperable tumors operable.
- Neoadjuvant chemotherapy converts 20–30% of patients initially ineligible for BCT to eligible.
- Complete clinical and pathologic response rates depend on the initial extent of disease.
- For advanced-stage disease, 20–40% achieve cCR after neoadjuvant chemotherapy and 10–20% achieve pCR.
- Clinical response frequently does not correlate with pathological response:
  - Approximately 1/3 with a cCR found to have pathological residual disease.
  - If initially cLN+, full ALND should be considered regardless of response to neoadjuvant chemo.
  - Diminished response noted in ER+, low-grade, or invasive lobular cancers.
- *Trastuzumab (Herceptin)*, a humanized monoclonal antibody for HER2/neu, indicated for most patients with HER2 overexpression to improve DFS:
- 12 months trastuzumab is standard as shorter duration is not as effective and longer duration has no added benefit.
- NCCN-preferred regimens are AC followed by paclitaxel with trastuzumab for 1 year or the TCH regimen (docetaxel, carboplatin, and trastuzumab).
- Concurrent administration with left-sided RT does not appear to increase cardiac risk.
- Perjeta (pertuzumab), a humanized monoclonal antibody targeting HER2 to inhibit dimerization, may be incorporated for dual anti-HER2 blockade in the neoadjuvant or adjuvant setting.
- Bisphosphonates may play a role in preventing skeletal events and improving DFS.
- Various other targeted therapies, such as antiangiogenic agents (bevacizumab), appear promising and are currently under investigation.

IN SITU DISEASE

Table 17.4 RECOMMENDED TREATMENT

Stage	Recommended treatment
DCIS	BCT with lumpectomy ± RT. RT generally indicated for all patients to reduce LR, but some patients may have small absolute benefit and may choose to omit RT [e.g., older women, with small (<0.5 cm), unicentric, low-grade tumors excised with wide (≥1 cm) negative margins]. Alternative is total mastectomy (TM) with or without SLN bx. TM indicated for diffuse malignant microcalcifications, multicentric disease, persistently +margins, or patient desire. Consider adjuvant tamoxifen for ER+ tumors
LCIS	Lifelong close observation ± tamoxifen for risk reduction (decrease invasive cancer rate by 56%). If young and strong FH, diffuse disease, or genetic predisposition, consider prophylactic bilateral mastectomy

V

- DCIS treatment is individualized based on clinical and pathological features, and patient preference.
- Margins ≤1–2 mm post-BCS require re-excision as up to 1/2 will have residual DCIS.
- Tamoxifen for ER + DCIS reduces local recurrence after lumpectomy and RT, although absolute benefit may be small and diminishes with increased follow-up:
  - NSABP B-24 (Wapnir JNCI 2011). 1804 patients with DCIS treated with lumpectomy and 50 Gy RT ± tamoxifen 20 mg daily × 5 years. 17.25-year follow-up: tamoxifen reduced IBTR from 16.6% to 13.2% (~50% invasive) and contralateral events from 8.1% to 4.9% (~67% invasive). No OS difference. On secondary analysis, benefit only seen for ER+ patients (50% risk reduction).
  - UK/ANZ (Cuzick Lancet Oncol 2011). See below for trial details. Tamoxifen reduced ipsilateral DCIS recurrences (HR 0.7) and contralateral tumors (HR 0.44).

RANDOMIZED DCIS TRIALS OF BCS ± RT

- Cochrane meta-analysis (Goodwin 2013). Four randomized trials of BCS ± RT, including 3925 patients, confirm benefit of RT on all ipsilateral breast events (HR 0.49) and ipsilateral DCIS recurrence (HR 0.61). All subgroups benefited from RT, with no significant long-term toxicity with RT. No OS difference noted:

- NSABP B-17 (Wapnir JNCI 2011). 818 pts underwent lumpectomy with +/- 50 Gy RT. At 17.25 years, RT reduced noninvasive LF from 15.4% to 9% and invasive LF from 19.6% to 10.7% (total LF: 35 → 19.8%).
- EORTC 10853 (Bijker JCO 2006). 1010 pts underwent lumpectomy with +/- 50 GyRT. RT reduced 10-yr noninvasive LF from 14% to 7% and invasive LF from 13% to 8% (total LF 26 → 15%).
- SweDCIS (Warnberg JCO 2014). 1046 pts underwent lumpectomy +/- RT (80% 50 Gy). RT reduced 20-yr recurrence by 12% (10% for in situ and 2% for invasive).
- UK/ANZ (Cuzick Lancet Oncol 2011). 1030 pts underwent lumpectomy with +/- 50 Gy RT +/- tamoxifen x 5 yrs (4-arm trial). At 12.7-yr follow-up, RT reduced IBTR on tamoxifen (9% to 3%) or off tamoxifen (12% to 4%).
- RTOG 9804 (McCormick, JCO 2015). 636 pts with mammographically detected "low risk" grade 1–2 DCIS <2.5 cm with margins ≥3 mm randomized to observation vs. RT. 62% received tamoxifen. At 7 yrs, RT reduced LF 6.7% to 0.9%. Of LF, 42% were invasive, and 58% were noninvasive. RT reduced cumulative mastectomy from 2.8% to 1.5%.

SELECT NONRANDOMIZED DCIS STUDIES OF BCS ± RT

- ECOG-ACRIN E1594 (Solin, JCO 2015). 665 pts with DCIS treated with lumpectomy with >3 mm margin, no RT. 30% got tamoxifen. Among 561 pts with grade 1–2 DCIS ≤ 2.5 cm, 12-yr IBTR rate was 14.4% (7.5% invasive). Among 104 pts with high-grade DCIS ≤ 1 cm, 12-yr IBTR rate was 24.6% (13.4% invasive).
- Wong (JCO 2006, Breast Cancer Res Treat 2014). Phase II trial of 158 women with predominantly grade 1–2 DCIS measuring ≤2.5 cm on mammography with final margins ≥1 cm observed after lumpectomy (no RT or Tamoxifen). 15.6% local failure at 10 years.

- VNPI (Silverstein, Am J Surg 2003, JNCI 2010). Retrospective review of 706 pts' status post-BCT with or without RT scored based on four parameters: tumor size ($\leq$1.5, 1.6–4.0, $\geq$4.0 cm); pathology (non-high grade without necrosis, non-high grade with necrosis, high grade); margins ($\geq$1, 0.1–0.9, <0.1 cm); and age (>60, 40–60, <40 years). For low risk (score 4, 5, 6), no significant difference in 12-year local RFS (>90–95%) with or without RT. For intermediate risk (score 7, 8, 9), addition of RT provided 12–15% 12-year local RFS benefit. For high risk (score 10, 11, 12, or score 8 with margins<3 mm, score 9 with margins <5 mm), mastectomy recommended due to high 5-year LR (~50%) with or without RT. New treatment recommendations were developed in 2010 to achieve LR of <20% at 12 years. Generalizability of study questioned given unique and intensive surgical/pathological specimen preparation techniques.

V

CLINICAL TOOLS FOR ESTIMATING RISK IN DCIS

- *Oncotype DCIS Score* (Solin, JNCI 2013): 12-gene OncotypeDx DCIS score validated in tissue from ECOG 5194 tumor specimens treated with surgery without radiotherapy. 10-year rates of IBE were 10.6%, 26.7%, and 25.9% for low-, intermediate-, and high-risk groups, respectively. Invasive IBE rates at 10 years for low-, intermediate-, and high-risk groups were 3.7%, 12.3%, and 19.2%, respectively.
- *MSKCC DCIS Nomogram* (Ruldoff JCO 2010): 1868 patients were treated with BCS for DCIS, adjuvant treatment according to clinical judgment and patient preference. Variables associated with risk include age, margin status, number of excisions, year of treatment, radiation therapy, and endocrine therapy. Externally validated by 4 separate studies (Yi 2012; Sweldens 2014; Wang 2014; Collins 2015). http://nomograms.mskcc.org/breast/DuctalCarcinoma InSituRecurrencePage.aspx

INVASIVE DISEASE ELIGIBLE FOR UPFRONT BREAST CONSERVING THERAPY

Table 17.5 RECOMMENDED TREATMENT

Stage	Recommended treatment
I–IIB (± T3 N0)	BCT with lumpectomy and surgical axillary staging + RT. Some consider RT optional for patients ≥70 years of age, with T1 N0, ER+, low grade, no LVI tumors in those who receive adjuvant hormone therapy (HT). Alternative: TM with surgical axillary staging ± RT as indicated. Adjuvant chemo, HT, and/or trastuzumab as indicated

- BCT is equivalent to mastectomy for early-stage disease in appropriately selected patients.
- BCT with lumpectomy + whole breast RT is considered standard of care.
- Repeat excision generally indicated for close/positive margins, especially in young, EIC+, ILC, multiple, or diffusely positive margins.
- Mastectomy reserved for patients ineligible for BCT due to medical or surgical contraindications, or patient preference.
  - See below for postmastectomy RT indications.
- Contraindications to BCT include multicentricity, ratio of tumor size to breast, diffuse microcalcifications, persistently close/positive margins despite reasonable number of repeat excisions (especially in the setting of EIC, ILCA, <35–40 years old, diffuse or multiple close/+ margins), previous breast RT, pregnancy, and scleroderma (lupus is a relative contraindication).
- Lymph node involvement not a contraindication to BCT.
- EIC is not an independent risk factor for recurrence post-BCT when margins are considered, but true negative margins may be more difficult to be achieved in the presence of EIC.
- Younger patients are generally at higher risk for LR.
- Positive margins, close margins (≤1–2 mm), and lymphatic invasions are associated with increased LR post-BCT.
- High grade associated with increased LR in some, but not all, series.

Table 17.6 PHASE III TRIALS HAVE DEMONSTRATED EQUIVALENT OS AND DFS WITH BCS + RT VS. MASTECTOMY FOR INVASIVE DISEASE. SELECT TRIALS

Study	Patients	Randomization	Outcome
NSABP B-06 (Fisher, NEJM, 2002)	1851 patients with stage I/II breast ca (<4 cm, negative margins)	Total mastectomy vs. lumpectomy alone vs. lumpectomy +50 Gy RT	20-year follow-up: no significant differences observed among three groups with respect to DFS, OS, or DM-free survival. Addition of RT to lumpectomy reduced LF 39 → 14% N+ patients had 5-FU based chemo
EORTC 10801 (van Dongen, JNCI 2000)	902 patients with stage I/II breast ca	Modified radical mastectomy vs. lumpectomy +50 Gy RT + boost	10-year follow-up: decreased LF with MRM (12 vs. 20%, $p = 0.01$). No difference in OS (66 vs. 65%). 48% in lumpectomy group had + margins
Milan I (NEJM 2002)	701 patients with T1N0 breast ca	Radical mastectomy vs. quadrantectomy +60 Gy RT	Median follow-up 20 years: LF 2.3 vs. 8.8% in favor of RM ($p < 0.001$). No difference in OS (59 vs. 58%) or breast ca-specific survival (76 vs. 74%). N+ patients had CMF chemo

PHASE III TRIALS OF BCS ± RT FOR INVASIVE DISEASE

Study	Patients	Randomization	Outcome
Oxford overview (Early Breast Cancer Trialists' Collaborative Group, Lancet 2011)	Meta-analysis of 10,801 women in 17 randomized trials with pN0 and pN+ disease	Randomized trials of radiotherapy vs. no RT after BCS	For all patients, RT decreased 10-year LR from 25% to 7.7% (pN0: 23% to 7.3%; pN+: 43% to 12.4%). RT produced similar proportional reduction in LR in all subgroups. RT reduced annual breast cancer death rate by 1/6

PHASE III TRIALS OF BCS AND TAMOXIFEN ± RT FOR INVASIVE DISEASE

Study	Pts	Randomization	Outcome
PMH/Canada	769 pts (median age 68 years), stage I/II pN0) ER/PR±)	Tamoxifen + RT vs. tamoxifen alone	RT reduced 8-year LR (12.2 vs. 4.1%) and improved DFS (82 vs. 76%). No difference in breast ca-specific survival or OS

continued

Study	Pts	Randomization	Outcome
PRIME II (Lancet oncology 2015)	1326 pts, age 65 or older with T1-T2 (up to 3 cm), N-, HR+ breast cancer. Grade 3 or LVI but not both	BCS+ endocrine therapy, randomized to RT (40–50 Gy in 15–25 fx) or no RT	5-year follow-up: ipsilateral breast tumor recurrence was 4.1% without RT, reduced to 1.3% with RT. No difference in regional recurrence, DM or OS
CALGB C9343/ INT trial (Hughes, NEJM 2004, JCO 2013).	636 pts (>70 years) pT1N0, ER+	Tamoxifen + RT vs. tamoxifen alone	Addition of RT to tamoxifen improved 10-year LR (2 vs. 10%,) No difference in breast ca-specific survival or OS
NSABP B-21 (Fisher et al, JCO 2002, Cancer 2007)	1009 pN0 patients with tumors ≤1 cm (both ER/PR ±)	Three arm trial: tamoxifen vs. RT + placebo vs. RT + tamoxifen	14-yr IBTR: Tam 19.5%, RT 10.8%, Tam + RT 10.1%. Tam decreased contralateral breast primaries by 3.2%. No difference in OS and DM

MANAGEMENT OF LOCALLY ADVANCED DISEASE

Table 17.7 RECOMMENDED TREATMENT

Stage	Recommended treatment
IIB (T3N0) and IIIA	Neoadjuvant chemo → surgery (mastectomy or BCT) with surgical axillary staging + RT as indicated Alternative: TM with surgical axillary staging + RT as indicated Adjuvant chemo, HT, and/or trastuzumab as indicated
IIIB–IIIC	Neoadjuvant chemo → surgery (mastectomy or BCT [except T4d: BCT contraindicated]) with surgical axillary staging + RT Adjuvant chemo, HT, and/or trastuzumab as indicated
IV	HT, chemo, and/or trastuzumab as indicated. Consider bisphosphonates for bone metastases. Palliative RT may be needed. Role of surgical resection of primary disease in selected stage IV patients is under investigation

POSTMASTECTOMY RT (PMRT)

- Early PMRT trials limited by selection, technique, and no systemic therapy. Survival detriment attributed to RT in early trials due to cardiac/pulmonary toxicity.
- Contemporary randomized trials have shown **OS** benefit for PMRT in patients receiving systemic therapy.
- Consensus PMRT indications (ASTRO, IJROBP 1999; Recht et al, JCO 2001):
  - T3/4 (T3N0 controversial)
  - +margins
  - Gross ECE
  - ≥4+ nodes
- ASCO/ASTRO/SSO Update (Recht et al, JCO 2016). PMRT reduces risk of LRF and breast cancer mortality for T1–2 N1 pts, but some subsets are likely to have such low risk of LRF that the absolute benefit of PMRT is outweighed by toxicities. In EBCTCG meta-analysis, PMRT reduced 10-yr isolated LRF from 21% to 4% and 20-yr breast cancer mortality from 49% to 41% (Lancet 2014). However, the LRF rates are higher than other modern studies with contemporary systemic therapy (4–20%):
  - Consider percent positive nodes (>20%; not applicable if SLNB only), size of nodal deposits, tumor size, receptor status, margins, LVSI, planned systemic therapy, patient age, histological grade, comorbidities, and life expectancy.
  - Percent nodes positive ≥20% may be better predictors of LR and OS than absolute number of positive nodes (Vinh-Hung JCO 2009; Truong IJROBP 2007).
- PMRT generally not indicated for T1–2N0 if adequate surgical axillary staging performed. Consider PMRT for close/positive margins, age ≤ 35 years, LVI + and/or grade 3.
- Three randomized trials using systemic therapy report decreased LR (~20%) and improved OS (~10%) with PMRT:

Table 17.8

Study	Patients	Randomization	Median follow-up	Outcome	Comment
Danish 82b (Overgaard et al. NEJM 1997)	1708 premenopausal patients status postmodified radical mastectomy	Adjuvant CMF chemo alone vs. chemo + RT	114 months	Postmastectomy RT reduced LRF (32 vs. 9%), 10-year DFS (34 vs. 48%), and OS (45 vs. 54%) Improvement in LC and OS in all subsets regardless of tumor size or number of involved LN	Study criticized for inadequate LN dissection (mean of 7 LN) Internal mammary irradiation used
Danish 82c (Lancet 1999)	1406 postmenopausal patients status postmodified radical mastectomy	Adjuvant tamoxifen alone vs. tamoxifen + RT (48–50 Gy)	10 years	RT improved LRF (35 vs. 8%), DFS (24 vs. 36%), and OS (36 vs. 45%) No survival benefit in N0 patients	Study criticized for inadequate LN dissection Internal mammary irradiation used
British-Columbia trial (JNCI 2005)	318 pLN+ premenopausal patients status postmodified radical mastectomy	CMF chemo alone vs. chemo + RT	20 years	RT reduced LRF (26 → 10%), and improved breast ca-specific survival (38 → 53%), and OS (37 → 47%)	Median 11 LN sampled

META-ANALYSIS AND SELECT NONRANDOMIZED STUDIES PMRT

- EBCTCG PMRT (Lancet 2014). Meta-analysis of 22 PMRT trials (8135 women). For pN0, the addition of RT did not impact LR or mortality, but for pN+ patients (irrespective of number of nodes involved), adding RT decreased LR at 10 years from 26% to 8.1%, which conferred an 8.1% benefit for 20-year breast cancer mortality.

- ECOG (Recht, JCO 1999). Retrospective review of 2016 pts treated with mastectomy and adjuvant CMF chemo without RT. 10-year LRF was 13% for 1–3 LN+ vs. 29% for ≥4 LN+.

- Taghian (JCO 2004). Patterns of LRF reviewed for 5758 patients enrolled on 5 NSABP trials treated with mastectomy and adjuvant chemotherapy (± tam) with no PMRT. 10-year LRF of 13%, 24%, and 32% for pts with 1–3, 4–9, and ≥10 + LN, and 15%, 21%, and 25%, and for pts with a tumor size of ≤2, 2.1–5.0, and >5.0 cm. Age, tumor size, premenopausal status, number of LN+, and number of dissected LN were significant predictors for LRF on multivariate analysis.

- CALGB 9741 (Citron, JCO 2003) patients with 1–3+ LNs postmastectomy and no PMRT had 5-year LR of 9.3% with AC and 5.2% with AC + T, as compared to 12.4% for patients with ≥4+ LN postmastectomy, no PMRT, and either chemo regimen.

- SUPREMO trial randomized about 1600 pts with high-risk node-negative or 1–3 positive nodes to PMRT or not. Results are pending.

- T1-T2N0 pts at high risk for LR without PMRT (Truong, IJROBP 2005a). 10-yr LR: grade 3 and LVI 21%; T2 grade 3 with no systemic therapy 23%.

- T1-2N1 pts at higher risk for LR without PMRT (Truong, IJROBP 2005b): 10-year LR for pts <45 was 29% (58% if >25% nodes involved). For pts >45, 10-year LR was 14% (27% if >25% nodes involved). Other significant predictors of LR on multivariate analysis included medial tumor location and ER negative status.

LR MANAGEMENT After NEOADJUVANT CHEMOTHERAPY

- Accuracy of SLNBx is likely not reduced after neoadjuvant chemotherapy (Buchholz JCO 2008); thus, it may be performed either pre or post neoadjuvant chemotherapy (at time of definitive surgery if post).
- BCT may be possible after neoadjuvant chemotherapy in properly selected patients:
  - Selection criteria for BCT after neoadjuvant chemotherapy remain to be defined.
  - BCT contraindicated if residual skin ulceration, edema, chest wall fixation, or inflammatory breast cancer.
- MRI to assess treatment response to neoadjuvant chemo often useful.
- Chen (JCO 2004). Retrospective review of 340 patients treated with neoadjuvant chemo + BCT demonstrated that acceptably low rates of LF (5% at 5 years) can be obtained when appropriate selection criteria are used.
- Huang (JCO 2004). Retrospective review of 679 patients treated with neoadjuvant chemo + mastectomy with or without postmastectomy RT. At 10-year follow-up, addition of RT reduced LRF (11 vs. 22%) and improved breast ca-specific survival for patients with clinical T3 tumors or stage III disease and for patients with ≥4 LN+.
- Huang (IJROBP 2006) MD Anderson Prognostic Index for patients treated with neoadjuvant chemo and LR risk based on local treatment (risk factors = cN2–3, LVI on bx or final pathology, multifocal residual disease, pathological tumor size >2 cm):

Table 17.9

Number of risk factors	10-year LR % with BCS + RT	10-year LR % with MRM + RT
0–1	9	5
2	28	12
3–4	61	19

- NSABP B-18/B-27 (Mamounas, JCO 2012). 3088 T1–3 N0–1 pts treated with neoadjuvant chemo. 10-year LR 12% for mastectomy pts. Predictors of LR were tumor size before chemo, clinical nodal status before chemo, and pathologic nodal status and tumor response. Nomograms for 10-yr LR generated based on age, tumor size, clinical node status, pathologic CR, and pathologic nodal status after chemo.

LOCOREGIONAL RECURRENCE AND ISOLATED AXILLARY DISEASE

V

Isolated axillary disease with occult breast primary	
Stage	**Recommended treatment**
TxN1–3	Workup: H&P, bilateral mammography, MRI of breast(s), PET–CT Treatment: TM with ALND ± RT. Systemic therapy as indicated

	Recommended treatment
Isolated chest wall recurrence	Resection. Consider SLN bx. If no prior RT, post-op RT to chest wall and SCV Adjuvant chemo, HT, and/or trastuzumab as indicated
Isolated axillary nodal recurrence	ALND + nodal RT if no prior RT, adjuvant chemo, HT and/or trastuzumab as indicated

RADIATION TECHNIQUES

- RT can usually begin within 2–4 weeks of surgery
- For patients receiving chemotherapy, RT begins 3–4 weeks after last cycle
- JCRT Sequencing (JCO 2005): 244 patients with stage I/II breast ca status post lumpectomy randomized to adjuvant doxorubicin-based chemo followed by RT vs. adjuvant RT followed by four cycles of same chemo. With 11-year follow-up, there are no differences in OS, DM, time to any event, or site of first failure. For close margins (<1 mm), crude LR was 32% with chemo first vs. 4% with RT first; for + margins, crude LR was 20–23% in both arms.

INTACT BREAST TECHNIQUE

SIMULATION AND FIELD DESIGN

- Patients usually treated in supine position with customized immobilization device.
- Bilateral arms abducted and externally rotated.
- Wire all surgical scars.
- Target volume is entire breast using tangential fields, and SCV fossa via third field as indicated (below).
- Mark estimated medial, lateral, cranial, and caudal field borders:
    - Medial border at midsternum.
    - Lateral border placed 2 cm beyond all palpable breast tissue (midaxillary line).
    - Inferior border is 2 cm from inframammary fold.
    - Superior border is at the head of clavicle or second intercostal space.
    - Deep (intrathoracic) field border must be nondivergent and edges made coplanar.
    - Use half-beam block techniques, or rotate gantry to make symmetric and align posterior edge of each tangent (gantry rotation angle = arctan ([0.5 × field width]/ SAD) ~ 3° for 10 cm field.
- Isocenter typically placed in the center of the treatment field.
- In general, 1–2 cm of underlying lung in the treatment field is acceptable.
- For left-sided lesions, minimize the amount of heart in tangential fields.
- CT planning allows for more accurate dose distribution and is recommended.
- Rarely need to treat completely dissected axilla (i.e., posterior axillary field) since axillary failure is uncommon.
- Tangential RT usually covers a large percentage of the level I and II axillary nodes.
- High tangent technique can be used to treat greater percentage of axilla if no axillary dissection performed. Best done with CT planning.
- When using third field (SCV), attention to geometric match with tangential fields is essential:
    - Half-beam block for caudal edge of supraclavicular field to eliminate divergence.

- Divergence of tangential fields superiorly can be eliminated with various techniques:
  - Couch-kick away from tangent field: arctan ([0.5 × tangent field length])/SAD), but can adjust with multi-leaf collimators.
  - The use of monoisocentric technique: SCV and tangent fields are half-beam blocked using same isocenter placed at edge of each respective field. Disadvantage: unable to collimate gantry for tangent fields, resulting in higher lung dose.
- Supraclavicular field is angled obliquely 10–15° laterally to keep off spinal cord.
- Inferior border of tangent field placed at inferior aspect of clavicular head.
- Superior border of supraclavicular field is above acromioclavicular joint, top of T1/first rib, short of flash.
- Medial border of supraclavicular field placed at the pedicles of vertebral bodies.
- Lateral border of supraclavicular field is coracoid process or lateral to humeral head.
- Boost field is delivered with appositional field using electrons to tumor bed.
- Each field should be treated on a daily basis, Monday through Friday.
- Bolus should not be used.

DOSE PRESCRIPTIONS

CONVENTIONAL FRACTIONATION WHOLE-BREAST TANGENTS ± SCV

- 45–50 Gy at 1.8–2 Gy/fx to whole breast with tangential fields
- 45–50 Gy at 1.8–2 Gy/fx to supraclavicular fossa (when included)

HYPOFRACTIONATION

- Hypofractionation (42.56 Gy in 2.66 Gyfx or 40.05 Gy in 2.67 Gyfx) may be recommended for many pts instead of standard fractionation regardless of laterality, tumor grade, hormone receptor status, HER2 receptor status, margin status, whether chemotherapy was received prior to radiotherapy, whether trastuzumab or endocrine therapy is received prior to or during radiotherapy, and regardless of breast size and central axis separation provided that dose homogeneity goals are met.

- There is no evidence of worse outcomes with hypofractionated RT for young pts with 10-yr follow-up in the randomized trials. However, only 6% of pts were <40 yrs old. The decision for or against hypofractionated RT should be individualized for young pts with very long life expectancy.

- Field-in-field technique is recommended to minimize volume of breast tissue receiving >105% of the prescription dose. Goal is for at least 95% of whole breast volume to receive 95% of the prescription dose:

- Whelan (IJROBP 2002; IJROBP 2008;NEJM 2010): 1234 pN0 patients treated with BCS randomized to whole-breast RT 50 Gy in 25 fxs over 5 wks vs. 42.5 Gy in 16 fxs over 3 wks. No boost. Large-breasted patients (>25 cm separation) not allowed. Only 11% of patients received chemotherapy in each arm, 25% <50 years old. No difference in 10-year LR (6.2 vs. 6.7%, respectively), DFS, OS, or good/excellent cosmetic outcome (70 vs. 71%).

- UK START A and B Trials (Lancet 2008a, Lancet Oncol 2008b, 2013). Two phase III trials randomized 2236 and 2215 pT1–3N0–1 patients to 50 Gy in 25 fxs vs. 41.6 Gy or 39 Gy in 13 fxs over 5 weeks (START A) or 50 Gy in 25 fxs vs. 40 Gy in 15 fxs over 3 weeks (START B), respectively. Twenty-one to twenty-three percent<50 years old, 22–35% of patients had chemotherapy, 23–29% were LN+, 43–60% of post-BCS patients had boost, and 8–15% of patients had mastectomy. No difference in 5-year or 10-year LR. Photographic and patient-assessed late adverse effects were lower with 39 vs. 50 Gy and with 40 vs. 50 Gy. Estimated α/β of 4.6 Gy for tumor control and 3.4 Gy for late breast appearance change.

- RMH/GO3 (Owen, Lancet Oncology 2006): 1410 T1–3 N01 patients randomized to 50 Gy in 25, 39 Gy in 13, or 42.9 Gy in 13 fractions over 5 weeks. Thirty percent of patients <50 year old, 14% had chemotherapy, and 75% had boost. Ten-year IBTR rates of 12.1%, 14.8%, and 9.6% (6.7–12.6) in each arm, respectively (difference between 39 and 42.9 Gy groups: $p = 0.027$). Estimated α/β of 4.0 Gy for tumor control.

- Hypofractionated RT may also be considered for pts with DCIS based on a number of published observational studies, case series, and population-based studies.

TUMOR BED BOOST

- For invasive disease, tumor bed boost is recommended for age ≤ 50 years (any grade), age 51–70 with high-grade, or positive margin. Boost may be omitted for pts with invasive disease who are > 70 years with low or intermediate grade and widely negative margins (≥2 mm). For other invasive pts, boost decision making should be individualized.
- For DCIS, tumor bed boost is recommended for age ≤ 50 years (any grade), high-grade, positive margin, or close (<2 mm) margin. Boost may be omitted for pts aged > 50 with screen-detected, low- to intermediate-grade DCIS, size ≤2.5 cm, with wide negative margins (≥3 mm). For other DCIS pts, boost decision making should be individualized.
- Sequential boost dose with electrons to tumor bed with 1–2 cm margin:
  - 10 Gy in 4–5 fractions recommended for most pts.
  - If positive margin or young age and close margin, 14–16 Gy in 7–8 fractions or 12.5 Gy in 5 fractions may be used.
  - Electron energy is selected to allow the 85–90% isodose line to encompass target with goal that tumor bed receives at least 95% of the prescription dose.
  - Re-simulation for boost planning may be considered for pts with large seroma at the time of whole breast planning.
- EORTC Boost Trial (Bartelink et al, NEJM 2001) and
- (Bartelink et al, JCO 2007) and (Bartelink et al, Lancet Oncol 2015): 5569 patients with stage I/II breast ca status post lumpectomy (negative invasive margins, DCIS margins ignored) randomized to 50 Gy RT vs. 50 Gy + 16 Gy boost. At 10-year follow-up, boost decreased LF from 10.2% to 6.2%, with largest benefit observed in patients≤40 years (23.9 → 13%). All age

groups benefited from boost, although benefit was small if >60 years old. Boost had slightly increased rates of severe fibrosis (4.4% vs. 1.6%).

▪ Lyon Boost Trial (JCO 1997): 1024 patients with early-stage breast ca status post lumpectomy (<3 cm tumor), ALND, and 50 Gy RT randomized to boost (10 Gy) vs. no boost. At median follow-up of 3 years, addition of boost reduced LF (3.6% vs. 4.5%). No difference in self-assessed cosmetic response between two arms.

ACCELERATED PARTIAL BREAST IRRADIATION (APBI)

▪ Ongoing APBI vs. whole breast RT trials include NSABP B-39/RTOG 0413, Ontario RAPID Trial, MRC Import Low, University of Florence.

▪ Techniques include intraoperative electron or X-rays, interstitial brachytherapy (HDR more common than LDR), balloon brachytherapy, or 3DCRT:
  ▪ HDR/balloon brachytherapy dose: 3.4 Gy b.i.d. × 5 days
  ▪ 3DCRT APBI dose: 3.85 Gy b.i.d. × 5 days

▪ Professional societies have varying recommendations for APBI criteria off-trial:

Table 17.10

	ASBS (2011)	ABS (Shah, Brachytherapy 2013)
Age (years)	≥45	≥50
Histology	Invasive carcinoma or DCIS	All invasive & DCIS
Tumor size	Total tumor size (invasive and DCIS) less than or equal to 3 cm	≤3 cm, including pure DCIS
Pathologic margins	Negative	Negative
Lymph node status	Sentinel lymph node negative	Node negative
ER status		ER+ or ER–
LVSI		LVSI not present

Table 17.11

ASTRO (Smith, IJRBOP 2009; Correa, Pract Radiat Oncol 2016)		
"Suitable" (meet all criteria)	**"Cautionary"** (meet any one criteria)	**"Unsuitable"** (meet any <u>one</u> criteria)
Age ≥ 50	Age 40–49 if all other "suitable" criteria met; age > 50 if patient has one factor below and no "unsuitable" factors	Age < 40; age 40–49 if do not meet cautionary criteria

continued

Table 17.11 (continued)

Pure DCIS if screen detected, grade 1–2, ≤2.5 cm, margins≥3 mm	Pure DCIS ≤3 cm if "suitable" criteria not fully met	Pure DCIS >3 cm
T1 invasive ≤2 cm	T2 invasive 2.1–3 cm*	T2 invasive >3cm, T3–4
Negative margins (>2mm)	Close margins (<2mm)	Positive margins
pN0 (i–, i+), Bx or ALND	–	pN+ or no nodal surgery
ER+	ER–	
No LVSI	Limited/focal LVSI	Extensive LVSI
Unicentric and unifocal		Multicentric, microscopically multifocal >3 cm in total size, or if clinically multifocal
No EIC	EIC ≤ 3 cm	EIC >3 cm
	Invasive lobular histology	–
BRCA1/2 mutation absent	–	BRCA1/2 mutation present
No neoadjuvant systemic tx	–	Received neoadjuvant systemic tx

*Microscopic multifocality allowed, provided the lesion is clinically unifocal and the total size of foci of multifocality and intervening normal parenchyma is between 2.1 and 3 cm

Table 17.12 SELECT APBI TRIALS

Study	Patients	Randomization or treatment	Outcome
Eliot (Veronesi et al, Lancet Oncol 2013)	1305 pts aged 48–75 with early breast cancer eligible for BCS and max tumor diameter 2.5 cm	EBRT (50 Gy + 10 Gy boost) vs. electron IORT (21 Gy single fx)	5-year IBTR rate for IORT was 4.4%, vs. 0.4% with external radiotherapy (p < 0.0001). Ipsilateral carcinomas higher too (1.9% vs. 0%). No OS difference
Targit-A (Vaidya et al, Lancet 2010; Vaidya et al, Lancet 2014)	3451 pts with early breast cancer, 45 years and older	EBRT 40–56 Gy +/–10–16 Gy boost vs. kV IORT 20 Gy to the surface of the tumor	5-yr LR for TARGIT vs. EBRT was 3.3% vs. 1.3% (p = 0.042). No difference in breast cancer mortality
GEC-ESTRO (Strnad, Lancet 2016)	1184 pts >40 yrs, pTis-T2a (≤3 cm), pN0/Nmi, neg. margins, no LVSI	EBRT (50–50.4 Gy + 10 Gy boost) vs. multi-catheter brachy to tumor bed (HDR 4.3 Gy × 7 or 4 Gy × 8 BID; or PDR 50 Gy)	5-yr LR EBRT 0.92% vs. APBI 1.4% (p = 0.42); regional recurrence EBRT 0.18% vs. APBI 0.48% (p = 0.39)
RTOG 95-17 (White, IJROBP 2016)	Phase II, 98 pts with stage I–II (<3 cm, unifocal, invasive nonlobular, no ECE)	Multi-catheter brachy to tumor bed only (60% LDR 45 Gy over 3.5–5 days, 40% HDR 3.4 Gy b.i.d. × 10fxs)	10-year in-breast recurrence 4.1%, regional recurrence 4.1%, contralateral breast failure 3.1%

POSTMASTECTOMY TECHNIQUE

SIMULATION AND FIELD DESIGN

- Patient simulated in similar manner to early-stage disease.
- Target volume includes chest wall and supraclavicular fossa as indicated (below).
- Wire all surgical scars and drain sites.
- Entire mastectomy scar, flaps, surgical clips, and drain sites included in the treatment field:
  - If outside of standard treatment field, drain site can be treated with local electron field if indicated.
- Attention to geometric match with SCV field to avoid junctional overdose.
- No boost is given to chest wall or scar with postmastectomy RT at UCSF, but it can be delivered using electrons in appositional field to high-risk area(s) of chest wall and skin.
- Each field should be treated on a daily basis, Monday through Friday.
- TLDs are used at UCSF to assess skin dose.
- 5–10 mm bolus typically used every other day for duration of RT at UCSF:
  - Bolus thickness is dependent on photon beam energy.
- Custom bolus may provide improved dose distribution over the reconstructed breast (i.e., the use of a form fitting Aquaplast cast and wax).

PMRT DOSE PRESCRIPTIONS

- 50–50.4 Gy at 1.8–2 Gy/fx to chest wall using tangential fields.
- 45–50.4 Gy at 1.8–2 Gy/fx to supraclavicular fossa as indicated.
- Electron boost can be used to bring total scar dose to 60–66 Gy in high-risk patients:
  - Electron energy selected to allow the 85–90% isodose line to encompass target

INDICATIONS FOR NODAL RT

- $\geq$4 involved axillary lymph nodes and inflammatory breast cancer are always indications for SCV RT.
- SCV RT is generally recommended for 1–3 involved axillary lymph nodes per updated ASCO/ASTRO/SSO recommendations, but there may be subgroups who will have limited, if any, benefit.
- SCV RT indications after good response to neoadjuvant chemotherapy are unclear.
- No axillary staging or no ALND in the case of +SLNB are relative indications for SCV RT.
- RT is given to internal mammary nodes if clinically or pathologically positive; otherwise, it is at the discretion of the treating radiation oncologist weighing potential incremental benefit vs. risks (see reviews by Chen JCO 2008; Freedman IJROBP 2000):
  - DBCG-IMN (Thorsen, JCO 2016). 3089 pts with early-stage N+ disease in Denmark treated with adjuvant RT to breast/chest wall and non-resected axilla and SCV. Right-sided disease also received IMN RT while left-sided did not. IMN RT improved 8-yr breast cancer mortality (20.9% vs. 23.4%) and DM (27.4% vs. 29.7%). Benefit greatest for node positive medial/central disease and pts with $\geq$4 nodes regardless of location. Pts with lateral lesions and 1–3 LN did not appear to benefit.
  - CT treatment planning should be utilized in all cases where RT is delivered to the internal mammary lymph nodes.
  - Internal mammary RT performed with partially wide tangential field or matched electron technique.
- Posterior axillary boost (PAB) is controversial with no proven benefit, not routinely done at UCSF.

V

DOSE LIMITATIONS

- Goal of treatment is to achieve homogeneous distribution throughout target volume.
- Careful attention must be paid to the amount of lung tissue and heart in treatment field.
- Wedging and weighting can achieve better dose distribution, although physical wedge increases scatter dose to contralateral breast (less so with virtual wedge or MLC).
- Field-in-field technique using static forward-planned IMRT often used to optimize dose distribution.
- At UCSF, ipsilateral lung V20 is limited to ≤10% with two-field tangents and ≤20% with three-field (SCV) technique.
- Left ventricle and combined bilateral ventricle limits: V5 ≤ 10% and V25 ≤ 5%. Also record and attempt to minimize whole heart dose.
- Deep inspiration breath hold respiratory gating, prone positioning, and/or MLC blocking may be used to minimize dose to lung and heart.
- ASTRO Consensus Statement dose constraints for 3DCRT APBI (*IJROBP 2009*): contralateral breast Dmax≤3%, ipsilateral lung V30% <15%, contralateral lung V5% <15%, heart V5% < 5% for R-sided tumors, and <40% for L-sided tumors.

COMPLICATIONS

- For complete skin care recommendations, please see reference *Skin Care in Radiation Oncology* (Fowble, Springer 2016).
- Acute skin reaction, treated with:
  - Erythema alone: moisturizing lotion or cream antifungal and hydrocortisone creams if evidence of topical fungal infection or pruritus
  - Dry desquamation: moisturizing and vitamins A&D creams
  - Wet desquamation: zinc oxide and Bacitracin
- Late cosmetic impairment (edema, fibrosis, telangiectasia), including risk of breast reconstruction complications and/or cosmetic impairment.

- Upper extremity lymphedema: 1–5% risk with RT alone, 4–10% with SLNB, 10% risk with ALND, 12% risk with ALND + RT, and 16–20% risk with ALND + SCV/axillary RT.
- Uncommon: brachial plexopathy, pneumonitis, and rib fracture.
- Risk of RT-induced cardiac toxicity can be minimized by modern techniques and cardiac risk modification (excellent review of cardiac risk: Harris 2008).
  - 50–70% of patients treated with L-sided tangents exhibit perfusion defect on SPECT 3–6 years post-RT (Prosnitz et al., 2007).
  - Increased risk of cardiac toxicity with doxorubicin, trastuzumab, and aromatase inhibitors.
  - Increased risk of acute coronary event or death from ischemic heart disease for patients with underlying risk factors for coronary artery disease receiving radiotherapy.
- Overall risk of second malignancies increased from <4 to 5%, sarcoma <0.5 risk in 20–30 years, lung cancer risk increased in smokers only, contralateral breast cancer risk increased from 15 to 16% with modern techniques, but may be higher in younger, positive family history, and BRCA1/2 patients.

FOLLOW-UP

- Monthly self-exam.
- H&P every 3 months for 1–2 years, then every 6 months for 5 years, and then annually.
- Bilateral breast mammograms annually. At UCSF, ipsilateral mammogram interval is 6 months for first 5 years.
- Cosmetic assessment.
- Median time to breast cancer recurrence is 5–7 years for women receiving adjuvant hormonal and/or chemotherapy, but is shorter for triple negative breast cancers (<3 years).

REFERENCES

American Society of Breast Surgeons. https://www.breastsurgeons.org/new_layout/about/statements/PDF_Statements/APBI.pdf. (2011).

Bartelink H, et al. Impact of a higher radiation dose on local control and survival in breast-conserving therapy of early breast cancer: 10-year results of the randomized boost versus no boost EORTC 22881-10882 trial. J Clin Oncol. 2007;25(22):3259–65.

Bartelink H, et al. Whole-breast irradiation with or without a boost for patients treated with breast-conserving surgery for early breast cancer: 20-year follow-up of a randomized phase 3 trial. Lancet Oncol. 2015;16(1):47–56.

Chen RC, et al. Internal mammary nodes in breast cancer: diagnosis and implications for patient managementDOUBLEHYPHENa systematic review. J Clin Oncol. 2008;26(30):4981–9.

Collins LC, et al. Risk prediction for local breast cancer recurrence among women with DCIS treated in a community practice: a nested, case-control study. Ann Surg Oncol. 2015;22:S502–8.

Correa C, et al. Accelerated partial breast irradiation: executive summary for the update of an ASTRO evidence based consensus statement. Pract Radiat Oncol. 2017;7(2):73–9.

Early Breast Cancer Trialists' Collaborative Group. Effect of radiotherapy after mastectomy and axillary surgery on 10-year recurrence and 20-year breast cancer mortality: meta-analysis of individual patient data for 8135 women in 22 randomized trials. Lancet. 2014;383:2127–35.

Fisher B, Bryant J, Dignam JJ, et al. Tamoxifen, radiation therapy, or both for prevention of ipsilateral breast tumor recurrence after lumpectomy in women with invasive breast cancers of one centimeter or less. J Clin Oncol. 2002;20(20):4141–9.

Freedman GM, et al. Should internal mammary lymph nodes in breast cancer be a target for the radiation oncologist? Int J Radiat Oncol Biol Phys. 2000;46(4):805–14.

Hughes KS, et al. Lumpectomy plus tamoxifen with or without irradiation in women 70 years of age or older with early breast cancer. NEJM. 2004;351:971–7.

Mamounas EP, et al. Predictors of locoregional recurrence after neoadjuvant chemotherapy: results from combined analysis of National Surgical Adjuvant Breast and bowel project B-18 and B-27. J Clin Oncol. 2012;30(32):3960–6.

Overgaard M, Hansen PS, Overgaard J, et al. Postoperative radiotherapy in high-risk premenopausal women with breast cancer who receive adjuvant chemotherapy. N Engl J Med. 1997;337:949–55.

Owen JR, et al. Effect of radiotherapy fraction size on tumor control in patients with early-stage breast cacer after local tumor excision: long-term results of a randomized trial. Lancet Oncol. 2006;7(6):467–71.

Recht A, et al. Postmastectomy radiotherapy: guidelines of the American Society of Clinical Oncology. J Clin Oncol. 2001;19(5):1539–69.

Recht A, et al. Postmastectomy radiotherapy: an American Society of Clinical Oncology, American Society for Radiation Oncology and Society of Surgical Oncology focused guideline update. J Clin Oncol. 2016;34(36):4431–42.

Rudloff U, et al. Nomogram for predicting the risk of local recurrence after breast-conserving surgery for ductal carcinoma in situ. J Clin Oncol. 2010;28(23):3762–9.

Shah C, et al. The American Brachytherapy Society Consensus statement for accelerated paratial breast irradiation. Brachytherapy. 2013;12(4):267–77.

Silverstein MJ, et al. The University of Southern California/Van Nuys prognostic index for ductal carcinoma in situ of the breast. Am J Surg. 2003;186(4):337–43.

Smith BD, et al. Accelerated partial breast irradiation consensus statement from the American Society for Radiation Oncology (ASTRO). Int J Radiat Oncol Biol Phys. 2009;74(4):987–1001.

Strnad V, et al. 5-year results of accelerated partial breast irradiation using sole interstitial multicatheter brachytherapy versus whole-breast irradiation with boost after breast-conserving surgery for low-risk invasive and in-situ carcinoma of the female breast: a randomised, phase 3, non-inferiority trial. Lancet. 2016;367(10015):229–38.

Sweldens C, et al. Local relapse after breast-conserving therapy for ductal carcinoma in situ: a European single-center experience and external validation of the Memorial Sloan-Kettering Cancer Center DCIS nomogram. Cancer J. 2014;20(1):1–7.

Thorsen LB, et al. DBCG-IMN: a population-basec cohort study on the effect of internal mammary node irradiation in early node-positive breast cancer. J Clin Oncol. 2016;34(4):314–20.

Vaidya JS, Joseph DJ, Tobias JS, et al. Targeted intraoperative radiotherapy versus whole breast radiotherapy for breast cancer (TARGIT-A trial): an international, prospective, randomized, non-inferiority phase 3 trial. Lancet. 2010;376:91–102.

Vaidya JS, Wenz F, Bulsara M, et al. Risk-adapted targeted intraoperative radiotherapy versus whole-breast radiotherapy for breast cancer: 5-year results for local control and overall survival from the TARGIT-A randomized trial. Lancet. 2014;383:603–13.

Van Dongen JA, Voogd AC, Fentiman IS, Legrand C, et al. Long-term results of a randomized trial comparing breast-conserving therapy with mastectomy: European organization for research and treatment of cancer 10801 trial. J Natl Cancer Inst. 2000;92:1143–50.

Veronesi U, et al. Intraoperative radiotherapy versus external radiotherapy early breast cancer (ELIOT): a randomized controlled equivalence trial. Lancet Oncol. 2013;14(13):1269–77.

Wang F, et al. Validation of a nomogram in the prediction of local recurrence risks after conserving surgery for Asian women with ductal carcinoma in situ of the breast. Clin Oncol (R Coll Radiol). 2014;26(11):684–91.

White J, et al. Long-term cancer outcomes from study NRG oncology/RTOG 9517: a phase 2 study of accelerated partial breast irradiation with multicatheter brachytherapy after lumpectomy for early-stage breast cancer. Int J Radiat Oncol Biol Phys. 2016;95(5):1460–5.

Yi M, et al. Evaluation of a breast cancer nomogram for predicting risk of ipsilateral breast tumor recurrences in patients with ductal carcinoma in situ after local excision. J Clin Oncol. 2012;30(6):600–7.

V

PART VI
Digestive System

VI

Chapter 18
Esophageal Cancer

Yao Yu, Hans T. Chung, and Mekhail Anwar

PEARLS

, Esophageal cancer accounts for 5% of all GI cancers. There are 16,910 new cases and 15,690 deaths from esophageal cancer each year in the USA (http://seer.cancer.gov/statfacts/html/esoph.html).

VI

, Incidence increases with age, peaks at sixth to seventh decade.
, Male/female = 4:1.
, Most common in China, Iran, South Africa, India, and the former Soviet Union.
, Risk factors: tobacco, EtOH, nitrosamines, Tylosis (congenital hyperkeratosis), Plummer-Vinson syndrome, achalasia, GERD, and Barrett's esophagus.
, Four regions of the esophagus: Cervical = cricoid cartilage to thoracic inlet (15–18 cm from the incisor). Upper thoracic = thoracic inlet to tracheal bifurcation (18–24 cm). Midthoracic = tracheal bifurcation to just above the GE junction (24–32 cm). Lower thoracic = GE junction (32–40 cm).
, Barrett's esophagus: metaplasia of the esophageal epithelial lining. The squamous epithelium is replaced by columnar epithelium, with 0.5% annual rate of neoplastic transformation.
, Adenocarcinoma: rapid rise in incidence. Comprises 60–80% of all new cases compared to 10–15% 10 years ago. Predominately white men. Associated with Barrett's,

© Springer International Publishing AG, part of Springer Nature 2018   **403**
Eric K. Hansen and M. Roach III (eds.), *Handbook of Evidence-Based Radiation Oncology*, https://doi.org/10.1007/978-3-319-62642-0_18

GERD, and hiatal hernia. Locations: 75% in the distal esophagus and 25% in the upper and mid-esophagus.

, Squamous cell carcinoma: associated with tobacco, alcohol, or prior history of head and neck cancers. Locations: 50% mid-esophagus and 50% distal esophagus.

, Patients with malignant fistula may be treated with a combination of stenting and chemoRT. Older studies reported that chemoRT yielded high rates of perforation, but more recent papers have reported fistula closure in a significant proportion of patients (Koike IJROBP 2008).

, Post-chemotherapy PET/CT response is prognostic (MUNICON II), but only a minority of patients with complete metabolic response have pCR. (zum Buschenfeld 2011, Lordick Lancet Oncol 2007). The feasibility of PET/CT guided neoadjuvant therapy was demonstrated in the CALGB 80803 trial.

WORKUP

, H&P: dysphagia, odynophagia, cough, hoarseness (laryngeal nerve involvement), weight loss, use of EtOH, tobacco, nitrosamines, history of GERD. Examine for cervical or supraclavicular adenopathy.

, Labs: CBC, chemistries, LFTs.

, EGD: direct visualization and biopsy.

, EUS: assess the depth of penetration and LN involvement. Limited by the degree of obstruction.

, Barium swallow: can delineate proximal and distal margins.

, CT chest and abdomen: assess adenopathy and metastasis.

, PET scan: can detect up to 15–20% of metastases not seen on CT and EUS.

, Bronchoscopy: rule out tracheoesophageal fistula for tumors at or above the carina.

, Pulmonary function test: to evaluate whether medically operable and serve as baseline lung function for chemoRT.

, Nutritional assessment.

, For operable patients unable to swallow enough to maintain nutrition, esophageal dilation, feeding jejunostomy, or nasogastric tube is preferred over gastrostomy tube due to potential compromise of gastric conduit reconstruction.

STAGING: ESOPHAGEAL CANCER

Editors' note: All TNM stage and stage groups referred to elsewhere in this chapter reflect the 2010 AJCC staging nomenclature unless otherwise noted as the new system below was published after this chapter was written.

Table 18.1 (AJCC 7TH ED., 2010)

Primary tumor (T)*

TX:	Primary tumor cannot be assessed
T0:	No evidence of primary tumor
Tis:	High-grade dysplasia**
T1:	Tumor invades lamina propria, muscularis mucosae, or submucosa
T1a:	Tumor invades lamina propria or muscularis mucosae
T1b:	Tumor invades submucosa
T2:	Tumor invades muscularis propria
T3:	Tumor invades adventitia
T4:	Tumor invades adjacent structures
T4a:	Resectable tumor invading pleura, pericardium, or diaphragm
T4b:	Unresectable tumor invading other adjacent structures, such as aorta, vertebral body, trachea, etc.

*(1) At least maximal dimension of the tumor must be recorded and (2) multiple tumors require the T(m) suffix
**High-grade dysplasia includes all noninvasive neoplastic epithelia that was formerly called carcinoma in situ, a diagnosis that is no longer used for columnar mucosae anywhere in the gastrointestinal tract.

Regional lymph nodes (N)*

NX:	Regional lymph nodes cannot be assessed
N0:	No regional lymph node metastasis
N1:	Metastasis in 1–2 regional lymph nodes
N2:	Metastasis in 3–6 regional lymph nodes
N3:	Metastasis in seven or more regional lymph nodes

*Number must be recorded for total number of regional nodes sampled and total number of reported nodes with metastasis

Distant metastasis (M)

M0:	No distant metastasis
M1:	Distant metastasis

VI

Table 18.1 (continued)

Anatomic stage/prognostic groups
*Squamous cell carcinoma**

Stage	T	N	M	Grade	Tumor location**
0:	Tis (HGD)	N0	M0	1, X	Any
IA:	T1	N0	M0	1, X	Any
IB:	T1	N0	M0	2–3	Any
	T2–3	N0	M0	1, X	Lower, X
IIA:	T2–3	N0	M0	1, X	Upper, middle
	T2–3	N0	M0	2–3	Lower, X
IIB:	T2–3	N0	M0	2–3	Upper, middle
	T1–2	N1	M0	Any	Any
IIIA:	T1–2	N2	M0	Any	Any
	T3	N1	M0	Any	Any
	T4a	N0	M0	Any	Any
IIIB:	T3	N2	M0	Any	Any
IIIC:	T4a	N1–2	M0	Any	Any
	T4b	Any	M0	Any	Any
IIIC:	T4a	N1–2	M0	Any	Any
	Any	N3	M0	Any	Any
IV:	Any	Any	M1	Any	Any

*Or mixed histology including a squamous component or NOS
**Location of the primary cancer site is defined by the position of the upper
(proximal) edge of the tumor in the esophagus. *Adenocarcinoma*

IIIC:	T4a	N1–2	M0	Any	Any
IIIC:	T4a	N1–2	M0	Any	Any
IIIC:	T4a	N1–2	M0	Any	Any
IIIC:	T4a	N1–2	M0	Any	Any
IIIC:	T4a	N1–2	M0	Any	Any
IIIC:	T4a	N1–2	M0	Any	Any

Used with permission of the American Joint Committee on Cancer (AJCC), Chicago,
Illinois. The original and primary source for this information is the AJCC Cancer Staging
Manual, Seventh Edition (2010) published by Springer Science + Business Media

Table 18.2 (AJCC 8TH ED., 2017)

Definitions of AJCC TNM

Definition of Primary Tumor (T)

Squamous Cell Carcinoma and Adenocarcinoma

T category	T criteria
TX	Tumor cannot be assessed
T0	No evidence of primary tumor
Tis	High-grade dysplasia, defined as malignant cells confined to the epithelium by the basement membrane
T1	Tumor invades the lamina propria, muscularis mucosae, or submucosa
T1a	Tumor invades the lamina propria or muscularis mucosae

continued

Table 18.2 (continued)

T1b	Tumor invades the submucosa
T2	Tumor invades the muscularis propria
T3	Tumor invades adventitia
T4	Tumor invades adjacent structures
T4a	Tumor invades the pleura, pericardium, azygos vein, diaphragm, or peritoneum
T4b	Tumor invades other adjacent structures, such as the aorta, vertebral body, or airway

DEFINITION OF REGIONAL LYMPH NODES (N)
Squamous Cell Carcinoma and Adenocarcinoma

N category	N criteria
NX	Regional lymph nodes cannot be assessed
N0	No regional lymph node metastasis
N1	Metastasis in one or two regional lymph nodes
N2	Metastasis in three to six regional lymph nodes
N3	Metastasis in seven or more regional lymph nodes

VI

DEFINITION OF DISTANT METASTASIS (M)
Squamous Cell Carcinoma and Adenocarcinoma

M category	M criteria
M0	No distant metastasis
M1	Distant metastasis

DEFINITION OF HISTOLOGIC GRADE (G)
Squamous Cell Carcinoma and Adenocarcinoma

G	G definition
GX	Grade cannot be assessed
G1	Well differentiated
G2	Moderately differentiated
G3	Poorly differentiated, undifferentiated

DEFINITION OF LOCATION (L)

Location category	Location criteria
X	Location unknown
Upper	Cervical esophagus to lower border of azygos vein
Middle	Lower border of azygos vein to lower border of inferior pulmonary vein
Lower	Lower border of inferior pulmonary vein to stomach, including gastroesophageal junction

Note: Location is defined by the position of the epicenter of the tumor in the esophagus

AJCC PROGNOSTIC STAGE GROUPS
CLINICAL (CTNM)

When cT is...	And cN is...	And M is...	Then the stage group is...
Tis	N0	M0	0
T1	N0–1	M0	I
T2	N0–1	M0	II
T3	N0	M0	II
T3	N1	M0	III
T1–3	N2	M0	III
T4	N0–2	M0	IVA
Any T	N3	M0	IVA
Any T	Any N	M1	IVB

PATHOLOGICAL (PTNM)

When pT is...	And pN is...	And M is	And G is...	And location is...	Then the stage group is...
Tis	N0	M0	N/A	Any	0
T1a	N0	M0	G1	Any	IA
T1a	N0	M0	G2–3	Any	IB
T1a	N0	M0	GX	Any	IA
T1b	N0	M0	G1–3	Any	IB
T1b	N0	M0	GX	Any	IB
T2	N0	M0	G1	Any	IB
T2	N0	M0	G2–3	Any	IIA
T2	N0	M0	GX	Any	IIA
T3	N0	M0	Any	Lower	IIA
T3	N0	M0	G1	Upper/middle	IIA
T3	N0	M0	G2–3	Upper/middle	IIB
T3	N0	M0	GX	Any	IIB
T3	N0	M0	Any	Location X	IIB
T1	N1	M0	Any	Any	IIB
T1	N2	M0	Any	Any	IIIA
T2	N1	M0	Any	Any	IIIA
T2	N2	M0	Any	Any	IIIB
T3	N1–2	M0	Any	Any	IIIB
T4a	N0–1	M0	Any	Any	IIIB
T4a	N2	M0	Any	Any	IVA
T4b	N0–2	M0	Any	Any	IVA
Any T	N3	M0	Any	Any	IVA
Any T	Any N	M1	Any	Any	IVB

POSTNEOADJUVANT THERAPY (YPTNM)

When yp T is...	And yp N is...	And M is...	Then the stage group is...
T0–2	N0	M0	I
T3	N0	M0	II
T0–2	N1	M0	IIIA
T3	N1	M0	IIIB
T0–3	N2	M0	IIIB
T4a	N0	M0	IIIB
T4a	N1–2	M0	IVA
T4a	*NX*	M0	IVA
T4b	N0–2	M0	IVA
Any T	N3	M0	IVA
Any T	Any N	M1	IVB

SURGICAL TECHNIQUES

VI

, Transhiatal esophagectomy (laparotomy and cervical anastomosis): for tumors anywhere in esophagus or gastric cardia. No thoracotomy. Blunt dissection of the thoracic esophagus. Left with cervical anastomosis. Limitations are lack of exposure of midesophagus and direct visualization and dissection of the subcarinal LN cannot be performed.

, Laparotomy and right thoracotomy (Ivor Lewis procedure): good for exposure of mid to upper esophageal lesions. Left with thoracic or cervical anastomosis.

, Left thoracotomy: appropriate for lower third of esophagus and gastric cardia. Left with low-to-midthoracic anastomosis.

, Radical (en block) resection: for tumor anywhere in esophagus or gastric cardia. Left with cervical or thoracic anastomosis. Benefit is more extensive lymphadenectomy and potentially better survival, but increased operative risk.

, No randomized trials have yet assessed whether minimally invasive esophagectomy approaches improve outcomes compared to open procedures.

, Endoscopic therapy [endoscopic mucosal resection (EMR) or endoscopic submucosal dissection (ESD) and ablation (RFA, photodynamic therapy, or cryoablation)] is recommended for <2 cm well-to-moderately differentiated Tis–T1a lesions, but lesions >2 cm have greater risk of complications.

TREATMENT RECOMMENDATIONS

Table 18.3 TREATMENT RECOMMENDATIONS

Stage, AJCC 7th edition	Recommended treatment
Tis–T1a	Endoscopic intervention preferred for <2 cm well-to-moderately differentiated lesions (e.g., EMR +/− ablation). Or esophagectomy for extensive disease
T1bN0 operable	Squamous: Esophagectomy Adeno: Endoscopic therapy for superficial T1b disease <2 cm, otherwise esophagectomy
Post-op chemoRT indications (no prior chemoRT)	Squamous: R1 or R2 resection Adenocarcinoma: LN+, T3–T4, close/positive margins
T1bN1-2, T2-4N0-2 resectable, medically fit	Pre-op chemoRT (41.4–50.4 Gy, carboplatin/paclitaxel)[†], followed by surgery. 5-year OS 40–50%, pCR 25–50% (depending on histology), LRF 20–25% (preferred). PET-CT, CT (chest and abdomen) and upper endoscopy to assess response and operability Definitive chemoRT (50.4 Gy, carboplatin/paclitaxel)[†] is an option for SCC; however, trimodality therapy is preferred provided the patient is a good operative candidate. Trimodality therapy including surgery is strongly recommended for adenocarcinoma. Three-year OS 20–30%. LF <45%. Higher doses can be considered in select cases Cervical esophagus: Definitive chemoRT (54–66 Gy in 1.8 Gy fx, carboplatin/paclitaxel) is preferred due to morbidity of surgery Resectable T4: involvement of pleura, pericardium, or diaphragm only
Stages I–III inoperable	Definitive chemoRT (50.4–54 Gy, carboplatin/paclitaxel)
Stage IV palliative	RT or chemoRT (concurrent carboplatin/paclitaxel)[†] can be used to palliate dysphagia, bleeding Radiation dose schedules include 50.4 Gy/28 fx, 35–40 Gy/15–16 fx, 30 Gy/10 fx Multidisciplinary support with systemic therapy, endoscopic therapy, stenting

[†]Carboplatin/paclitaxel, cisplatin/5-FU, and oxaliplatin/5-FU are NCCN preferred concurrent chemoRT regimens.

STUDIES

PRE-OP AND POST-OP RT

- Five randomized trials of pre-op RT vs surgery alone demonstrate no difference in LF and OS.
- Phase III data from outside the USA demonstrate decreased LF, but no difference in OS or DM with post-op RT.

POSTOPERATIVE CHEMORT

, The role of postoperative chemoradiotherapy for adeno-carcinomas of the GEJ was established by Intergroup 0116, which showed benefit over surgery alone. There is limited evidence for adjuvant therapy for squamous cell carcinomas; however, patients with positive margins or gross residual likely benefit.

, Intergroup 0116 (Macdonald NEJM 2001, Smalley JCO 2012). See gastric chapter for complete details. Patients with ≥ T3 or N+ gastric or GEJ adenocarcinoma s/p R0 resection were randomized to observation vs adjuvant chemoRT. HR for OS and RFS were 1.32 and 1.51, favoring adjuvant chemoRT.

, ARTIST (Lee JCO 2012). See gastric chapter for complete details. Patients with ≥ stage II gastric cancer treated with R0 gastrectomy and D2 lymph node dissection were randomized to adjuvant chemotherapy vs chemoRT. In post hoc analysis, patients with N+ disease benefited from chemoRT.

, Adelstein (J Thorac Oncol 2009). Phase II: 50 patients with T3, N1, or M1a disease were treated with surgery and chemoradiotherapy (50.4–59.4 Gy) with concurrent 5-FU and cisplatin. 86% adenocarcinoma and 86% node positive. 4-year OS 51%, DMFS 56%, LC 86%.

VI

NEOADJUVANT THERAPY

, *Meta-analysis* (Sjoquist, Lancet Oncol 2011). 24 studies including 4188 patients evaluating neoadjuvant chemo and neoadjuvant chemoRT vs surgery alone, including early results from CROSS trial. Pre-op chemoRT reduced mortality overall (HR 0.78) and in both histologic subgroups. Pre-op chemo reduced mortality overall (HR 0.87), but only in adenocarcinoma subgroup (HR 0.83, $p = 0.01$). A trend for reduced mortality with chemoRT was observed over pre-op chemo alone (HR 0.88, $p = 0.07$).

PRE-OP CHEMO VERSUS SURGERY ALONE

, *RTOG 8911/INT 0133* (Kelsen NEJM 1998; JCO 2007). Phase III: 467 patients with resectable T1-2NxM0 SCC and adenocarcinoma randomized to surgery ± neoadjuvant chemo (cisplatin, 5-FU). Pre-op chemo did not improve MS or 4-year OS (26% vs 23%). 12% cCR and 2.5% pCR. No difference between histologies. Update 2007: only R0 resection resulted in significant long-term survival advantage. Five-year OS R0 32%, R1 5%.

- *MRC OE2* (MRC Lancet 2002; Allum JCO 2009). Phase III: 802 patients with resectable SCC (30%) and adenocarcinoma (66%) randomized to surgery ± neoadjuvant chemo (5-FU, cisplatin). Nine percent of patients from each arm received pre-op RT. Pre-op chemo improved 5-year OS (17% vs 23%) and complete resection rate (54% vs 60%). Survival advantage was seen in adenocarcinoma (17% vs 24%) and SCC (18% vs 23%).
- See MAGIC (Cunningham NEJM 2006) in the Gastric Chapter.

PRE-OP CHEMORT VERSUS SURGERY ALONE

- *CROSS* (van Hagen NEJM 2012; Oppedijk JCO 2014; Shapiro Lancet Oncol 2015). Phase III: 368 patients (75% adenocarcinoma) with T1N1 or T2-3 N0-1 esophagus or GEJ randomized to surgery ± neoadjuvant chemoRT (41.4 Gy/23 fx, carboplatin + paclitaxel). pCR 29% (23% adeno, 49% SCC). *ChemoRT improved 5-yr OS (47% vs 33%)*, PFS (44% vs 27%), and reduced locoregional progression (22% vs 38%) and distant progression (39% vs 48%). Postoperative mortality was similar in both arms (5% vs 3%).
- *FFCD 9901* (Mariette JCO 2014). Phase III, revised due to poor accrual, closed due to futility: 195 patients with early stage (I–II, 72% N0) esophageal cancer (70% squamous cell carcinoma), randomized surgery ± neoadjuvant chemoRT (45 Gy/25 fx, cisplatin + 5-FU). ChemoRT reduced pathologic tumor stage; however, the rate of R0 resection was 92% in both arms. In-hospital mortality was higher than expected in the chemoRT arm (11.1% vs 3.4). No difference in overall survival. *Caveats: early stage, high postoperative mortality.*
- *CALGB 9781* (Tepper JCO 2008). Phase III: closed due to poor accrual: 56 patients with resectable SCC and adenocarcinoma (T1-3N1M0) randomized to surgery ± neoadjuvant chemoRT (50.4 Gy/28 fx, cisplatin + 5-FU). *ChemoRT improved 5-year survival (16% vs 39%), median survival (1.8 vs 4.5 years)*. 40% pCR in patients with pre-op chemoRT.

, *TROG/AGITG* (Burmeister Lancet Oncol 2005). Phase III: 256 patients with T1-3N0-1 SCC or adenoCA (61%) randomized to surgery ± neoadjuvant chemoRT (35 Gy/15 fx, cisplatin + 5-FU). No difference in 3-year DFS (~30–35%) or OS (~35%), but chemoRT improved R0 resection rate (60% vs 80%). Subgroup analysis showed SCC had improved DFS and OS with chemoRT. No difference in patterns of failure. Thirteen percent of patients with pCR had 3-year OS 49%. Caveats: single cycle of chemotherapy.

, *Michigan* (Urba JCO 2001). Phase III: 100 patients, localized CA, 75% adenocarcinoma, 25% SCC randomized to surgery ± neoadjuvant chemoRT (45 Gy/30 bid fractions, cisplatin + vinblastine + 5-FU). Pre-op chemoRT significantly decreased LR (19% vs 42%). Improved 3-year OS (30% vs 15%) did not reach statistical significance ($p = 0.07$).

, *Walsh* (NEJM 1996). Phase III: 113 patients, *adenocarcinoma only*, randomized to surgery ± neoadjuvant chemoRT (40 Gy/15 fx; cisplatin + 5-FU). Pre-op chemoRT improved OS at 1 year (52% vs 44%) and 3 years (32% vs 6%) and MS (16 vs 11 months). Twenty-five percent pCR rate in chemoRT arm. Positive LN or mets at surgery: 42% chemoRT, 82% surgery alone. Caveats: small patient number, poor outcome of surgery alone arm, unconventional fractionation, and short follow-up (11 months).

, *EORTC* (Bosset NEJM 1997). Phase III: 282 patients, T1-3N0 and T1-2N1M0, *SCC only*, randomized to surgery ± neoadjuvant chemoRT (split-course 37 Gy/10 fx, cisplatin 0–2 days prior to RT). Surgery was en bloc esophagectomy and proximal gastrectomy. pCR 26%. No difference in OS (~25% at 5 years). Pre-op chemoRT improved DFS (~40% vs 28%), R0 resection rate ($p = 0.017$). A lower proportion of mortality was attributable to cancer chemoRT arm (67% vs 86%). The chemoRT arm had higher post-op mortality (12% vs 3%).

PRE-OP CHEMO VERSUS PRE-OP CHEMO + CHEMORT

, *German POET* (Stahl JCO 2009). Phase III: 126 patients with locally advanced (uT3/4NxM0) but resectable *adenocarcinoma* of the lower esophagus or gastric cardia randomized to induction chemo (cisplatin + leucovorin +

VI

5-FU x 2.5 c) + surgery vs induction chemo (PLF x 2 c) + chemoRT (30 Gy with cisplatin + etoposide) + surgery. Study closed due to poor accrual. 3-yr OS (27.7% vs 47.4%, p = 0.07), pCR rate (2% vs 15.6%), and N0 rate (37.7% vs 64.4%) favored chemoRT.

- Burmeister (Eur J Cancer 2011). Phase II: 75 patients with adenocarcinoma of the GEJ randomized to neoadjuvant chemo (cisplatin + 5-FU) vs neoadjuvant chemoRT (35 Gy/15 fx, cisplatin + 5-FU), both followed by surgery. Toxicity was similar. ChemoRT conferred improved response rate (31% vs 8%), reduced R1 resection rate (0 vs 11%). Median PFS (14 vs 26 mo), and OS (29 vs 32 mo) higher in chemoRT, but not statistically different.

DEFINITIVE CHEMORT

- RTOG 8501 (Herskovic NEJM 1992, al-Sarraf JCO 1997, Cooper JAMA 1999). Phase III: 121 patients, T1-3N0-1M0, adenocarcinoma and SCC, randomized to RT alone (64 Gy/32 fx) vs chemoRT (50 Gy, 5-FU + cisplatin). Interim analysis showed improved OS with chemoRT. 69 additional patients were treated according to the chemoRT protocol and followed prospectively. Five-year OS for RT alone was 0%, for chemoRT (randomized) 27%, and for chemoRT (nonrandomized) 14%. No differences in OS based on histology. Persistent disease was identified in 26% vs 37%, favoring chemoRT.

- RTOG 9405, INT 0123 (Minsky, JCO 2002). Phase III: 236 patients, T1-4N0-1M0, SCC and adenocarcinoma, randomized to low-dose (50.4 Gy) vs high-dose (64.8 Gy) chemoRT (concurrent 5-FU + cisplatin). Trial was stopped after an interim analysis. High-dose arm had higher treatment-related death (10% vs 2%). *Of the 11 deaths in high-dose arm, 7 occurred at $\leq$ 50.4 Gy*. No differences in MS (13 vs 18 months), 2-year OS (31 vs 40%), or LRF (56 vs 52%) between high-dose and low-dose arms.

- PRODIGE5/ACCORD17 (Conroy Lancet Oncol 2014). Phase II/III: 134 patients randomized to definitive chemoRT (50 Gy) with concurrent FOLFOX vs cisplatin + 5-FU. Oncologic outcomes were similar: 71% vs 76% completed treatment; 3-year PFS was 18.2% vs 17.4%; 3-year OS was 19.9% vs 26.9%, however (HR 0.94 log-rank

$p = 0.7$). One and six toxic deaths occurred in the FOLFOX and Cis-5-FU arms, respectively.

ₔ *RTOG 9207* (Gaspar IJROBP 2000). Phase I/II: 49 patients T1-2N0-1M0, 92% SCC, 8% adenocarcinoma treated with concurrent chemo (5-FU, cisplatin) + RT (EBRT 50 Gy/25 fx + HDR 5 Gy × 3 or LDR 20 Gy × 1). Twenty-four percent Grade 4 toxicity, 12% fistula, 10% treatment-related deaths with MS 11 months. Three-year OS 29% and LF 63%. Brachytherapy not recommended due to high toxicity.

ₔ *CALGB 80803* (Goodman, ASCO GI 2017). Randomized phase II trial of patients with esophageal adenocarcinoma, treated with induction chemo, either FOLFOX or carboplatin + paclitaxel (CP), followed by PET-directed chemoRT (50.4 Gy/28 fx). Metabolic responders (SUVmax reduction ≥ 35%) continued the same chemotherapy during chemoRT, while metabolic non-responders switched over to the alternative chemotherapy during chemoRT. 257 patients were randomized. Overall, the pCR rate was higher among patients randomized to FOLFOX 30% (0.2–0.38) vs CP 12.5% (0.05–0.19). After induction chemo PET-R was achieved in 57% and 50%, respectively, corresponding to pCR rates of 38% vs 10.7%. Among metabolic nonresponders (30% and 38%), the complete response rate with alternate chemo was 16.2% vs 15%.

ₔ *RTOG 1010* (Ongoing). Phase III trial for patients with esophageal adenocarcinoma, evaluating addition of trastuzumab to neoadjuvant chemoRT, followed by surgery. This trial is based upon the findings of the ToGA trial, which showed HER2 amplification in 32.2% of patients with GEJ adenocarcinoma (Bang 2010, Van Cutsem 2015).

VI

DEFINITIVE CHEMORT VERSUS TRIMODALITY THERAPY

ₔ Two randomized trials evaluating trimodality therapy vs chemoRT for patients with SCC have failed to show a survival benefit, but had ~ 10% treatment-related mortality in the surgical arms.

ₔ Stahl (JCO 2005). Phase III: 172 patients, T3–4 N0–1 M0, SCC, treated with induction chemo (5-FU, leucovorin, etoposide, cisplatin) and then randomized to trimodality therapy (chemoRT 40 Gy/20 fx, cisplatin + etoposide, followed by surgery) vs definitive chemoRT (50 Gy/25 fx + hyperfractionated or HDR boost to 64–65 Gy, cisplatin + etoposide). pCR was 35% at surgery. No difference in MS (16 vs 15 months) or 5-year/10-year OS (28/19% vs 17/12%). Surgery improved 2-year FFLP (64% vs 41%), but led to increased postoperative mortality (13% vs 4%). Trial closed early due to lack of accrual.

- *FFCD 9102* (Bonnetain Ann Onc 2006, Bedenne JCO 2007, Crehange JCO 2007). Phase III: 444 patients with potentially resectable T3–4 N0–1 SCC (90%) or adenoCA (10%) were treated with chemoRT (46 Gy/23 fx or split-course 30 Gy/15 fx, concurrent cisplatin + 5-FU). 75% of patients had ≥PR, and 259 patients were randomized to surgery vs additional chemoRT (20 Gy/10 fx or split-course 15 Gy/5 fx, cisplatin + 5-FU). No difference in 2-year OS (34–40%) or MS (18–19 months). Surgery was associated with higher post-op mortality (9% vs 1%) and worse early QOL, but decreased LF (43% vs 34%) and stent requirement (32% vs 5%). Split-course RT had worse local RFS (57% vs 77%).

- *RTOG 0246* (Swisher IJROBP 2012, Swisher J Thorac Oncol 2017). Phase II study of 36 patients with resectable T1-4N0-1M0 esophageal carcinoma (73% adenocarcinoma) treated with induction chemo (5-FU, cisplatin, paclitaxel x 2c) → chemoRT (50.4 Gy, 5-FU, cisplatin). Selective esophagectomy was considered only for patients with residual disease after chemoRT (by EGD, EUS, CT) or for recurrent disease on surveillance. Clinical CR achieved in 42% of patients after chemoRT with 5/7-yr OS 53%/47% vs 33%/29% for patients with nonclinical CR (but 41%/35% if had resection). 3 of 15 clinical CR patients developed LRR on surveillance and had resection. Esophageal resection was not required in 49% of patients on trial.

SALVAGE SURGERY

- *Sudo* (JCO 2014). 276 patients treated with chemoRT for esophageal carcinoma. 70% of patients achieved clinical CR by EGD biopsies and PET/CT (70% adeno/72% squamous), of whom 52% experienced relapse (23% local only; 20% DM only; 9% local + DM). 23% of entire cohort had local only relapse as first site of failure. Of 64 patients with local only relapse 36% underwent salvage surgery with MS 58.6 mo vs 9.5 mo for 41 patients who did not have salvage surgery.

PALLIATION

- TROG 03.01/NCIC CTG ES2 (Penniment, ASCO GI 2015). 220 patients randomized to RT alone (35 Gy/15 fx or 30 Gy/10 fx) or with concurrent cisplatin/5-FU chemo. No difference in dysphagia response (RT 68%, chemoRT 74%), maintained swallowing improvement (41%, 47%), QOL, or MS (203 days, 210 days) but increased toxicity with chemoRT. Nearly 10% of patients alive at 2 yrs.
- Li (ASTRO 2016 abstr 1). 60 patients with stage IV esophageal squamous cell carcinoma randomized to at 2 cycles cisplatin docetaxel alone or with concurrent RT 50–60 Gy/25–30 fx. ChemoRT improved median PFS (9.3 vs 4.7 months), MS (18.3 vs 10.2 months), and 1/2-yr survival (73/43% vs 47/27%).

VI

RADIATION TECHNIQUES

GENERAL PRINCIPLES
Simulation
- Simulate supine with arms up.
- Wing board or Vac-Lok bag may be used for immobilization.
- Oral and/or IV contrast may aid target localization.
- 4D-CT may be helpful in quantifying target motion, particularly for distal or GEJ lesions.
- Fusion with PET/CT can be useful for target delineation.
- Incorporate endocopy findings.

Field Design
- IMRT should be considered for cancers of the cervical esophagus or when sparing of normal tissues (e.g., heart, lungs) cannot be achieved with 3D planning.
- Consensus IMRT contouring guidelines for definitive/pre-op target volumes have been published (Wu, IJROBP 2015).
- GTV is primary and involved regional nodes identified by endoscopy, EUS, CT, and/or PET.
- CTV for primary includes 1 cm radial and 3–4 cm superior/inferior margin along esophagus and cardia.
  - For proximal lesions, superior border should not extend above cricoid cartilage unless there is gross disease.

- For distal esophageal or GEJ tumors, distal border should include at least 3 cm margin along clinically uninvolved gastric mucosa.
- May limit radial border to 0.5 cm if abutting uninvolved heart or liver. Vertebral bodies may be excluded in absence of invasion.
- CTV for involved nodes includes 0.5–1.5 cm margin.
- CTV for elective nodes depends on location of the primary.
  - Cervical esophagus: supraclavicular nodes +/– higher cervical nodes especially if LN+ (We recomend extension of coverage of 1 echelon of nodes above involved nodal region).
  - Upper 1/3 tumors above the carina: include SCV and mediastinal and paraesophageal lymph nodes.
  - Middle 1/3: include paraesophageal nodes.
  - Distal 1/3 and GE junction: include paraesophageal, celiac, para-aortic and gastrohepatic (lesser curvature) nodes, with coverage extending to the celiac axis.
  - Elective nodal coverage improves survival. (Wu ASCO 2016).
- PTV includes 0.5–1 cm expansion.
- Volumes should be adapted to individual patient anatomy.
- Post-op target volumes:
  - For gastric and GEJ tumors, please refer to the gastric cancer chapter.
- Refer to gastric cancer target volumes for Siewert III tumors or those extending ≥5 cm into stomach.
- 3D field design options:
  - SCV and primary tumor treated in one field. 6MV AP field and 18MV field with off-cord boost to the primary after 41.4 Gy.
  - Single-isocenter split-field, matching the SCV with primary esophagus fields. SCV treated with 6MV AP field with spinal cord block. Primary tumor treated with AP/PA and oblique beam arrangement.
  - AP/PA with lightly weighted lateral.
  - AP and off-cord obliques.

DOSE PRESCRIPTIONS
- Pre-op: 41.4–50.4 Gy in 1.8 Gy fractions.
- Definitive: 50.4 Gy–54 Gy in 1.8 Gy fractions.

, Post-op: 45–50.4 Gy in 1.8 Gy fractions. Higher doses for gross residual disease.
, Cervical esophagus: 54 Gy–66 Gy in 1.8–2 Gy fractions (strongly consider higher dose if surgery not planned).

DOSE LIMITATIONS (CONVENTIONAL FRACTIONATION)
, Spinal cord: Dmax ≤45 Gy
, Lung: V20 ≤ 25%, V5 ≤ 50%
, Heart: Mean ≤ 32 Gy, V40 ≤ 33–50%
, Liver: Mean liver ≤21 Gy, V30 < 30%
, Kidneys: V20 ≤ 30%

COMPLICATIONS
, Acute side effects: esophagitis, weight loss, fatigue, and anorexia.
, Esophageal perforation may present with substernal chest pain, increased heart rate, fever, and hemorrhage.
, Pneumonitis: subacute, occurs <6 weeks after RT. Presents with cough, dyspnea, hypoxia, and fever. Depending on severity, treat with NSAIDs or steroids.
, Late strictures possible, half are due to LR. For benign strictures, dilation results in palliation in the majority of patients. For malignant strictures, dilation does not work as well.
, Pericarditis, coronary artery disease.
, With brachytherapy and/or EBRT, tumor involvement of the trachea can lead to fistula formation during RT (5–10%), secondary to tumor necrosis or natural progression of the disease.

VI

FOLLOW-UP

, H&P every 4 months for 1 year, then every 6 months for 5 years, then annually thereafter. CBC, metabolic panel, endoscopy, CT chest/abdomen, and PET should be considered when clinically indicated.
, For locally advanced esophageal cancers undergoing combined chemoRT, metabolic response as determined by FDG-PET imaging before and after treatment is a strong predictor of OS (Lordick Lancet Oncol 2007).[3]

Acknowledgment We thank Charlotte Dai Kubicky MD, PhD, and Marc B. Nash MD for their work on the prior edition of this chapter.

REFERENCES

Adelstein DJ, Rice TW, Rybicki LA, et al. Mature Results from a Phase II Trial of Postoperative Concurrent Chemoradiotherapy for Poor Prognosis Cancer of the Esophagus and Gastroesophageal Junction.J Thor Oncol. 2009;4(10):1264–69.

Allum WH, Stenning SP, Bancewicz J, Clark PI, Langley RE. Long-term results of a randomized trial of surgery with or without preoperative chemotherapy in esophageal cancer. J Clin Oncol. 2009;27:5062–7.

Al-Sarraf M, Martz K, Herskovic A, et al. Progress report of combined chemoradiotherapy versus radiotherapy alone in patients with esophageal cancer: an intergroup study. J Clin Oncol. 1997;15:277–84.

Bang Y-J, Van Cutsem E, Feyereislova A, et al. Trastuzumab in combination with chemotherapy versus chemotherapy alone for treatment of HER2-positive advanced gastric or gastro-oesophageal junction cancer (ToGA): a phase 3, open-label, randomised controlled trial. Lancet. 2010;376:687–97.

Bedenne L, Michel P, Bouché O, et al. Chemoradiation followed by surgery compared with chemoradiation alone in squamous cancer of the esophagus: FFCD 9102. J Clin Oncol. 2007;25:1160–8.

Bonnetain F, Bouche O, Michel P, et al. A comparative longitudinal quality of life study using the Spitzer quality of life index in a randomized multicenter phase III trial (FFCD 9102): chemoradiation followed by surgery compared with chemoradiation alone in locally advanced squamous resectable thoracic esophageal cancer. Ann Oncol. 2006;17:827–34.

Bosset JF, Gignoux M, Triboulet JP, et al. Chemoradiotherapy followed by surgery compared with surgery alone in squamous-cell cancer of the esophagus. N Engl J Med. 1997;337:161–7.

Burmeister BH, Smithers BM, Gebski V, et al. Surgery alone versus chemoradiotherapy followed by surgery for resectable cancer of the oesophagus: a randomised controlled phase III trial. Lancet Oncol. 2005;6:659–68.

Burmeister BH, Thomas JM, Burmeister EA, et al. Is concurrent radiation therapy required in patients receiving preoperative chemotherapy for adenocarcinoma of the oesophagus? A randomised phase II trial. Eur J Cancer. 2011;47:354–60.

Büschenfelde zum CM, Herrmann K, Schuster T, et al. (18)F-FDG PET-guided salvage neoadjuvant radiochemotherapy of adenocarcinoma of the esophagogastric junction: the MUNICON II trial. J Nucl Med. 2011;52:1189–96.

Conroy T, Galais M-P, Raoul J-L, et al. Definitive chemoradiotherapy with FOLFOX versus fluorouracil and cisplatin in patients with oesophageal cancer (PRODIGE5/ACCORD17): final results of a randomised, phase 2/3 trial. Lancet Oncol. 2014;15:305–14.

Cooper JS, Guo MD, Herskovic A, et al. Chemoradiotherapy of locally advanced esophageal cancer: long-term follow-up of a prospective randomized trial (RTOG 85-01). Radiation therapy oncology group. *JAMA*. 1999;281:1623–7.

Créhange G, Maingon P, Peignaux K, et al. Phase III trial of protracted compared with split-course chemoradiation for esophageal carcinoma: federation francophone de Cancerologie digestive 9102. J Clin Oncol. 2007;25:4895–901.

Cunningham D, Allum WH, Stenning SP, et al. Perioperative chemotherapy versus surgery alone for resectable gastroesophageal cancer. N Engl J Med. 2006;355:11–20.

Gaspar LE, Winter K, Kocha WI, Coia LR, Herskovic A, Graham M. A phase I/II study of external beam radiation, brachytherapy, and concurrent chemotherapy for patients with localized carcinoma of the esophagus (radiation therapy oncology Group study 9207): final report. Cancer. 2000;88:988–95.

Goodman KA, Niedzwiecki D, Hall N, et al. 2017. Initial results of CALGB 80803 (alliance): a randomized phase II trial of PET scan-directed combined modality therapy for esophageal cancer. *ASCO GI*.

Herskovic A, Martz K, Al-Sarraf M, et al. Combined chemotherapy and radiotherapy compared with radiotherapy alone in patients with cancer of the esophagus. N Engl J Med. 1992;326:1593–8.

Kelsen DP, Ginsberg R, Pajak TF, et al. Chemotherapy followed by surgery compared with surgery alone for localized esophageal cancer. N Engl J Med. 1998;339:1979–84.

Kelsen DP, Winter KA, Gunderson LL, et al. Long-term results of RTOG trial 8911 (USA intergroup 113): a random assignment trial comparison of chemotherapy followed by surgery compared with surgery alone for esophageal cancer. J Clin Oncol. 2007;25:3719–25.

Koike R, Nishimura Y, Nakamatsu K, Kanamori S, Shibata T. Concurrent chemoradiotherapy for esophageal cancer with malignant fistula. Int J Radiat Oncol Biol Phys. 2008;70:1418–22.

Lee J, Lim D-H, Kim S, et al. Phase III trial comparing capecitabine plus cisplatin versus capecitabine plus cisplatin with concurrent capecitabine radiotherapy in completely resected gastric cancer with D2 lymph node dissection: the ARTIST trial. J Clin Oncol. 2012;30:268–73.

Li T, Lv J, Li F, et al. Prospective randomized phase II study of concurrent chemoradiotherapy versus chemotherapy alone in stage IV esophageal squamous cell carcinoma. Int J Radiat Oncol Biol Phys. 2016;96(Suppl 2):S1.

Lordick F, Ott K, Krause B-J, et al. PET to assess early metabolic response and to guide treatment of adenocarcinoma of the oesophagogastric junction: the MUNICON phase II trial. Lancet Oncol. 2007;8:797–805.

Macdonald JS, Smalley SR, Benedetti J, et al. Chemoradiotherapy after surgery compared with surgery alone for adenocarcinoma of the stomach or gastroesophageal junction. N Engl J Med. 2001;345:725–30.

Mariette C, Dahan L, Mornex F, et al. Surgery alone versus chemoradiotherapy followed by surgery for stage I and II esophageal cancer: final analysis of randomized controlled trial FFCD 9901. J Clin Oncol. 2014;32:2416–22.

Medical Research Council Oesophageal Cancer Working Group. Surgical resection with or without preoperative chemotherapy in oesophageal cancer: a randomised controlled trial. Lancet. 2002;359:1727–33.

Minsky BD, Pajak TF, Ginsberg RJ, et al. INT 0123 (radiation therapy oncology Group 94-05) phase III trial of combined-modality therapy for esophageal cancer: high-dose versus standard-dose radiation therapy. J Clin Oncol. 2002;20:1167–74.

Oppedijk V, van der Gaast A, van Lanschot JJB, et al. Patterns of recurrence after surgery alone versus preoperative chemoradiotherapy and surgery in the CROSS trials. J Clin Oncol. 2014;32:385–91.

Penniment MG, Harvey JA, Wong R, et al. A randomized phase III study in advanced esophageal cancer (OC) to compare the quality of life (QoL) and palliation of dysphagia in patients treated with radiotherapy (RT) or chemoradiotherapy (CRT) TROG 03.01 NCIC CTG ES.2. J Clin Oncol. 2015;33(suppl 3; abstr 6)

Shapiro J, van Lanschot JJB, Hulshof MCCM, et al. Neoadjuvant chemoradiotherapy plus surgery versus surgery alone for oesophageal or junctional cancer (CROSS): long-term results of a randomised controlled trial. Lancet Oncol. 2015;16:1090–8.

Sjoquist KM, Burmeister BH, Smithers BM, et al. Survival after neoadjuvant chemotherapy or chemoradiotherapy for resectable oesophageal carcinoma: an updated meta-analysis. Lancet Oncol. 2011;12:681–92.

Smalley SR, Benedetti JK, Haller DG, et al. Updated analysis of SWOG-directed intergroup study 0116: a phase III trial of adjuvant radiochemotherapy versus observation after curative gastric cancer resection. J Clin Oncol. 2012;30:2327–33.

Stahl M. Chemoradiation with and without surgery in patients with locally advanced squamous cell carcinoma of the esophagus. J Clin Oncol. 2005;23:2310–7.

VI

Stahl M, Walz MK, Stuschke M, et al. Phase III comparison of preoperative chemotherapy compared with Chemoradiotherapy in patients with locally advanced adenocarcinoma of the Esophagogastric junction. J Clin Oncol. 2009;27:851–6.

Sudo K, Xiao L, Wadhwa R, et al. Importance of surveillance and success of salvage strategies after definitive chemoradiation in patients with esophageal cancer. J Clin Oncol. 2014;32:3400–5.

Swisher SG, Winter KA, Komaki RU, et al. A phase II study of a paclitaxel-based chemoradiation regimen with selective surgical salvage for resectable locoregionally advanced esophageal cancer: initial reporting of RTOG 0246. Int J Radiat Oncol Biol Phys. 2012;82:1967–72.

Swisher SG, Moughan J, Komaki RU, et al. Final results of NRG oncology RTOG 0246: an organ-preserving selective resection strategy in esophageal cancer patients treated with definitive Chemoradiation. J Thorac Oncol. 2017;12:368–74.

Tepper J, Krasna MJ, Niedzwiecki D, et al. Phase III trial of trimodality therapy with cisplatin, fluorouracil, radiotherapy, and surgery compared with surgery alone for esophageal cancer: CALGB 9781. J Clin Oncol. 2008;26:1086–92.

Urba SG, Orringer MB, Turrisi A, Iannettoni M, Forastiere A, Strawderman M. Randomized trial of preoperative chemoradiation versus surgery alone in patients with locoregional esophageal carcinoma. J Clin Oncol. 2001;19:305–13.

Van Cutsem E, Bang Y-J, Feng-Yi F, et al. HER2 screening data from ToGA: targeting HER2 in gastric and gastroesophageal junction cancer. Gastric Cancer. 2015;18:476–84.

van Hagen P, Hulshof MCCM, van Lanschot JJB, et al. Preoperative Chemoradiotherapy for esophageal or junctional cancer. N Engl J Med. 2012;366:2074–84.

Walsh TN, Noonan N, Hollywood D, Kelly A, Keeling N, Hennessy TP. A comparison of multimodal therapy and surgery for esophageal adenocarcinoma. N Engl J Med. 1996;335:462–7.

Wu AJ, Bosch WR, Chang DT, et al. Expert Consensus Contouring Guidelines for Intensity Modulated Radiation Therapy in Esophageal and Gastroesophageal Junction Cancer. Int J Radiat Oncol Biol Phys. 2015;92(4):911–20.

Wu SX, Luo H, Wang L, et al. Phase III randomized study of elective nodal irradiation plus erlotinib combined with chemotherapy for esophageal squamous cell carcinoma. J Clin Oncol. 2016;34:2016. (suppl; abstr 4048)

Chapter 19
Gastric Cancer

Jennifer S. Chang, Mekhail Anwar,
and Hans T. Chung

PEARLS

- 26,370 new cases and 10,730 deaths from gastric cancer estimated in 2016 in the USA, with both decreasing over time.
- Highest death rates are reported in Chile, Costa Rica, Japan, China, and the former Soviet Union.
- Median age of diagnosis is 69.
- Male/female = 1.5:1.
- Environmental risk factors: low fruits and vegetables, high salts and nitrates, salted fish, smoked meats, *Helicobacter pylori*, hypochlorhydria, pernicious anemia, polyps, previous radiation, gastrectomy, obesity, smoking.
- Predisposing genetic mutations: CDH1 mutation, Lynch syndrome, familial adenomatous polyposis, Peutz-Jeghers, juvenile polyposis.
- Tumor location.
  - GE junction, cardia, and fundus 35% (diffuse subtype, incidence rising).
  - Body 25%.
  - Antrum and distal stomach 40% (intestinal subtype, incidence falling).
  - Siewert type III tumors (tumor center is 2–5 cm below GEJ, infiltrates GEJ) are treated as gastric cancer.

VI

© Springer International Publishing AG, part of Springer Nature 2018   **423**
Eric K. Hansen and M. Roach III (eds.), *Handbook of Evidence-Based Radiation Oncology*, https://doi.org/10.1007/978-3-319-62642-0_19

- Intestinal subtype: more commonly seen in patients >40 years, less aggressive.
- Diffuse subtype: affects younger patients, more aggressive.
- Seven primary LN groups:
  - Perigastric LN along greater and lesser curvatures, gastroduodenal, para-aortics, celiac axis, porta-hepatic, suprapancreatic group, and splenic hilum. If GE junction, also distal paraesophageal.
- Histology: 90% adenocarcinoma. Others: sarcoma, GIST, carcinoid, small-cell, undifferentiated, MALT lymphoma, and leiomyosarcoma.

WORKUP

- H&P: dysphagia, indigestion, early satiety, loss of appetite, nausea, abdominal pain, weight loss, obstruction (pyloric lesion), anemia, hematemesis (10–15%), melena. Check for cervical, SCV, axillary, and periumbilical adenopathy.
- Labs: CBC, liver and renal function tests, CEA (elevated in 1/3), *H. pylori*.
- Upper endoscopy (for direct visualization and biopsy), EUS (assess depth of penetration and LN involvement), CT chest/abdomen/pelvis with contrast (assess adenopathy and metastasis).
- PET scan if clinically indicated; may not be appropriate for T1 disease.
- HER2-neu testing if metastatic adenocarcinoma.
- Laparoscopy with cytology: consider to assess the extent of disease, peritoneal implants, and resectability in cT1b or higher stage, especially if cT3 and/or cN+. May also consider if planning pre-op chemoRT.
- Consider preradiation quantitative renal perfusion study to evaluate relative bilateral renal function, which may affect radiation planning and dose constraints.

STAGING: GASTRIC CANCER

Editors' note: All TNM stage and stage groups referred to elsewhere in this chapter reflect the 2010 AJCC staging nomenclature unless otherwise noted, as the new system below was published after this chapter was written.

Table 19.1 (AJCC 7TH ED., 2010)

Primary tumor (T)

TX:	Primary tumor cannot be assessed
T0:	No evidence of primary tumor
Tis:	Carcinoma in situ: intraepithelial tumor without invasion of the lamina propria
T1:	Tumor invades lamina propria, muscularis mucosae, or submucosa
T1a:	Tumor invades lamina propria or muscularis mucosae
T1b:	Tumor invades submucosa
T2:	Tumor invades muscularis propria*
T3:	Tumor penetrates subserosal connective tissue without invasion of visceral peritoneum or adjacent structures** and ***
T4:	Tumor invades serosa (visceral peritoneum) or adjacent structures** and ***
T4a:	Tumor invades serosa (visceral peritoneum)
T4b:	Tumor invades adjacent structures

*Note: A tumor may penetrate the muscularis propria with extension into the gastrocolic or gastrohepatic ligaments, or into the greater or lesser omentum, without perforation of the visceral peritoneum covering these structures. In this case, the tumor is classified T3. If there is perforation of the visceral peritoneum covering the gastric ligaments or the omentum, the tumor should be classified T4.

**The adjacent structures of the stomach include the spleen, transverse colon, liver, diaphragm, pancreas, abdominal wall, adrenal gland, kidney, small intestine, and retroperitoneum.

***Intramural extension to the duodenum or esophagus is classified by the depth of the greatest invasion in any of these sites, including the stomach.

Regional lymph nodes (N)

NX:	Regional lymph node(s) cannot be assessed
N0:	No regional lymph node metastasis*
N1:	Metastasis in 1–2 regional lymph nodes
N2:	Metastasis in 3–6 regional lymph nodes
N3:	Metastasis in seven or more regional lymph nodes
N3a:	Metastasis in 7–15 regional lymph nodes
N3b:	Metastasis in 16 or more regional lymph nodes

*Note: A designation of pN0 should be used if all examined lymph nodes are negative, regardless of the total numbervremoved and examined.

Distant metastasis (M)

M0:	No distant metastasis
M1:	Distant metastasis

continued

VI

Table 19.1 (continued)

Anatomic stage/prognostic groups	
0:	Tis N0 M0
IA:	T1 N0 M0
IB:	T2 N0 M0
	T1 N1 M0
IIA:	T3 N0 M0
	T2 N1 M0
	T1 N2 M0
IIB:	T4a N0 M0
	T3 N1 M0
	T2 N2 M0
	T1 N3 M0
IIIA:	T4a N1 M0
	T3 N2 M0
	T2 N3 M0
IIIB:	T4b N0 M0
	T4b N1 M0
	T4a N2 M0
	T3 N3 M0
IIIC:	T4b N2 M0
	T4b N3 M0
	T4a N3 M0
IV:	Any T any N M1

Used with permission from the American Joint Committee on Cancer (AJCC), Chicago, Illinois. The original source for this material is the AJCC Cancer Staging Manual, Seventh Edition (2010), published by Springer Science+Business Media

Table 19.2 (AJCC 8TH ED., 2017)

Definitions of AJCC TNM	
Definition of Primary Tumor (T)	
T category	**T criteria**
TX	Primary tumor cannot be assessed
T0	No evidence of primary tumor
Tis	Carcinoma in situ: intraepithelial tumor without invasion of the lamina propria and high grade dysplasia
T1	Tumor invades the lamina propria, muscularis mucosae, or submucosa
T1a	Tumor invades the lamina propria or muscularis mucosae
T1b	Tumor invades the submucosa
T2	Tumor invades the muscularis propria*
T3	Tumor penetrates the subserosal connective tissue without invasion of the visceral peritoneum or adjacent structures**,***
T4	Tumor invades the serosa (visceral peritoneum) or adjacent structures**,***
T4a	Tumor invades the serosa (visceral peritoneum)
T4b	Tumor invades adjacent structures/organs

*A tumor may penetrate the muscularis propria with extension into the gastrocolic or gastrohepatic ligaments or into the greater or lesser omentum, without perforation of the visceral peritoneum covering these structures. In this case, the tumor is classified as 13. If there is perforation of the visceral peritoneum covering the gastric ligaments or the omentum, the tumor should be classified as T4

**The adjacent structures of the stomach include the spleen, transverse colon, liver, diaphragm, pancreas, abdominal wall, adrenal gland, kidney, small intestine, and retroperitoneum

***Intramural extension to the duodenum or esophagus is not considered invasion of an adjacent structure but is classified using the depth of the greatest invasion in any of these sites

DEFINITION OF REGIONAL LYMPH NODE (N)

N category	N criteria
NX	Regional lymph node(s) cannot be assessed
N0	No regional lymph node metastasis
N1	Metastasis in one or two regional lymph nodes
N2	Metastasis in three to six regional lymph nodes
N3	Metastasis in seven or more regional lymph nodes
N3a	Metastasis in seven or more regional lymph nodes
N3b	Metastasis in 16 or more regional lymph nodes

DEFINITION OF DISTANT METASTASIS (M)

M category	M criteria
M0	No distant metastasis
M1	Distant metastasis

AJCC PROGNOSTIC STAGE GROUPS
CLINICAL (CTNM)

When T is...	And N is...	And M is...	Then the stage group is...
Tis	N0	M0	0
T1	N0	M0	I
T2	N0	M0	I
T1	N1, N2,or N3	M0	IIA
T2	N1,N2,or N3	M0	IIA
T3	N0	M0	IIB
T4a	N0	M0	IIB
T3	N1, N2,or N3	M0	**III**
T4a	N1, N2,or N3	M0	**III**
T4b	Any N	M0	IVA
Any T	Any N	M1	IVB

VI

PATHOLOGICAL (PTNM)

When T is...	And N is...	And M is...	Then the stage group is...
Tis	N0	M0	0
T1	N0	M0	IA
T1	N1	M0	IB
T2	N0	M0	IB
T1	N2	M0	IIA
T2	N1	M0	IIA
T3	N0	M0	IIA
T1	N3a	M0	IIB
T2	N2	M0	IIB
T3	N1	M0	IIB
T4a	N0	M0	IIB
T2	N3a	M0	IIIA
T3	N2	M0	IIIA
T4a	N1	M0	IIIA
T4a	N2	M0	IIIA
T4b	N0	M0	IIIA
T1	N3b	M0	IIIB
T2	N3b	M0	IIIB
T3	N3a	M0	IIIB
T4a	N3a	M1	IIIB
T4b	N1	M0	IIIB
T4b	N2	M0	IIIB
T3	N3b	M0	IIIC
T4a	N3b	M0	IIIC
T4b	N3a	M0	IIIC
T4b	N3b	M0	IIIC
Any T	Any N	M1	IV

POSTNEOADJUVANT THERAPY (YPTNM)

When T is...	And N is...	And M is...	Then the stage group is...
T1	N0	M0	I
T2	N0	M0	I
T1	N1	M0	I
T3	N0	M0	II
T2	N1	M0	II
T1	N2	M0	II
T4a	N0	M0	II
T3	N1	M0	II
T2	N2	M0	II
T1	N3	M0	II
T4a	N1	M0	III
T3	N2	M0	III
T2	N3	M0	III
T4b	N0	M0	III

T4b	N1	M0	III
T4a	N2	M0	III
T3	N3	M0	III
T4b	N2	M0	III
T4b	N3	M0	III
T4a	N3	M0	III
Any T	Any N	M1	IV

Used with permission of the American Joint Committee on Cancer (AJCC), Chicago, Illinois. The original and primary source for this information is the AJCC Cancer Staging Manual, Eighth Edition (2017) published by Springer International Publishing

SURGERY

- General guidelines:
  - For proximal (cardia): total or proximal gastrectomy.
  - For distal (body and antrum): prefer subtotal gastrectomy.
  - For palliation: gastrectomy without LN dissection or consider palliative radiation if symptomatic (i.e., bleeding, obstruction).
  - Avoid splenectomy unless spleen/hilum involvement.
  - Aim for ≥ 5 cm proximal and distal margins whenever possible.
  - Remove minimum of 15 LNs. D2 nodal dissection is preferred.
  - Consider placing feeding jejunostomy tube.
  - For gastric outlet obstruction, gastrojejunostomy is preferable over endoluminal stenting.
- D1 dissection: removes involved proximal or distal or entire stomach; right/left cardiac, lesser and greater curvature, suprapyloric (along right gastric artery) and infrapyloric LN.
- D2 dissection: D1 plus left gastric, common hepatic, celiac, splenic artery, splenic hilum LN.
- D3 dissection: D2 plus hepatoduodenal ligament, superior mesenteric vein, retropancreatic.
- Billroth I = end-to-end gastrojejunal anastomosis, gastric resection margin used for anastomosis.
- Billroth II = end-to-side gastrojejunal anastomosis, closure of the duodenal stump, and the lesser curvature of the stomach. Gastric resection margin is usually NOT used for anastomosis.
- Sites of LF after surgery.
  - Gastric bed ~50%, LN ~40%, anastomosis or stumps ~25%.

VI

TREATMENT RECOMMENDATIONS

Table 19.3 TREATMENT RECOMMENDATIONS

2010 stage	Recommended treatment
T1N0	Surgery alone (partial or total gastrectomy with at least D1 LN dissection). Selected T1a patients, or those medically unfit to tolerate major surgery, may be candidates for endoscopic mucosal resection at experienced centers

T2–4 and/or LN+ resectable and operable	Pre-op chemo x3c (FLOT: docetaxel, oxaliplatin, fluorouracil/leucovorin or MAGIC: epirubicin, cisplatin, 5-FU) → surgery → post-op chemo x3c (same as pre-op chemo) in patients with good KPS
	 Surgery (without pre-op therapy) followed by adjuvant therapy
	   pT2N0: surveillance for selected pts with R0 resection and without high-risk features (poorly differentiated, high grade, LVSI, PNI, age <50 years). Otherwise, adjuvant therapy as below:
	   pT3–4, pN+, or R1/2 resection: post-op 5-FU/leucovorin (LV) or capecitabine × 1c → concurrent infusional 5-FU or capecitabine with RT (45 Gy) → 5-FU/leucovorin (LV) or capecitabine x 2c
	 Pre-op chemoRT may be considered and is the subject of ongoing trials for resectable gastric cancer

T2–4 and/or LN+ unresectable or inoperable	Concurrent chemoRT (5-FU or taxane-based and 45–50.4 Gy). If not an RT candidate: chemo alone (5-FU, cisplatin, oxaliplatin, taxane, or irinotecan based) Poor PS: best supportive care. RT alone may provide some palliation, but no survival benefit
M1	Palliative chemo ± RT (5-FU or capecitabine + 45 Gy). 50-75% experience improvement of symptoms such as gastric outlet obstruction, pain, bleeding, or biliary obstruction. Duration of palliation 4–18 months. Alternatively, palliative surgery or best supportive care. Trastuzumab should be added to chemo for HER2-neu overexpressing metastatic adenocarcinoma

STUDIES

EXTENT OF LYMPHADENECTOMY

- Gastrectomy with D2 dissection is standard in Asian countries. In Western countries, extended lymph node dissection is less commonly used. Removal of 15 or more nodes is recommended for staging. Technical aspects of extended node dissection required training and expertise. Prophylactic pancreatectomy and splenectomy are no longer recommended with D2 dissection.
- *Dutch trial* (Bonenkamp, NEJM 1999; Hartgrink, JCO 2004; Songun, Lancet Onc 2010): 711 patients with resectable gastric CA randomized to D1 vs. D2 lymph node

dissection. D2 dissection led to a significantly higher rate of complications (43% vs. 25%), more post-op deaths (10% vs. 4%). D1 with higher local recurrence (22% vs. 12%) and gastric cancer-related death (48% vs. 37%) but similar 15-year OS (29% vs. 21%).

, *MRC trial* (Cuschieri, Br J Cancer 1999): 400 patients randomized to D1 vs. D2 lymph node dissection. D2 dissection with significantly increased postoperative morbidity (46% vs. 28%) and mortality (13% vs. 6.5%).

, *Italian Gastric Cancer Study Group* (Degiuli, Eur J Surg Oncol 2004): 162 patients randomized to D1 or pancreas-sparing D2 dissection. No difference in morbidity (10.5% vs. 16.3%) and mortality (0% vs. 1.3%). Reported morbidity and mortality may be lower than MRC and Dutch trials because those studies included resection of the distal pancreas and spleen.

VI

, *JCOG trial* (Sano, JCO 2004, Sasako, JCO 2008): 523 patients with resectable gastric cancer randomized to standard D2 vs. D2 + para-aortic nodal dissection. Similar 5-year OS (69.2% D2 vs. 70.3% D2 + PALND) and RFS. Overall morbidity was higher in the extended surgery group (28.1% vs. 20.9%; $p = 0.067$). No difference in major complication rate.

, *Taiwanese trial* (Wu, Lancet Oncol 2006): 221 patients with resectable gastric adenocarcinoma randomized to D1 vs. D3 lymphadenectomy. Single institution with experienced surgeons. D3 dissection improved 5-year OS (54% → 60%) and DFS (58% → 63%). No pre-op or post-op chemo or RT.

PERI-OP CHEMO

, *MAGIC trial* (Cunningham, NEJM 2006): 503 patients with resectable adenocarcinoma of stomach (74%), GE junction, lower esophagus, randomized to surgery alone vs. pre-op ECF × 3 cycles → surgery → post-op ECF × 3 cycles. Similar post-op morbidity and mortality. Perioperative chemo improved rates of downstaging, R0 resection, OS (36% vs. 23%), PFS (HR 0.66). ECF (epirubicin, cisplatin, and continuous infusion 5-FU).

, *FNCLCC/FFCD* (Ychou, JCO 2011): 224 patients with resectable adenocarcinoma of the lower esophagus (11%), GEJ (64%), or stomach (25%) randomized to surgery alone vs. pre-op chemo (cisplatin + continuous 5-FU) × 2–3 cycles → surgery → post-op chemo × 3–4 cycles. Closed early due to poor accrual. Chemo with better 5-year OS (38% vs. 24%) and 5-year DFS (34% vs. 19%). Chemo with 38% grade 3–4 toxicity. Similar post-op morbidity, mortality.

, *EORTC 40954* (Schuhmacher, JCO 2009): 144 patients with locally advanced adenocarcinoma of the stomach or GEJ randomized to surgery alone vs. pre-op chemo (cisplatin, folinic acid, continuous 5-FU) x 2 cycles. Stopped early due to poor accrual. Chemo with better R0 resection rate (81.9% vs. 66.7%) and fewer LN mets (61.4% vs. 76.5%) but similar 2-year OS (72.7% vs. 69.9%).

, *CLASSIC* (Bang, Lancet 2012): 1035 patients with D2 resection for gastric cancer, randomized to adjuvant capecitabine + oxaliplatin x 8 cycles vs. no chemo. Chemo with improved 3-year DFS (74% vs. 59%) but increased grade 3–4 toxicity (56% vs. 6%).

, *MAGIC-B* (phase III): Histologically confirmed, previously untreated stage IB–IV (M0) resectable disease of the stomach or GE junction randomized to pre-op ECX × 3c → surgery → ECX × 3c, or pre-op ECX-B → surgery → ECX-B × 3c. ECX (epirubicin, cisplatin, and capecitabine), B (bevacizumab). Results not yet reported.

, *MAGIC-B study FLOT4* (Al-Batran, JCO 2017): 716 patients with ≥cT2 or node-positive resectable gastric or GEJ adenocarcinoma were randomized to either 3 pre-op and 3 post-op cycles of ECF/ECX (epirubicin, cisplatin, infusional 5-FU or capecitabine) or 4 pre-op and 4 post-op cycles of FLOT(docetaxel, oxaliplatin, leucovorin, 5-FU). FLOT significantly improved median OS (35 vs 50 months) and PFS (18 vs 30 months). There was more grade 3-4 nausea and vomiting with ECF/ECX and more grade 3-4 neutropenia with FLOT.

PRE-OP CHEMORT

, *RTOG 9904* (Ajani, JCO 2006) *Phase II*: 43 operable patients with localized gastric cancer treated with pre-op chemo × 2c (5-FU, leucovorin, and cisplatin) → concurrent chemoradiation (45 Gy and infusional 5-FU and weekly paclitaxel) → surgery (with D2 dissection in 50%). 77% R0 resection rate, 26% pCR rate. OS 82% at 1 year for pCR vs. 69% if <pCR. Patterns of failure: DM (30%) vs. tumor bed failure (19%) vs. nodal and regional failure (2%).

, *TOPGEAR* (Leong, BMC Cancer 2015; Leong, Ann Surg Oncol 2017): Ongoing phase III trial of pre-op ECF x3 → surgery → post-op ECF x3 vs. ECF x2 with pre-op chemoRT → surgery → post-op ECF x3. Primary endpoint is OS. Interim results of the first 120 patients showed that the addition of pre-op chemoradiation was feasible and tolerable, with 92% receiving the planned pre-op treatment and no difference in grade 3 or higher surgical complications or GI toxicities.

POST-OP CHEMORT

, *INT0116/SWOG* 9008 (Macdonald, NEJM 2001; Smalley, JCO 2012): 559 patients with resected stage IB–IV M0 stomach and gastroesophageal junction tumors (20%) randomized to observation vs. post-op chemo × 1c → concurrent chemo × 2c + RT → chemo × 2c. 54% had D0 dissection and 10% had D2 dissection. Chemo was bolus 5-FU + leucovorin. RT was 45 Gy/25 fx to tumor bed, regional nodes, and 2 cm proximal and distal margin. 41% Grade 3 and 30% Grade 4 toxicity with chemoRT. Post-op chemoRT with better OS (median 35 vs. 27 months) and relapse-free survival (median 27 vs. 19 months). All subtypes except diffuse histology benefited. Criticism: extent of surgery suboptimal.

, *CALGB 80101* (Fuchs, ASCO 2011 abstract): Resected adenocarcinoma of stomach or GEJ randomized to adjuvant bolus 5-FU/leucovorin → concurrent chemoradiation (45 Gy with infusional 5-FU) → 5-FU/leucovorin × 2c vs. adjuvant ECF (epirubicin, cisplatin, infusional 5-FU) → concurrent chemoradiation (45 Gy with infusional 5-FU) → ECF × 2c. Grade 4 toxicity 40% with 5-FU/leucovorin vs. 26% with ECF. Similar median OS (37 vs. 38 months), median DFS (30 vs. 28 months).

, *RTOG 0114 randomized phase II* (Schwartz, JCO 2009): 78 patients with resected gastric cancer, randomized to chemoRT with concurrent paclitaxel/cisplatin/5-FU (PCF) vs. concurrent paclitaxel/cisplatin (PC). Compared to INT0116 results. PCF with 59% grade 3 or higher toxicity vs. 41% in INT0116; PCF arm was closed. 2-year DFS for PC was 52%, which did not exceed the lower bound of 52.9% for the targeted 67% DFS.

, *ARTIST* (Park, JCO 2015): 458 patients with gastrectomy and D2 dissection, randomized to capecitabine and cisplatin (XP) x 6 cycles vs. XP x 2 cycles → chemoRT (45 Gy with concurrent capecitabine) → XP x 2 cycles. Similar

5-year OS (73% vs. 75%), DFS. Exploratory subgroup analysis showed OS benefit for chemoRT with node-positive (HR 0.7) and intestinal type (HR 0.442) subsets.

， *Dutch CRITICS* (Verheij, ESMO World Congress Abstract 2016): 788 patients with stage Ib–IVa (M0) resectable gastric cancer randomized to pre-op ECX (epirubicin, cisplatin or oxaliplatin, capecitabine) × 3c → surgery → concurrent chemoradiation (45 Gy with cisplatin and capecitabine) vs. pre-op ECX × 3c → surgery → ECX × 3c. Similar 5-year OS (40.9 chemoRT vs. 40.8% chemo). Grade 3+ heme toxicity higher with chemo (34% vs. 44%) but GI toxicity higher with chemoRT (42% vs. 37%). High percentage in both arms did not complete rx: 52% of chemo, 47% of chemoRT.

， *ARTIST II*: Ongoing phase III. Stage II–III gastric/GEJ, node-positive, adenocarcinoma with gastrectomy and at least D2 dissection, randomized to 1) S-1 x 8 vs. 2) SOX x 8 vs. 3) SOX x2 -> chemoRT to 45 Gy with S-1 - > SOX x4. SOX (S-1, oxaliplatin).

RADIATION TECHNIQUES

SIMULATION AND FIELD DESIGN

， Ensure adequate nutrition prior to radiation. Arrange for a nutrition consult. Recommend at least 1500 Cal/day.

， Patient may require feeding tube (preferable if placed at the time of surgery).

， Patient should fast for 3 h before simulation and all treatments.

， Simulate supine; immobilize with wing board or alpha cradle with arms above head.

， Use pre-op CT, post-op CT, PET, surgical clips, operative report, pathology report, and upper GI studies to guide target definition.

， Traditionally, celiac axis is located at approximately T12–L1. Porta-hepatis LN are covered by a field that extends 2 cm to the right of T11–L1.

， Recommend CT simulation and 3D treatment planning. Oral contrast may aid delineation of post-operative anatomy. IV contrast not used. 4D CT for ITV generation is recommended. 4D CT planning or other motion management strategies may be considered.

, At UCSF, we use IMRT to help reduce dose to normal tissues, such as small bowel, spinal cord, liver, and kidneys.

, General target volume.

  , Initial tumor bed: all patients. Exception is proximal T1–2aN0 patients with margin >5 cm.

  , Remaining stomach: all patients. Exception is proximal T1–3N0 patients with margin >5 cm.

  , Anastomotic site: all patients. Exception is proximal T1–2aN0 patients with margin >5 cm.

  , Residual disease: all patients.

, Adjacent structures: see tables below.

, Regional LN (depends on location and TN stage; see tables below).

  , Perigastric LN: always included, except proximal T1–2aN0 with margins >5 cm and >10–15 LN resected.

  , Celiac and suprapancreatic LN: For T4, LN+, or T3 N0 with <15 LN resected.

  , Porta-hepatic LN: for all T4 or LN+. Exception: proximal lesions with only 1–2 involved LN and >15 LN resected.

Table 19.4 GE junction tumors

Site/stage	Remaining stomach	Tumor bed**	Nodes
T2N0 with invasion of subserosa	Variable dependent on surgical-pathologic findings*	Medial left hemidiaphragm; adjacent body of pancreas	None or perigastric, periesophageal***
T3N0	Variable dependent on surgical-pathologic findings*	Medial left hemidiaphragm; adjacent body of pancreas	None or perigastric, periesophageal, mediastinal, or celiac***
T4N0	Preferable, but dependent on surgical-pathologic findings*	As for T3N0 plus site(s) of adherence with 3–5 cm margin	Nodes related to site(s) of adherence, ±perigastric, periesophageal, mediastinal, and celiac
T1–2N+	Preferable	Not indicated for T1 As above for T2 into subserosa	Periesophageal, mediastinal, proximal perigastric, and celiac
T3–4N+	Preferable	As for T3–4N0	As for T1–2N+ and T4N0

Tolerance organ structures: heart, lung, spinal cord, and kidneys

*For tumors with wide (>5 cm) surgical margins confirmed pathologically, treatment of residual stomach is optional, especially if this would result in substantial increase in normal tissue morbidity

**Use pre-op imaging (CT, barium swallow), surgical clips, and post-op imaging (CT, barium swallow)

***Optional node inclusion for T2–3N0 lesions if there has been an adequate surgical node dissection (D2 dissection) and at least 10–15 nodes have been examined pathologically

Table 19.5 Cardia/proximal one-third of the stomach tumors

Site/stage	Remaining stomach	Tumor bed**	Nodes
T2N0 with invasion of subserosa	Variable dependent on surgical-pathologic findings*	Medial left hemidiaphragm, adjacent body of pancreas (±tail)	None or perigastric
T3N0	Variable dependent on surgical-pathologic findings*	Medial left hemidiaphragm, adjacent body of pancreas (±tail)	None or perigastric, optional: periesophageal, and mediastinal, celiac****
T4N0	Variable dependent on surgical-pathologic findings*	As for T3N0, plus site(s) of adherence with 3–5 cm margin	Nodes related to site(s) of adherence, ±perigastric, periesophageal, mediastinal, and celiac
T1–2N+	Preferable	Not indicated for T1 As above for T2 into subserosa	Perigastric, celiac, splenic, suprapancreatic, ±periesophageal, mediastinal pancreaticoduodenal, and porta-hepatis***
T3–4N+	Preferable	As for T3–4N0	As for T1–2N+ and T4N0

10–15 nodes have been examined pathologically
Tolerance organ structures: kidneys, spinal cord, liver, heart, and lung
*For tumors with wide (>5 cm) surgical margins confirmed pathologically, treatment of residual stomach is not necessary, especially if this would result in substantial increase in normal tissue morbidity
**Use pre-op imaging (CT, barium swallow), surgical clips, and post-op imaging (CT, barium swallow)
***Pancreaticoduodenal and porta-hepatis nodes are at low risk if nodal positivity is minimal (i.e., 1–2 positive nodes with 10–15 nodes examined), and this region does not need to be irradiated. Periesophageal and mediastinal nodes are at risk if there is esophageal extension
****Optional node inclusion for T2–3 N0 lesions if there has been an adequate surgical node dissection (D2 dissection) and at least

Table 19.6 Body/middle one-third of the stomach tumors

Site/stage	Remaining stomach	Tumor bed*	Nodes
T2N0 with invasion of subserosa – especially post wall	Yes	Body of pancreas (±tail)	None or perigastric; optional: celiac, splenic, suprapancreatic, pancreaticoduodenal, and porta-hepatis**
T3N0	Yes	Body of pancreas (±tail)	None or perigastric, optional: celiac, splenic, suprapancreatic, pancreaticoduodenal, and porta-hepatis**

continued

Table 19.6 (continued)

T4N0	Yes	As for T3N0, plus site(s) of adherence with 3–5 cm margin	Nodes related to site(s) of adherence, ±perigastric, celiac, splenic, suprapancreatic, pancreaticoduodenal, and porta-hepatis
T1–2N+	Yes	Not indicated for T1	Perigastric, celiac, splenic, suprapancreatic, pancreaticoduodenal, and porta-hepatis
T3–4N+	Yes	As for T3–4N0	As for T1–2N+ and T4N0

Tolerance organ structures: kidneys, spinal cord, liver
*Use pre-op imaging (CT, barium swallow), surgical clips, and post-op imaging (CT, barium swallow)
**Optional node inclusion for T2–3 N0 lesions if there has been an adequate surgical node dissection (D2 dissection) and at least 10–15 nodes have been examined pathologically

Table 19.7 Antrum/pylorus/distal one-third of the stomach tumors

Site/stage	Remaining stomach	Tumor bed**	Nodes
T2 N0 with invasion of subserosa	Variable dependent of surgical-pathologic findings*	Head of pancreas (±body), first and second part of the duodenum	None or perigastric; optional: pancreaticoduodenal, porta-hepatis, celiac, and suprapancreatic***
T3 N0	Variable dependent of surgical-pathologic findings*	Head of pancreas (±body), first and second part of the duodenum	None or perigastric; optional: pancreaticoduodenal, porta-hepatis, celiac, and suprapancreatic***
T4 N0	Preferable, but dependent on surgical-pathologic findings*	As for T3 N0 plus site(s) of adherence with 3–5 cm margin	Nodes related to site(s) of adherence, ±perigastric, pancreaticoduodenal, porta-hepatis, celiac, and suprapancreatic
T1–2 N+	Preferable	Not indicated for T1	Perigastric, pancreaticoduodenal, porta-hepatis, celiac, suprapancreatic, and optional splenic hilum***
T3–4 N+	Preferable	As for T3–4 N0	As for T1–2 N+ and T4 N0

Tolerance organ structures: kidneys, liver, and spinal cord
*For tumors with wide (>5 cm) surgical margins confirmed pathologically, treatment of residual stomach is optional if this would result in substantial increase in normal tissue morbidity
**Use pre-op imaging (CT, barium swallow), surgical clips, and post-op imaging (CT, barium swallow)
***Optional node inclusion for T2–3 N0 lesions if there has been an adequate surgical node dissection (D2 dissection) and at least 10–15 nodes have been examined pathologically
While post op chemoradiation is standard of care, pre operative chemoradiation can be considered.

> Splenic LN: for all T4 or LN+. Exception: distal lesions with only 1–2 involved LN and >15 LN resected.
> Distal paraesophageal LN: for lesions with esophageal extension.
> The following are guidelines for target volume definition depending on the site of involvement [reprinted from Tepper and Gunderson (2002)].

DOSE PRESCRIPTIONS
> 1.8 Gy/fx to 45–50.4 Gy depending on margin status and presence/absence of residual disease.

DOSE LIMITATIONS
> Spinal cord $D_{max} \le 45$ Gy.
> Heart: V30Gy<20% mean <30Gy.
> Liver: V30Gy≤33%, mean dose ≤25 Gy.
> Kidneys: each V20Gy<33% mean <18Gy.
> Small Bowel V45Gy<195cc.

COMPLICATIONS
> Acute complications include nausea, anorexia, fatigue, and myelosuppression with chemo.
> Consider H2-blocker or proton pump inhibitor for ulcer prophylaxis.
> For severe nausea, recommend ondansetron 8 mg 1 h before RT daily and every 8 h prn.
> 25% of patients have persistent decrease in acid production for >1–5 years.
> Late complications: dyspepsia, radiation gastritis, and gastric ulcers.
> Gastric late effects are rare with 40–52 Gy. Incidence of late effects rises with higher doses.

FOLLOW-UP

> H&P every 4 months for 1 year, then every 6 months for 2 years, then annually. CBC, metabolic panel, endoscopies, CT as clinically indicated.

, Long-term parenteral vitamin B12 supplementation for all patients who undergo proximal or total gastrectomy.

Acknowledgment We thank Charlotte Dai Kubicky MD, PhD, and Jennifer S. Yu, MD, for their work on the prior edition of this chapter.

REFERENCES

Ajani JA, Winter K, Okawara GS, et al. Phase II trial of preoperative chemoradiation in patients with localized gastric adenocarcinoma (RTOG9904): quality of combined modality therapy and pathologic response. J Clin Oncol. 2006;24:3953–8.

Al-Batran S-E, Homann N, Schmalenberg H, et al. Perioperative chemotherapy with docetaxel, oxalipatin, and fluorouracil/leucovorin (FLOT) versus epirubicin, cisplatin, and fluorouracil or capecitabine (ECF/ECX) for resectable gastric or gastroesophageal junction (GEJ) adenocarcinoma (FLOT4-AIO): a multicenter, randomized phase 3 trial. J Clin Oncol. 2017;35(15_suppl):4004.

Bang Y-J, Kim Y-W, Yang H-K, et al. Adjuvant capecitabine and oxaliplatin for gastric cancer after D2 gastrectomy (CLASSIC): a phase 3 open-label, randomized controlled trial. Lancet. 2012;379:315–21.

Bonenkamp JJ, Hermans J, Sasako M, et al. Extended lymph-node dissection for gastric cancer. N Engl J Med. 1999 Mar 25;340(12):908–14.

Cunningham D, Alum WH, Stenning SP, et al. Perioperative chemotherapy versus surgery alone for resectable gastroesophageal cancer. N Engl J Med. 2006;355:11–20.

Cuschieri A, Weeden S, Fielding J, et al. Patient survival after D1 and D2 resections for gastric cancer: long-term results of the MRC randomized surgical trial. Surgical Co-operative Group. Br J Cancer. 1999;79:1522–30.

Degiuli M, Sasako M, Calgaro M, et al. Morbidity and mortality after D1 and D2 gastrectomy for cancer: interim analysis of the Italian Gastric Cancer Study Group (IGCSG) randomised surgical trial. Eur J Surg Oncol. 2004;30:303–8.

Fuchs CS, Tepper JE, Niedzwiecki D, et al. Postoperative adjuvant chemoradiation for gastric or gastroesophageal junction (GEJ) adenocarcinoma using epirubicin, cisplatin, and infusional (CI) 5-FU (ECF) before and after CI 5-FU and radiotherapy (CRT) compared with bolus 5-FU/LV before and after CRT: intergroup trial CALGB 80101. J Clin Oncol. 2011. ASCO Annual Meeting Abstracts Part 1;29:4003.

Hartgrink HH, van de Velde CJ, Putter H, et al. Extended lymph node dissection for gastric cancer: who may benefit? Final results of the randomized Dutch gastric cancer group trial. J Clin Oncol. 2004;22:2069–77.

Leong T, Smithers BM, Haustermans K, et al. TOPGEAR: a randomized, phase III trial of perioperative ECF chemotherapy with or without preoperative chemoradiation for resectable gastric cancer: interim result from an international, intergroup trial of the AGITG, TROG, EORT and CCTG. Ann Surg Oncol. 2017;24(8):2252–8.

Leong T, Smithers BM, Michael M, et al. TOPGEAR: a randomized phase III trial of perioperative ECF chemotherapy versus preoperative chemoradiation plus perioperative ECF chemotherapy for resectable gastric cancer (an international, intergroup trial of the AGITG/TROG/EORTC/NCIC CTG). BMC Cancer. 2015;15:532.

Macdonald JS, Smalley SR, Benedetti J, et al. Chemoradiotherapy after surgery compared with surgery alone for adenocarcinoma of the stomach or gastroesophageal junction. N Engl J Med. 2001;345:725–30.

National Comprehensive Cancer Network. Clinical practice guidelines in oncology: gastric cancer. Available at: http://www.nccn.org/professionals/physician_gls/PDF/gastric.pdf. Accessed 15 Jan 2017.

Park SH, Son TS, Lee J, et al. Phase III trial to compare adjuvant chemotherapy with capecitabine and cisplatin versus concurrent chemoradiotherapy in gastric cancer:

final report of the adjuvant chemoradiotherapy in stomach tumors trial, including survival and subset analyses. J Clin Oncol. 2015;33:3130–6.

Sano T, Sasako M, Yamamoto S, et al. Gastric cancer surgery: morbidity and mortality results from a prospective randomized controlled trial comparing D2 and extended para-aortic lymphadenectomy – Japan clinical oncology group study 9501. J Clin Oncol. 2004;22:2767–73.

Sasako M, Sano T, et al. D2 lymphadenectomy alone or with para-aortic nodal dissection for gastric cancer – JCOG 9501. N Engl J Med. 2008;359:453–62.

Schuhmacher C, Gretschel S, Lordick F, et al. Neoadjuvant chemotherapy compared with surgery alone for locally advanced cancer of the stomach and cardia: European Organisation for Research and Treatment of Cancer randomized trial 40954. J Clin Oncol. 2009;28(35):5210–8.

Schwartz GK, Winter K, Minsky BD, et al. Randomized phase II trial evaluating two paclitaxel and cisplatin-containing chemoradiation regimens as adjuvant therapy in resected gastric cancer (RTOG- 0114). J Clin Oncol. 2009;27(12):1956–62.

Smalley SR, Benedetti JK, Haller DG, et al. Updated analysis of SWOG-directed intergroup study 0116: a phase III trial of adjuvant radiochemotherapy versus observation after curative gastric resection. J Clin Oncol. 2012;31(19):2327–33.

Songun I, Putter H, Kranenbarg EM-K, et al. Surgical treatment of gastric cancer: 15-year follow-up results of the randomized nationwide Dutch D1D2 trial. Lancet Oncol. 2010;11:439–49.

Tepper JE, Gunderson LL. Radiation treatment parameters in the adjuvant postoperative therapy of gastric cancer. Semin Radiat Oncol. 2002;12:187–95.

Verheij M, Cats A, Jansen EPM, et al. A multicenter randomized phase III trial of neoadjuvant chemotherapy followed by surgery and chemotherapy or by surgery and chemoradiotherapy in resectable gastric cancer: first results from the CRITICS study. ESMO World Congress on Gastrointestinal Cancer. Abstract LBA-02. Presented June 30, 2016.

Wu CW, Hsiung CA, Lo SS, et al. Nodal dissection for patients with gastric cancer: a randomised controlled trial. Lancet Oncol. 2006 Apr;7(4):309–15.

Ychou M, Boige V, Pignon J-P, et al. Perioperative chemotherapy compared with surgery alone for resectable gastroesophageal adenocarcinoma: an FNCLCC and FFCD multicenter phase III trial. J Clin Oncol. 2011;29:1715–21.

Chapter 20
Pancreatic Cancer

Jennifer S. Chang and Mekhail Anwar

PEARLS

- Estimated 53,070 cases diagnosed in the USA in 2016, with 41,780 deaths.
- Found primarily in Western countries. Known risks include tobacco use, diet high in animal fat, ionizing radiation, chemotherapy, and exposure to 2-naphthylamine, benzene, and gasoline. Possible links with alcohol use, coffee use, chronic pancreatitis, and diabetes are less clear.
- Increased hereditary risk with mutations in *BRCA1*, *BRCA2*, *PALB2*, *ATM*, and *CDKN2A* and with Peutz-Jeghers syndrome and Lynch syndrome.
- Four parts of pancreas: head (including uncinate process), neck, body, and tail. 2/3 of cancers present in the head.
- Most common presenting symptoms: jaundice (common bile duct obstruction), weight loss (malabsorption from exocrine dysfunction), diabetes (related to endocrine dysfunction), gastric outlet obstruction, and abdominal pain. Jaundice is most common with lesions in the head. Lesions arising in the body or tail typically present with midepigastric or back pain. May infrequently present with Trousseau's sign (migratory thrombophlebitis) or Courvoisier's sign (palpable gallbladder).

- Primary LN drainage includes the pancreaticoduodenal, suprapancreatic, pyloric, and pancreaticosplenic LN with the porta hepatic, infrapyloric, subpyloric, celiac, superior mesenteric, and para-aortic areas being involved in advanced disease.
- Most common type is of ductal origin. Cystadenocarcinomas, intraductal carcinomas, and solid and cystic papillary neoplasms (also known as *Hamoudi tumors*) have a more indolent course. Acinar cell cancers and giant cell tumors are aggressive and have poor survival. 5% are tumors of the endocrine pancreas – these tumors are rare, slow growing, and have a long natural history.
- Mutant k-*ras* oncogene present in 70–100%. TP53 mutation present in approximately 50%.
- Pancreatic cancer has four molecular subtypes: squamous, pancreatic progenitor, immunogenic, and aberrantly differentiated endocrine exocrine (ADEX).
- Peritoneal and liver mets are most common. Lung is most common location outside the abdomen.
- Post-resection CA19-9 level is prognostic in patients treated with postop chemoRT, per RTOG 9704 (Berger, JCO 2008).

WORKUP

- Main purposes: determine resectability, establish histologic diagnosis, reestablish biliary tract outflow, and circumvent gastric outlet obstruction.
- H&P, pancreas protocol (multiphase, thin slice, no skip) CT, and endoscopic US.
- Pathology: EUS, ERCP, laparoscopy, or CT-guided biopsy.
- Labs: CBC, CEA, CA19-9, glucose, amylase, lipase, bilirubin, alkaline phosphatase, LDH, and LFTs.
- Endoscopy of the upper GI tract is extremely valuable with endobiliary stent placement as needed. Endoscopic ultrasound can also be performed to aid T- and N-stage.
- Pancreatic neuroendocrine tumors (including carcinoid tumors) are staged by the same pancreatic staging system.

Table 20.1 STAGING (AJCC 7TH ED., 2010)

Primary tumor (T)

TX: Primary tumor cannot be assessed

T0: No evidence of primary tumor

Tis: Carcinoma in situ*

T1: Tumor limited to the pancreas, 2 cm or less in greatest dimension

T2: Tumor limited to the pancreas, more than 2 cm in greatest dimension

T3: Tumor extends beyond the pancreas but without involvement of the celiac axis or the superior mesenteric artery

T4: Tumor involves the celiac axis or the superior mesenteric artery (unresectable primary tumor)

Regional lymph nodes (N)

NX: Regional lymph nodes cannot be assessed

N0: No regional lymph node metastasis

N1: Regional lymph node metastasis

Distant metastasis (M)

M0: No distant metastasis

M1: Distant metastasis

Anatomic stage/prognostic groups

0: Tis N0 M0

IA: T1 N0 M0

IB: T2 N0 M0

IIA: T3 N0 M0

IIB: T1-T3 N1 M0

III: T4 Any N M0/

IV: Any T Any N M1

Used with the permission from the American Joint Committee on Cancer (AJCC), Chicago, Illinois. The original source for this material is the AJCC Cancer Staging Manual, Seventh Edition (2010), published by Springer Science+Business Media
*This also includes the "PanInIII" classification

Table 20.2 (AJCC 8TH ED., 2017)

Definitions of AJCC TNM

Definition of Primary Tumor (T)

T category	T criteria
TX	Tumor cannot be assessed
T1	Tumor limited to the pancreas,* <2 cm
T2	Tumor limited to the pancreas,* 2–4 cm

continued

Table 20.2 (continued)

T3	Tumor limited to the pancreas,* >4 cm or tumor invading the duodenum or bile duct
T4	Tumor invading the adjacent organs (stomach, spleen, colon, adrenal gland) or the wall of the large vessels (celiac axis or the superior mesenteric artery)

Limited to the pancreas means there is no invasion of adjacent organs (stomach, spleen, colon, adrenal gland) or the wall of large vessels (celiac axis or the superior mesenteric artery). Extension of tumor into peripancreatic adipose tissue is *not* a basis for staging

Note: Multiple tumors should be designated as such (the largest tumor should be used to assign T category):

If the number of tumors is known, use T(#), e.g., pT3(4) N0 M0

If the number of tumors is unavailable or too numerous, use the *m* suffix, T(m), e.g., pT3(m) N0 M0

DEFINITION OF REGIONAL LYMPH NODE (N)

N category	N criteria
NX	Regional lymph nodes cannot be assessed
N0	No regional lymph node involvement
N1	Regional lymph node involvement

DEFINITION OF DISTANT METASTASIS (M)

M category	M criteria
M0	No distant metastasis
M1	Distant metastases
M1a	Metastasis confined to the liver
M1b	Metastases in at least one extrahepatic site (e.g., lung, ovary, nonregional lymph node, peritoneum, bone)
M1c	Both hepatic and extrahepatic metastases

AJCC PROGNOSTIC STAGE GROUPS

When T is...	And N is...	And M is...	Then the stage group is...
T1	N0	M0	I
T2	N0	M0	II
T3	N0	M0	II
T4	N0	M0	III
Any T	N1	M0	III
Any T	Any N	M1	IV

Used with permission of the American Joint Committee on Cancer (AJCC), Chicago, Illinois. The original and primary source for this information is the AJCC Cancer Staging Manual, Eighth Edition (2017) published by Springer International Publishing

- For practical purposes, tumors are generally classified as resectable (Stages I and II), unresectable (Stage III), and metastatic (Stage IV).
- Resectable disease includes:
  - No arterial contact with celiac axis, superior mesenteric artery (SMA), or common hepatic artery.
  - ≤180° contact with the superior mesenteric vein (SMV) or portal vein, without vein contour irregularity.
- Definition of unresectable varies by institution but generally includes:
  - Distant metastasis, including non-regional nodes.
  - >180° contact with celiac axis or SMA.
  - Solid tumor contact with 1st jejunal SMA branch (for head/uncinate).
  - Aortic involvement(for body/tail).
  - Inability to reconstruct SMV/portal vein due to occlusion or tumor involvement.
- Prognostic markers: surgical margins (R0 resection), nodal status, and tumor grade.

VI

TREATMENT RECOMMENDATIONS

Table 20.3 TREATMENT RECOMMENDATIONS

Stage	Recommended treatment

Resectable (~10–20% of patients)	Pancreaticoduodenectomy (Neoadjuvant chemotherapy can be considered for high risk tumors). Surgical mortality <5% when performed by experienced surgeons. Pylorus-preserving pancreaticoduodenectomy may be considered. Body/tail cancers should undergo distal pancreatectomy often with en bloc splenectomy
	Adjuvant treatment options include:
	  Clinical trial
	  Chemotherapy alone (gemcitabine/capecitabine, gemcitabine, or 5-FU based)
	  ChemoRT, particularly if R1 resection or node positive.
	  ChemoRT may be with concurrent 5-FU, capecitabine, or gemcitabine and may be delivered immediately, sandwiched between chemo cycles, or after 2–6 cycles of chemo

Borderline resectable	Consider staging laparoscopy. If negative, neoadjuvant therapy (FOLFIRINOX or gemcitabine + albumin-bound paclitaxel, followed by restaging and concurrent gemcitabine +/– 5-FU-based chemoRT), followed by restaging and surgical resection if feasible. If resected, consider additional chemo or chemoRT (particularly if R1 or node positive)

continued

Table 20.3 (continued)

Stage	Recommended treatment

Unresectable	Options:
	  Clinical trial preferred
	    Initial chemo (FOLFIRINOX or gemcitabine based), then restaging and if negative, then definitive chemoRT (SBRT can be considered in select cases.)
	      Definitive concurrent chemoRT (5-FU or gemcitabine based)
	    Palliation with stents or surgical bypass

Metastatic	Palliation with stents, surgical bypass, chemo, RT, supportive care, or combination. FOLFIRINOX or gemcitabine + albumin-bound paclitaxel preferred for good PS. If poor PS, gemcitabine alone and best supportive care Celiac nerve block may be an effective palliative tool for pain
Endocrine	Surgical treatment. Chemo for unresectable or metastatic disease. Effects of RT unknown, although anecdotal responses exist

STUDIES

RESECTABLE ADJUVANT TREATMENT

- No definite standard has been established for adjuvant treatment of resected pancreas cancer. Recurrence risk is very high even after R0 resection, so all eligible patients should be offered adjuvant therapy. Median survival is typically about 20–25 months.

- *ASCO guideline* (Khorana, JCO 2016): Recommends 6-month adjuvant chemo for all eligible patients who did not receive preoperative therapy. ChemoRT may be considered in patients with no preoperative therapy who had either R1 resection or node-positive disease after 4–6 mo of systemic chemo.

- A number of studies report that post-op chemo improves survival. For example:
  - ESPAC-1 (Neoptolemos, Lancet 2001, NEJM 2004): 2×2 factorial design, 541 patients with resected pancreatic or periampullary carcinoma (only 289 of which were randomized). Arms were chemoRT (40 Gy split course with 5-FU), adjuvant chemo alone (5-FU/leucovorin), both chemoRT and chemo, or observation alone. In final analysis (2004) of randomized patients, chemo improved 5-yr OS (21% vs. 8%), while chemoRT was detrimental (5-yr OS 10% vs. 20%). Caveats: no RT quality assurance. Only 128 patients with RT details available, of whom only 90 patients received the prescribed dose of split course 40 Gy. Progressive disease in 19% of patients precluded RT.

, CONKO-001 (Oettle, JAMA 2007, JAMA 2013): 368 patients with R0/R1 resection randomized to observation vs. gemcitabine × 6c. Adjuvant gemcitabine improved DFS (13.4 vs. 6.7 mo), and OS (5-yr 20.7% vs. 10.4%, 10-yr 12.2% vs. 7.7%). Excluded patients with post-op CEA/CA19-9 levels ≥2.5× upper limit of normal.

, ESPAC-3 (Neoptolemos, JAMA 2010): 428 patients with resected periampullary adenocarcinoma randomized to adjuvant 5-FU/folinic acid vs. gemcitabine. Observation arm eliminated after CONKO results. No difference in MS 23–23.6 mo between chemo arms.

, ESPAC-4 (Neoptolemos, Lancet 2017): 730 patients with R0 or R1 resection of ductal pancreatic adenocarcinoma randomized to adjuvant gemcitabine x 6 cycles +/– capecitabine. Gemcitabine/capecitabine improved median OS vs. gemcitabine alone (28 mo vs. 25.5 mo). Increased neutropenia and hand-foot syndrome.

, A number of studies also report benefit of post-op chemoRT. For example:

, GITSG 91-73 (Kalser, Arch Surg 1985): 43 patients with resectable pancreatic cancer were randomized to surgery, followed by EBRT (40 Gy split course) with concurrent 5-FU vs. surgery alone. Adjuvant chemoRT improved OS (2-year/5-year OS 43%/14% vs. 18%/5%). Update (Cancer, 1987): additional 30 nonrandomized patients entered into adjuvant therapy group. Two-year OS 46%. Note: few radiation oncologists currently use this split-course regimen.

, EORTC-30013-22012/FFCD-9203/GERCOR (Van Laethem, JCO 2010): 90 patients with R0 resection of pancreatic head cancer, treated with gemcitabine 2c, then randomized to gemcitabine x 2 additional cycles vs. chemoRT to 50.4 Gy with weekly gemcitabine. Median DFS 11 months for chemo, 12 months for chemoRT. First local recurrence decreased with chemoRT (11% vs. 24%). Median OS 24 months in both arms.

, Johns Hopkins-Mayo Clinic Collaborative (Hsu, Ann Surg Oncol 2010): Retrospective study of 1092 patients with resected pancreatic adenocarcinoma who were observed or received adjuvant 5-FU-based chemoRT (median 50.4 Gy). ChemoRT improved MS (21.1 mo vs. 15.5 mo; 2-/5-year OS 44.7/22.3% vs. 34.6/16.1%). Matched-pair analysis confirmed improved OS with chemoRT vs. observation (MS 21.9 mo vs. 14.3 mo; 2-/5-year OS 45.5/25.4% vs. 31.4/12.2%).

, Multi-institutional (Morganti, IJROBP 2014): Retrospective review of 955 patients with R0/R1 resection of pancreatic cancer without IORT. Median OS was improved with chemoRT (39.9 mo vs. 27.8 mo with chemo vs. 24.8 mo with no adjuvant treatment). Adverse prognostic factors: R1 resection, higher pT stage, positive nodes, tumor >2 cm.

, NCDB (Kooby, Ann Surg Onc 2013): Analysis of 11,526 patients who underwent resection for pancreatic adenocarcinoma and were treated with adjuvant chemo (9%), adjuvant chemoRT (46%), or no adjuvant treatment (45%). ChemoRT had best OS (HR 0.70) compared to chemo only (HR 1.04) and no adjuvant treatment.

, SEER (Hazard, Cancer 2007): 3008 patients with resected pancreas cancer. 1148 patients received post-op RT, 76 received pre-op RT. Pts who received RT had improved survival (MS 17 mo vs. 12 mo, 5-year OS 13% vs. 9.7%). RT improved OS for T3–4 or node-positive patients, but not T1-2N0 patients. RT improved CSS in patients with positive nodes.

, RTOG 97-04 (Regine, JAMA 2008): 451 patients with resected pancreatic cancer randomized to weekly gemcitabine vs. protracted venous infusion 5-FU for 3 weeks before and for 12 weeks after concurrent chemoRT (5-FU, 50.4 Gy). Trend for improved MS (20.5 vs. 16.9 months) and 3-year OS (31 vs. 22%, p = 0.09) with gemcitabine. Patterns of failure similar in both arms: distant (71–77%) more common than local (23–28%) more common than regional nodes associated with tumor site (7–8%).

, The ESPAC-1 and EORTC trials do not support adjuvant chemoRT, but there are significant criticisms of these trials:

, ESPAC-1 criticisms: see above.

, EORTC 40891 (Klinkenbijl, Ann Surg 1999; Smeenk, Ann Surg 2007): 218 patients with resected pancreatic or periampullary cancer randomized to chemoRT (40 Gy split course with 5-FU) vs. observation. Adjuvant treatment resulted in no significant difference in 10-year OS (18% overall, 8% pancreatic head group, 29% periampullary group) or PFS (median PFS 1.2 years in observation arm vs. 1.5 years in treatment arm). Criticisms: only 119 patients had pancreatic cancer, no maintenance therapy was given, and the study included patients with positive margins without stratification. No RT quality assurance.

, Ongoing studies will further clarify the role of adjuvant chemoRT. For example:

, RTOG 0848. Patients with R0/R1 resected pancreatic adenocarcinoma with CA 19-9 < 180 first randomized to gemcitabine alone or combination chemo x 5 mo +/− erlotinib x 5 cycles (erlotinib arm closed in 4/2014 due to negative LAP-07 results). Then, if no progression patients are randomized to 1 more cycle of chemo alone or followed by chemoRT (50.4 Gy with concurrent capecitabine or 5-FU).

VI

NEOADJUVANT TREATMENT

, Potential benefits of neoadjuvant therapy: downsize borderline resectable tumors to resectable; increase likelihood of R0 resection in resectable patients; increase proportion of resectable patients who will receive chemo and/or RT; select patients with stable or disease responsive to therapy.

, There is no standard neoadjuvant regimen. Acceptable chemo regimens include FOLFIRINOX or gemcitabine/albumin-bound paclitaxel.

, A number of phase II trials have evaluated neoadjuvant chemoRT. For example:

, Multi-institutional (Kim, Cancer 2013). Phase II trial of 68 patients (23 resectable, 39 borderline resectable, 6 unresectable) treated with 2 cycles gemcitabine and oxaliplatin with concurrent 30 Gy/15 fx RT during cycle 1. 63% of patients resected, of which 84% were R0. MS for resected patients was 27 mo vs. not resected 11 mo.

, MDACC (Evans, JCO 2008): Phase II, 86 patients with potentially resectable disease treated with chemoRT (30 Gy/10 fx and weekly gemcitabine × 7 weeks) → surgery. RT included pancreaticoduodenal, porta hepatic, superior mesenteric, and celiac axis LN. All patients restaged after chemoRT. 10% were found to have extrapancreatic disease, 85% went on to surgery. Overall MS 22.7 months, 5-year OS 27%, but MS 34 mo for resected patients vs. 7 months for unresectable patients.

- ˌ Krishnan (Cancer 2007): 247 patients with unresectable disease received neoadjuvant chemoRT (30 Gy/10 fx or 50.4 Gy/28 fx with 5-FU, gemcitabine, or capecitabine), whereas 76 patients received induction gemcitabine-based chemo, followed by chemoRT if no progression. RT included regional nodes in 69% patients. Induction chemo improved MS (12 mo vs. 4 mo) by selecting out patients with rapid progression.
- ˌ MDACC (Cloyd, Cancer 2016). Retrospective review of 472 patients. 47.5% received 30 Gy/10 fx, 46.8% received 50.4 Gy/28 fx, and 5.7% received chemo alone. On multivariate analysis, absence of RT increased local recurrence risk (odds ratio 2.21). No survival differences. LRR 22% for both RT regimens vs. 33% with chemo alone.
- ˌ Alliance A021101 (Katz, JAMA Surg 2016). 22 borderline resectable patients treated with modified FOLFIRINOX x 4 cycles, followed by 50.4 Gy RT with concurrent capecitabine. 68% underwent resection, 33% had <5% residual cancer cells, 13% had pCR, MS 21.7 months. 64% grade ≥ 3 toxicity.
- ˌ Ongoing randomized trials will clarify the role of neoadjuvant therapy:
  - ˌ NEOPAC (NCT01521702). Phase III trial of resectable patients randomized to surgery and adjuvant gemcitabine x 6c with or without neoadjuvant gemcitabine and oxaliplatin x 4. Results pending.
  - ˌ NEOPA (NCT01900327). Phase III trial of resectable patients randomized to surgery and adjuvant chemo (preferably gemcitabine x 6c) with or without neoadjuvant chemoRT (weekly gemcitabine for 6 wks with concurrent 50.4 Gy RT).
  - ˌ Alliance A021501 (NCT02839343). Phase II trial of borderline resectable patients treated with mFOLFIRINOX x 8c + surgery + FOLFOX x 4c vs. mFOLFIRINOX x 7c + SBRT/hypofx RT + surgery + FOLFOX x 4c.

UNRESECTABLE

- ˌ *ASCO guideline for unresectable* (Balaban, JCO 2016): Initial systemic therapy with combination regimen is recommended for patients with good PS, limited comorbidities.

ChemoRT or SBRT may be offered up front at physician or pt preference. Or, chemoRT or SBRT may be offered for patients with response or stable disease after 6 months chemo, if unacceptable chemo-related toxicity, or local-only progression. SBRT may be offered, but additional prospective and/or randomized trials are needed. Consider palliative RT for symptoms.

, Initial chemotherapy may identify patients with rapid progression allowing selection of patients most likely to benefit from subsequent chemoRT.

, Some studies support a role of chemoRT for unresectable disease, while others do not. Selected studies include:

, GERCOR (Huguet, JCO 2007): reviewed 181 patients with locally advanced disease treated with 5-FU- or gemcitabine-based chemo × 3 months without evidence of progression who then received either additional chemo or chemoRT (physician choice). ChemoRT improved median PFS (7.4 → 10.8 months) and OS (11.7 → 15 months).

, ECOG E4201 (Loehrer, JCO 2011): 74 patients with localized unresectable pancreas cancer randomized to gemcitabine alone vs. chemoRT (50.4 Gy with concurrent gemcitabine). Closed early due to poor accrual. Better OS with chemoRT (median 11.1 vs. 9.2 months). Worse grade 4/5 toxicity with chemoRT (41 vs. 9%) but similar grade 3/4 toxicity (79 vs. 77%) and QoL.

, SCALOP (Mukherjee, Lancet Oncol 2013): 114 patients with locally advanced pancreatic cancer <7 cm were treated with 12-wk gemcitabine/capecitabine. 74 patients with stable/improved disease were then randomized to chemoRT (50.4 Gy in 28 fx) with either concurrent gemcitabine or concurrent capecitabine. OS better with capecitabine chemoRT (median 15.2 mo vs. 13.4 mo, 1-year OS 79.2% vs. 64.2%). Lower grade 3–4 toxicity with capecitabine, similar QoL.

, LAP 07 (Hammel, JAMA 2016): 2x2 randomization for locally advanced disease: 442 patients randomized to 4 cycles induction gemcitabine vs. gemcitabine and erlotinib; if stable/improved and progression-free after 4 months (269 patients), then randomize to 2 months of continued chemo vs. chemoRT with 54 Gy and concurrent capecitabine. No survival benefit of erlotinib. While there was no median OS difference (16.5 months chemo

VI

vs. 15.2 months chemoRT), chemoRT reduced locoregional progression (32% vs. 46%) with no increase in grade 3–4 toxicity except for nausea.

- GITSG 9273 (Moertel, Cancer 1981): 194 patients with unresectable pancreatic cancer randomized to split-course EBRT (40 Gy) with concomitant bolus 5-FU vs. split-course EBRT (60 Gy) with concomitant bolus 5-FU vs. EBRT (60 Gy) alone. Both concomitant chemo arms prolonged MS vs. EBRT alone (42.2, 40.3, and 22.9 weeks, respectively).

- RTOG 9812 (Tyvin, Am J Clin Oncol 2004): Phase II study of 109 patients with unresectable pancreatic cancer treated with EBRT 50.4 Gy and weekly paclitaxel. All patients were restaged 6 weeks after completion of chemoRT. If marked shrinkage, resection was attempted. MS 11.2 months with 1-year OS 43% and 2-year OS 13%. 40% grade 3 and 5% grade 4 toxicity with 1 death due to treatment.

- Murphy (IJROBP 2007): 74 patients with locally advanced pancreatic cancer treated with chemoRT (36 Gy/15 fx) with full-dose gemcitabine (1000 mg/m2 on days 1, 8, and 15). PTV = GTV + 1 cm. Six-month OS 46%/13%, median OS 11.2 months.

- FFCD/SFRO (Chauffert, Ann Oncology 2008): 119 patients with locally advanced pancreatic cancer randomized to induction chemoRT (60 Gy with 5-FU infusion and cisplatin) vs. induction gemcitabine. All patients received maintenance gemcitabine. In the chemo arm, 73% received 75% or more of the planned total dose, but in the chemoRT arm, only 42% received at least 75% of the planned dose for both chemo and RT. Better OS with chemo alone (median 8.6 vs. 13 mo), felt to be related to higher grade 3–4 toxicity with this particular chemoRT regimen (36% vs. 22%).

SBRT

- SBRT is an emerging treatment option for unresectable or borderline resectable pancreas cancer based on retrospective and prospective data. So far, there is no randomized data supporting its use. It may offer local control with minimal interruption of systemic chemotherapy and without the need for up to 6 weeks of daily treatments.

, So far there is no established standard or consensus on optimal SBRT total dose, dose per fraction, or number of fractions, although 33Gy in 5 fractions is commonly used.

, The optimal sequencing of SBRT and chemotherapy remains unknown, either upfront, sandwiched, or after chemotherapy.

, Selected studies of pancreatic SBRT include:

  , Petrelli (IJROBP 2017). Pooled analysis of 1009 patients treated with SBRT for locally advanced pancreatic cancer. No randomized studies, 6 prospective studies, 13 retrospective studies. Chemo was given before or after SBRT in 18/19 studies. Pooled 1-yr OS 52% in 13 trials. Median OS ranged 5.7–47 mo (median 17 mo). One-yr LRC 72%. Acute severe toxicity 0–36%, late grade ¾ toxicity 0–11%.

  , Mellon (Acta Oncol 2015). 110 borderline resectable and 49 locally advanced pancreatic cancer patients treated with neoadjuvant chemo, followed by SBRT. Median OS was 19 mo for borderline resectable, 15 mo for locally advanced patients, 34 mo if resected vs. 14 mo if unresected. For patients not resected, 1-yr LRC 78%. Grade >3 radiation toxicity 7%.

  , Pollom (IJROBP 2014). 167 patients with unresectable pancreatic adenocarcinoma treated with SBRT. 87.5% received chemo. 45.5% received 1-fx and 54.5% received 5-fx SBRT. No difference 1-yr LR (10–12%) or OS (31–35%) between 1- and 5-fx schedule, but single fx increased 1-yr grade 3 GI toxicity (12% vs. 6%).

RADIATION TECHNIQUES

SIMULATION AND FIELD DESIGN

, Sim supine, arms up with IV and oral contrast.

, Treat tumor (or tumor bed) +/– nodal groups at risk using pre-op and post-op imaging studies, as well as findings at surgery.

- Traditionally, pancreas is at L1–L2. Celiac axis is at T12, SMA is at L1.
- Recommend 3D CT planning. 4D CT may be considered to construct ITV to account for respiratory motion. Respiratory gating or breathhold technique, may also be considered.
- GTV should be contoured for intact pancreatic tumors
- CTV for adjuvant cases includes pancreatic tumor bed, high-risk peripancreatic nodes, and anastomoses. See RTOG 0848 for post-op pancreas contouring guidelines (Goodman, IJROBP 2012). Elective nodal irradiation is commonly used for adjuvant cases but is controversial for unresectable, neoadjuvant, and borderline resectable cases.
- CTV for unresectable cases routinely includes GTV plus 0.5–1.5 cm margin. For SBRT cases, there is no CTV. Additional 0.5–2 cm PTV margin is added for setup error and tumor/breathing motion.
- Traditional elective nodal regions include:
  - Pancreatic head lesions: pancreaticoduodenal, suprapancreatic, celiac nodes, porta hepatis, entire duodenal loop.
  - Body/tail lesions: treat pancreaticoduodenal, portal hepatic, lateral suprapancreatic nodes, splenic hilum nodes. Porta hepatis and duodenal bed do not need to be covered.
- Historically, patients were treated with a three- or four-field design – AP (50–80% of dose), two laterals or slightly off-axis superior/inferior obliques (20% of dose), +/– posterior field. High-energy photon fields (e.g., 18 MV) are useful particularly for the lateral/oblique fields.
- IMRT may reduce grade 3–4 nausea and vomiting (e.g., 0% IMRT vs. 11% with 3D in RTOG 97-04) and diarrhea (3% vs. 18%) (Yovino, IJROBP 2011).
- For SBRT, recommend 4D CT and/or respiratory motion management. Internal fiducials may be implanted in the tumor for motion monitoring. Smaller PTV margins are used (0.2–0.5 cm) and there is no elective nodal treatment.

DOSE PRESCRIPTIONS

- Adjuvant: Treat to 45 Gy at 1.8 Gy/fx to tumor bed, anastomosis, and nodes, followed by conedown to tumor bed/involved margins to 50.4 Gy paying close attention to dose to bowel and stomach.

, Unresectable: Consider boost to 54–59.4 Gy if feasible, respecting normal tissue tolerance.
, Hypofractionated regimens with chemo are also an option for locally advanced (e.g., 36 Gy in 15 fx of 2.4 Gy or 30 Gy in 10 fx of 3 Gy).
, For SBRT, 33 Gy in 5 fractions is commonly used, however other dose and fractionation regimens have been reported or are under investigation. Multifraction SBRT has similar LC but lower toxicity (Pollom, IJROBP 2014).
, For IORT, treat with 10–20 Gy in 1 fraction, alone or with external beam.
, Multiple dose escalation studies with hyperfractionation, brachytherapy, IORT, radiosurgery, hypofractionation, and other methods are under investigation.

VI

DOSE LIMITATIONS

, Conventional fractionation:
  , Doses up to 50 Gy are tolerated by small volumes of stomach and intestine. Bowel Dmax <55 Gy. Keep volume receiving 45–55 Gy <30%. Most common late effects are mucosal ulceration and bleeding. Perforation is rare.
  , Kidneys: <30% of total kidney volume over 18 Gy. Mean total kidney dose <18 Gy. If only 1 kidney functional, limit <10–15% over 18 Gy and <30% over 14 Gy.
  , Limit the mean liver dose to <25–30 Gy to prevent radiation hepatitis. Small volumes of liver can be treated to high doses.
  , Spinal cord Dmax <45 Gy.
  , See RTOG 1102 (unresectable) and RTOG 0848 (postop) protocols.
, SBRT constraints: Protocol specific.

COMPLICATIONS

, Pancreas has both exocrine and endocrine secretions, and both can decrease following treatment. Monitor for diabetes and supplement with pancreatic enzymes if exocrine insufficiency is suspected (pancrelipase with each meal).
, Acute – nausea, vomiting, gastritis (use antiemetics, proton pump inhibitor or H2 blocker). Diarrhea less

common. If jaundice develops during RT or following treatment, ascending cholangitis must be considered as a potential etiology.

₃ Late – ulceration, stricture formation, obstruction, and (less commonly) perforation of GI tract.

FOLLOW-UP

₃ H&P, labs, and abdominal CT as often as every 3 months to evaluate for disease recurrence/progression.

Acknowledgment We thank Jennifer S. Yu MD, PhD, Joy Coleman MD, and Jeanne Marie Quivey MD, FACR, for their work on the prior edition of this chapter.

REFERENCES

Balaban EP, Mangu PB, Khorana AA, et al. Locally advanced, unresectable pancreatic cancer: American Society of Clinical Oncology clinical practice guideline. J Clin Oncol. 2016;34(22):2654–68.

Berger AC, Garcia M Jr, Hoffman JP, et al. Postresection CA 19-9 predicts overall survival in patients with pancreatic cancer treated with adjuvant chemoradiation: a prospective validation by RTOG 9704. J Clin Oncol. 2008;26(36):5918–22.

Chauffert B, Momex F, Bonnetain F, et al. Phase III trial comparing intensive induction chemoradiotherapy (60 Gy, infusional 5-FU and intermittent cisplatin) followed by maintenance gemcitabine with gemcitabine alone for locally advanced unresectable pancreatic cancer. Definitive results of the 2000-01 FFCD/SFRO study. Ann Oncol. 2008;19:1592–9.

Cloyd JM, Crane CH, Koay EJ, et al. Impact of hypofractionated and standard fractionated chemoradiation before pancreatoduodenectomy for pancreatic ductal adenocarcinoma. Cancer. 2016;122(17):2671–9.

Evans DB, Varadhachary GR, Crane CH, et al. Preoperative gemcitabine-based chemoradiation for patients with resectable adenocarcinoma of the pancreatic head. J Clin Oncol. 2008;26(21):3496–502.

GITSG. Further evidence of effective adjuvant combined radiation and chemotherapy following curative resection of pancreatic cancer. Gastrointestinal Tumor Study Group. Cancer. 1987;59(12):2006–10.

Goodman KA, Regine WF, Dawson LA, et al. Radiation therapy Oncology group consensus panel guidelines for the delineation of the clinical target volume in the postoperative treatment of pancreatic head cancer. Int J Radiat Oncol Biol Phys. 2012;83(3):901–8.

Hammel P, Huguet F, van Laethem JL, et al. Effect of Chemoradiotherapy vs chemotherapy on survival in patients with locally advanced pancreatic cancer controlled after 4 months of gemcitabine with or without Erlotinib: the LAP07 randomized clinical trial. JAMA. 2016;315(17):1844–53.

Hazard L, Tward JD, Szabo A, et al. Radiation therapy is associated with improved survival in patients with pancreatic adenocarcinoma: results of a study from the surveillance, epidemiology, and end results (SEER) registry data. Cancer. 2007;11(10):2191–201.

Hsu CC, Herman JM, Corsini MM, et al. Adjuvant chemoradiation for pancreatic adeno-carcinoma: the Johns Hopkins Hospital-Mayo Clinic collaborative study. Ann Surg Oncol. 2010;17(4):981–90.

Huguet F, Andre T, Hammel P, et al. Impact of chemoradiotherapy after disease control with chemotherapy in locally-advanced pancreatic adenocarcinoma in GERCOR Phase II and III studies. J Clin Oncol. 2007;25:326–31.

Kalser M, Ellenberg S. Pancreatic cancer. Adjuvant combined radiation and chemother-apy following curative resection. Arch Surg. 1985;120(8):899–903. Erratum in: Arch Surg 1986;121(9):1045

Katz SJ. Jama Surg. 2016;151(8):e161(3).

Khorana AA, Mangu PB, Berlin J, et al. Potentially curable pancreatic cancer: American Society of Clinical Oncology clinical practice guidelines. J Clin Oncol. 2016;34(21):2541–56.

Kim EJ, Ben-Josef E, Herman JM. A multi-institutional phase 2 study of neoadjuvant gemcitabine and oxaliplatin with radiation therapy in patients with pancreatic can-cer. Cancer. 2013;119(15):2692–700.

Klinkenbijl JH, Jeekel J, Sahmoud T, et al. Adjuvant radiotherapy and 5-fluorouracil after curative resection of cancer of the pancreas and periampullary region: phase III trial of the EORTC gastrointestinal tract cancer cooperative group. Ann Surg. 1999;230(6):776–82. discussion 782-784

Kooby DA, Gillespie TW, Liu Y, et al. Impact of adjuvant radiotherapy on survival after pancreatic cancer resection: an appraisal of data from the national cancer data base. Ann Surg Oncol. 2013;20(11):3634–42.

Krishnan S, Rana V, Janjan NA, et al. Induction chemotherapy selects patients with locally advanced, unresectable pancreatic cancer for optimal benefit from consolida-tive chemoradiation therapy. Cancer. 2007;110(1):47–55.

Loehrer PJ, Feng Y, Cardenes H, et al. Gemcitabine alone versus gemcitabine plus radio-therapy in patients with locally advanced pancreatic cancer: an eastern cooperative Oncology group trial. J Clin Oncol. 2011;29:4105–12.

Mellon EA, Hoffe SE, Springett GM, et al. Long-term outcomes of induction chemo-therapy and neoadjuvant stereotactic body radiotherapy for borderline resectable and locally advanced pancreatic adenocarcinoma. Acta Oncol. 2015;54(7):979–85.

Moertel CG, Frytak S, Hahn RG, et al. Therapy of locally unresectable pancreatic carci-noma: a randomized comparison of high dose (6000 rads) radiation alone, moderate dose radiation (4000 rads + 5-fluorouracil), and high dose radiation + 5-fluorouracil: the gastrointestinal tumor study group. Cancer. 1981;48(8):1705–10.

Morganti AG, Falconi M, van Stiphout RGPM, et al. Multi-institutional pooled analysis on adjuvant chemoradiation in pancreatic cancer. Int J Radiat Oncol Biol Phys. 2014;90(4):911–7.

Mukherjee S, Hurt CN, Bridgewater J, et al. Gemcitabine-based or capecitabine-based chemoradiotherapy for locally advanced pancreatic cancer (SCALOP): a multicenter, randomized, phase 2 trial. Lancet Oncol. 2013;14:317–26.

Murphy JD, Adusumilli S, Griffith KA, et al. Full dose gemcitabine and concurrent radio-therapy for unresectable pancreatic cancer. Int J Radiat Oncol Biol Phys. 2007;68:801–8.

Neoptolemos JP, Dunn JA, Stocken DD, et al. Adjuvant chemoradiotherapy and chemo-therapy in resectable pancreatic cancer: a randomised controlled trial. Lancet. 2001;358(9293):1576–85.

Neoptolemos JP, Stocken DD, Friess H, et al.; European Study Group for Pancreatic Cancer. A randomized trial of chemoradiotherapy and chemotherapy after resection of pancreatic cancer. N Engl J Med. 2004;350(12):1200–10. Erratum in: N Engl J Med 2004; 351(7):726.

Neoptolemos JP, Stocken DD, Bassi C, et al. Adjuvant chemotherapy with fluorouracil plus folinic acid vs gemcitabine following pancreatic cancer resection: a randomized controlled trial. JAMA. 2010;304(10):1073–81.

VI

Neoptolemos JP, Palmer DH, Ghaneh P, et al. Comparison of adjuvant gemcitabine and capecitabine with gemcitabine monotherapy in patients with resected pancreatic cancer (ESPAC-4): a multicenter, open-label, randomized, phase 3 trial. Lancet. 2017. https://doi.org/10.1016/S0140-6736(16)32409-6.

Oettle H, Post S, Neuhaus P, et al. Adjuvant chemotherapy with gemcitabine vs observation in patients undergoing curative-intent resection of pancreatic cancer (CONKO-001). JAMA. 2007;297(3):267–76.

Oettle H, Neuhaus P, Hochhaus A, et al. Adjuvant chemotherapy with gemcitabine and long-term outcomes among patients with resected pancreatic cancer: the CONKO-001 randomized trial. JAMA. 2013;310(14):1473–81.

Petrelli F, Comito T, Ghidini A, et al. Stereotactic body radiation therapy for locally advanced pancreatic cancer: a systematic review and pooled analysis of 19 trials. Int J Radiat Oncol Biol Phys. 2017;97(2):313–22.

Pollom EL, Alagappan M, von Eyben R, et al. Single- versus multifraction stereotactic body radiation therapy for pancreatic adenocarcinoma: outcomes and toxicity. Int J Radiat Oncol Biol Phys. 2014;90(4):918–25.

Regine WF, Winter KA, Abrams RA, et al. Fluorouracil vs gemcitabine chemotherapy before and after fluorouracil-based chemoradiation following resection of pancreatic adenocarcinoma. JAMA. 2008;299(9):1019–26.

Smeenk HG, van Eijck CHJ, Hop WC, et al. Long-term survival and metastatic pattern of pancreatic and periampullary cancer after adjuvant chemoradiation or observation: long-term results of the EORTC trial 40891. Ann Surg. 2007;246(5):734–40.

Tyvin R, Harris J, Abrams R, et al. Phase II study of external irradiation and weekly paclitaxel for nonmetastatic, unresectable pancreatic cancer: RTOG-98-12. Am J Clin Oncol. 2004;27:51–6.

Van Laethem J-L, Hammel P, Mornex F, et al. Adjuvant gemcitabine alone versus gemcitabine-based chemoradiotherapy after curative resection for pancreatic cancer: a randomized EORTC-40013-22012/FFCD-9203/GERCOR phase II study. J Clin Oncol. 2010;28(29):4450–6.

Yovino S, Poppe M, Jabbour S, et al. Intensity-modulated radiation therapy significantly improves acute gastrointestinal toxicity in pancreatic and ampullary cancers. Int J Radiat Oncol Biol Phys. 2011;79(1):158–62.

Chapter 21
Hepatobiliary Cancer

Jennifer S. Chang and Mekhail Anwar

GENERAL PEARLS

- ~39,000 cases and 27,000 deaths for liver and intrahepatic bile duct cancers in 2016 in the USA.
- ~11,000 cases and 3700 deaths for gallbladder and other biliary cancers in 2016 in the USA.
- Frequency: hepatocellular carcinoma (most common) > gallbladder cancer > extrahepatic cholangiocarcinoma > intrahepatic cholangiocarcinoma (least common).

VI

LIVER (HEPATOCELLULAR)

PEARLS

- 100–250× more common in patients with chronic hepatitis B.
- Cirrhosis, chronic liver disease, hepatitis C, hereditary hemochromatosis, and aflatoxin B exposure are also risk factors.
- ~3–4× more common in men.
- Prevention: Hepatitis B vaccine, treatment of hepatitis B and C (reduces but does not eliminate risk).
- Milano/Mazzaferro criteria for liver transplantation: solitary tumor ≤5 cm or up to 3 tumors all ≤3 cm.
- UCSF criteria for liver transplanation: solitary tumor < or = 6.5 cm, or < or = 3 nodules with the largest lesion < or = 4.5 cm and total tumor diameter < or = 8 cm

© Springer International Publishing AG, part of Springer Nature 2018   **459**
Eric K. Hansen and M. Roach III (eds.), *Handbook of Evidence-Based Radiation Oncology*, https://doi.org/10.1007/978-3-319-62642-0_21

WORKUP

- Screening tools frequently used in high-risk patients every 6–12 months: serum alpha-fetoprotein, liver ultrasound.
- H&P: jaundice, diarrhea, bone pain or dyspnea (metastases), hepatosplenomegaly, ascites.
- Labs: CBC, LFTs (including bilirubin, transaminases, alk phos), chemistries, coagulation panel, albumin, serum AFP (10–15% false negative), hepatitis B/C panels.
- 3-phase liver protocol CT and/or MRI with IV contrast, including late arterial and portal venous phase.
- Chest CT; bone scan if clinically indicated.
- Assess liver reserve (Child-Pugh score, portal HTN).
- Consider indocyanine green clearance test to assess liver function, if resection is being considered.
- FNA can be performed but is not always needed, if radiographic characteristics are diagnostic.

STAGING: HEPATOCELLULAR

Editors' note: All TNM stage and stage groups referred to elsewhere in this chapter reflect the 2010 AJCC staging nomenclature unless otherwise noted, as the new system below was published after this chapter was written.

Table 21.1 (AJCC 7TH ED., 2010)

Primary tumor (T)

TX:	Primary tumor cannot be assessed
T0:	No evidence of primary tumor
T1:	Solitary tumor without vascular invasion
T2:	Solitary tumor with vascular invasion or multiple tumors not more than 5 cm
T3a:	Multiple tumors more than 5 cm
T3b:	Single tumor or multiple tumors of any size involving a major branch of the portal vein or hepatic vein
T4:	Tumor(s) with direct invasion of adjacent organs other than the gallbladder or with perforation of visceral peritoneum

Regional lymph nodes (N)

NX:	Regional lymph nodes cannot be assessed
N0:	No regional lymph node metastasis
N1:	Regional lymph node metastasis

Table 21.1 (continued)

Distant metastasis (M)	
M0:	No distant metastasis
M1:	Distant metastasis

Anatomic stage/prognostic groups	
I:	T1 N0 M0
II:	T2 N0 M0
IIIA:	T3a N0 M0
IIIB:	T3b N0 M0
IIIC:	T4 N0 M0
IVA:	Any T N1 M0
IVB:	Any T Any N M1

Used with the permission from the American Joint Committee on Cancer (AJCC), Chicago, Illinois. The original source for this material is the AJCC Cancer Staging Manual, Seventh Edition (2010), published by Springer Science + Business Media

VI

Table 21.2 (AJCC 8TH ED., 2017)

Definitions of AJCC TNM

Definition of primary tumor (T)

T category	T criteria
TX	Primary tumor cannot be assessed
T0	No evidence of primary tumor
T1	Solitary tumor ≤ 2cm or >2 cm without vascular invasion
T1a	Solitary tumor ≤ 2 cm
T1b	Solitary tumor >2 cm without vascular invasion
T2	Solitary tumor >2 cm with vascular invasion or multiple tumors, not >5 cm
T3	Multiple tumors, at least one of which is >5 cm
T4	Single tumor or multiple tumors of any size involving a major branch of the portal vein or hepatic vein or tumor(s) with direct invasion of adjacent organs other than the gallbladder or with perforation of visceral peritoneum

DEFINITION OF REGIONAL LYMPH NODE (N)

N category	N criteria
NX	Regional lymph nodes cannot be assessed
N0	No regional lymph node metastasis
N1	Regional lymph node metastasis

DEFINITION OF DISTANT METASTASIS (M)

M category	M criteria
M0	No distant metastasis
M1	Distant metastasis

AJCC PROGNOSTIC STAGE GROUPS

When T is...	And N is...	And M is...	Then the stage group is...
T1a	N0	M0	IA
T1b	N0	M0	IB
T2	N0	M0	II
T3	N0	M0	IIIA
T4	N0	M0	IIIB
Any T	N1	M0	IVA
Any T	Any N	M1	IVB

Used with permission of the American Joint Committee on Cancer (AJCC), Chicago, Illinois. The original and primary source for this information is the AJCC Cancer Staging Manual, Eighth Edition (2017) published by Springer International Publishing

TREATMENT RECOMMENDATIONS

Table 21.3 TREATMENT RECOMMENDATIONS

Presentation	Recommended treatment
Resectable	Partial hepatectomy
Unresectable, medically operable	Liver transplant Bridging therapy can be used while awaiting transplant
Unresectable, medically inoperable	Ablation (radiofrequency, cryotherapy, percutaneous ethanol or acetic acid, microwave) Arterially directed (bland embolization, transarterial chemoembolization, radioembolization) Conformal RT +/− chemo SBRT Systemic therapy alone Supportive care

SURGERY

- Child-Pugh score is used to assess prognosis of chronic liver disease.
  - Score 1–3 each for total bilirubin, albumin, prothrombin time or INR, ascites, hepatic encephalopathy categories.
  - Class A = 5–6 points, good operative risk, 2-yr OS 85%.
  - Class B = 7–9 points, moderate operative risk, 2-yr OS 57%.
  - Class C = 10–15 points, poor operative risk, 2-yr OS 35%.
- Partial hepatectomy is a treatment of choice if tumor can be resected with negative margins and patient has enough functional reserve. Generally, Child-Pugh Class A without

portal hypertension; solitary mass without major vascular invasion; adequate future liver remnant.

  » Five-year overall survival ~35–40%.
» Total hepatectomy with liver transplant is an option for patients with advanced cirrhosis and either a single tumor <5 cm or up to 3 lesions up to 3 cm each, without vascular invasion.
  » Five-year overall survival as high as ~70% in selected patients.
» MELD score is used to assess severity of liver disease and prioritize allocation of liver transplants. Calculated based on bilirubin, creatinine, and INR to predict survival.

ABLATIVE PROCEDURES

» Consider ablative therapy for pts who are not surgical candidates as it may cure tumors <3 cm and may prolong survival for tumors 3–5 cm. Lesions >5 cm should be considered for arterially directed or systemic therapy.
» Radiofrequency ablation (RFA) is typically used for tumors <4 cm. Usually performed percutaneously by US or CT guidance.
» Technically challenging areas for ablation include subdiaphragmatic location, subcapsular lesions, and proximity of major biliary or vascular structures that could cause biliary injury or heat-sink effect.
» 5-yr local progression after ablation is about 5–15%, but intrahepatic recurrence is 60–75%.

ARTERIALLY DIRECTED AND SYSTEMIC THERAPY

» Arterially directed therapy is potentially indicated if arterial blood supply to tumor may be isolated without excessive nontarget treatment.
  » Relatively contraindicated if bilirubin > 3 or if main portal vein thrombosis and Child-Pugh class C.
  » Transarterial chemoembolization (TACE) involves intra-arterial injection of chemotherapy, often with lipiodol and/or chemotherapeutics.
  » Chemoembolization and intrahepatic artery chemotherapy have response rates of 40–50% but may not improve survival.

- ˒ Transarterial radioembolization (TARE) Y-90 microspheres have increased risk of radiation-induced liver disease in pts with bilirubin > 2. Randomized trials of TARE are ongoing.
- ˒ Sorafenib may have survival benefit over supportive care for advanced HCC, although response rates are low (SHARP trial, Llovet NEJM 2008).
- ˒ Antiviral therapy for patients with chronic hepatitis.

RADIATION THERAPY
- ˒ *Definitive EBRT (3D, IMRT, or preferably SBRT)*
  - ˒ Option for unresectable tumors or as an alternative to ablation/embolization techniques or when they have failed or are contraindicated. There must be sufficient uninvolved liver and liver radiation tolerance must be respected. There should be no or minimal extrahepatic disease. Most data includes Child-Pugh class A disease, with more limited data for Child-Pugh class B or poorer liver function.
  - ˒ Use highly conformal radiotherapy techniques for each lesion, typically with SBRT or protons with modern immobilization, respiratory motion management, and image guidance.
  - ˒ Higher doses may improve local control and survival.
  - ˒ Concurrent FUDR hepatic arterial chemotherapy may be considered with fractionated conformal radiotherapy.
  - ˒ SBRT may be an alternative or adjunct to RFA and TACE as a bridge for pts waiting for a liver transplant because delay to transplant contributes to about 20% of potentially curable pts being delisted before surgery.
- ˒ *Palliative EBRT*
  - ˒ Consider for lung, brain, node, and bone metastases with about 70–80% response rate. There is little published data on the role of low-dose palliative whole liver RT for patients with multiple small lesions and liver-related symptoms who are not candidates for other therapies.

STUDIES
- ˒ *Huo (JAMA Oncol 2015)*: Meta-analysis of unresectable HCC treated with TACE alone vs. TACE + RT (including SBRT). 25 trials with 2577 patients showed better

complete response (OR 2.73), 1-year OS (OR 1.36) with addition of RT, with survival benefit more pronounced with longer follow-up. Increased incidence of ulcers, transaminitis, elevated TBili with TACE + RT.

CONVENTIONALLY FRACTIONATED EBRT

- *Dawson (JCO 2000):* University of Michigan method for treating with high-dose 3DCRT, delivered 1.5 Gy BID. 68% response rate. Survival improved with tumor doses of 70 Gy or higher.
- *Dawson (IJROBP 2002):* Liver tolerance histograms. No radiation-induced liver disease (RILD) with mean liver dose <31 Gy. Whole organ TD_{50} for mets 45.8 Gy, for primary hepatobiliary 39.8 Gy.
- *French RTF-1 trial (Mornex, IJROBP 2006):* Prospective phase II trial including 25 patients with small HCC (1 nodule ≤5 cm or 2 nodules ≤3 cm) received 66 Gy in 2 Gy/fraction 3DCRT. CR achieved in 80% and PR in 12%. Stable disease in 8%. Grade 4 toxicities occurred only in Child-Pugh B patients.
- *Seong (IJROBP 2007):* Retrospective analysis of 305 patients undergoing radiotherapy for HCC. Median survival was 11 months. 1-, 2-, and 5-year OS were 45%, 24%, and 6%, respectively.
- *Zeng (Cancer J 2004):* Retrospective analysis of 203 patients with unresectable hepatocellular carcinoma received transcatheter arterial chemoembolization (TACE) or combination therapy with external beam radiotherapy. 1-/2-/3-yr OS for RT and non-RT groups was 72%/60%/42% vs. 26%/24%/11%, respectively.

SBRT

- See excellent review by McPartlin and Dawson (The Cancer Journal 2016).
- *TRIAL 1/2 (Bujold, JCO 2013):* Phase I (50 patients) and phase II (52 patients) trials of SBRT for Child-Pugh A HCC not suitable for resection, RFA, or TACE. Received 24–54 Gy in 6 fractions, based on RILD model and proximity to GI. 1-year local control 87%, median OS 17 months. Grade ≥ 3 toxicity in 30%. Tumor vascular thrombosis correlated with worse OS.

VI

- *Lasley (Practic Radiat Oncol 2015).* Phase I/II trial of 38 Child-Pugh A and 26 Child-Pugh B HCC pts treated with SBRT (48 Gy in 3 fx or 40 Gy in 5 fx). 3-yr LC/OS: Child-Pugh A 91%/61%, Child-Pugh B 82%/26%.
- *Wahl (JCO 2016):* Prospective single-institution database of inoperable, nonmetastatic HCC treated with RFA (249 lesions, 161 patients) or SBRT (83 lesions, 63 patients). Larger tumor correlated with worse freedom from local progression for RFA but not SBRT. Lesions ≥2 cm had increased freedom from local progression with SBRT; no difference for smaller lesions. Similar acute grade 3+ complications and 1- and 2-yr overall survival.
- *Sanuki (Acta Oncol 2014).* 185 pts with single HCC ≤5 cm treated with SBRT. 40 Gy/5 fx for Child-Pugh A, 35 Gy/5 fx for Child-Pugh B. 3-yr LC 89–91%, OS 66–72%. Acute grade ≥ 3 toxicity 13%.

RADIATION TECHNIQUES
SIMULATION AND FIELD DESIGN

- Supine with arms out of field.
- Use Vac-Lok or SBRT body fixation.
- 3D treatment planning. IV contrast with planning CT to visualize tumor. Consider MRI fusion.
- Recommend 4D-CT imaging and/or respiratory gating motion management.
- CTV is typically the gross tumor.
- PTV = CTV + 0.5–1 cm margin (Often 5mm axially, and 8mm joint).

DOSE PRESCRIPTIONS

Mean Liver Dose (Liver-GTV)	
50 Gy/5	13 Gy
45 Gy/5	15 Gy
40 Gy/5	15 Gy
35 Gy/5	15.5 Gy
30 Gy/5	16 Gy
27.5 Gy/5	17 Gy

DOSE LIMITATIONS

- QUANTEC (Pan, IJROBP 2010) estimates <5% risk of radiation-induced liver disease (RILD):
  - Palliative whole liver: <28 Gy at 2 Gy/fx or <21 Gy at 3 Gy/fx.

   , Partial liver: mean dose (minus GTV) <28 Gy in 2 Gy fx.
   , SBRT: mean dose (minus GTV) <13 Gy/3fx, <18 Gy/6 fx,
     <6 Gy Child-Pugh B at 4–6 Gy/fx; >700 ml normal liver
     should receive <15 Gy in 3–5 fx.
  , Other SBRT dose constraints are evolving. Recommend
   following established constraints in published prospective
   or large retrospective studies.

COMPLICATIONS
  , Fatigue, nausea/vomiting, gastritis/esophagitis, further
   decline in liver function, uncommonly GI bleeding or
   ulceration.
  , RILD typically occurs 4–8 weeks after treatment but can
   be as early as 2 weeks or as late as 7 months later.
  , Classical RILD (pts without underlying liver disease) may
   present with fatigue, abdominal pain, hepatomegaly, ascites, and elevated alkaline phosphatase out of proportion
   to liver enzymes.
  , Nonclassical RILD (pts with underlying liver disease)
   present with elevated transaminase or jaundice.
  , There is no specific RILD treatment. Supportive care
   with paracentesis for ascites and correction of coagu-
   lopathy, and consider steroids to reduce hepatic
   congestion.

VI

FOLLOW-UP
  , Office visit, MRI or multiphase CT, and labs (LFTs, AFP)
   every 3–4 months for 2 years, then every 6 months. Chest
   CT as clinically indicated.

GALLBLADDER

PEARLS
  , <5000 cases per year in the USA.
  , Most are asymptomatic and found incidentally during
   cholecystectomy.
  , Chronic gallbladder inflammation is a risk factor, often
   from gallstones or chronic infection.

- Other risk factors: anomalous pancreaticobiliary duct junction, gallbladder polyps, primary sclerosing cholangitis, porcelain gallbladder.
- Resectable disease in ~30% of patients.
- Frequently advanced stage at presentation; generally poor prognosis.
- Jaundice is associated with more advanced disease and worse prognosis.

WORKUP

- Labs: CBC, LFTs, chemistries, coagulation panel.
- Consider baseline serum CEA, CA 19–9.
- Ultrasound (RUQ or endoscopic) and/or abdominal CT scan and/or MRI.
- If suspicious mass is present, a biopsy is not necessary and can lead to peritoneal spread.
- Consider staging laparoscopy, especially for ≥T3, poorly differentiated, or positive margin on cholecystectomy.
- CT chest.

STAGING: GALLBLADDER

Editors' note: All TNM stage and stage groups referred to elsewhere in this chapter reflect the 2010 AJCC staging nomenclature unless otherwise noted as the new system below was published after this chapter was written.

Table 21.4 (AJCC 7TH ED., 2010)

Primary tumor (T)	
TX:	Primary tumor cannot be assessed
T0:	No evidence of primary tumor
Tis:	Carcinoma in situ
T1:	Tumor invades lamina propria or muscular layer
T1a:	Tumor invades lamina propria
T1b:	Tumor invades muscular layer
T2:	Tumor invades perimuscular connective tissue; no extension beyond serosa or into liver
T3:	Tumor perforates the serosa (visceral peritoneum) and/or directly invades the liver and/or another adjacent organ or structure, such as the stomach, duodenum, colon, pancreas, omentum, or extrahepatic bile ducts
T4:	Tumor invades main portal vein or hepatic artery or invades two or more extrahepatic organs or structures

Table 21.4 (continued)

Regional lymph nodes (N)

NX: Regional lymph nodes cannot be assessed

N0:   No regional lymph node metastasis

N1:   Metastases to nodes along the cystic duct, common bile duct, hepatic artery, and/or portal vein

N2:   Metastases to periaortic, pericaval, superior mesenteric artery, and/or celiac artery lymph nodes

Distant metastasis (M)

M0:   No distant metastasis

M1:   Distant metastasis

Anatomic stage/prognostic groups

0:	Tis N0 M0
I:	T1 N0 M0
II:	T2 N0 M0
IIIA:	T3 N0 M0
IIIB:	T1-3 N1 M0
IVA:	T4 N0-1 M0
IVB:	Any T N2 M0
	Any T Any N M1

Used with the permission from the American Joint Committee on Cancer (AJCC), Chicago, Illinois. The original source for this material is the AJCC Cancer Staging Manual, Seventh Edition (2010), published by Springer Science + Business Media.

VI

Table 21.5 (AJCC 8TH ED., 2017)

Definitions of AJCC TNM

Definition of primary tumor (T)

T category	T criteria
TX	Primary tumor cannot be assessed
T0	No evidence of primary tumor
Tis	Carcinoma in situ
T1	Tumor invades the lamina propria or muscular layer
T1a	Tumor invades the lamina propria
T1b	Tumor invades the muscular layer
T2	Tumor invades the perimuscular connective tissue on the peritoneal side, without involvement of the serosa (visceral peritoneum) or tumor invades the perimuscular connective tissue on the hepatic side, with no extension into the liver
T2a	Tumor invades the perimuscular connective tissue on the peritoneal side, without involvement of the serosa (visceral peritoneum)
T2b	Tumor invades the perimuscular connective tissue on the hepatic side, with no extension into the liver
T3	Tumor perforates the serosa (visceral peritoneum) and/ or directly invades the liver and/or one other adjacent organ or structure, such as the stomach, duodenum, colon, pancreas, omentum, or extrahepatic bile ducts
T4	Tumor invades the main portal vein or hepatic artery or invades two or more extrahepatic organs or structures

DEFINITION OF REGIONAL LYMPH NODE (N)

N category	N criteria
NX	Regional lymph nodes cannot be assessed
N0	No regional lymph node metastasis
N1	Metastases to one to three regional lymph nodes
N2	Metastases to four or more regional lymph nodes

DEFINITION OF DISTANT METASTASIS (M)

M category	M criteria
M0	No distant metastasis
M1	Distant metastasis

AJCC PROGNOSTIC STAGE GROUPS

When Tis...	And Nis...	And M is...	Then the stage group is...
Tis	N0	M0	0
T1	N0	M0	I
T2a	N0	M0	IIA
T2b	N0	M0	IIB
T3	N0	M0	IIIA
T1–3	N1	M0	IIIB
T4	N0–1	M0	IVA
Any T	N2	M0	IVB
Any T	Any N	M1	IVB

Used with permission of the American Joint Committee on Cancer (AJCC), Chicago, Illinois. The original and primary source for this information is the AJCC Cancer Staging Manual, Eighth Edition (2017) published by Springer International Publishing

TREATMENT RECOMMENDATIONS

Table 21.6 TREATMENT RECOMMENDATIONS

Presentation	Recommended treatment
Incidental finding on cholecystectomy, pT1a	If negative margins, observe
Incidental finding on cholecystectomy, pT1b or greater; resectable	Lymphadenectomy with hepatic resection ± bile duct excision to obtain clear margins No standard adjuvant regimen. Consider adjuvant RT and concurrent 5FU- based chemo, or adjuvant chemo alone
Jaundice or mass on imaging, resectable	Resection with lymphadenectomy No standard adjuvant regimen. Consider adjuvant RT and concurrent 5FU-based chemo, or adjuvant chemo alone

Table 21.6 (continued)

Presentation	Recommended treatment
Unresectable	Biliary drainage if needed
	Gemcitabine/cisplatin combination chemo
	Consider RT with concurrent 5FU based chemo
	Clinical trial
	Supportive care
Metastatic	Biliary drainage if needed
	Gemcitabine/cisplatin combination chemotherapy
	Clinical trial
	Best supportive care

SURGERY
- Radical cholecystectomy with partial hepatectomy for node-negative patients with invasion of perimuscular connective tissue.
- Before definitive resection, consider staging laparoscopy for poorly differentiated, T3, or positive margin to rule out disseminated disease.

ADJUVANT THERAPY
- Combination gemcitabine/cisplatin improved survival compared to single-agent chemo for locally advanced/metastatic disease.
- Role of chemoRT uncertain but generally recommended for T2 N1, T3/4, +margins, or residual disease after surgery.

STUDIES
- Cubertafond (Hepatogastroenterol 1999): Review of surgical data for 724 patients with gallbladder cancer, treated with simple cholecystectomy. Five-year survival for node negative: Tis 93%, T1 18%, T2 10%. No 3-year survivors with T3/4 disease.
- SEER (Wang, JCO 2008): 4180 patients with resected gallbladder cancer, 18% received adjuvant RT. Adjuvant RT improved MS for ≥T2 N+ disease from 8 to 15 months. Some patients with ≥T2 N0 disease may benefit, but to a smaller degree. Nomogram derived in paper.
- SEER (Pollom, Cancer Medicine 2016): 2343 patients with unresectable biliary tract cancer (444 with gallbladder cancer). Longer median survival with RT (10 vs. 9.3 months, $P = 0.02$). Among patients who received chemo, RT was associated with improved survival (HR 0.82). For patients

not receiving chemo, no RT benefit was seen. RT has declined since 1998.

- *NCDB* (Mantripragada, JNCI 2016): National Cancer Data Base analysis of 4775 patients with T2–3 or node-positive, nonmetastatic gallbladder cancer s/p resection with grossly negative margins. 29% received adjuvant chemo, 13.5% received adjuvant concurrent chemoRT. ChemoRT associated with a 6.7% improvement in 2-year OS for T3 or node-positive disease, but no difference by 5 years. No OS difference in overall cohort.

- Kim (Ann Surg Onc 2016): Retrospective multi-institutional analysis of 291 patients with gallbladder cancer undergoing R0 or R1 resection. 46% with T2 disease, 39% with T3, 38% with positive nodes. 21% with adjuvant chemo, 15% with adjuvant chemoRT. Improved OS with adjuvant chemo (HR 0.38) or chemoRT (HR 0.26). Only those with high-risk features (T3/T4, positive nodes, R1 resection) showed a benefit.

- Engineer (Ann Surg Onc 2016): Prospective study of 28 patients with stage III disease, treated with neoadjuvant chemoRT with 57 Gy in 25 fractions to gross disease and 45 Gy in 25 fractions to nodes with concurrent gemcitabine. 89% completed chemoRT, 71% with partial/complete response. 18 patients underwent surgery, and 14 patients had R0 resections. Median OS 20 months. 5-year OS 24% for entire group and 47% for those with R0 resection.

- *SWOG S0809* (Ben-Josef, JCO 2015): Phase II with 79 patients with resected gallbladder carcinoma or extrahepatic cholangiocarcinoma, stages pT2-4 or node positive. Received gemcitabine/capecitabine x 4 cycles, then chemoRT with 45 Gy to regional nodes and 54–59.4 Gy to tumor bed with concurrent capecitabine. 52% with grade 3 and 11% with grade 4 adverse effects. Overall 2-year survival 65%; median OS 35 months.

- *ABC-02* (Valle, NEJM 2010): Phase III RCT of 410 patients with locally advanced or metastatic cholangiocarcinoma, gallbladder, or ampullary cancer. Randomized to cisplatin and gemcitabine vs. gemcitabine alone. Combination chemo with better median OS for (11.7 vs. 8.1 mo), median PFS (8 vs. 5 months). More neutropenia with combination chemo but similar neutropenia-associated infection rate.

RADIATION TECHNIQUES
SIMULATION AND FIELD DESIGN
, Supine with arms up out of field.
, Use Vac-Lok or alpha cradle to stabilize torso.
, CT scan for treatment planning. Consider IV and/or oral contrast.
, Cover tumor bed and regional lymph nodes including porta hepatis, pericholedochal, celiac, and pancreaticoduodenal.
, Consider 4D-CT and/or respiratory gating.

DOSE PRESCRIPTION
, 45 Gy/25 fx followed by boost to reduced fields, 50.4–54 Gy to tumor bed/+margins, up to 54–55.8 Gy to gross disease (respecting normal tissue tolerance).

DOSE LIMITATIONS
, Small bowel <45–50.4 Gy/25–28 fx.
, Spinal cord <45 Gy/25 fx.
, Liver (see previous section).
, Kidney ≤1/3 receiving ≥20 Gy.

COMPLICATIONS
, Fatigue, nausea, vomiting, loose bowel movements, gastritis.
, Small risk of RILD.
, Uncommon: bowel ulceration or necrosis, small bowel obstruction, rarely fistula formation.

FOLLOW-UP
, Consider exam and imaging every 6 months for 2 years if clinically indicated, then annually up to 5 years, with CEA and CA 19-9 as clinically indicated.

BILE DUCT

PEARLS

- Divided into intrahepatic (IHCC, ~20%) and extrahepatic (EHCC) cholangiocarcinoma.
- Intrahepatic includes small or large ducts proximal to the bifurcation of the common hepatic duct.
- Extrahepatic includes perihilar (Klatskin) tumors and distal segments.
- Risk factors: primary sclerosing cholangitis (~10% lifetime risk), congenital biliary tree abnormalities, hepatolithiasis, chronic tapeworm infection, Thorotrast. Possible association with cholecystitis.
- Cholecystectomy decreases risk of cholangiocarcinoma.
- Can present concurrently with hepatocellular carcinoma.
- ~55% of patients are lymph node positive at diagnosis.

WORKUP

- H&P: For extrahepatic – jaundice, hepatomegaly, pruritis, dark urine, clay-colored stool, pain, weight loss, fever. Intrahepatic may have RUQ pain, weight loss, may be asymptomatic.
- Labs: CBC, LFTs, chemistries, coagulation panel, CA 19–9, CEA, AFP (rule out HCC), hepatitis B/C.
- Right upper quadrant US and/or abdominal multiphasic CT and possibly MRI/MRCP.
- EUS/ERCP with biopsy.
- EGD and colonoscopy.
- Chest CT.
- Consider staging laparoscopy before or in conjunction with resection to rule out disseminated disease.
- Biopsy not necessary for suspicious mass on imaging.
- If potential transplant candidate, refer to transplant center prior to biopsy.

Table 21.7 STAGING (AJCC 7TH ED., 2010): INTRAHEPATIC BILE DUCT

Primary tumor (T)

TX: Primary tumor cannot be assessed

T0:   No evidence of primary tumor

Tis: Carcinoma in situ (intraductal tumor)

T1:   Solitary tumor without vascular invasion

T2a: Solitary tumor with vascular invasion

T2b: Multiple tumors, with or without vascular invasion

T3:   Tumor perforating the visceral peritoneum or involving the local extra hepatic structures by direct invasion

T4:   Tumor with periductal invasion

Regional lymph nodes (N)

NX: Regional lymph nodes cannot be assessed

N0:   No regional lymph node metastasis

N1:   Regional lymph node metastasis present

Distant metastasis (M)

M0:   No distant metastasis

M1:   Distant metastasis present

Anatomic stage/prognostic groups

0:     Tis N0 M0

I: T1 N0 M0

II: T2 N0 M0

III: T3 N0 M0

IVA: T4 N0 M0

       Any T N1 M0

IVB: Any T any N M1

Used with the permission from the American Joint Committee on Cancer (AJCC), Chicago, Illinois. The original source for this material is the AJCC Cancer Staging Manual, Seventh Edition (2010), published by Springer Science + Business Media

Table 21.8 STAGING (AJCC 7TH ED., 2010): PERIHILAR BILE DUCT

Primary tumor (T)

TX: Primary tumor cannot be assessed

T0:   No evidence of primary tumor

Tis: Carcinoma in situ

T1:   Tumor confined to the bile duct, with extension up to the muscle layer or fibrous tissue

T2a: Tumor invades beyond the wall of the bile duct to surrounding adipose tissue

T2b: Tumor invades adjacent hepatic parenchyma

T3:   Tumor invades unilateral branches of the portal vein or hepatic artery

T4:   Tumor invades main portal vein or its branches bilaterally; or the common hepatic artery; or the second-order biliary radicals bilaterally; or unilateral second-order biliary radicals with contralateral portal vein or hepatic artery involvement

VI

continued

Table 21.8   (continued)

Regional lymph nodes (N)

NX: Regional lymph nodes cannot be assessed

N0:   No regional lymph node metastasis

N1:   Regional lymph node metastasis (including nodes along the cystic duct, common bile duct, hepatic artery, and portal vein)

N2:   Metastasis to periaortic, pericaval, superior mesenteric artery, and/or celiac artery lymph nodes

Distant metastasis (M)

M0:   No distant metastasis

M1:   Distant metastasis

Anatomic stage/prognostic groups

0:   Tis N0 M0

I: T1 N0 M0

II: T2a-b N0 M0

IIIA: T3 N0 M0

IIIB: T1-3 N1 M0

IVA: T4 N0-1

IVB: Any T N2 M0

 Any T any N M1

Used with the permission of the American Joint Committee on Cancer (AJCC), Chicago, Illinois. The original source for this material is the AJCC Cancer Staging Manual, Seventh Edition (2010) published by Springer Science + Business Media

Table 21.9 STAGING (AJCC 7TH ED., 2010): DISTAL BILE DUCT

Primary tumor (T)

TX: Primary tumor cannot be assessed

T0:   No evidence of primary tumor

Tis: Carcinoma in situ

T1:   Tumor confined to the bile duct histologically

T2:   Tumor invades beyond the wall of the bile duct

T3:   Tumor invades the gallbladder, pancreas, duodenum, or other adjacent organs without involvement of the celiac axis, or the superior mesenteric artery

T4:   Tumor involves the celiac axis, or the superior mesenteric artery

Regional lymph nodes (N)

NX: Regional lymph nodes cannot be assessed

N0:   No regional lymph node metastasis

N1:   Regional lymph node metastasis

Distant metastasis (M)

M0:   No distant metastasis

M1:   Distant metastasis

Table 21.9 (continued)

Anatomic stage/prognostic groups

0:	Tis N0 M0
IA:	T1 N0 M0
IB:	T2 N0 M0
IIA:	T3 N0 M0
IIB:	T1-T3 N1 M0
III:	T4 Any N M0
IV:	Any T any N M1

Used with the permission of the American Joint Committee on Cancer (AJCC), Chicago, Illinois. The original source for this material is the AJCC Cancer Staging Manual, Seventh Edition (2010), published by Springer Science + Business Media

Table 21.10 STAGING (AJCC 7TH ED., 2010): AMPULLA OF VATER

VI

Primary tumor (T)

TX:	Primary tumor cannot be assessed
T0:	No evidence of primary tumor
Tis:	Carcinoma in situ
T1:	Tumor limited to ampulla of Vater or sphincter of Oddi
T2:	Tumor invades duodenal wall
T3:	Tumor invades pancreas
T4:	Tumor invades peripancreatic soft tissues or other adjacent organs or structures other than the pancreas

Regional lymph nodes (N)

NX:	Regional lymph nodes cannot be assessed
N0:	No regional lymph node metastasis
N1:	Regional lymph node metastasis

Distant metastasis (M)

M0:	No distant metastasis
M1:	Distant metastasis

Anatomic stage/prognostic groups

0:	Tis N0 M0
IA:	T1 N0 M0
IB:	T2 N0 M0
IIA:	T3 N0 M0
IIB:	T1-T3 N1 M0
III:	T4 Any N M0
IV:	Any T Any N M1

Used with the permission of the American Joint Committee on Cancer (AJCC), Chicago, Illinois. The original source for this material is the AJCC Cancer Staging Manual, Seventh Edition (2010) published by Springer Science + Business Media

STAGING (AJCC 8TH ED., 2017)

Table 21.11 INTRAHEPATIC BILE DUCT

Definitions of AJCC TNM
Definition of primary tumor (T)

T category	T criteria
TX	Primary tumor cannot be assessed
T0	No evidence of primary tumor
Tis	Carcinoma in situ (intraductal tumor)
T1	Solitary tumor without vascular invasion, ≤5 cm or >5 cm
T1a	Solitary tumor ≤5 cm without vascular invasion
T1b	Solitary tumor >5 cm without vascular invasion
T2	Solitary tumor with intrahepatic vascular invasion or multiple tumors, with or without vascular invasion
T3	Tumor perforating the visceral peritoneum
T4	Tumor involving local extrahepatic structures by direct invasion

DEFINITION OF REGIONAL LYMPH NODE (N)

N category	N criteria
NX	Regional lymph nodes cannot be assessed
N0	No regional lymph node metastasis
N1	Regional lymph node metastasis present

DEFINITION OF DISTANT METASTASIS (M)

M category	M criteria
M0	No distant metastasis
M1	Distant metastasis present

AJCC PROGNOSTIC STAGE GROUPS

When T is...	And N is...	And M is...	Then the stage group is...
Tis	N0	M0	0
T1a	N0	M0	IA
T1b	N0	M0	IB
T2	N0	M0	II
T3	N0	M0	IIIA
T4	N0	M0	IIIB
Any T	N1	M0	IIIB
Any T	Any N	M1	IV

Table 21.12 PERIHILAR BILE DUCT

Definition of AJCC TNM
Definition of primary tumor (T)

T category	T criteria
TX	Primary tumor cannot be assessed
T0	No evidence of primary tumor
Tis	Carcinoma in situ/high-grade dysplasia
T1	Tumor confined to the bile duct, with extension up to the muscle layer or fibrous tissue
T2	Tumor invades beyond the wall of the bile duct to surrounding adipose tissue or tumor invades adjacent hepatic parenchyma
T2a	Tumor invades beyond the wall of the bile duct to surrounding adipose tissue
T2b	Tumor invades adjacent hepatic parenchyma
T3	Tumor invades unilateral branches of the portal vein or hepatic artery
T4	Tumor invades the main portal vein or its branches bilaterally, the common hepatic artery, or the unilateral second-order biliary radicals with contralateral portal vein or hepatic artery involvement

VI

DEFINITION OF REGIONAL LYMPH NODE (N)

N category	N criteria
NX	Regional lymph nodes cannot be assessed
N0	No regional lymph node metastasis
N1	One to three positive lymph nodes typically involving the hilar, cystic duct, common bile duct, hepatic artery, posterior pancreaticoduodenal, and portal vein lymph nodes
N2	Four or more positive lymph nodes from the sites described for N1

DEFINITION OF DISTANT METASTASIS (M)

M category	M criteria
M0	No distant metastasis
M1	Distant metastasis

AJCC PROGNOSTIC STAGE GROUPS

When T is...	And N is...	And M is...	Then the stage group is...
Tis	N0	M0	0
T1	N0	M0	I
T2a–b	N0	M0	II
T3	N0	M0	IIIA
T4	N0	M0	IIIB
Any T	N1	M0	IIIC
Any T	N2	M0	IVA
Any T	Any N	M1	IVB

Table 21.13 DISTAL BILE DUCT

Definitions of AJCC TNM

Definition of primary tumor (T)

T category	T criteria
TX	Primary tumor cannot be assessed
T0	No evidence of primary tumor
Tis	Carcinoma in situ
T1	Tumor limited to ampulla of Vater or sphincter of Oddi or tumor invades beyond the sphincter of Oddi (perisphincteric invasion) and/or into the duodenal submucosa
T1a	Tumor limited to ampulla of Vater or sphincter of Oddi
T1b	Tumor invades beyond the sphincter of Oddi (perisphincteric invasion) and/or into the duodenal submucosa
T category	**T criteria**
T2	Tumor invades into the muscularis propria of the duodenum
T3	Tumor directly invades the pancreas (up to 0.5 cm) or the tumor extends more than 0.5 cm into the pancreas or extends into peripancreatic or periduodenal tissue or duodenal serosa without involvement of the celiac axis or superior mesenteric artery
T3a	Tumor directly invades pancreas (up to 0.5 cm)
T3b	Tumor extends more than 0.5 cm into the pancreas or extends into peripancreatic tissue or duodenal serosa without involvement of the celiac axis or superior mesenteric artery
T4	Tumor involves the celiac axis, superior mesenteric artery, and/or common hepatic artery, irrespective of size

DEFINITION OF REGIONAL LYMPH NODE (N)

N category	N criteria
NX	Regional lymph nodes cannot be assessed
N0	No regional lymph node metastasis
N1	Metastasis to one to three regional lymph nodes
N2	Metastasis to four or more regional lymph nodes

DEFINITION OF DISTANT METASTASIS (M)

M category	M criteria
M0	No distant metastasis
M1	Distant metastasis

AJCC PROGNOSTIC STAGE GROUPS

When T is...	And N is...	And M is...	Then the stage group is...
Tis	N0	M0	0
T1a	N0	M0	IA
T1a	N1	M0	IIIA
T1b	N0	M0	IB
T1b	N1	M0	IIIA
T2	N0	M0	IB
T2	N1	M0	IIIA
T3a	N0	M0	IIA
T3a	N1	M0	IIIA
T3b	N0	M0	IIB
T3b	N1	M0	IIIA
T4	Any N	M0	IIIB
Any T	N2	M0	IIIB
Any T	Any N	M1	IV

VI

Table 21.14 AMPULLA OF VATER

Definitions of AJCC TNM	
Definition of primary tumor (T)	
T category	**T criteria**
TX	Primary tumor cannot be assessed
T0	No evidence of primary tumor
Tis	Carcinoma in situ
	This includes high-grade pancreatic intraepithelial neoplasia (PanIn-3), intraductal papillary mucinous neoplasm with high-grade dysplasia, intraductal tubulopapillary neoplasm with high-grade dysplasia, and mucinous cystic neoplasm with high-grade dysplasia
T1	Tumor ≤2 cm in greatest dimension
T1a	Tumor ≤0.5 cm in greatest dimension
T1b	Tumor >0.5 cm and <1 cm in greatest dimension
T1c	Tumor 1–2 cm in greatest dimension
T2	Tumor >2 cm and ≤4 cm in greatest dimension
T3	Tumor >4 cm in greatest dimension
T category	**T criteria**
T4	Tumor involves celiac axis, superior mesenteric artery, and/or common hepatic artery, regardless of size

DEFINITION OF REGIONAL LYMPH NODE (N)

N category	N criteria
NX	Regional lymph nodes cannot be assessed
N0	No regional lymph node metastases
N1	Metastasis in one to three regional lymph nodes
N2	Metastasis in four or more regional lymph nodes

DEFINITION OF DISTANT METASTASIS (M)

M category	M criteria
M0	No distant metastasis
M1	Distant metastasis

AJCC PROGNOSTIC STAGE GROUPS

When T is...	And N is...	And M is...	Then the stage group is...
Tis	N0	M0	0
T1	N0	M0	IA
T1	N1	M0	IIB
T1	N2	M0	III
T2	N0	M0	IB
T2	N1	M0	IIB
T2	N2	M0	III
T3	N0	M0	IIA
T3	N1	M0	IIB
T3	N2	M0	III
T4	Any N	M0	III
Any T	Any N	M1	IV

Used with permission of the American Joint Committee on Cancer (AJCC), Chicago, Illinois. The original and primary source for this information is the AJCC Cancer Staging Manual, Eighth Edition (2017) published by Springer International Publishing

TREATMENT RECOMMENDATIONS

Table 21.15 TREATMENT RECOMMENDATIONS

Presentation	Recommended treatment
Intrahepatic cholangiocarcinoma	
Resectable, no residual disease	Surgery alone Consider adjuvant chemo

Table 21.15 (continued)

Presentation	Recommended treatment
Resectable, microscopic positive margins (R1) or node positive	No standard adjuvant therapy Consider RT with concurrent 5FU-based chemo Consider gemcitabine- or cisplatin-based chemo
Resectable, gross residual disease (R2)	No standard adjuvant therapy Consider repeat resection if possible Consider ablative procedure Consider adjuvant gemcitabine/cisplatin chemo Consider RT with concurrent 5FU-based chemo
Unresectable	No standard treatment regimen Gemcitabine/cisplatin chemo Consider locoregional therapy Supportive care
Extrahepatic cholangiocarcinoma	
Resectable, no residual disease	Surgery Consider adjuvant 5FU-based chemoRT Consider adjuvant 5FU/gemcitabine-based chemo
Resectable, residual disease or positive nodes	Surgery followed by RT with concurrent 5FU-based chemo, then adjuvant chemo Or surgery with adjuvant 5FU-/gemcitabine-based chemo for positive nodes
Unresectable	Biliary drainage, if needed Consider for transplant Consider gemcitabine/cisplatin chemo Consider RT with concurrent 5FU-based chemo Supportive care

VI

SURGERY

, Complete surgical resection is the most effective treatment.

, Surgical procedure depends on tumor location and extent of disease.

  , Partial hepatectomy or lobectomy for intrahepatic tumors.

  , Roux-en-y hepaticojejunostomy for hilar tumors.

  , Pancreaticoduodenectomy for distal lesions.

  , Liver transplant.

, Include portal lymphadenectomy.

, Contraindications to resection: lymph nodes beyond porta hepatis, distant metastases. Highly selected cases of multifocal disease can be considered for resection.

, Palliative options – biliary enteric bypass, percutaneous transhepatic biliary drainage, stents.

ADJUVANT THERAPY

- Limited data; no standard adjuvant regimen.
- Risk factors for local recurrence: lymphovascular invasion, perineural invasion, positive node(s), primary ≥5 cm.

STUDIES

- Todoroki (IJROBP 2000): 63 patients. Treatment: surgical resection. RT given to 28/47 with microscopic disease and 13/14 with gross residual disease. 5-year OS with RT 32 months vs. surgery alone 13.5 months. RT group OS: IORT + EBRT 39%, IORT alone 17%, EBRT alone 0%. LRC with RT 79% vs. with surgery alone 31.2%. IORT dose recommendations - 20 Gy, 8 MeV electrons, 6 cm cone.
- Schoenthaler (Ann Surg 1994): UCSF experience. 129 patients, retrospective, extrahepatic ducts only. Treatment: 62 patients surgery alone, 45 patients surgery + conventional RT (46 Gy median), 22 patients surgery + charged particles (60 GyE median). MS: 6.5 months with surgery, 11 months with surgery + EBRT, 14 months with surgery + particles, 7 months with gross residual disease, 19 months with microscopic residual disease, and 39 months with negative margins.
- Alden (IJROBP 1994): Unresectable disease. Higher RT doses improve survival. MS: 44 Gy = 4.5 months, 45–54 Gy = 18 months, >54 Gy = 24 months. Recommended dose is 45 Gy EBRT with a 25 Gy intraluminal brachytherapy boost.
- Crane (IJROBP 2002): 52 patients, locally advanced, unresectable treated with RT + chemo (73% of patients, PVI 5FU). Median time to local progression: 9 months after 30 Gy, 11 months after 36–50.4 Gy, 15 months after 54–85 Gy (p = ns). MS 10 months. Grade 3 toxicity similar in all groups.
- Borghero (Ann Surg Oncol 2008): Retrospective analysis of 65 patients with extrahepatic bile duct adenocarcinoma treated with curative-intent resection (S). For those with high-risk of local regional recurrence (42 patients), adjuvant chemoradiation (S-CRT) was implemented. Five-year OS and LRR for S- vs. S-CRT groups were 36% vs. 42% and 38% vs. 37%, respectively.

, Nelson (IJROBP 2009): Retrospective analysis of 45 patients undergoing resection followed by concurrent chemoradiation. Thirty-three patients underwent adjuvant radiotherapy and 12 neoadjuvant radiotherapy. Five-year OS, DFS, and LRC were 33%, 37%, and 78%, respectively. Median survival was 34 months. Patients treated neoadjuvantly showed a trend toward longer 5-year OS (53% vs. 23%) but was not statistically significant.

, Tse (JCO 2008): Phase I trial with 41 patients (31 with HCC and 10 with intrahepatic cholangiocarcinoma), unresectable Child-Pugh class A treated with 6-fraction SBRT. Median dose 36 Gy. 12% with grade 3 liver enzymes, no grade 4/5 toxicity. Median survival of IHC was 15 months.

, Ben-David (IJROBP 2006): Retrospective single-institution experience of 81 patients with extrahepatic cholangiocarcinoma or gallbladder cancer, all treated with surgery (35% R0/R1) and adjuvant 3D RT to mean dose 58.4 Gy. 54% with concurrent chemo. Median OS 14.7 months, median PFS 11 months. R0 resection was only predictive factor; R1 and R2 outcomes similar. 69% of failures were locoregional.

, Wang (JCO 2013): Nomogram for intrahepatic cholangiocarcinoma treated with partial hepatectomy. Independent factors for survival: CEA, CA 19-9, tumor diameter and number, vascular invasion, lymph node involvement, direct invasion, local extrahepatic metastasis.

, Al-Adra (Eur J Surg Oncol 2015): Systematic review of 12 retrospective studies involving 298 patients treated with Y-90 microspheres for unresectable intrahepatic cholangiocarcinoma. Most had undergone prior treatment. Median overall survival 15.5 months. Stable disease in 54%, partial response in 28%.

, Tao (JCO 2015): Single-institution retrospective analysis of 79 patients with inoperable intrahepatic cholangiocarcinoma, treated with RT +/− chemo. Median OS 30 months, no significant treatment-related toxicities. RT dose correlated with 3-year OS: 73% for BED >80.5 Gy vs. 38% with lower doses.

, Horgan (JCO 2012): Analysis of 20 studies including 6712 patients with gallbladder and bile duct tumors who underwent surgery with curative intent. Nonsignificant improvement in overall survival with any adjuvant therapy compared to surgery (pooled odds ratio 0.74, P = 0.06). Chemo or chemoRT with more benefit than RT alone (OR 0.39, 0.61, and 0.98, respectively). Greatest benefit of adjuvant therapy in node-positive disease (OR 0.49).

ᶾ *SWOG S0809* (Ben-Josef JCO 2015): Phase II with 79 patients with resected gallbladder carcinoma or extrahepatic cholangiocarcinoma, stages pT2-4 or node positive. Received gemcitabine/capecitabine x 4 cycles, then chemoRT with 45 Gy to regional nodes and 54–59.4 Gy to tumor bed with concurrent capecitabine. 52% with grade 3 and 11% with grade 4 adverse effects. Overall 2-year survival 65%; median OS 35 months.

ᶾ *ACTICCA-1*: Ongoing phase III trial of adjuvant gemcitabine and cisplatin vs. observation for resected colangiocarcinoma or muscle-invasive gallbladder carcinoma.

RADIATION TECHNIQUES
SIMULATION AND FIELD DESIGN

ᶾ Supine with arms up out of field.
ᶾ Use Vac-Lok or alpha cradle to stabilize torso.
ᶾ CT scan for treatment planning. Consider IV and/or oral contrast.
ᶾ Cover tumor bed, porta hepatis, celiac axis + 1–2 cm margin.
ᶾ Consider extending field up to 3–5 cm into liver to cover additional intrahepatic bile duct length for margin as indicated, respecting liver tolerance.
ᶾ Add additional margins as needed to account for organ motion secondary to breathing, or perform 4D CT to define ITV. Consider respiratory gating.

DOSE PRESCRIPTION

ᶾ 45 Gy/25 fx to large field described above.
ᶾ Additional boost dose should be given. Options include EBRT with conedown to tumor bed up to 54–60 Gy total; ^{192}Ir intraluminal brachytherapy (20–25 Gy); IORT at time of surgery.

DOSE LIMITATIONS
, See liver section.

COMPLICATIONS
, Fatigue, nausea, vomiting, loose bowel movements, gastritis.
, RILD uncommon as much of the liver can be excluded from the field.
, Cholangitis after brachytherapy.
, Small bowel damage (ulcer, bleeding, obstruction).

FOLLOW-UP
, No data to support aggressive surveillance imaging.
, Consider imaging every 6 months for 2 years if clinically indicated, then annually up to 5 years.

VI

Acknowledgment We thank Chien Peter Chen MD, Kim Huang MD, and Mack Roach III MD, for their work on the prior edition of this chapter.

REFERENCES
Al-Adra DP, Gill RS, Axford SJ, et al. Treatment of Unresectable intrahepatic cholangio-carcinoma with yttrium-90 Radioembolization: a Systematic review and pooled analysis. Eur J Surg Oncol. 2015;41(1):120–7.

Alden ME, Mohiuddin M. The impact of radiation dose in combined external beam and intraluminal Ir-192 brachytherapy for bile duct cancer. Int J Radiat Oncol Biol Phys. 1994;28:945–51.

Ben-David MA, Griffith KA, Abu-Isa E, et al. External-beam radiotherapy for localized extrahepatic cholangiocarcinoma. Int J Radiat Oncol Biol Phys. 2006;66(3):772.

Ben-Josef E, Guthrie KA, El-Khoueiry AB, et al. SWOG S0809: a phase II intergroup trial of adjuvant capecitabine and gemcitabine followed by radiotherapy and concurrent capecitabine in extrahepatic cholangiocarcinoma and gallbladder carcinoma. J Clin Oncol. 2015;33(24):2617–22.

Borghero Y, Crane CH, Szklaruk J, et al. Extrahepatic bile duct adenocarcinoma: patients at high-risk for local recurrence treated with surgery and adjuvant chemo-radiation have an equivalent overall survival to patients with standard-risk treated with surgery alone. Ann Surg Oncol. 2008;15:3147–56.

Bujold A, Massey CA, Kim JJ, et al. Sequential phase I and II trials of stereotactic body radiotherapy for locally advanced hepatocellular carcinoma. J Clin Oncol. 2013;31(13):1631–9.

Crane CH, MacDonald KO, Vauthey JN, et al. Limitations of conventional doses of chemoradiation for unresectable biliary cancer. Int J Radiat Oncol Biol Phys. 2002;53:969–74.

Cubertafond P, Mathonnet M, Gainant A, et al. Radical surgery for gallbladder cancer. Results of the French surgical association survey. Hepatogastroenterology. 1999;46:1567–71.

Dawson LA, McGinn CJ, Normolle D, et al. Escalated focal liver radiation and concurrent hepatic artery fluorodeoxyuridine for unresectable intrahepatic malignancies. J Clin Oncol. 2000;18:2210–8.

Dawson LA, Normolle D, Balter JM, et al. Analysis of radiation-induced liver disease using the Lyman NTCP model. Int J Radiat Oncol Biol Phys. 2002;53:810–21.

Engineer R, Goel M, Chopra S, et al. Neoadjuvant chemoradiation followed by surgery for locally advanced gallbladder cancers : a new paradigm. Ann Surg Onc. 2016;23(9):3009–15.

Horgan AM, Amir E, Walter T, Knox JJ. Adjuvant therapy in the treatment of biliary tract cancer : a systematic review and meta-analysis. J Clin Oncol. 2012;30(16):1934–40.

Huo YR, Eslick GD. Transcatheter arterial chemoembolization plus radiotherapy compared with chemoembolization alone for hepatocellular carcinoma: a systematic review and meta-analysis. JAMA Oncol. 2015;1(6):756–65.

Kim Y, Amini N, Wilson A, et al. Impact of chemotherapy and external-beam radiation therapy on outcomes among patients with resected gallbladder cancer : a multi-institutional analysis. Ann Surg Onc. 2016;23(9):2998–3008.

Lasley FD, Mannina EM, Johnson CS, et al. Treatment variables related to liver toxicity in patients with hepatocellular carcinoma, Child-Pugh class A and B enrolled in a phase 1-2 trial of stereotacti body radiation therapy. Pract Radiat Oncol. 2015;5(5):e443–9.

Mantripragada KC, Hamid F, Shafgat H, Olszewski AJ. Adjuvant therapy for resected gallbladder cancer: analysis of the national cancer data base. J Natl Cancer Inst. 2016;109(2):pii. djw202

McPartlin AJ, Dawson LA. Stereotactic body radiotherapy for hepatocellular carcinoma. Cancer J. 2016;22(4):296–301.

Mornex F, Girarda N, Beziat C, et al. Feasibility and efficacy of high-dose three-dimensional radiotherapy in cirrhotic patients with small-size hepatocellular carcinoma non-eligible for curative therapies – mature results of the French phase II RTF-1 trial. Int J Radiat Oncol Biol Phys. 2006;66:1152–8.

National Comprehensive Cancer Network. Clinical practice guidelines in oncology: hepatobiliary cancers. Available at: https://www.nccn.org/professionals/physician_gls/pdf/hepatobiliary.pdf. Accessed on 25 Jan 2017.

Nelson JW, Ghafoori AP, Willett CG, et al. Concurrent chemoradiotherapy in resected extrahepatic cholangiocarcinoma. Int J Radiat Oncol Biol Phys. 2009;73:148–53.

Pan CC, Kavanagh BD, Dawson LA, et al. Radiation-associated liver injury. Int J Radiat Oncol Biol Phys. 2010;76(3):S94–S100.

Pollom EL, Alagappan M, Park LS, et al. Does radiotherapy still have a role in Unresected biliary tract cancer? Cancer Med. 2016. https://doi.org/10.1002/cam4.975.

Sanuki N, Takeda A, Oku Y, et al. Stereotactic body radiotherapy for small hepatocellular carcinoma: a retrospective outcome analysis in 185 patients. Acta Oncol. 2014;53(3):399–404.

Seong J, Shim SJ, Lee IJ, et al. Evaluation of the prognostic value of Okuda, cancer of the liver Italian program, and Japan integrated staging systems for hepatocellular carcinoma patients undergoing radiotherapy. Int J Radiat Oncol Biol Phys. 2007;67:1037–42.

Schoenthaler R, Phillips TL, Efrid JT, et al. Carcinoma of the extrahepatic bile ducts, the University of California at San Francisco experience. Ann Surg. 1994;219:267–74.

Tao R, Krishnan S, Bhosale PR, et al. Ablative radiotherapy doses lead to a substantial prolongation of survival in patients with inoperable intrahepatic cholangiocarcinoma: a retrospective dose response analysis. J Clin Oncol. 2015;34(3):219–26.

Tse RV, Hawkins M, Lockwood G, et al. Phase I study of individualized Stereotactic body radiotherapy for hepatocellular carcinoma and intrahepatic cholangiocarcinoma. J Clin Oncol. 2008;26:657–64.

Todoroki T, Ohara K, Kawamoto T, et al. Benefits of adjuvant radiotherapy after radical resection of locally advanced main hepatic duct carcinoma. Int J Radiat Oncol Biol Phys. 2000;46:581–7.

Valle JW, Hasan HS, Palmer DD, et al. Cisplatin plus gemcitabine versus gemcitabine for biliary tract cancer. N Engl J Med. 2010;362:1273–81.

Wahl DR, Stenmark MH, Tao Y, et al. Outcomes after stereotactic body radiotherapy or radiofrequency ablation for hepatocellular carcinoma. J Clin Oncol. 2016;34(5):452–9.

Wang SJ, Fuller CD, Kim JS, et al. Prediction model for estimating the survival benefit of adjuvant radiotherapy for gallbladder cancer. J Clin Oncol. 2008;26:2116–7.

Wang Y, Li J, Xia Y, et al. Prognostic Nomogram for intrahepatic cholangiocarcinoma after partial hepatectomy. J Clin Oncol. 2013;31(9):1188–95.

Zeng ZC, Tang ZY, Fan J, et al. A comparison of chemoembolization combination with and without radiotherapy for unresectable hepatocellular carcinoma. Cancer J. 2004;10:307–16.

VI

Chapter 22
Colorectal Cancer

Yao Yu, Mekhail Anwar, and Hans T. Chung

PEARLS

- Third most frequently diagnosed cancer and second leading cause of cancer death in the USA (Siegel 2016).
- Estimated annual incidence (2016): 95,270 colon cancers, 39,220 rectal cancers. Estimated annual cancer mortality (2016): 49,190 combined colon and rectal cancers.
- 3% of cases are attributable to HNPCC /Lynch syndrome.
- Microsatellite instability is detected in approximately 15% of sporadic cases.
- The rectum begins at the rectosigmoid junction at level of S3 vertebra. It is divided into three ~5 cm segments by transverse folds: upper, mid, and lower rectum. Cancer of the rectum is defined as those straddling or inferior to the peritoneal reflection.
- Rectal nodal drainage: superior half rectum drains to pararectal, sacral, sigmoidal, inferior mesenteric; inferior half rectum drains to internal iliacs; lower rectal tumors crossing the dentate line in the anal canal may drain to superficial inguinal nodes.
- Rectal metastases travel along portal drainage to liver via the superior rectal vein; pulmonary metastases can result from drainage via the middle and inferior rectal veins to the systemic circulation.
- Colon nodal drainage: left colon to inferior mesenteric; right colon to superior mesenteric. Periaortic nodes are at risk if cancer invades the retroperitoneum and external iliac nodes at risk if cancer invades adjacent pelvic organs.

VI

SCREENING

˒ Average risk persons (beginning age 50–75): colonoscopy q 10 years. Alternatives include guaiac fecal occult blood (annual), fecal immunochemical testing (annual), CT colonography (q5 years), flexible sigmoidoscopy (q5 years), combined flexible sigmoidoscopy + fecal immuno-chemical testing (USPSTF 2016).

˒ Inflammatory bowel disease: colonoscopy q1–2 years, initiate 8 years after symptom onset if pancolitis or 15 years after symptom onset if L-sided colitis (American Gastrointestinal Association).

˒ Family Hx (non-FAP/HNPCC): colonoscopy q1–5 years, initiate at age 40 years or 10 years prior to earliest cancer diagnosis in the family.

˒ FAP (lifetime cancer risk ~100% by age 50): APC genetic testing, early screening, colectomy, or proctocolectomy after onset of polyposis.

˒ HNPCC (lifetime colorectal cancer risk 10–70%, depending on mismatch repair status): colonoscopy q1–2 years, initiate at age 20–25 or 10 years younger than earliest cancer diagnosis in the family (Syngal 2015).

WORKUP

˒ H&P including DRE and complete pelvic exam in women. Note size, location, ulceration, mobile vs tethered vs fixed, and sphincter function on rectal exam.

˒ Labs including CBC, LFTs, CEA.

˒ Complete colonoscopy with endoscopic biopsy, pathology review.

˒ CT chest/abdomen/pelvis.

˒ MRI pelvis to assess T stage, distance from anal verge/sphincter, tumor location (low/mid/high), relationship to anterior peritoneal reflection (straddles/below), clock face involvement of tumor, mucinous, extramural depth of invasion, shortest distance to mesorectal fascia, extramural venous invasion, mesorectal nodes, and extramesorectal nodes. (Endoscopic ultrasound can also be used for determining T stage).

, For patients at high risk for obstruction, consider diversion surgery prior to neoadjuvant chemoRT.

STAGING: COLORECTAL CANCER

Editors' note: All TNM stage and stage groups referred to elsewhere in this chapter reflect the 2010 AJCC staging nomenclature unless otherwise noted as the new system below was published after this chapter was written.

VI

Table 22.1 (AJCC 7TH ED., 2010)

Primary tumor (T)

TX:	Primary tumor cannot be assessed
T0:	No evidence of primary tumor
Tis:	Carcinoma in situ: intraepithelial or invasion of lamina propria[a]
T1:	Tumor invades submucosa
T2:	Tumor invades muscularis propria
T3:	Tumor invades through the muscularis propria into pericolorectal tissues
T4a:	Tumor penetrates to the surface of the visceral peritoneum[b]
T4b:	Tumor directly invades or is adherent to other organs or structures[b, c]

[a]*Note*: Tis includes cancer cells confined within the glandular basement membrane (intraepithelial) or mucosal lamina propria (intramucosal) with no extension through the muscularis mucosae into the submucosa

[b]Note: Direct invasion in T4 includes invasion of other organs or other segments of the colorectum as a result of direct extension through the serosa, as confirmed on microscopic examination (e.g., invasion of the sigmoid colon by a carcinoma of the cecum) or, for cancers in a retroperitoneal or subperitoneal location, direct invasion of other organs or structures by virtue of extension beyond the muscularis propria (i.e., respectively, a tumor on the posterior wall of the descending colon invading the left kidney or lateral abdominal wall or a mid or distal rectal cancer with invasion of prostate, seminal vesicles, cervix, or vagina)

[c]*Note*: Tumor that is adherent to other organs or structures, grossly, is classified cT4b. However, if no tumor is present in the adhesion, microscopically, the classification should be pT1-4a depending on the anatomical depth of wall invasion. The V and L classifications should be used to identify the presence or absence of vascular or lymphatic invasion, whereas the PN site-specific factor should be used for perineural invasion

continued

Table 22.1 (continued)

Regional lymph nodes (N)

NX:	Regional lymph nodes cannot be assessed
N0:	No regional lymph node metastasis
N1:	Metastasis in 1–3 regional lymph nodes
N1a:	Metastasis in one regional lymph node
N1b:	Metastasis in 2–3 regional lymph nodes
N1c:	Tumor deposit(s) in the subserosa, mesentery, or nonperitonealized pericolic or perirectal tissues without regional nodal metastasis
N2:	Metastasis in four or more regional lymph nodes
N2a:	Metastasis in 4–6 regional lymph nodes
N2b:	Metastasis in seven or more regional lymph nodes

Note: A satellite peritumoral nodule in the pericolorectal adipose tissue of a primary carcinoma without histologic evidence of residual lymph node in the nodule may represent discontinuous spread, venous invasion with extravascular spread (V1/2), or a totally replaced lymph node (N1/2)

Replaced nodes should be counted separately as positive nodes in the N category, whereas discontinuous spread or venous invasion should be classified and counted in the site-specific factor category tumor deposits (TD)

Distant metastasis (M)

M0:	No distant metastasis
M1:	Distant metastasis
M1a:	Metastasis confined to one organ or site (e.g., liver, lung, ovary, nonregional node)
M1b:	Metastases in more than one organ/site or the peritoneum

Anatomic stage/prognostic groups

Stage	T	N	M	Dukes*	MAC*
0	Tis	N0	M0	–	–
I:	T1	N0	M0	A	A
IIA:	T2	N0	M0	A	B1
IIB:	T3	N0	M0	B	B2
IIC:	T4a	N0	M0	B	B2
IIIA:	T4b	N0	M0	B	B3
IIIB:	T1–T2	N1/N1c	M0	C	C1
IIIC:	T1	N2a	M0	C	C1
IVA:	T3–T4a	N1/N1c	M0	C	C2
IVB:	T2–T3	N2a	M0	C	C1/C2
	T1–T2	N2b	M0	C	C1
	T4a	N2a	M0	C	C2
	T3–T4a	N2b	M0	C	C2
	T4b	N1–N2	M0	C	C3
	Any T	Any N	M1a	–	–
	Any T	Any N	M1b	–	–

Note: cTNM is the clinical classification, pTNM is the pathologic classification. The *y* prefix is used for those cancers that are classified after neoadjuvant pretreatment (e.g., ypTNM). Patients who have a complete pathologic response are ypT0N0cM0 that may be similar to Stage Group 0 or I. The *r* prefix is to be used for those cancers that have recurred after a disease-free interval (rTNM)

˙Dukes B is a composite of better (T3 N0 M0) and worse (T4 N0 M0) prognostic groups, as is Dukes C (any TN1 M0 and any T N2 M0). MAC is the modified Astler-Coller classification˙

Used with the permission from the American Joint Committee on Cancer (AJCC), Chicago, Illinois. The original source for this material is the AJCC Cancer Staging Manual, Seventh Edition (2010), published by Springer Science+Business Media

Table 22.2 (AJCC 8TH ED., 2017)

Definitions of AJCC TNM

Definition of primary tumor (T)

T category	T criteria
TX	Primary tumor cannot be assessed
T0	No evidence of primary tumor
Tis	Carcinoma in situ and intramucosal carcinoma (involvement of lamina propria with no extension through muscularis mucosae)
T1	Tumor invades the submucosa (through the muscularis mucosa but not into the muscularis propria)
T2	Tumor invades the muscularis propria
T3	Tumor invades through the muscularis propria into pericolorectal tissues

T category	T criteria
T4	Tumor invades the visceral peritoneum or invades or adheres to adjacent organ or structure
T4a	Tumor invades through the visceral peritoneum (including gross perforation of the bowel through tumor and continuous invasion of tumor through areas of inflammation to the surface of the visceral peritoneum)
T4b	Tumor directly invades or adheres to adjacent organs or structures

DEFINITION OF REGIONAL LYMPH NODE (N)

N category	N criteria
NX	Regional lymph nodes cannot be assessed
N0	No regional lymph node metastasis
N1	One to three regional lymph nodes are positive (tumor in lymph nodes measuring ≥0.2 mm), or any number of tumor deposits is present, and all identifiable lymph nodes are negative
N1a	One regional lymph node is positive
N1b	Two or three regional lymph nodes are positive
N1c	No regional lymph nodes are positive, but there are tumor deposits in the: • subserosa • mesentery • or nonperitonealized pericolic or perirectal/mesorectal tissues

continued

VI

N2	Four or more regional nodes are positive
N2a	Four to six regional lymph nodes are positive
N2b	Seven or more regional lymph nodes are positive

DEFINITION OF DISTANT METASTASIS (M)

M category	M criteria
M0	No distant metastasis by imaging, etc.; no evidence of tumor in distant sites or organs (this category is not assigned by pathologists)
M1	Metastasis to one or more distant sites or organs, or peritoneal metastasis is identified

M category	M criteria
M1a	Metastasis to one site or organ is identified without peritoneal metastasis
M1b	Metastasis to two or more sites or organs is identified without peritoneal metastasis
M1c	Metastasis to the peritoneal surface is identified alone or with other site or organ metastases

AJCC PROGNOSTIC STAGE GROUPS

When T is...	And N is...	And M is...	Then the stage group is...
Tis	N0	M0	0
T1, T2	N0	M0	I
T3	N0	M0	IIA
T4a	N0	M0	IIB
T4b	N0	M0	IIC
T1–T2	N1/N1c	M0	IIIA
T1	N2a	M0	IIIA
T3–T4a	N1/N1c	M0	IIIB
T2–T3	N2a	M0	IIIB
T1–T2	N2b	M0	IIIB
T4a	N2a	M0	IIIC
T3–T4a	N2b	M0	IIIC
T4b	N1–N2	M0	IIIC
Any T	Any N	M1a	IVA
Any T	Any N	M1b	IVB
Any T	Any N	M1c	IVC

TREATMENT RECOMMENDATIONS

SURGICAL PRINCIPLES

ˌ Transanal excision may be considered for favorable cT1N0 patients. Criteria: <3 cm size, <30% circumferential involvement, within 8 cm of anal verge, well-moderately differentiated, not fixed, margin >3 mm, no LVSI or PNI.

ˌ Transabdominal resection of rectal cancers

   ˌ Total mesorectal excision and sharp dissection of the entire mesorectum are the standard of care to reduce positive radial margin rate and to remove draining nodes. It generally extends 4–5 cm below distal edge of tumor, but for distal tumors <5 cm from the anal verge, 1–2 cm negative bowel margin may be acceptable.

   ˌ Low-anterior resection is used for mid-upper lesions and selected lower lesions; otherwise abdominoperineal resection is used for lower lesions.

   ˌ Biopsy or resection of clinically suspicious nodes beyond the field of resection is indicated when possible.

   ˌ Surgery is generally performed 5–12 weeks following neoadjuvant chemoRT.

ˌ For colon cancers, colectomy with en bloc removal of regional nodes is preferred. Minimum 12 LN should be examined to establish N stage. Consider more extensive colectomy for patients with a strong family history of colon cancer or young age < 50 years.

VI

Table 22.3 TREATMENT RECOMMENDATIONS

Stage	Rectal cancer	~5-year LF/OS
I	Favorable T1N0 lesions may be treated with transanal minimally invasive surgery alone. See criteria above Following local excision, favorable T1 lesions may be observed, whereas high-risk features (T2, positive margins, LVI, poorly differentiated) should receive adjuvant chemoRT (45–50.4 Gy in 1.8 Gy fractions) or LAR or APR If not appropriate for transanal excision, TME with APR (low lesions) or LAR (mid-upper lesions). If pT1-2N0, no adjuvant treatment	<5% LF 90% OS
II/III pre-op	Pre-op chemoRT (50.4 Gy/28 fx + capecitabine or infusional 5-FU) → LAR/APR → adjuvant 5-FU-based therapy (FOLFOX or CAPEOX preferred) Pre-op RT (25 Gy/5 fx) → LAR/APR → adjuvant 5-FU-based therapy (FOLFOX or CAPEOX preferred) Pre-op chemo and then chemoRT (FOLFOX or CAPEOX → chemoRT) → LAR or APR Ongoing clinical trials (PROSPECT) are investigating neoadjuvant chemotherapy alone for patients with high tumors with intermediate risk for LR, as well nonoperative management for patients who would be ineligible for sphincter preservation	pCR ~10% pCR vs no pCR[a] 2.8 vs 9.7% LF 87.6 vs 76.4% OS
II/III post-op	Adjuvant FOLFOX or CAPEOX x 2 cycles → chemoRT (50.4-55.8 Gy + capecitabine or infusional 5-FU) → additional FOLFOX or CAPEOX x 2 cycles	T3N0, T1-2N1: 5–10% LF 75–80% OS T4N0, T3N1, T1-2N2: 10–15% LF 50–60% OS T4N1, T3/4N2: 15–20% LF 40% OS
T4 unresectable	Consider diverting colostomy if near or total obstruction Consider induction FOLFOX ChemoRT (55.8 – 59.4 Gy + capecitabine or 5-FU) → resection (if possible) At the time of resection, consider IORT or brachytherapy boost for gross residual disease All patients should receive adjuvant FOLFOX or CAPEOX as tolerated	

Table 22.3 (continued)

IV oligometastatic	Care should be individualized with coordination between systemic, locally directed, and metastasis-directed therapy Induction chemotherapy (e.g., CAPEOX, FOLFOX, FOLIRI) followed by response assessment with restaging Often treat primary with chemoRT and/or resection Staged or synchronous treatment of liver or lung metastasis (resection preferred, or SBRT) Adjuvant systemic therapy
Pelvic recurrence	Individualized options. If no prior pelvic RT, then pre-op chemoRT (50.4 Gy/28 fx + capecitabine or 5-FU), followed by surgery ± IORT or brachytherapy. If prior pelvic RT, then surgery or pre-op chemoRT (30 Gy in 1.2 Gy bid or 30.6 Gy/17 fx + capecitabine or 5-FU) → surgery ± IORT or brachytherapy as appropriate

VI

Stage	Colon cancer[b]
I	Colectomy + LND
II	Colectomy + LND. For adverse pathologic features, consider adjuvant chemo for 0-5% survival benefit (e.g., <12 LN analyzed, LVSI, PNI, close/+ margins). Stage II patients with high microsatellite instability have good prognosis and do not benefit from adjuvant chemo
III	Colectomy + LND followed by adjuvant chemo (FOLFOX or CAPEOX preferred)
IV	Individualize treatment. Consider resection and neoadjuvant/adjuvant chemo

[a]Maas 2010
[b]No clear OS/LC benefit with post-op RT in colon CA. May consider post-op RT if close/+ margins and tumor bed can be clearly identified

STUDIES

RECTAL

Pre-op RT vs Surgery Alone

- Pre-operative RT improves survival for patients with locally advanced disease treated without total mesorectal excision.
- For patients treated with total mesorectal excision, the baseline risk for local recurrence is reduced and pre-op RT improves local control but not survival.
- *Dutch TME* (Kapiteijn NEJM 2001, Peeters JCO 2005, Peeters Ann Surg 2007, van Gijn Lancet Oncol 2011): Phase III. 1861 patients with resectable rectal CA randomized to pre-op RT (25 Gy/5 fx) and surgery vs surgery alone (TME surgery). Pre-op RT improved 5-year LR (5.6% vs 10.9%) and 10-year LR (5% vs 11%). RT reduced cancer-specific survival but not overall survival. Subset analyses showed improved survival for patients with stage III disease and negative circumferential resection margins. At 5 years, RT increased fecal incontinence (62% vs 38%), pad wearing, bleeding (11% vs 3%), and mucous discharge.
- *Swedish Rectal Cancer Trial* (NEJM 1997; Folkesson JCO 2005): Phase III. 1168 patients with resectable rectal CA randomized to pre-op RT (25 Gy/5 fx) and surgery vs surgery alone (non-TME). Pre-op RT improved 5-year LR (11% vs 27%) and 5-year OS (58% vs 48%). Thirteen-year OS was 38% vs 30% favoring RT.

Pre-op vs Post-op ChemoRT

- Compared with post-op RT, pre-op RT reduces risk of local recurrence, increases sphincter preservation, and decreases toxicity. However, some patients may receive unnecessary radiation, as up to 20% of patients are overstaged.
- *German Rectal Cancer Study Group* (Sauer NEJM 2004, JCO 2012): Phase III. 823 patients with T3/4 or N+ rectal CA randomized to pre-op (50.4 Gy + 5-FU) vs post-op chemoRT (54 Gy + 5-FU). All patients received an additional 4 cycles of bolus 5-FU. Pre-op chemoRT improved 5-year LR rate (6% vs 13%), increased sphincter

preservation (39% vs 19%), and decreased grade 3–4 acute and late toxicity and late anastomotic strictures. Twenty-five percent of pre-op group compared to 40% post-op had positive LN, and there was pCR in 8% of pre-op group. In post-op arm, 18% of initially eligible patients were over-staged and excluded due to finding of pT1-2N0 disease at time of surgery. No difference in survival.

, *MRC CR07/NCIC-CTG C016* (Sebag-Montefiore Lancet 2009, Quirke Lancet 2009): Phase III. 1350 patients with resectable rectal CA randomized to short-course pre-op RT (25 Gy/5fx) + surgery vs surgery + selective post-op chemoRT (45 Gy and 5-FU) for patients with positive radial margins. Pre-op RT reduced 3-year LR (4.4% vs 10.6%). No difference in OS. In a substudy, patients were stratified by the surgical plane. 3-year LRR was 4% (meso-rectal), 7% (intramesorectal), and 13% (muscularis pro-pria). All groups benefited from pre-op RT.

, *NSABP R-03* (Roh JCO 2009): Phase III, closed early due to poor accrual. Confirmed findings of the German Rectal Cancer Study. 267 patients with T3/4 or N+ rectal cancer randomized to pre-op chemoRT or post-op RT (50.4 Gy + 5-FU/LV). Both arms received TME and addi-tional adjuvant chemo. 5-year DFS was improved with pre-op chemoRT (64.7% vs 53.4%), and there was a trend toward improved OS (74.5% vs 65.6%). Among node-pos-itive patients, 5-year OS was improved (66.7% vs 52.5%). 15% pCR rate with pre-op chemoRT. Risk of local recur-rence was 10% in both arms with long-term follow-up.

Pre-op RT vs Pre-op ChemoRT

, Pre-op chemoRT increased the rate of pCR (~5 vs 15%) and LC (~80–85% vs 90%), but not sphincter preservation (~50%) or OS (~65%) compared with pre-op RT alone.

, *French FFCD 9203* (Gerard, JCO 2006): 733 eligible patients with T3-4 N0 resectable adenocarcinoma of the rectum randomized to pre-op RT (45 Gy/25 fx) vs pre-op concurrent RT + bolus 5-FU and LV d1–5 weeks 1 and 5. All patients had adjuvant 4c of FU-LV chemo. Pre-op chemoRT increased pCR (4% vs 11%) and LC (83% vs 92%), but also grade 3–4 toxicity (3% vs 15%). No differ-ence in sphincter saving surgery (52%), EFS, or OS (67%).

VI

, *EORTC 22921* (Bosset, JCO 2005, NEJM 2006, Lancet Oncol 2014): 1011 patients with resectable T3/4 rectal CA randomized in 2x2 fashion to pre-op RT vs pre-op chemoRT, adjuvant chemo vs observation. RT consisted of 45 Gy and chemo consisted of 5-FU and leucovorin (pre-op chemo x 2 cycles, post-op chemo x 4 cycles). 5-year LRR reduced for chemoRT groups (10.7–13.7%) vs RT alone group (21.9%); chemoRT increased the likelihood of pCR (5% vs 14%). With long-term follow-up post-operative chemotherapy did not improve 10-year DFS or OS.

Pre-op Short-Course vs Pre-op Long-Course ChemoRT

, Although three randomized trials failed to show a significant difference, these trials had modest sample sizes, which limit their ability to detect small differences between groups. In the USA, long-course chemoRT remains favored due to their ability to give concurrent chemotherapy, improved sphincter preservation, and tumor regression. New trials evaluating sequential neoadjuvant short-course RT and chemotherapy are ongoing.

, *Polish* (Bujko Br J Surg 2006, Pietrzak Radiother Oncol 2007): Phase III trial. 312 patients with T3/4 resectable rectal CA randomized to pre-op RT (25 Gy/5fx) + surgery vs pre-op chemoRT (50.4 Gy with bolus 5-FU and leucovorin) + surgery. Early toxicity was higher in the chemoRT group (18.2% vs 3.2%). ChemoRT did not increase OS, LC, or late toxicity compared to short-course RT alone. Patients treated with chemoRT were likely to have higher pCR rates and lower pathologic stage and had lower rates of radial margin involvement.

, *TROG 01.04* (Ngan JCO 2012): Phase III. 326 patients with T3N0-2 low rectal cancer randomized between short-course RT vs long-course chemoRT. All patients received adjuvant chemotherapy. 3-year LR rates were nonsignificantly reduced with long-course CRT (7.5% vs 4.4%, p = 0.24). There was no difference in distant recurrence or overall survival.

, *Stockholm III* (Pettersson BJS 2010, BJS 2015): Phase III. 303 patients randomized to short-course RT (25 Gy/5 fx) and early surgery (within 1 week), short-course and delayed surgery (after 4–8 weeks), and long-course RT (50 Gy/2 fx). The post-op complication rates were 46%, 40%, and 32% for the arms, respectively (p = 0.164).

Among patients receiving short-course RT, patients in the delayed surgery arm had lower ypT stages, higher rates of pCR (11.8% vs 1.7%), and higher likelihood of tumor regression (10.1% vs 1.7%).

- *Polish* (Bujko Ann Onc 2016): Phase III. 515 patients randomized to pre-op sequential short-course RT (25 Gy/5 fx) + FOLFOX4 vs pre-op long-course chemoRT (50.4 Gy/28 fx with 5-FU). Short-course RT-FOLFOX was associated with lower rates of acute toxicity (75% vs 83%; driven by grade I–II toxicity), higher rates of R0 resection (77% vs 71%, p = 0.07). pCR rates were 16% vs 12% (p = 0.17). 3-year OS higher with short-course RT (73% vs 65%, p = 0.046); however, DFS, LR, and DM were not different. Post-op complication (29% vs 25%, p = 0.18) and late complications (20% vs 22%) were not different.

VI

Post-op Chemo, RT, and/or ChemoRT

- Post-op RT improves LC. Post-op chemo improves LC and OS. Infusional 5-FU during RT improves OS compared with bolus 5-FU.
- *GITSG 7175* (Thomas Radiother Oncol 1988): 227 patients with stage B2-C rectal CA randomized post-operatively to no adjuvant therapy vs chemo alone vs RT alone vs concurrent chemoRT. ChemoRT arm improved 5-year DFS and OS over control.
- *NSABP R01* (Fisher JNCI 1988): 555 patients with B–C (II–III) rectal cancer treated with surgery alone vs post-op RT (46–47 Gy) vs post-op chemo (5-FU, semustine, vincristine). RT improved LF (25% vs 16%), but did not improve DFS or OS. Post-op chemo improved DFS (30% vs 42%) and OS (43% vs 53%) compared with observation.
- *NCCTG 79-47-51* (Krook NEJM 1991): 204 patients with T3/4 or LN+ (B2-C) randomized to post-op RT (45–50.4 Gy) vs chemoRT (bolus 5-FU concurrent). ChemoRT improved LF (14% vs 25%), DM, DFS, and OS (58% vs 48%) vs RT alone.
- *Intergroup/NCCTG* (O'Connell NEJM 1994): 660 patients with stage II or III rectal CA underwent chemo, chemoRT, and further adjuvant chemo. 2x2 randomization of bolus vs infusional 5-FU during radiation and 5-FU ± semustine. Infusional 5-FU improved 4-year OS (70% vs 60%)

and relapse-free rate (63% vs 53%). No benefit with semustine.

, *NSABP R02* (Wolmark JNCI 2000): 694 patients with Dukes' B–C (II–III) treated with surgery, randomized to post-op chemo (5-FU/LV vs MOF) vs chemoRT. Post-op RT reduced 5-year LF (8% vs 14%), but there was no difference in DFS or OS. 5-FU/LV improved DFS but not OS compared with MOF.

, *Pooled analysis* (Gunderson, JCO 2004): Pooled rectal analysis of 3791 patients on NCCTG trials, Int 0144, NSABP R01, and R02. Increasing T and N stage negatively impacted survival, but N stage alone does not determine survival. For intermediate-risk patients, post-op chemo appeared to improve OS after surgery (to ~85%), similar to post-op chemoRT. For moderately high-risk and high-risk patients, DFS, OS, and LF tended to be better with chemoRT than with chemo alone.

Table 22.4 Outcomes by Stage

Pooled analysis risk groups	~5-year OS	~DFS	~LR	~DM
Low T1-2N0	90%	90%	<5%	10%
Intermediate T1-2N1, T3N0	80% (75–85%)	75% (65–80%)	5–10%	15–20%
Moderately high T1-2N2, T3N1, T4N0	60% (40–80%)	55% (45–60%)	10–20% C only > 15% CRT 10–15%	30–35%
High T3N2, T4N+	40% (25–60%)	30–35%	15–20% C only > 20% CRT <20%	> 40%

FUTURE DIRECTIONS

ORGAN PRESERVATION/NONOPERATIVE THERAPY

, Limited clinical series report favorable results with nonoperative management among select patients who achieve a clinical CR with chemoradiotherapy. Local recurrence risk after chemoRT without surgery is about 26–38%. Many, but not all, patients can be salvaged with subsequent surgery. Additional clinical trials are ongoing (e.g., OPRA NCT02008656).

, *Sao Paulo* (Habr-Gama IJROBP 2014): Single-institution retrospective. 183 patients with cT2-4 or N+ disease were treated with neoadjuvant chemoRT (50.4–54 Gy + 5-FU), with planned response assessment at 8 weeks. Patients with less than cCR underwent TME surgery; those with cCR were enrolled on a nonoperative management arm, reserving surgery for salvage. 90 (49%) patients achieved cCR. Of these, the 5-year LRFS rate was 69% and salvage therapy was possible in 93% of failures (primarily R0 resection).

, *Danish* (Appelt Lancet Oncol 2015): Single-institution phase I/II trial. 55 patients treated with high-dose chemoRT (60Gy/30 fx to tumor, 50 Gy/30 fx to elective nodes, 5 Gy endorectal brachytherapy boost + oral tegafur-uracil). 40 patients achieved cCR at 6-week response assessment and were allocated watchful waiting, the remainder underwent surgery. 2-year LR was 25.9% (9 patients), and all underwent successful salvage surgery with clear margins.

, *UK* (Renehan, Lancet Oncol 2016). 129 patients treated with pre-op chemoRT 45 Gy with fluoropyrimidine-based chemo had clinical CR and were observed. 3-year LR 38%. 88% of nonmetastatic local failures were salvaged. Compared to matched cohort who had surgical resection, a greater portion of patients watched after CR after chemoRT were colostomy free at 3 years (74% vs 47%).

VI

SELECTIVE RADIATION

, Early clinical data suggest high rates of response following full-dose neoadjuvant chemotherapy with modern systemic agents (FOLFOX, FOLFOX + Bev). A multi-institutional phase II/III clinical trial of neoadjuvant FOLFOX with selective radiation is underway for patients with high rectal tumors (PROSPECT, NCT01515787).

, *MSKCC Pilot (Schrag JCO 2014):* Phase II. 32 patients with stage II–III rectal cancer treated with neoadjuvant FOLFOX + Bev x 6 cycles. 2 patients who could not complete chemo received neoadjuvant chemoRT (50.4 Gy + 5-FU); the remaining 30 patients had treatment response and didn't receive RT. 25% of patients achieved pCR. No patients experienced LR, and 4-year DFS was 84%.

- *GEMCAD 0801 (Fernandez-Martos Oncologist 2014):* Phase I/II multi-institutional. 46 patients with intermediate-risk T3N0 disease were treated with neoadjuvant FOLFOX + Bev x 4 cycles. Two patients died during neoadjuvant chemotherapy (PE, diarrhea), and one died post-operatively due to anastomotic leak. The rate of anastomotic leak was 13%. 44 patients underwent R0 resection. At 2-years, LR was 2% and DFS was 75%. High rate of toxicity in multi-institutional setting.

LOCAL EXCISION

- Local excision can be considered for sphincter preservation in patients with low-risk cT1 N0 low-lying rectal cancers (<8 cm from anal verge). Patients with pT1 disease with high-risk pathologic features (positive margins, LVI, poorly differentiated, or more than 2/3 of submucosal invasion) or pT2 after WLE should receive adjuvant therapy due to high risk of LR (> 15%) and pelvic nodal involvement, or LAR/APR.
- *RTOG 89-02* (Russell, IJROBP 2000): 65 patients in phase II trial of sphincter-sparing local excision for low-lying rectal tumors ≤4 cm, ≤40% circumference, mobile, N0 status. 51 higher-risk patients also received post-op chemoRT. RT dose 45–50 Gy with boost to total 50–65 Gy. Five-year OS 78%, 11 patients failed. LRF correlated with T stage (T1 4%, T2 16%, T3 23%) and percentage of rectal circumference involved. DM correlated with T stage.
- *MDACC* (Bonnen, IJROBP 2004): 26 patients with T3 rectal cancer refused APR after pre-op chemoRT and were treated with WLE. 54% had pCR, 35% had micro residual, and 12% had gross residual disease. Only 2/26 (6%) pelvic failures.
- Cochrane Review (Borstlap BJS 2016): Meta-analysis of patients with cT1/2 rectal adenocarcinomas treated with local excision followed by completion TME vs adjuvant (chemo-)radiation. 14 studies with 405 patients treated with excision followed by (chemo-) radiation and 7 studies with 130 patients treated with completion TME were included. Local recurrence rates for adjuvant (chemo-) radiation vs completion TME were 10% vs 6% for T1 tumors and 15% vs 10% for T2 tumors (nonsignificant).

, MSKCC (Nash Dis Rec Col 2009): Single-institution retrospective study of 145 radical resections and 137 transanal excisions for T1 rectal cancer (1985–2004). Transanal excision was used more often for older patients, smaller tumors, and tumors closer to the anal verge. 20% of radical resections harbored subclinical nodal metastases. Compared with radical surgery, transanal surgery was associated with inferior local control (13.2% vs 2.7%), 5-year DFS (87% vs 96%). The authors concluded that transanal excision should only be offered for very selected patients with major contraindications.

RECURRENT DISEASE

, Kentucky (Mohiuddin, Cancer 2002): Single-institution retrospective series of 103 patients with rectal cancer, who had previously received 5-FU + 50.4 Gy to the pelvis, who were subsequently treated with reirradiation, 34.8 Gy (range 15–49.2 Gy), following median interval of 19 months. 34 patients also subsequently underwent resection for residual disease. 5-year survival was 19%. 22 patients developed late complications: 18 developed persistent severe diarrhea, 15 developed small bowel obstruction, 4 developed fistulas, 2 developed coloanal strictures.

, Pooled analysis (Holman, Eur J Surg Oncol 2017). Results of 256 patients with locally recurrent rectal cancers (previously received neoadjuvant chemoradiation for their primary tumors) treated with intra-operative electron radiation therapy (IOERT) and surgical resection at the Mayo Clinic Rochester and the Catharina Hospital Eindhoven were pooled. The median reirradiation dose was 30 Gy (range 5–39.6 Gy), with most receiving concurrent 5-FU-based chemotherapy. Mean interval between completion of neoadjuvant therapy and surgery with IOERT was 41 days. The IOERT dose ranged from 15 to 20 Gy, using 8–12 MeV electrons. 3-year local re-recurrence rate was 46%.

COLON

, Surgical resection and adjuvant chemotherapy is the standard of care as distant metastases are the dominant mode of failure (Moertel 1969, André 2009). Patients with T4

VI

disease represent a subset at high risk of local failure. However, a single randomized trial enrolling primarily patients with T4 disease did not demonstrate a benefit.

- *INT0130 Trial* (Martenson JCO 2004): 222 patients with resected T3N1-N2 or T4 (80%) colon CA randomized to chemo vs chemoRT. RT given as 45 Gy ± 5.4 boost to tumor bed. No difference in survival or local recurrence. Underpowered, 80% chance to detect a 75% decrease in death.
- *MGH* (Willett JCO 1993): Retrospective. 203 patients with high-risk colon cancer treated with surgery and post-op RT ± 5-FU, compared with 395 patients treated with surgery alone. Patients with B3, C3, and cancer and those with abscess or fistula had improved LF and RFS.

RADIATION TECHNIQUES

RECTAL CANCER

Simulation

- Supine. Radio-opaque marker to identify anus. Wire perineal scar if present; small bowel contrast optional, ensure bladder full. Historically, prone positioning was used to reduce small bowel dose; however supine treatment may be more reproducible, particularly if using IMRT. Consider prone position with belly board for obese patients with low-lying small bowel loops.
- Vac-Lok bag immobilization to ensure daily positioning.
- May consider vaginal dilator during simulation and treatment to reduce vaginal wall dose, but stable and reproducible position must be ensured.

TRADITIONAL FIELD DESIGN

- Rectal field designed to cover tumor or tumor bed with margin, mesorectal, presacral, and internal iliac nodes (if T4, external iliac nodes also included).
- 3D conformal technique is standard, generally with 3–4 fields.
- Please consult the RTOG anorectal contouring atlas for CTV.

- 3DCRT:
  - Whole pelvis (PA field) borders: superior = L5-S1; inferior = 3 cm below initial tumor volume or inferior obturator foramen, whichever most inferior; lateral = 1.5 cm outside pelvic inlet.
  - Whole pelvis (lateral fields) borders: posterior = behind bony sacrum; anterior = posterior pubic symphysis if T3 vs anterior pubic symphysis if T4. Corner blocks as needed.
  - Avoid flashing posterior skin, unless s/p APR (include perineal scar in all fields).
  - Tumor bed boost borders: tumor +2–3 cm margin superior/inferior/anterior; posterior border includes sacral hollow. Corner blocks used to protect small bowel.
- IMRT/VMAT technique may be considered as an option specially for the pelvic kidney and reirradiation for recurrent disease, unresectable/inoperable disease or need to cover inguinal nodes.
- For rectal cancers extending inferior to dentate line, inguinal nodes may be at risk and IMRT may be considered in this situation to decrease dose to the genitalia. There is no widespread consensus on whether elective inguinal RT is routinely necessary;

VI

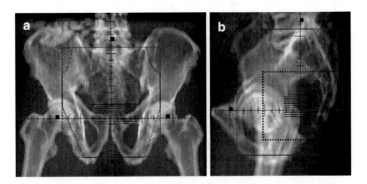

Fig. 22.1 (**a**) PA and (**b**) lateral DRRs of fields used to treat a T3 N0 rectal primary. The lateral boost field is indicated by the black dotted line. *Note*: radio-opaque markers not shown

> Yeo (Radiat Oncol 2014). Retrospective review of 189 patients with anal canal invasion (tumor within 3 cm of anal verge) vs 1057 patients without. All patients received pre-op or post-op chemoRT and surgery. Inguinal LN were not irradiated. 5 year inguinal recurrence 3.5% for anal canal invasion vs 0.2% if not present.

> IMRT may also be considered for patients requiring dose escalation or simultaneous integrated boost. However prospective data have not shown toxicity benefit.

> IORT: consider for close/+ microscopic margins, especially for T4 or recurrent CA.

> Brachytherapy: consider for macroscopic residual after pre-op chemoRT and resection.

CHEMO DURING RADIATION

> Concurrent infusional 5-FU-based therapy is given as 5-FU 225 mg/m^2 over 24 hrs 7 days/week during RT.

> Capecitabine 825 mg/m^2 twice daily is an acceptable alternative based upon randomized non-inferiority data (Hofheinz 2012, O'Connell 2014).

DOSE PRESCRIPTIONS

> Pre-op chemoRT:
>> Pelvis: 45 Gy/25 fx.
>> Tumor bed boost: 5.4 Gy/3 fx.
>> Alternatively, IMRT with simultaneous integrated boost, 45 Gy to pelvis and 50 Gy to tumor + margin in 25 fx.

> Pre-op short-course pelvic RT: 25 Gy in 5 fx.

> Post-op chemoRT: 45–50.4 Gy to pelvis, boost tumor bed additional 5.4–9 Gy.

> Unresectable/inoperable chemoRT:
>> Pelvis to 45 Gy, boost primary to 55.8–59.4 Gy.
>> Consider IMRT to limit small bowel dose. 45 Gy to the whole pelvis, 50.4 Gy to the primary and sacral hollow, 55.8–59.4 Gy to the primary tumor.

> IORT: Dose individualized. After 45–54 Gy, typically 10–12.5 Gy IORT for R0–R1 resection or 15–20 Gy for R2 resection.

DOSE LIMITATIONS (STANDARD FRACTIONATION)
- Small bowel <45–50 Gy
- Femoral head and neck <42 Gy
- Bladder <65 Gy
- Rectum <60 Gy
- IMRT dose constraints per RTOG 0822 (Hong 2015)

RADIATION TECHNIQUES: COLON CANCER
- No clear evidence of benefit with RT. However, RT may be useful in the setting of node-negative disease with close/+ microscopic margins at the primary site, where a target can be clearly demarcated. If RT is included in treatment regimen, field should include margin around tumor bed based on pre-op imaging and/or surgical clips.
- Dose 45–50.4 Gy in 25–28 fx.

VI

COMPLICATIONS
- Potential side effects include diarrhea, dysuria, fatigue, skin irritation, and hematologic toxicity. Long-term GI complications include change in bowel habits, rectal urgency, diarrhea, anastomotic stricture, and small bowel obstruction. Women are at risk for sterility, early menopause, and vaginal stenosis. Men should be counseled about infertility and given information about sperm banking.
- Check weekly CBC and skin reaction on treatment.

FOLLOW-UP
- HP, CEA every 3 months x 2 years, then every 6 months x5 years.
- Consider CT scan if high risk of recurrence approximately every 4–6 months. Recurrence commonly occurs within 2 years after initial therapy. However, late failures even beyond 5 years have been noted after local excision.
- Colonoscopy in 1 year, then every 2–3 years if negative.

Acknowledgment We thank Marc B. Nash MD, Kavita K. Mishra MD, MPH, and Richard Krieg, MD, for their work on prior editions of this chapter.

REFERENCES

André T, et al. Improved overall survival with oxaliplatin, fluorouracil, and leucovorin as adjuvant treatment in stage II or III colon cancer in the MOSAIC trial. J Clin Oncol. 2009;27:3109–16.

Appelt AL, et al. High-dose chemoradiotherapy and watchful waiting for distal rectal cancer: a prospective observational study. Lancet Oncol. 2015;16:919–27.

Bonnen M, et al. Long-term results using local excision after preoperative chemoradiation among selected T3 rectal cancer patients. Int J Radiat Oncol Biol Phys. 2004;60:1098–105.

Borstlap WAA, et al. Meta-analysis of oncological outcomes after local excision of pT1-2 rectal cancer requiring adjuvant (chemo)radiotherapy or completion surgery. Br J Surg. 2016;103:1105–16.

Bosset J-F, et al. Enhanced tumorocidal effect of chemotherapy with preoperative radiotherapy for rectal cancer: preliminary results--EORTC 22921. J Clin Oncol. 2005;23:5620–7.

Bosset J-F, et al. Chemotherapy with preoperative radiotherapy in rectal cancer. N Engl J Med. 2006;355:1114–23.

Bosset J-F, et al. Fluorouracil-based adjuvant chemotherapy after preoperative chemoradiotherapy in rectal cancer: long-term results of the EORTC 22921 randomised study. Lancet Oncol. 2014;15:184–90.

Bujko K, et al. Long-term results of a randomized trial comparing preoperative short-course radiotherapy with preoperative conventionally fractionated chemoradiation for rectal cancer. Br J Surg. 2006;93:1215–23.

Bujko K, et al. Long-course oxaliplatin-based preoperative chemoradiation versus 5 × 5 Gy and consolidation chemotherapy for cT4 or fixed cT3 rectal cancer: results of a randomized phase III study. Ann Oncol. 2016;27:834–42.

Fernández-Martos C, et al. Preoperative chemotherapy in patients with intermediate-risk rectal adenocarcinoma selected by high-resolution magnetic resonance imaging: the GEMCAD 0801 Phase II Multicenter Trial. Oncologist. 2014;19:1042–3.

Fisher B, et al. Postoperative adjuvant chemotherapy or radiation therapy for rectal cancer: results from NSABP protocol R-01. J Natl Cancer Inst. 1988;80:21–9.

Folkesson J, et al. Swedish Rectal Cancer Trial: long lasting benefits from radiotherapy on survival and local recurrence rate. J Clin Oncol. 2005;23:5644–50.

Gerard JP. Preoperative radiotherapy with or without concurrent fluorouracil and leucovorin in T3-4 rectal cancers: results of FFCD 9203. J Clin Oncol. 2006;24:4620–5.

Gunderson LL, et al. Impact of T and N stage and treatment on survival and relapse in adjuvant rectal cancer: a pooled analysis. J Clin Oncol. 2004;22:1785–96.

Habr-Gama A, et al. Local recurrence after complete clinical response and watch and wait in rectal cancer after neoadjuvant chemoradiation: impact of salvage therapy on local disease control. Int J Radiat Oncol Biol Phys. 2014;88:822–8.

Hofheinz R-D, et al. Chemoradiotherapy with capecitabine versus fluorouracil for locally advanced rectal cancer: a randomised, multicentre, non-inferiority, phase 3 trial. Lancet Oncol. 2012;13:579–88.

Holman FA, et al. Results of a pooled analysis of IOERT containing multimodality treatment for locally recurrent rectal cancer: results of 565 patients of two major treatment centres. Eur J Surg Oncol. 2017;43:107–17.

Hong TS, et al. NRG oncology radiation therapy oncology group 0822: a phase 2 study of preoperative chemoradiation therapy using intensity modulated radiation therapy in combination with capecitabine and oxaliplatin for patients with locally advanced rectal cancer. Int J Radiat Oncol Biol Phys. 2015;93:29–36.

Kapiteijn E, et al. Preoperative radiotherapy combined with total mesorectal excision for resectable rectal cancer. N Engl J Med. 2001;345:638–46.

Krook JE, et al. Effective surgical adjuvant therapy for high-risk rectal carcinoma. N Engl J Med. 1991;324:709–15.

Maas M, et al. Long-term outcome in patients with a pathological complete response after chemoradiation for rectal cancer: a pooled analysis of individual patient data. Lancet Oncol. 2010;11:835–44.

Martenson JA, et al. Phase III study of adjuvant chemotherapy and radiation therapy compared with chemotherapy alone in the surgical adjuvant treatment of colon cancer: results of intergroup protocol 0130. J Clin Oncol. 2004;22:3277–83.

Moertel CG, Childs DS, Reitemeier RJ, Colby MY, Holbrook MA. Combined 5-fluorouracil and supervoltage radiation therapy of locally unresectable gastrointestinal cancer. Lancet. 1969;2:865–7.

Mohiuddin M, Marks G, Marks J. Long-term results of reirradiation for patients with recurrent rectal carcinoma. Cancer. 2002;95:1144–50.

Nash GM, et al. Long-term survival after transanal excision of T1 rectal cancer. Dis Colon Rectum. 2009;52:577–82.

Ngan SY, et al. Randomized trial of short-course radiotherapy versus long-course chemoradiation comparing rates of local recurrence in patients with T3 rectal cancer: trans-tasman radiation oncology group trial 01.04. J Clin Oncol. 2012;30:3827–33.

O'Connell MJ, et al. Improving adjuvant therapy for rectal cancer by combining protracted-infusion fluorouracil with radiation therapy after curative surgery. N Engl J Med. 1994;331:502–7.

O'Connell MJ, et al. Capecitabine and oxaliplatin in the preoperative multimodality treatment of rectal cancer: surgical end points from National Surgical Adjuvant Breast and Bowel Project trial R-04. J Clin Oncol. 2014;32:1927–34.

Peeters KCMJ, et al. Late side effects of short-course preoperative radiotherapy combined with total mesorectal excision for rectal cancer: increased bowel dysfunction in irradiated patients--a Dutch colorectal cancer group study. J Clin Oncol. 2005;23:6199–206.

Peeters KCMJ, et al. The TME trial after a median follow-up of 6 years: increased local control but no survival benefit in irradiated patients with resectable rectal carcinoma. Ann Surg. 2007;246:693–701.

Pettersson D, et al. Interim analysis of the Stockholm III trial of preoperative radiotherapy regimens for rectal cancer. Br J Surg. 2010;97:580–7.

Pettersson, D. et al. Tumour regression in the randomized Stockholm III trial of radiotherapy regimens for rectal cancer. Br J Surg. 2015;102:972–8–discussion 978.

Pietrzak L, et al. Quality of life, anorectal and sexual functions after preoperative radiotherapy for rectal cancer: report of a randomised trial. Radiother Oncol. 2007;84:217–25.

Quirke P, et al. Effect of the plane of surgery achieved on local recurrence in patients with operable rectal cancer: a prospective study using data from the MRC CR07 and NCIC-CTG CO16 randomised clinical trial. Lancet. 2009;373:821–8.

Renehan AG, et al. Watch-and-wait approach versus surgical resection after chemoradiotherapy for patients with rectal cancer (the OnCoRe project): a propensity-score matched cohort analysis. Lancet Oncol. 2016;17:174–83.

Roh MS, et al. Preoperative multimodality therapy improves disease-free survival in patients with carcinoma of the rectum: NSABP R-03. J Clin Oncol. 2009;27:5124–30.

Russell AH, et al. Anal sphincter conservation for patients with adenocarcinoma of the distal rectum: long-term results of radiation therapy oncology group protocol 89-02. Int J Radiat Oncol Biol Phys. 2000;46:313–22.

VI

Sauer R, et al. Preoperative versus postoperative chemoradiotherapy for rectal cancer. N Engl J Med. 2004;351:1731–40.

Sauer R, et al. Preoperative versus postoperative chemoradiotherapy for locally advanced rectal cancer: results of the German CAO/ARO/AIO-94 randomized phase III trial after a median follow-up of 11 years. J Clin Oncol. 2012;30:1926–33.

Schrag D, et al. Neoadjuvant chemotherapy without routine use of radiation therapy for patients with locally advanced rectal cancer: a pilot trial. J Clin Oncol. 2014;32:513–8.

Sebag-Montefiore D, et al. Preoperative radiotherapy versus selective postoperative chemoradiotherapy in patients with rectal cancer (MRC CR07 and NCIC-CTG C016): a multicentre, randomised trial. Lancet. 2009;373:811–20.

Siegel RL, Miller KD, Jemal A. Cancer statistics, 2016. CA Cancer J Clin. 2016;66:7–30. 5.

Swedish Rectal Cancer Trial. Improved survival with preoperative radiotherapy in resectable rectal cancer. N Engl J Med. 1997;336:980–7.

Syngal, S. et al. ACG clinical guideline: genetic testing and management of hereditary gastrointestinal cancer syndromes. Am J Gastroenterol. 2015;110: 223–62–quiz 263.

Thomas PR, Lindblad AS. Adjuvant postoperative radiotherapy and chemotherapy in rectal carcinoma: a review of the gastrointestinal tumor study group experience. Radiother Oncol. 1988;13:245–52.

US Preventive Services Task Force, et al. Screening for solorectal cancer: US Preventive Services Task Force recommendation statement. JAMA. 2016;315:2564–75.

van Gijn W, et al. Preoperative radiotherapy combined with total mesorectal excision for resectable rectal cancer: 12-year follow-up of the multicentre, randomised controlled TME trial. Lancet Oncol. 2011;12:575–82.

Willett CG, Fung CY, Kaufman DS, Efird J, Shellito PC. Postoperative radiation therapy for high-risk colon carcinoma. J Clin Oncol. 1993;11:1112–7.

Wolmark N, et al. Randomized trial of postoperative adjuvant chemotherapy with or without radiotherapy for carcinoma of the rectum: National Surgical Adjuvant Breast and Bowel Project Protocol R-02. J Natl Cancer Inst. 2000;92:388–96.

Yeo SG, et al. Is elective inguinal radiotherapy necessary for locally advanced rectal adenocarcinoma invading anal canal? Radiat Oncol. 2014;9:296.

Chapter 23
Anal Cancer

Serah Choi, Hans T. Chung, and Mekhail Anwar

PEARLS

- 8,080 estimated new cases and 1,080 estimated deaths in the United States in 2016.
- 75–80% are squamous cell carcinoma (SCC); others are adenocarcinoma or melanoma.
- HPV: found in 85–95% and strongly associated with SCC and may be requisite for disease formation. High-grade anal intraepithelial lesions (HSIL) are precursors. In particular HPV-16, 18 as in cervical cancer.
- HPV vaccines in the United States: quadrivalent vaccine (HPV 6, 11, 16, and 18); 9-valent vaccine (HPV 6, 11, 16, 18, 31, 33, 45, 52, and 58); and bivalent vaccine (HPV 16 and 18).
- 11% of untreated HSIL progress to SCC; 50% progress with extensive disease of immunosuppression; with treatment, progression is reduced to 0.4%.
  - HIV positivity increases risk, likely through an association with immunodeficiency in the setting of HPV coinfection. Increased risk if CD4 < 200.
- Additional risk factors: >10 sexual partners, history of genital warts, receptive anal intercourse, chronic immunosuppression, and cigarette smoking.
- Anatomy: anal canal is 3–5 cm long. Extends from anal verge to the anorectal ring. The dentate line lies within the

anal canal and divides it by histology. Proximal to the dentate line is colorectal mucosa, distal to it is nonkeratinizing squamous epithelium. The dentate line contains transitional mucosa. Anal margin is a 5 cm ring of skin around the anus. Use CT to measure depth of inguinal nodes using the femoral vessels as a surrogate due to large variations.

ᵔ Anal margin tumors: may behave like skin cancers, and can be treated as skin cancers as long as there is no involvement of the anal sphincter, tumor is <2 cm, and moderately or well-differentiated, and resected with adequate margins

ᵔ Adenocarcinoma: higher local and distant recurrence rates with chemo-RT compared to SCC. Treatment similar to that of rectal cancer. Use 5-FU chemo-RT pre-op followed by APR.

ᵔ Lymph node drainage: superiorly (above dentate line) along hemorrhoidal vessels to perirectal and internal iliac nodes; inferior canal (below dentate line) and anal verge to inguinal nodes.

ᵔ Presentation: bleeding, anorectal pain/sensation of mass, altered bowel movements/rectal urgency, genital warts/condyloma, pruritus, asymptomatic.

WORKUP

ᵔ H&P. Include inguinal LN evaluation. Note anal sphincter tone, pain, bleeding, HIV risk factors, inflammatory bowel disease, prior RT. For women, a comprehensive gynecological exam should be performed. On DRE, note anal sphincter tone and tumor location (clock location prone or supine position, distance from verge, circumferential involvement, size, and superior extent).

ᵔ Labs: CBC, HIV test if any risk factors. CD4 count if HIV-positive.

ᵔ Proctoscopy with biopsy.

ᵔ May biopsy inguinal nodes if clinically suspicious. Only FNA, avoid open biopsy.

⌐ CT chest/abdomen and pelvic CT or MRI.

⌐ PET/CT is recommended as it is better than CT at detecting the primary tumor and is more sensitive at staging nodal disease (Winton, Br J Cancer 2009; Mistrangelo, IJROBP 2012; Cotter, IJROBP 2006; Schwarz, IJROBP 2008; Trautmann, Mol Imaging Biol 2005).

Table 23.1 STAGING (AJCC 7TH ED., 2010): ANAL CANAL

Primary tumor (T)

TX: Primary tumor cannot be assessed

T0: No evidence of primary tumor

Tis: Carcinoma in situ (Bowen's disease, high-grade squamous intraepithelial lesion (HSIL), anal intraepithelial neoplasia II–III (AIN II–III))

T1: Tumor 2 cm or less in greatest dimension

T2: Tumor more than 2 cm, but not more than 5 cm in greatest dimension

T3: Tumor more than 5 cm in greatest dimension

T4: Tumor of any size invades adjacent organ(s), e.g., vagina, urethra, and bladder[a]

[a]*Note*: Direct invasion of the rectal wall, perirectal skin, subcutaneous tissue, or the sphincter muscle(s) is not classified as T4

Regional lymph nodes (N)

NX: Regional lymph nodes cannot be assessed

N0: No regional lymph node metastasis

N1: Metastasis in perirectal lymph node(s)

N2: Metastasis in unilateral internal iliac and/or inguinal lymph node(s)

N3: Metastasis in perirectal and inguinal lymph nodes and/or bilateral internal iliac and/or inguinal lymph nodes

Distant metastasis (M)

M0: No distant metastasis

M1: Distant metastasis

Anatomical stage/prognostic groups

0: Tis N0 M0

I: T1 N0 M0

II: T2 N0 M0

  T3 N0 M0

IIIA: T1–T3 N1 M0

  T4 N0 M0

IIIB: T4 N1 M0

  Any T N2 M0

  Any T N3 M0

IV: Any T Any N M1

Used with the permission from the American Joint Committee on Cancer (AJCC), Chicago, Illinois. The original source for this material is the AJCC Cancer Staging Manual, Seventh Edition (2010), published by Springer Science+Business Media

VI

TABLE 23.2 (AJCC 8TH ED., 2017)
DEFINITION OF PRIMARY TUMOR (T)

T category	T criteria
TX	Primary tumor not assessed
T0	No evidence of primary tumor
Tis	High-grade squamous intraepithelial lesion (previously termed carcinoma in situ, Bowen disease, anal intraepithelial neoplasias II—III, high-grade anal intraepithelial neoplasia)
T1	Tumor <2 cm
T2	Tumor >2 cm but <5 cm
T3	Tumor >5 cm
T4	Tumor of any size invading adjacent organ(s), such as the vagina, urethra, or bladder

Used with permission of the American Joint Committee on Cancer (AJCC), Chicago, Illinois. The original and primary source for this information is the AJCC Cancer Staging Manual, Eighth Edition (2017) published by Springer International Publishing

Definition of Regional Lymph Node (N)	
N category	N criteria
NX	Regional lymph nodes cannot be assessed
N0	No regional lymph node metastasis
N1	Metastasis in inguinal, mesorectal, internal iliac, or external iliac nodes
N1a	Metastasis in inguinal, mesorectal, or internal iliac lymph nodes
N1b	Metastasis in external iliac lymph nodes
N1c	Metastasis in external iliac with any N1a nodes

DEFINITION OF DISTANT METASTASIS (M)

M category	M criteria
M0	No distant metastasis
M1	Distant metastasis

AJCC PROGNOSTIC STAGE GROUPS

When T is...	And N is...	And M is...	Then the stage group is...
Tis	N0	M0	0
T1	N0	M0	I
T1	N1	M0	IIIA
T2	N0	M0	IIA
T2	N1	M0	IIIA
T3	N0	M0	IIB

T3	N1	M0	IIIC
T4	N0	M0	IIIB
T4	N1	M0	IIIC
Any T	Any N	M1	IV

TREATMENT RECOMMENDATIONS

Table 23.3 **TREATMENT RECOMMENDATIONS**

Situations	Recommended treatments
Anal canal, stage I–III with intact sphincter	Concurrent chemo-RT with 5-FU/mitomycin C
Anal canal, recurrence	Abdominoperineal resection. Salvage rate ~50% after chemo-RT Inguinal node recurrence: groin dissection
Distant metastasis	5FU/cisplatin chemo. Consider local RT for palliation, in particular for pts with good PS and limited metastatic disease
Anal margin tumors	Wide local excision with ≥1 cm margin. Well-differentiated T1N0 can be observed with close follow-up. All others get definitive chemo-RT to primary with elective inguinal LN RT for T2-4 and poorly differentiated tumors. Include pelvic LN if involvement of anal canal above dentate line or node positive. Alternative is post-op RT or chemo-RT with inguinal management as above. Dose 45 Gy elective, 60 Gy to gross disease

VI

TRIALS

CHEMO-RT VS. RT

UKCCCR ACT I (Lancet 1996; Northover, Br J Cancer 2010): 585 pts with epidermoid cancer of anal canal or margin. RT: 45 Gy + boost (15 Gy EBRT or 25 Gy brachy) ± 5-FU + mitomycin C (MMC). 6-wk break in RT. Chemo-RT improved 3-yr LC (59% vs. 36%), but no significant change in 3-yr OS (65% vs. 58%). Poorer results with RT alone may be due to mandatory 6-wk break. 13-yr median follow-up: for every 100 pts treated with chemo-RT, 25.3 fewer pts with LRR and 12.5 fewer anal cancer deaths vs. 100 pts treated with RT alone. There was a 9.1% increase in nonanal cancer deaths in the first 5 yrs of chemo-RT, which disappeared by 10 yrs.

- *EORTC* (Bartelink, JCO 1997): 110 pts. T3-4N0-3 or T1-2N1-3. RT (45 Gy + 15–20 Gy boost) + concurrent chemo (bolus 5-FU + MMC) vs. RT alone. 6-wk break in RT, prior to boost. Chemo-RT improved CR rate (80% vs. 54%), 5-yr LC (68% vs. 50%), colostomy-free survival (72% vs. 40%), and PFS (61% vs. 43%). No difference in OS (57% vs. 52%). Poorer results with RT alone may again be due to mandatory 6-wk break.
- For pts ineligible for concurrent chemo, good results are achievable with RT alone:
  - Deniaud-Alexandre (IJROBP 2003). 305 pts treated with 45 Gy EBRT, 4–6 wk break, then boost of 20 Gy EBRT (279 pts) or brachy (17 pts). Only 19 pts received concurrent chemo. Complete response rate: T1 96%, T2 87%, T3 79%, and T4 44%. Salvage APR was used successfully for 44% of locally progressive tumors and 54% of local recurrences.

ROLE OF MITOMYCIN (MMC)

- *RTOG 87-04* (Flam, JCO 1996): 291 pts treated with 45 Gy + 5FU ± MMC. Median follow-up of 36 mos. If no CR at 6 wks, gave 9 Gy boost +5-FU/cisplatin. 5-FU given as bolus × 4 day starting d1, d29 (1000 mg/m^2/day). MMC given as 10 mg/m^2 bolus d1, d29. MMC improved CR rate (92% vs. 85%) and decreased 4-yr colostomy rate (9% vs. 22%). No difference in 4-yr OS (75 vs. 70%).

ROLE OF CISPLATIN

- *ACT II* (James, Lancet Oncol 2013): 940 pts with anal cancer [stage T1–T2 (50%), T3–T4 (43%); LN-(62%), LN+ (30%)] treated with 5-FU (1,000 mg/m^2/day on d1-4 and 29–32) and RT (50.4 Gy in 28 fx), randomized to either concurrent MMC (12 mg/m^2, d1) or cisplatin (60 mg/m^2 on d1 and 29), and also randomized to maintenance therapy (2c of cisplatin/5-FU weeks 11 and 14) 4 wks after chemo-RT or no maintenance therapy. No significant difference in complete response at 26 wks between MMC (90.5%) and cisplatin (89.6%) groups. Similar toxicity between the MMC (71%) and cisplatin (72%) groups. No significant difference in PFS between maintenance (74%) vs. nonmaintenance (73%) groups.

, Based on the above results and RTOG 98-11 (see below), 5-FU/MMC chemotherapy remains the standard of care.

, It remains unclear whether the 2nd dose of MMC improves efficacy or merely increases toxicity. Some phase III trials have used 2 cycles, while others have used 1 cycle. Retrospective series suggests similar outcomes with less toxicity with only 1 cycle (Yeung, Curr Oncol 2014; White, Radiother Oncol 2015).

VI

ROLE OF INDUCTION CHEMO

, No proven advantage to induction chemo exists; Results to 98-11 may indicate a disadvantage with neoadjuvant chemo.

, *RTOG 98-11* (Ajani, JAMA 2008; Gunderson, JCO 2012; Gunderson, IJROBP 2013): 644 pts, T2–T4, any N. Neoadjuvant cisplatin + 5-FU × 2 followed by concurrent cisplatin +5-FU × 2 and 45–59 Gy vs. concurrent 5-FU + mitomycin and 45–59 Gy. Worse colostomy rate in cisplatin arm (19%) vs. mitomycin arm (10%). At long-term FU, upfront RT + 5FU/MCC improved 5-yr DFS (68% vs. 58%) and OS (78% vs. 71%) vs. induction/concurrent 5FU/cisplatin + RT. T- and N-stage impacted outcomes. In 5FU/MMC arm:

, 3-yr colostomy: T2N0 9%, T3N0 12%, T4N0 20%, T2N+ 4%, T3N+ 19%, T4N+ 28%.

, 3-yr LRF: T2N0 10%, T3N0 22%, T4N0 27%, T2N+ 18%, T3N+ 38%, T4N+ 61%.

, 5-yr DFS: T2N0 80%, T3N0 60%, T4N0 65%, T2N+ 68%, T3N+ 43%, T4N+ 27%.

, *ACCORD 03 Trial* (Peiffert, JCO 2012): 283 pts with locally advanced anal cancer randomized to: (1) two induction chemo cycles (5-FU 800 mg/m²/d IV infusion, days 1–4 and 29–32; and cisplatin 80 mg/m² IV, on days 1 and 29), concomitant chemo-RT (45 Gy in 25 fxs/5 wks, 5-FU and cisplatin during wks 1–5), and standard-dose boost (15 Gy); (2) two induction chemo cycles, concomitant chemo-RT and high-dose boost (20–25 Gy); (3) concomitant chemo-RT and standard dose boost; and (4) concomitant chemo-RT and high-dose boost. Induction chemo or high-dose radiation boost did not improve 5-yr colostomy-free survival rates.

INFUSIONAL 5-FU VS. CAPECITABINE

- ˒ Capecitabine is a promising alternative to 5FU for anal cancer, but phase III data are needed.
- ˒ Phase II data with oral capecitabine concurrently with mitomycin and RT in anal cancer report overall low toxicity (Glynne-Jones, IJROBP 2008).
- ˒ BC Cancer Agency (Peixoto, J Gastrointest Oncol 2016): retrospective single institution study of 300 pts who received either 5-FU/MMC (64.6%) vs. capecitabine/MMC (35.3%) in combination with RT for locally advanced anal cancer. No difference in disease-free survival or anal cancer-specific survival.

HIV

- ˒ Oehler-Jänne (J Clin Oncol 2008): retrospective, multicentric cohort comparison of 40 HIV+ pts with HAART and 81 HIV- pts treated with RT or CRT. 55% of HIV+ pts had AIDS-defining clinical conditions. CR was 92% of HIV+ and 96% of HIV- cases. 5-yr OS was 61% in HIV+ and 65% in HIV- pts at a median follow-up of 36 mos. 5-yr LC worse in HIV+ pts (38%) vs. HIV- pts (87%), compromising cancer-specific survival and sphincter preservation. Increased grade 3/4 acute skin and hematological in HIV+ pts.
- ˒ White (Am J Clin Oncol 2017): single institution retrospective cohort study of 53 consecutive HIV+ pts treated between 1987 and 2013 vs. 205 consecutive HIV- pts treated between 2003 and 2013. Median RT dose was 54 Gy (28–60 Gy), concurrent chemo was 2 cycles of 5-FU/MMC on day 1 ± day 29. 70% of the HIV+ pts were on HAART at the time of treatment, 65% of pts had an undetectable HIV viral load, and the mean CD4 count was 455. At 3 yrs, no significant difference in PFS (75% vs. 76%),

colostomy-free survival (85% vs. 85%), or cancer-specific survival (79% vs. 88%, $P = 0.36$), respectively.

BRACHYTHERAPY

- Not frequently used in North America due to higher complication rates, including risk of necrosis. Rates of necrosis in the range of 7–15% (Sandhu, IJROBP 1998; Gerard, Radiother Oncol 1999), 6% complication requiring surgery (Ng, IJROBP 1988).

IMRT

- Multiple studies have reported similar LRC, DFS, colostomy rates, but comparable or lower toxicity with IMRT vs. traditional planning techniques.
- RTOG 0529 (Kachnic, IJROBP 2013): phase II multi-institutional trial. 52 pts, 54% with stage II, 25% IIIA, and 21% IIIB. 77% experienced grade 2+ GI/GU acute AEs (vs. RTOG 9811 77%). There were significant reductions in acute adverse events (AEs): grade 2+ hematologic (73% vs. 85% in RTOG 9811), grade 3+ GI (21% vs. 36% in RTOG 9811), and grade 3+ dermatological (23% vs. 49% in RTOG 9811).
- Call (Am J Clin Oncol 2016). Multi-institutional retrospective review of 152 pts treated with IMRT. 3-yr OS 87%, CFS T1-2 96% vs. T3-4 84%, LC T1-2 90% vs. T3-3 79%. Severe acute toxicity: skin 20%, GI 11%, and hematological 41%.

RT DOSE

- Optimal dose of RT continues to be explored.
- Multi-institutional and retrospective analyses report improved LC for doses >54–55 Gy (e.g., Huang, World J Gastroenterol 2007; Widder, Radiother Oncol 2008).
- ACCORD 03 trial (above) reported nonsignificant trend for improved colostomy-free survival with increased RT boost dose 20–25 Gy vs. 15 Gy (78% vs. 74%, $p = 0.067$).
- Elevated dose with a treatment break does not appear to improve disease outcomes. For example, RTOG 92-08

VI

(John, Cancer J Sci Am 1996) treated pts with 5-FU/ MMC + 59.6 Gy with 2 wk planned break included and colostomy rate at 2 yrs was 30%.

POST-TREATMENT BIOPSY
- Cummings (IJROBP 1991): no benefit to routine rebiopsy at 6 weeks post chemo-RT. Continued regression of tumor for up to 12 months, mean time to regression 3 months. ACT II trial reported optimal time point for evaluation of disease response is at 26 weeks because 72% of pts who did not show a CR at 11 weeks had achieved a CR by 26 weeks (Glynne-Jones, Lancet Oncol 2017).
- Follow pts clinically. Biopsy for clinically suspicious lesions.

SALVAGE APR
- Several studies report that salvage APR can achieve 30–77% LC after chemo-RT.
- Ellenhorn (Ann Surg Oncol 1994): retrospective review of 38 pts treated with RT + 5-FU/MMC. 5-yr OS was 44% when salvage APR used for chemo-RT failure.

RADIATION TECHNIQUES

GENERAL POINTS
- IMRT is favored over 3D conformal RT to reduce toxicity. It is critical to follow detailed target volumes as used in RTOG 0529.
- Minimize treatment breaks (try to keep under 2 weeks). Overall treatment time, but not duration of RT, has a detrimental effect on local failure and colostomy rate (Ben-Josef, JCO 2010).
- HIV+ pts with CD4 < 50–150.
  - Consider weekly 5FU/Cisplatin.
  - Consider RT alone 4.
  - (Re)institute HAART.
- HIV+ pts with CD4 < 150–200.

, Personalize treatment, but consider standard of care treatment with 5FU/MMC/RT.
, Consider cycle 2 dose reduction or omission of 2nd cycle MMC.
, HIV+ pts: post-therapy, rigorous HIV management is needed.

SIMULATION AND PLANNING

, Simulate patient supine, frog leg in vac lock bag immobilization.
, Anal marker to mark anal verge.
, Consider bolus on superficial large palpable groin nodes and any exposed tumor
, Treat with full bladder to minimize small bowel toxicity and use oral contrast 1–1.5 h before simulation. For patients who have trouble keeping a consistent full bladder, an empty bladder should be considered for reproducibility.
, Use PET-CT findings in treatment planning.

VI

CONVENTIONAL PLANNING (RTOG 98-11 TECHNIQUE)

, Targets: primary tumor, grossly enlarged LN, internal/external iliac LN, inguinal LN.
, Initial large field (all patients) treated AP/PA, energy 18 MV AP, 6 MV PA, dose 30.6 Gy at 1.8 Gy/fx.
  , Borders: superior = L5/S1. Inferior = 2.5 cm margin on anus and tumor. AP field includes lateral inguinal nodes. PA field = 2 cm lateral to greater sciatic notch (not including lateral inguinal LN).
  , Supplementary RT delivered to inguinal nodes with anterior electron fields matched with exit of PA field. Alternatively, may use modified segmental boost photon technique (Moran, IJROBP 2004).
, Reduced field #1 (all patients) drops AP/PA superior border to inferior border of sacroiliac joints and is treated 14.4 Gy at 1.8 Gy/fx (total 45 Gy). If N0, field is also reduced off inguinal nodes after 36 Gy.
, Reduced field #2 (for T3–T4, LN+, and T2 lesions with residual disease after 45 Gy).

ˌ Boost original tumor plus 2–2.5 cm margin 9–14 Gy at 1.8–2 Gy/fx (total 54–59 Gy) using either a multifield technique or laterals or a direct photon or electron perineal field.

ˌ Involved inguinal and/or pelvic LN should be included if small bowel can be avoided, boost 9–14 Gy (total 54–59 Gy) with electrons.

RTOG 0529 IMRT TECHNIQUE

ˌ Follow RTOG anorectal contouring atlas (Myerson, IJROBP 2008).

ˌ Uses dose painting (all PTVs treated simultaneously).

ˌ GTVA = gross primary tumor.

ˌ GTVN50 = all involved nodal regions with macroscopic disease <3 cm greatest dimension.

ˌ GTVN54 = all nodal regions containing macroscopic disease >3 cm greatest dimension.

ˌ CTVA: 2.5 cm expansion around gross primary disease and anal canal.

ˌ CTV45, CTV50, CTV54 includes the nodal regions (respectively, uninvolved, involved with nodes <3 cm, and involved with nodes >3 cm) and a 1.0 cm expansion (except into uninvolved bone, genitourinary structures, muscles, or bowel).

ˌ For T2N0:
  ˌ PTVA (primary tumor): 50.4 Gy in 28 fx of 1.8 Gy.
  ˌ PTV42 (all nodal regions receives): 42 Gy in 28 fx of 1.5 Gy.

ˌ For T3-4N0:
  ˌ PTVA: 54 Gy in 30 fx of 1.8 Gy (but for large T3 or T4 tumors, we recommend a subsequent cone-down to 55.8 to 59.4 Gy at 1.8 Gy/fx).
  ˌ PTV45: 45 Gy in 30 fx of 1.5 Gy.

ˌ For N+:
  ˌ PTVA: 54 Gy in 30 fx of 1.8 Gy.
  ˌ PTV45 (uninvolved LN): 45 Gy in 30 fx of 1.5 Gy.
  ˌ PTV50 (LN ≤ 3 cm): 50.4 Gy in 30 fx of 1.68 Gy.
  ˌ PTV54 (LN > 3 cm): 54 Gy in 30 fx of 1.8 Gy.

ˌ For further details, see http://www.rtog.org/members/protocols/0529/0529.pdf

UCSF IMRT DOSES

- We use dose-painting (all PTVs treated simultaneously).
- Primary tumor doses:
  - T1: 50.4–53.2 Gy/28 fx.
  - T2: 53.2 Gy/28 fx.
  - T3: 56–58.8 Gy/28 fx.
  - T4: 58.8 Gy/28 fx.
- Involved lymph nodes:
  - 50.4 Gy/28 fx if ≤2 cm.
  - 54–58.8 Gy if >2 cm.
- High-risk lymph nodes (perirectal, presacral, internal iliacs):
  - 47.6 Gy/28 fx.
- Low-risk lymph nodes (external iliacs and inguinals):
  - 44.8 Gy/28 fx.

DOSE LIMITATIONS

- See RTOG 0529 constraints. UCSF constraints:
- Small bowel: Dmax < 54 Gy, ≤ 30% volume > 45 Gy
- Bladder: Dmax < 54 Gy; ≤ 30% volume > 45 Gy
- Femoral Neck: Dmax < 45 Gy
- Gluteal folds: minimize dose, < 36 Gy if possible
- Skin (0.5 cm rind): minimize dose, < 20 Gy

COMPLICATIONS

- Acute complications: skin reaction/desquamation, leukopenia, thrombocytopenia, proctitis, diarrhea, and cystitis.
- Subacute and late complications include chronic diarrhea, rectal urgency, sterility, impotence, vaginal dryness, and vaginal fibrosis/stenosis (use vaginal dilator status post-XRT to help avoid), and possibly decreased testosterone.
- Increased risk of late pelvic fracture, particularly among older women.

FOLLOW-UP

- H&P with anal & inguinal LN exam q8–12 wks until CR, then every 3–6 mos × 5 yrs. Examine more frequently if persistent disease (e.g., monthly).

ﾠ On exam if mass increases in size, or new clinical symptoms develop (pain, bleeding, incontinence) → biopsy. If locally recurrent → salvage APR. If metastatic disease → 5-FU/cisplatin. If tumor decreasing in size, continue to follow. Median time to regression ~3 months, but tumor response can still be observed up to 6 months.

ﾠ Anoscopy q6–12 mos × 3 yrs.

ﾠ For T3–T4 or inguinal LN+: annual CT chest/abdomen/pelvis for 3 yrs.

ﾠ Most recurrences occur within 2 yrs.

ﾠ Anal pap, if available, is useful for follow-up.

ﾠ Recommend vaginal dilator and pelvic floor physical therapy in women to help reduce stenosis/narrowing, starting at 4 weeks post-therapy.

ﾠ Male pts may notice decrease in ejaculate; testosterone levels may be checked for sexual difficulties.

Acknowledgment The authors thank Amy Gillis MD and Gautam Prasad MD, PhD for their work on the prior edition of this chapter.

REFERENCES

Ajani JA, Winter KA, Gunderson LL, et al. Fluorouracil, mitomycin, and radiotherapy vs fluorouracil, cisplatin, and radiotherapy for carcinoma of the anal canal: a randomized controlled trial. JAMA. 2008;299(16):1914–21.

Bartelink H, Roelofsen F, et al. Concomitant radiotherapy and chemotherapy is superior to radiotherapy alone in the treatment of locally advanced anal cancer: results of a phase III randomized trial of the European Organization for Research and Treatment of Cancer Radiotherapy and Gastrointestinal Cooperative Groups. J Clin Oncol. 1997;15:2040–9.

Ben-Josef E, Moughan J, Ajani JA, et al. Impact of overall treatment time on survival and local control in patients with anal cancer: a pooled data analysis of Radiation Therapy Oncology Group trials 87-04 and 98-11. J Clin Oncol. 2010;28(34):5061–6.

Boman BM, Moertel CG, et al. Carcinoma of the anal canal. A clinical and pathological study of 188 cases. Cancer. 1984;54:114–25.

Call JA, Prendergast BM, Jensen LG, et al. Intensity-modulated radiation therapy for anal cancer: results from a multi-institutional retrospective cohort study. Am J Clin Oncol. 2016;39(1):8–12.

Cotter SE, Grigsby PW, Siegel BA, et al. FDG-PET/CT in the evaluation of anal carcinoma. Int J Radiat Oncol Biol Phys. 2006;65:720–5.

Cummings BJ, Keane TJ, O'Sullivan B, et al. Epidermoid anal cancer: treatment by radiation alone or by radiation and 5-fluorouracil with and without mitomycin-c. Int J Radiat Oncol Biol Phys. 1991;21(5):1115–25.

Deniaud-Alexandre E, Touboul E, Tiret E, et al. Results of definitive irradiation in a series of 305 epidermoid carcinomas of the anal canal. Int J Radiat Oncol Biol Phys. 2003;56(5):1259–73.

Ellenhorn JD, Enker WE, Quan SH. Salvage abdominoperineal resection following combined chemotherapy and radiotherapy for epidermoid carcinoma of the anus. Ann Surg Oncol. 1994;1:105–10.

Flam M, Madhu J, et al. Role of mitomycin in combination with fluorouracil and radiotherapy, and of salvage chemoradiation in the definitive nonsurgical treatment of epidermoid carcinoma of the anal canal: results of a Phase III Randomized Intergroup Study. J Clin Oncol. 1996;14:2527–39.

Gerard JP, Ayzac L, et al. Treatment of anal canal carcinoma with high dose radiation therapy and concomitant fluorouracil-cisplatinum. Long-term results in 95 patients. Radiother Oncol. 1998;46(3):249–56.

Glynne-Jones R, Meadows H, Wan S, et al. Extra – a multicenter phase ii study of chemoradiation using a 5 day per week oral regimen of capecitabine and intravenous mitomycin c in anal cancer. Int J Radiat Oncol Biol Phys. 2008;72(1):119–26.

Glynne-Jones R, Sebag-Montefiore D, Meadows HM, et al. Best time to assess complete clinical response after chemoradiotherapy in squamous cell carcinoma of the anus (ACT II): a post-hoc analysis of randomised controlled phase 3 trial. Lancet Oncol. 2017;S1470-2045(17):30071–2.

Greenall MJ, Quan HQ, Decosse JJ. Epidermoid cancer of the anus. Br J Surg. 1985;72:S97.

Gunderson LL, Winter KA, Ajani JA, et al. Long-term update of US GI intergroup RTOG 98-11 phase III trial for anal carcinoma: survival, relapse, and colostomy failure with concurrent chemoradiation involving fluorouracil/mitomycin versus fluorouracil/cisplatin. J Clin Oncol. 2012;30(35):4344–51.

Gunderson LL, Moughan J, Ajani JA, et al. Anal carcinoma: impact of TN category of disease on survival, disease relapse, and colostomy failure in US Gastrointestinal Intergroup RTOG 98-11 phase 3 trial. Int J Radiat Oncol Biol Phys. 2013;87(4):638–45.

Hatfield P, Cooper R, Sebag-Montefiore D. Involved-field, low-dose chemoradiotherapy for early-stage anal carcinoma. Int J Radiat Oncol Biol Phys. 2008;70(2):419–24.

Hoffman R, Welton ML, et al. The significance of pretreatment CD4 count on the outcome and treatment tolerance of HIV-positive pts with anal cancer. Int J Radiat Oncol Biol Phys. 1999;44:127–31.

Huang K, Haas-Kogan D, Weinberg V, et al. Higher radiation dose with a shorter treatment duration improves outcome for locally advanced carcinoma of anal canal. World J Gastroenterol. 2007;13(6):895–900.

James R, Glynne-Jones D, Meadows HM, et al. Mitomycin or cisplatin chemoradiation with or without maintenance chemotherapy for treatment of squamous-cell carcinoma of the anus (ACT II): a randomised, phase 3, open-label, 2 × 2 factorial trial. Lancet Oncol. 2013;14:516–24.

John M, Pajak T, et al. Dose escalation in chemoradiation for anal cancer: preliminary results of RTOG 92-08. Cancer J Sci Am. 1996;2(4):205.

Kachnic LA, Winter K, Myerson RJ, et al. RTOG 0529: a phase 2 evaluation of dose-painted intensity modulated radiation therapy in combination with 5-fluorouracil and mitomycin-C for the reduction of acute morbidity in carcinoma of the anal canal. Int J Radiat Oncol Biol Phys. 2013;86:27–33.

Koh WJ, Chiu M, Stelzer KJ, et al. Femoral vessel depth and the implications for groin node radiation. Int J Radiat Oncol Biol Phys. 1993;27:969–74.

Martenson JA, Gunderson LL. External radiation therapy without chemotherapy in the management of anal cancer. Cancer. 1993;71(5):1736–40.

Meropol NJ, Niedzwiecki D, Shank B, et al. Induction therapy for poor-prognosis anal canal carcinoma: a phase II study of the Cancer and Leukemia Group B (CALGB 9281). J Clin Oncol. 2008;26(19):3229–34.

VI

Milano MT, Jani AB, Farrey KJ, et al. Intensity-modulated radiation therapy (IMRT) in the treatment of anal cancer: toxicity and clinical outcome. Int J Radiat Oncol Biol Phys. 2005;63:354–61.

Mistrangelo M, Pelosi E, Bellò M, et al. Role of positron emission tomography-computed tomography in the management of anal cancer. Int J RadiatOncolBiol Phys. 2012;84(1):66–72.

Moran M, Lund MW, Ahmad M, et al. Improved treatment of pelvis and inguinal nodes using modified segmental boost technique: dosimetric evaluation. Int J Radiat Oncol Biol Phys. 2004;59(5):1523–30.

Myerson RJ, et al. Elective clinical target volumes for conformal therapy in anorectal cancer: an Radiation Therapy Oncology Group consensus panel contouring atlas. Int J Radiat Oncol Biol Phys. 2008;74:824–30.

National Cancer Institute Surveillance, Epidemiology, and End Results Program (SEER). https://www.seer.cancer.gov/statfacts/html/anus.html. Accessed 5 Dec 2016.

National Comprehensive Cancer Network. Clinical Practice Guidelines in Oncology: Anal Carcinoma (Version 1.2017). https://www.nccn.org/professionals/physician_gls/pdf/anal.pdf. Accessed 5 Dec 2016.

Ng Y, Ying Kin NY, Pigneux J, et al. Our experience of conservative treatment of anal cancal carcinoma combining external irradiation and interstitial implants. Int J Radiat Oncol Biol Phys. 1988;14:253–9.

Northover J, Glynne-Jones R, Sebag-Montefiore D, et al. Chemoradiation for the treatment of epidermoid anal cancer: 13-year follow-up of the first randomised UKCCCR Anal Cancer Trial (ACT I). Br J Cancer. 2010;102:1123–8.

Oehler-Jänne C, Huguet F, Provencher S, et al. HIV-specific differences in outcome of squamous cell carcinoma of the anal canal: a multicentric cohort study of HIV-positive patients receiving highly active antiretroviral therapy. J Clin Oncol. 2008;26:2550–7.

Papagikos M, Crane CH, et al. Chemoradiation for adenocarcinoma of the anus. Int J Radiat Oncol Biol Phys. 2003;55:669–78.

Papillon J, Montbarbon JF. Epidermoid carcinoma of the anal canal. A series of 276 cases. Dis Colon Rectum. 1987;30:324–33.

Peiffert D, Bey P, Pernot M, et al. Conservative treatment by irradiation of epidermoid carcinomas of the anal margin. Int J Radiat Oncol Biol Phys. 1997;39:57–66.

Peiffert D, Tournier-Rangeard L, Gérard JP, et al. Induction chemotherapy and dose intensification of the radiation boost in locally advanced anal canal carcinoma: final analysis of the randomized UNICANCER ACCORD 03 trial. J Clin Oncol. 2012;30:1941–8.

Peixoto RD, Wan DD, Schellenberg D, et al. A comparison between 5-fluorouracil/mitomycin and capecitabine/mitomycin in combination with radiation for anal cancer. J Gastrointest Oncol. 2016;7:665–72.

Salama JK, Mell LK, Schomas DA, et al. Concurrent chemotherapy and intensity-modulated radiation therapy for anal canal cancer patients: a multicenter experience. J Clin Oncol. 2007;29:4851–6.

Sandhu APS, Symonds RP, et al. Interstitial Iridium-192 implantation combined with external radiotherapy in anal cancer: ten yrs experience. Int J Radiat Oncol Biol Phys. 1998;40:575–81.

Schwarz JK, Siegel BA, Dehdashti F, et al. Tumor response and survival predicted by post-therapy FDG-PET/CT in anal cancer. Int J Radiat Oncol Biol Phys. 2008;71(1):180–6.

Trautmann TG, Zuger JH. Positron emission tomography for pretreatment staging and post-treatment evaluation in cancer of the anal canal. Mol Imaging Biol. 2005;7:309–13.

UKCCCR Anal Cancer Trial Working Party. Epidermoid anal cancer: results from the UKCCCR randomized trial of radiotherapy alone versus radiotherapy, 5-fluorouracil, and mitomycin. Lancet. 1996;348:1049–54.

Widder J, Kastenberger R, Fercher E, et al. Radiation dose associated with local control in advanced anal cancer: retrospective analysis of 129 patients. Radiother Oncol. 2008;87(3):367–75.

Winton Ed, Heriot AG, Ng M, et al.The impact of 18-fluorodeoxyglucose positron emission tomography on the staging, management and outcome of anal cancer. Br J Cancer. 2009;100(5):693–700.

White EC, Goldman K, Aleshin A, et al. Chemoradiotherapy for squamous cell carcinoma of the anal canal: comparison of one versus two cyclesmitomycin-C. Radiother Oncol. 2015;117(2):240–5.

White EC, Khodayari B, Erickson KT, et al. Comparison of toxicity and treatment outcomes in HIV-positive versus HIV-negative patients with squamous cell carcinoma of the anal canal. Am J Clin Oncol. 2017;40(4):386–92.

Wo JY, Hong TS, Callister MD, et al. Anal carcinoma. In: Gunderson LL, Tepper JE, editors. Clinical radiation oncology. 4th ed. Philadelphia: Churchill Livingstone; 2015. p. 1019–34.e4.

Yeung R, McConnell Y, Roxin G, et al. One compared with two cycles of mitomycin C in chemoradiotherapy for anal cancer: analysis of outcomes and toxicity. Curr Oncol. 2014;21(3):e449–56. https://doi.org/10.3747/co.21.1903.

VI

PART VII

Genitourinary Sites

VII

Chapter 24
Renal Cell Carcinoma

Michael A. Garcia and Alexander R. Gottschalk

PEARLS

- Renal cell carcinoma (RCC) constitutes 80–95% of primary renal neoplasms.
- Estimated 63,000 new cases and 14,000 deaths from RCC in the United States in 2016.
- Male predominance (M:F 1.5:1).
- Most common in 6th–8th decades; median age at diagnosis is 64.
- At presentation, 65% RCC localized, 16% regional lymph node involvement, and 16% metastatic. Slow decrease in size of tumors at presentation likely due to greater number of incidental tumors found on abdominal imaging (SEER data).
- Ninety-five percent diagnoses made with imaging (solid, hypervascular renal mass).
- RCC subtypes: clear cell (75–85%), chromophilic/papillary (10–15%), chromophobic (5–10%), oncocytic (3–5%), and collecting duct (very rare).
- Fuhrman grading system: I–IV based on nuclear size and shape, nucleoli presence, and the presence of clumped chromatin.
- Risk factors: tobacco, occupational exposure to cadmium/asbestos/petrols, obesity, acquired cystic disease of the kidney, and phenacetin-containing analgesics exposure.

VII

© Springer International Publishing AG, part of Springer Nature 2018   **535**
Eric K. Hansen and M. Roach III (eds.), *Handbook of Evidence-Based Radiation Oncology*, https://doi.org/10.1007/978-3-319-62642-0_24

- *Von Hippel–Lindau (VHL)* tumor suppressor gene, found on chromosome 3p25.
  - 50% of sporadic RCC have a silencing *VHL* mutation.
  - VHL disease is inherited in autosomal dominant manner and associated with:
    - >70% risk of developing RCC.
    - Retinal hemangioblastomas, CNS hemangioblastomas, pheochromocytoma, and pancreatic neuroendocrine tumors.
- RCC is a radioresistant tumor and has low response rates to cytotoxic chemotherapies, though targeted molecular agents and stereotactic ablative radiotherapy are redefining management of disease.

WORKUP

- H&P:
  - Classic triad: hematuria (80%), flank pain (45%), and flank mass (15%).
    - Triad only present in 10% of patients.
    - Other signs and symptoms include normocytic/normochromic anemia, fever, weight loss, high alk phos without mets (Stauffer syndrome), polycythemia, and hypercalcemia.
  - Labs: CBC, comprehensive metabolic panel, and urinalysis.
  - Imaging: Abdominal CT or MRI with or without contrast depending on renal function.
  - Metastatic evaluation: Chest CT, bone scan, and/or MRI brain if clinically indicated.

STAGING: RENAL CELL CARCINOMA

Editors' note: All TNM stage and stage groups referred to elsewhere in this chapter reflect the 2007 AJCC staging nomenclature unless otherwise noted as the new system below was published after this chapter was written.

Table 24.1 (AJCC 7TH ED., 2010)

Primary tumor (T)

TX:	Primary tumor cannot be assessed
T0:	No evidence of primary tumor
T1:	Tumor 7 cm or less in greatest dimension, limited to the kidney
T1a:	Tumor 4 cm or less in greatest dimension, limited to the kidney
T1b:	Tumor more than 4 cm, but not more than 7 cm in greatest dimension, limited to the kidney
T2:	Tumor more than 7 cm in greatest dimension, limited to the kidney
T2a:	Tumor more than 7 cm, but less than or equal to 10 cm in greatest dimension, limited to the kidney
T2b:	Tumor more than 10 cm, limited to the kidney
T3:	Tumor extends into major veins or perinephric tissues, but not into the ipsilateral adrenal gland and not beyond Gerota's fascia
T3a:	Tumor grossly extends into the renal vein or its segmental (muscle-containing) branches, or tumor invades perirenal and/or renal sinus fat, but not beyond Gerota's fascia
T3b:	Tumor grossly extends into the vena cava below the diaphragm
T3c:	Tumor grossly extends into the vena cava above the diaphragm or invades the wall of the vena cava
T4:	Tumor invades beyond Gerota's fascia (including contiguous extension into the ipsilateral adrenal gland)

Regional lymph nodes (N)

NX:	Regional lymph nodes cannot be assessed
N0:	No regional lymph node metastasis
N1:	Metastasis in regional lymph node(s)

Distant metastasis (M)

M0:	No distant metastasis
M1:	Distant metastasis

Anatomical stage/prognostic groups

I:	T1 N0 M0
II:	T2 N0 M0
III:	T1 or T2 N1 M0
	T3 N0 or N1 M0
IV:	T4 Any N M0
	Any T Any N M1

Used with the permission from the American Joint Committee on Cancer (AJCC), Chicago, Illinois. The original source for this material is the AJCC Cancer Staging Manual, Seventh Edition (2010), published by Springer Science+Business Media.

Table 24.2 (AJCC 8TH ED., 2017)

Definitions of AJCC TNM

Definition of Primary Tumor (T)

T category	T criteria
TX	Primary tumor cannot be assessed
T0	No evidence of primary tumor
Ta	Papillary noninvasive carcinoma
Tis	Carcinoma in situ

continued

Table 24.2 (continued)

T1	Tumor invades subepithelial connective tissue
T2	Tumor invades the muscularis
T3	For the renal pelvis only: tumor invades beyond muscularis into peripelvic fat or into the renal parenchyma. For the ureter only: tumor invades beyond muscularis propria into periureteral fat
T4	Tumor invades adjacent organs or through the kidney into the perinephric fat

DEFINITION OF REGIONAL LYMPH NODE (N)

N category	N criteria
NX	Regional lymph nodes cannot be assessed
N0	No regional lymph node metastasis
N1	Metastasis in a single lymph node, ≤2 cm in greatest dimension
N2	Metastasis in a single lymph node, >2 cm, or multiple lymph nodes

DEFINITION OF DISTANT METASTASIS (M)

M category	M criteria
M0	No distant metastasis
M1	Distant metastasis

AJCC PROGNOSTIC STAGE GROUPS

When T is...	And N is...	And M is...	Then the stage group is...
Ta	N0	M0	0a
Tis	N0	M0	0is
T1	N0	M0	I
T2	N0	M0	II
T3	N0	M0	III
T4	N0	M0	IV
Any T	N1	M0	IV
Any T	N2	M0	IV
Any T	Any N	M1	IV

Used with permission of the American Joint Committee on Cancer (AJCC), Chicago, Illinois. The original and primary source for this information is the AJCC Cancer Staging Manual, Eighth Edition (2017), published by Springer International Publishing

TREATMENT RECOMMENDATIONS

Table 24.3 TREATMENT RECOMMENDATIONS

2002 Stages	Recommended treatments

I–III	Nephrectomy
	    Partial nephrectomy if feasible
	    Radical nephrectomy if partial not feasible or central location
	    May spare adrenal gland if uninvolved
	    Regional LN dissection recommended for radiographic or palpable adenopathy
	No established role for adjuvant systemic therapy
	No established role for neoadjuvant or adjuvant radiotherapy
	Consider cryosurgery, radiofrequency ablation, or SBRT for inoperable patients

IV	Cytoreductive nephrectomy is generally recommended for potentially resectable primary site in patients with solitary metastasis, good performance status, and/or limited metastatic burden
	    Adding nephrectomy to interferon alpha improved survival in randomized trials, but has not yet been demonstrated with targeted therapies
	First-line systemic therapies (NCCN 2016)
	    Molecularly targeted agents
	        Bevacizumab, axitinib (VEGF receptor inhibitor)
	        Sunitinib, pazopanib, and sorafenib (tyrosine kinase inhibitors)
	        Temsirolimus (mTOR inhibitor)
	    Immunotherapy (IL-2, interferon alpha, or combination)
	Treatment of metastases
	    Focal palliation of metastases
	    Radiotherapy (SBRT or EBRT)
	    Metastasectomy.

VII

TRIALS

RADIOTHERAPY

, There is no clear OS or PFS benefit with postoperative RT after nephrectomy or partial nephrectomy, but there may be a role for LC among high-risk patients.

, Early trials showed no benefit to post-op RT, though they did not select a population likely to benefit from PORT and used now obsolete RT techniques.

, LR in most radical nephrectomy series is ~5%, driven mainly by completely resected stage I/II tumors. However, with incomplete resection or nodal involvement, LR rises to 20–30%. Retrospective studies and a meta-analysis support a potential role for post-op RT among high-risk patients:

> Stein (Radiother Oncol 1992): Retrospective, 147 patients treated with PORT (median 46 Gy) vs. observation. Among T3N0 patients, LR was 10% vs. 37% favoring PORT. Three of 19 recurrences were at the scar.

> Kao (Radiology 1994): Retrospective, 12 patients with perinephric invasion or + margins who received PORT 41–63 Gy (1.8–2 Gy fx). 5-yr LC was 100% and 5-yr actuarial PFS was 75% compared with 30% in 12 patients of similar stage treated with surgery alone.

> Meta-analysis (Tunio, Ann Oncol 2010) of 7 trials with 735 patients with localized RCC comparing PORT vs. nephrectomy alone. Locoregional failure improved if PORT added (HR 0.47, $p < 0.0001$), though no difference in OS or PFS.

- Radiofrequency ablation and cryotherapy may be considered for small tumors away from the ureter and renal pelvis.

- For larger or other inoperable tumors, SBRT may be considered for primary tumor control.

  > Siva (BJUI 2012). Systematic review of 10 publications with 126 patients treated with SBRT with a variety of techniques for primary RCC. Weighted LC 94% (range 84–100%) and weighted severe grade 3 toxicity 3.8% (range 0–19%).

  > A number of subsequent series report similarly high LC and acceptable toxicity (e.g., Chang, Clin Oncol 2016; Staehler, J Urol 2015; Pham, IJROBP 2014; McBride IJROBP 2013).

  > IROCK (Siva, Future Oncol 2016). International Radiosurgery Oncology Consortium for Kidney, consisting of 8 international institutions, provides a review of patient selection, SBRT dose and fractionation, technical details of SBRT delivery, and clinical FU parameters.

  > SBRT may also contribute to systemic antitumor activity through abscopal response (Wersäll, Acta Oncol 2006).

  > Prospective SBRT trials for RCC are ongoing.

TREATMENT OF METASTATIC DISEASE

- A number of retrospective studies report improved survival with complete metastasectomy compared to incomplete or no metastasectomy (Dabestani, Lancet Oncol 2014). Potential candidates have primary RCC with solitary metastasis or oligometastatic recurrence after prolonged disease-free interval in the lung, bone, or brain. While long-term PFS has been reported, most patients who have resection of solitary metastasis develop recurrence.

ˌ In contrast to conventional fractionation, SRS and SBRT provide excellent LC at metastatic RCC sites with adequate dose and dose per fraction.

ˌ Kothari (Acta Oncol 2015). Systematic review of SRS and SBRT for RCC metastasis, including 810 intracranial patients with 2433 targets and 389 extracranial patients with 730 targets. Weighted LC 92% intracranial, 89% extracranial, with 0–6% risk of grade 3–4 toxicity.

ˌ Zelefsky (IJROBP 2012): 105 RCC spine mets treated with 18–24 Gy × 1 or 20–30 Gy in 3–5 fx. Median f/u 12 months. 3-yr local PFS for all lesions was 44%. The 3-yr local PFS for high single-dose (24 Gy), low single-dose (<24 Gy), or hypofractionation regimens were 88%, 21%, and 17%, respectively.

RADIATION TECHNIQUES

VII

SIMULATION AND FIELD DESIGN
Primary Site

ˌ CT simulation, supine, arms up to allow visualization of lateral isocenter marks, immobilize with wing-board, alpha cradle, or SBRT body fixation device. 4D CT recommended to account for tumor respiratory motion. Consider MRI fusion. Wire scar in post-op cases.

ˌ Volume:

ˌ Inoperable: GTV = gross disease; CTV = GTV + 0–5 mm; PTV = ITV + 0–5 mm.

ˌ Post-op: Nephrectomy bed +/− high-risk LN drainage sites, surgical clips. Consider treating scar in treatment volume or with electrons to full dose if indicated due to limited reports of scar failures.

Metastatic Site (Non-CNS)

ˌ Proper immobilization technique based on site.

ˌ Planning CT and/or MRI if 3DCRT/SBRT to be used.

ˌ Volume: Focal treatment of metastasis with limited margin depending on treatment setup.

ˌ See Chap. 42 for management of CNS metastases.

DOSE PRESCRIPTIONS

- Primary site:
  - A variety of SBRT fractionation schemes have been utilized ranging from 23–26 Gy in 1 fx, 30–54 Gy in 3 fx, 32–48 Gy in 4 fx, and 40–50 Gy in 5 fx. We recommend treating on prospective study until there is more consensus on dose fractionation.
- Post-op: 45–50 Gy in 1.8–2 Gy fx with 10–16 Gy boost to close or positive margins.
- Metastases:
  - SBRT may be preferred for many patients due to improved LC. A variety of SBRT fractionation regimens have been utilized ranging from 15–24 Gy in 1 fx, 24–45 Gy in 3 fx, 32–40 Gy in 4 fx, and 40–50 Gy in 5 fx. We recommend treating on prospective study until there is more consensus on dose fractionation.
  - Conventional 30 Gy in 10 fx can offer pain relief in many patients, but local recurrence can be problematic. With standard EBRT, we may consider escalating dose to 45–50 Gy or hypofractionation when SBRT is not available or appropriate.

DOSE LIMITATIONS

- For primary site conventional EBRT:
  - Contralateral kidney: limit to ≤20 Gy in 2–3 weeks.
  - Liver: limit to <30% receiving >36–40 Gy.
  - Spinal cord: <45 Gy.
  - Small bowel: <45 Gy.
- For primary site SBRT, dose constraints dependent on fractionation. See IROCK dose constraints for 1–5 fraction SBRT (Siva, Future Oncol 2016).

Acknowledgment The authors thank Sunanda Pejavar MD and James Rembert MD for their work on the prior edition of this chapter.

REFERENCES

Amin MB, Edge S, Greene F, Byrd DR, Brookland RK, Washington MK, Gershenwald JE, Compton CC, Hess KR, Sullivan DC, Jessup JM, Brierley JD, Gaspar LE, Schilsky RL, Balch CM, Winchester DP, Asare EA, Madera M, Gress DM, Meyer LR (editos). AJCC cancer staging manual, 8th edition. Springer; 2017

Dabestani S, Marconi L, Hofmann F, et al. Local treatments for metastases of renal cell carcinoma: a systematic review. Lancet Oncol. 2014;15(12):e549–61.

Edge SB, American Joint Committee on Cancer, American Cancer Society. AJCC cancer staging manual. 7th ed. New York: Springer; 2010.

Edge SB, Byrd DR, Compton CC, Fritz AG, Greene FL, Trotti A, (editors). AJCC cancer staging manual, 7th edition. Springer; 2010

Kao GD, Malkowicz SB, Whittington R, et al. Locally advanced renal cell carcinoma: low complication rate and efficacy of postnephrectomy planned with CT. Radiology. 1994;193(3):725–30.

Kothari G, Foroudi F, Gill S, Corcoran NM, Siva S. Outcomes of stereotactic radiotherapy for cranial and extracranial metastatic renal cell carcinoma: a systematic review. Acta Oncol. 2015;54(2):148–57.

National Comprehensive Cancer Network. Clinical practice guidelines in oncology: kidney cancer. Available at: http://www.nccn.org/professionals/physician_gls/PDF/kidney.pdf. Accessed 3 Aug 2016.

Siva S, Pham D, Gill S, Corcoran NM, Foroudi F. A systematic review of stereotactic radiotherapy ablation for primary renal cell carcinoma. BJU Int. 2012;110(11 Pt B):E737–43.

Siva S, Ellis RJ, Ponsky L, et al. Consensus statement from the International Radiosurgery Oncology Consortium for Kidney for primary renal cell carcinoma. Future Oncol. 2016;12(5):637–45.

Stein M, Kuten A, Halpern J, et al. The value of postoperative irradiation in renal cell cancer. Radiother Oncol. 1992;24(1):41–4.

Tunio MA, Hashmi A, Rafi M. Need for a new trial to evaluate postoperative radiotherapy in renal cell carcinoma: a meta-analysis of randomized controlled trials. Ann Oncol. 2010;21(9):1839–45.

Wersäll PJ, Blomgren H, Pisa P, Lax I, Kälkner K-M, Svedman C. Regression of non-irradiated metastases after extracranial stereotactic radiotherapy in metastatic renal cell carcinoma. Acta Oncol. 2006;45(4):493–7.

Zelefsky MJ, Greco C, Motzer R, et al. Tumor control outcomes after hypofractionated and single-dose stereotactic image-guided intensity-modulated radiotherapy for extracranial metastases from renal cell carcinoma. Int J Radiat Oncol Biol Phys. 2012;82(5):1744–8.

VII

Chapter 25
Bladder Cancer

Michael A. Garcia and Albert J. Chang

PEARLS

- Epidemiology:
  - ACS estimates for the United States in 2016: 76,500 new bladder cancers and 16,390 deaths.
  - Men 3–4x higher risk than women (1 in 26 men vs. 1 in 88 women).
  - Risk factors: cigarette smoke, naphthylamines, dyes, arsenic, cyclophosphamide chronic irritation (nephrolithiasis, chronic UTI, and chronic indwelling catheter).
  - Urothelial carcinoma (formally transitional cell carcinoma) constitutes 90% of bladder cancers in the United States.
  - In developing countries, squamous cell carcinoma (SCC) is more common (associated with Schistosome infection).
  - In the United States, SCC comprises 3% cases, adenocarcinoma 2%, and small cell 1%
- Bladder lymphatics:
  - 1^0 drainage: hypogastric → obturator → iliac (internal and external) → perivesical → sacral → presacral nodes.
  - 2^0 drainage: common iliac.
- Most common sites: bladder trigone, lateral/posterior walls, and bladder neck
  - Most tumors tend to be multifocal in nature.

VII

‚ At presentation, 75% bladder cancers are nonmuscle invasive.

‚ Presenting symptoms: painless hematuria, irritative voiding, pelvic pain, obstructive uropathy, and hydronephrosis.

WORKUP

‚ H&P including gynecological exam for women; Labs: CBC, chemistries, BUN, Cr, alkaline phosphatase, UA with urine cytology.

‚ Urine cytology (low sensitivity, improves with higher grade tumors, but 95% specific).

‚ Office cystoscopy.

‚ Imaging of upper urinary tracts (CT urography, renal U/S, retrograde ureteropyelogram, ureteroscopy, or MRI urogram).

‚ Abdominal/pelvic CT or MRI before TURBT.

‚ Maximal TURBT with random biopsies of normal appearing mucosa to exclude multifocal disease and Tis. If trigone involved, prostatic urethra biopsy.

    ‚ Fluorescence cystoscopy-guided transurethral resection may reduce nonmuscle invasive recurrence compared to white-light cystoscopy, but not progression to muscle invasive disease (Yuan PLoS One 2013).

‚ Chest imaging if muscle invasive; bone scan if clinical suspicion for bone mets.

STAGING: BLADDER CANCER

Editors' note: All TNM stage and stage groups referred to elsewhere in this chapter reflect the 2007 AJCC staging nomenclature unless otherwise noted as the new system below was published after this chapter was written.

Table 25.1   AJCC 7TH ED., (2010)

Primary tumor (T)

TX: Primary tumor cannot be assessed
T0:   No evidence of primary tumor
Ta: Noninvasive papillary carcinoma
Tis: Carcinoma in situ: "flat tumor"
T1:   Tumor invades subepithelial connective tissue
T2:   Tumor invades muscularis propria
pT2a: Tumor invades superficial muscularis propria (inner half)
pT2b   Tumor invades deep muscularis propria (outer half)
T3:   Tumor invades perivesical tissue
pT3a: Microscopically
pT3b: Macroscopically (extravesical mass)
T4:   Tumor invades any of the following: prostatic stroma, seminal vesicles, uterus, vagina, pelvic wall, and abdominal wall
T4a: Tumor invades prostatic stroma, uterus, and vagina
T4b: Tumor invades pelvic wall and abdominal wall

Regional lymph nodes (N)

Regional lymph nodes include both primary and secondary drainage regions. All other nodes above the aortic bifurcation are considered distant lymph nodes.

NX: Lymph nodes cannot be assessed
N0:   No lymph node metastasis
N1:   Single regional lymph node metastasis in the true pelvis (hypogastric, obturator, external iliac, or presacral lymph node)
N2:   Multiple regional lymph node metastasis in the true pelvis (hypogastric, obturator, external iliac, or presacral lymph node metastasis)
N3:   Lymph node metastasis to the common iliac lymph nodes

VII

Distant metastasis (M)

M0:   No distant metastasis
M1:   Distant metastasis

Anatomical stage/prognostic groups

0a: Ta N0 M0
0is: Tis N0 M0
I: T1 N0 M0
II: T2a N0 M0
        T2b N0 M0
III: T3a N0 M0
        T3b N0 M0
        T4a N0 M0
IV: T4b N0 M0
        Any T N1-3 M0
        Any T Any N M1

Used with the permission from the American Joint Committee on Cancer (AJCC), Chicago, Illinois. The original source for this material is the AJCC Cancer Staging Manual, Seventh Edition (2010), published by Springer Science+Business Media.

Table 25.2 AJCC 8TH ED., (2017) STAGING

Definitions of AJCC TNM

Definition of Primary Tumor (T)

T category	T criteria
TX	Primary tumor cannot be assessed
T0	No evidence of primary tumor
Ta	Noninvasive papillary carcinoma
Tis	Urothelial carcinoma in situ: "flat tumor"
T1	Tumor invades the lamina propria (subepithelial connective tissue)
T2	Tumor invades the muscularis propria
pT2a	Tumor invades the superficial muscularis propria (inner half)
pT2b	Tumor invades the deep muscularis propria (outer half)
T3	Tumor invades perivesical soft tissue
pT3a	Microscopically
pT3b	Macroscopically (extravesical mass)
T4	Extravesical tumor directly invades any of the following: prostatic stroma, seminal vesicles, uterus, vagina, pelvic wall, and abdominal wall
T4a	Extravesical tumor invades directly into the prostatic stroma, uterus, and vagina
T4b	Extravesical tumor invades the pelvic wall, and abdominal wall

DEFINITION OF REGIONAL LYMPH NODE (N)

N category	N criteria
NX	Lymph nodes cannot be assessed
N0	No lymph node metastasis
N1	Single regional lymph node metastasis in the true pelvis (perivesical, obturator, internal and external iliac, or sacral lymph node)
N2	Multiple regional lymph node metastasis in the true pelvis (perivesical, obturator, internal and external iliac, or sacral lymph node metastasis)
N3	Lymph node metastasis to the common iliac lymph nodes

DEFINITION OF DISTANT METASTASIS (M)

M category	M criteria
M0	No distant metastasis
M1	Distant metastasis
M1a	Distant metastasis limited to lymph nodes beyond the common iliacs
M1b	Non-lymph node distant métastases

AJCC PROGNOSTIC STAGE GROUPS

When T is...	And N is...	And M is...	Then the stage group is...
Ta	N0	M0	Oa
Tis	N0	M0	Ois
T1	N0	M0	I
T2a	N0	M0	II
T2b	N0	M0	II
T3a, T3b, T4a	N0	M0	IIIA
T1-T4a	N1	M0	IIIA
T1-T4a	N2, N3	M0	IIIB
T4b	N0	M0	IVA
Any T	Any N	M1a	IVA
Any T	Any N	M1b	IVB

Used with permission of the American Joint Committee on Cancer (AJCC), Chicago, Illinois. The original and primary source for this information is the AJCC Cancer Staging Manual, Eighth Edition (2017) published by Springer International Publishing

VII

TREATMENT RECOMMENDATIONS

Table 25.3 TREATMENT RECOMMENDATIONS

Stages	Recommended treatments
Nonmuscle invasive (Ta, Tis, T1)	Indications for adjuvant intravesical chemo (IVC) after TURBT: multifocality, residual disease, grade II/III, Tis, T1, persistent abnormal cytology **Low-grade cTa**: TURBT alone or with IVC (commonly mitomycin) **High-grade cTa**: TURBT (repeat TURBT if incomplete resection or no muscle in initial TURBT) followed by IVC (BCG or mitomycin). May consider observation **Low-grade or high-grade cT1**: Strongly consider repeat TURBT. Adjuvant IVC (BCG or mitomycin). Consider cystectomy for residual disease or multifocality. May consider bladder conservation with chemoradiation for high-grade cT1 (Weiss 2006) **Tis**: TURBT followed by BCG

continued

Table 25.3 (continued)

Muscle invasive (T2–T4)	Treatment options:
	    Neoadjuvant cisplatin-based chemo → radical cystectomy
	    Neoadjuvant cisplatin-based chemo → partial cystectomy (selected patients with small solitary lesion in suitable location and no Tis)
	    Bladder preservation with chemo-RT after maximal TURBT
	        Optimal candidate: Unifocal, <5 cm, no hydronephrosis, good bladder function, visibly complete TURBT
	        Consider bladder preservation as a option for all appropriate patients
	    RT alone (if nonsurgical/not a chemo candidate)

Persistent disease
or
local recurrence
	For nonmuscle invasive after initial treatment:
	    If (+) cytology after adjuvant IVC → Cystectomy or change IVC agent
	    If cystoscopy positive → repeat TURBT followed by adjuvant IVC
	    If LR after 2x IVC → repeat TURBT
	        If no residual disease → maintenance BCG
	        If Tis or cTa → change IVC agent or cystectomy or chemo-RT
	        If cT1 or high grade → cystectomy or chemo-RT (preferably on clinical study, i.e., RTOG 0926)
	For muscle invasive:
	    After bladder preservation with chemo-RT (among initial CR patients, 20% ultimately develop superficial LR and 10–20% develop invasive LR).
	        Tis, Ta, or T1 → TURBT with BCG or cystectomy
	        Invasive → cystectomy or palliative TURBT with supportive care
	        (+) cytology with (−) cystoscopy/biopsies → retrograde selective washings of upper tract, prostate urethral biopsy
	    After radical cystectomy → chemo-RT (usually cisplatin-based):
	        40–45 Gy to pelvis, 50–54 Gy to sidewall if clinical recurrence, 60–64 Gy to LR.

Table 25.3 (continued)

Treatments	Descriptions
Radical cystectomy	Procedure:
	En bloc removal of bladder, perivesical tissue, urethra, and prostate/seminal vesicles or uterus/fallopian tubes/ovaries/anterior vaginal wall, with urinary diversion:
	Ileal conduit (noncontinent diversion): External bag at skin surface collects urine
	Indiana pouch (continent diversion): Internal nonorthotopic reservoir is catheterized by patient to drain urine
	Studer pouch (continent diversion): Orthotopic neobladder created by intestinal detubularized segment anastomosed to urethra, allows volitional voiding
	Bilateral pelvic lymphadenectomy should include the common, internal and external iliac, obturator nodes
	23% of all patients have LN+ disease (5% for pT0–T1, 18% for pT2, 26% for pT3a, 46% for T3b, and 42% for pT4) (Stein et al., JCO 2001).
	Neoadjuvant therapy:
	2016 NCCN guidelines recommends neoadjuvant chemo for muscle invasive disease. Pre-op RT not routinely used.
	Postoperative RT:
	If (+) margins, consider post-op chemo-RT with concurrent cisplatin (mitomycin or 5-FU if low renal function) or chemo alone if no neoadjuvant chemo given
Bladder preservation	Maximal TURBT
	Continuous course: Complete chemo-RT (60–65 Gy) → 3mo → cystoscopy
	If no tumor → observe, if tumor → cystectomy
	Split course: Induction chemo-RT (40–45 Gy) → 3 wk → cystoscopy
	If no tumor → complete chemo-RT (to 60–65 Gy), if tumor → cystectomy.

VII

STUDIES

- RT for Tis and Ta disease is generally not supported by available evidence.
- RT, or preferably chemo-RT, may be considered for high-risk T1 bladder cancers.
  - Harland (J Urol 2007): 210 patients with T1 grade 3 disease. Group 1 (unifocal, no Tis) randomized to RT alone (no

chemo) vs. observation after TURBT. Group 2 (multifocal and/or Tis) randomized to IVC vs. RT after TURBT. Median follow-up 44 mos. No difference in PFS, OS, or cystectomy rates among Group 1 or Group 2. Relatively poor LC rates may be due to the lack of concurrent chemo.

- Weiss (JCO 2006): T1 high-risk lesions without prior BCG therapy received RT or chemo-RT after TURBT. 141 patients (81 T1 grade 3). 88% achieved complete response with 5-yr PFS 81%, 10-yr PFS 70%, 5-yr DSS 82%, 10-yr DSS 73%, and >80% bladder preservation.

- RTOG 0926: Phase II trial of operable high-grade T1 disease that has failed or is ineligible for IVC. Patients receive TURBT →RT (61.2 Gy) with concurrent chemo (cisplatin or 5FU/mitomycin) → cystoscopic surveillance. Results pending.

- RT for muscle-invasive bladder cancer.
  - No randomized trials have compared radical cystectomy vs. bladder preservation.
  - For eligible patients, concurrent chemo-RT is superior to RT alone.
    - BC2001 (James, NEJM 2012): 360 patients with T2-T4aN0M0 randomized to definitive RT ± concurrent 5FU/mitomycin. Adding chemo improved 2-yr RFS (67% vs. 54%), LRF (18% vs. 32%), cystectomy rate (11% vs. 17%), and 5-yr OS (48% vs. 35%). Isolated pelvic node recurrences occurred in 5% of chemo-RT and 7% of RT groups.
  - Long-term outcomes of chemo-RT bladder preservation protocols report that about 70% of patients achieve CR and maintain their bladder with survival rates similar to surgical series.
    - Pooled RTOG analysis (Mak, JCO 2014): 468 patients with clinical T2–T4a on 6 RTOG chemo-RT bladder preservation studies. 69% achieved CR. 5/10-yr OS 57%/36%, DSS 71%/65%, muscle invasive LF 13%/14%, noninvasive LF 31%/36%, and DM 31%/35%.
    - MGH (Efstathiou, Eur Urol 2012): Single-institution retrospective. 348 patients with T2–T4a disease received maximal TURBT followed by concurrent cisplatin-based chemo-RT. 72% achieved CR. 5/10-yr OS 52/35%, DSS, 64/59%. Among CR patients, 10-yr noninvasive LR 29%, invasive LR 16%, pelvic

recurrence 11%, and DM 32%. Among visibly complete TURBT patients, only 22% required cystectomy (vs. 42% with incomplete TURBT).

- May use reduced high-dose volume RT.

  BC2001 (Huddart, IJROBP 2013): 219 patients were randomized to whole-bladder RT vs. reduced high-dose volume RT (80% of dose to whole bladder instead of 100% dose). RT was 64 Gy in 32 fx (64%) or 55 Gy in 20 fx (36%). No significant difference in 2-yr LRR-free (61% whole bladder vs. 64% reduced high-dose volume) or cumulative grade 3/4 toxicity (13%).

- Preoperative RT is not recommended to improve survival, but can improve downstaging (Granfors, Scand J Urol Nephrol 2009). Adding concurrent chemo with preoperative RT improves outcomes (Coppin, JCO 1996).

- Postoperative RT may be considered for pT3-pT4a pN0-2.

  Pelvic failure risk estimates after cystectomy (Christodouleas, IJROBP 2016). Low (pT0-2): 8%; intermediate (pT3-4, −margins, ≥10 LN removed): 18–21%; and high (pT3-4 with +margin or <10 LN removed): 41–46%.

  Consensus postoperative contouring guidelines have been published describing coverage of pelvic nodes, cystectomy bed (for +margins), and organs at risk (Baumann, IJROBP 2016).

  NRG-GU001 is a phase II trial of pT3/pT4 pN0–2 urothelial bladder cancer following radical cystectomy with ileal conduit randomized to no RT vs. postoperative 50.4 Gy IMRT.

VII

RADIATION TECHNIQUES

SIMULATION AND FIELD DESIGN

- Radiation treatment should begin within 8 weeks after maximal TURBT.
- CT simulation: Patient supine with immobilization and empty bladder.

       , Refer to bladder map from TURBT for planning. Placement of fiducial markers may be utilized to delineate the tumor bed.

       , Use of fiducials (if available) and daily image-guided RT (IGRT) help ensure setup reproducibility and accuracy of tumor targeting for boost.

       , Treat with empty bladder to ensure reproducibility of bladder volume.

    , 3D/IMRT volumes.

       , GTV_{tumor}: Any residual tumor seen on CT/MRI/cystoscopy.

       , $CTV_{tumor\ bed}$: GTV_{tumor} + tumor bed.

       , $CTV_{bladder}$: $CTV_{tumor\ bed}$ + whole bladder; use for whole bladder boost.

       , CTV_{nodal}:

           Regional lymph nodes: obturator, external iliac, and internal iliac with 0.7 cm expansion around vessels.

       , CTVpelvis: CTVbladder + CTVnodal + prostate and prostatic urethra (men).

       , PTVtumor bed: CTVtumor bed + 1.25–1.5 cm expansion.

       , PTVbladder: CTVbladder + 1.25–1.5 cm expansion.

       , PTVnodal: CTVnodal + 0.5–0.7 cm expansion.

       , PTVpelvis: PTVtumor bed + PTVbladder + PTVnodal.

    , Traditional field design.

       , Whole pelvis.

           AP/PA borders: S2–S3, lower pole of obturator foramen, widest bony pelvis margin +1.5–2 cm. Block medial border of femoral heads.

           Lateral borders: 2 cm beyond CTV_{pelvis}, same inferior and superior borders as for AP/PA field. Block rectum, small bowel.

    , Post-op for pT3-4 pN0-2 (see Baumann, IJROBP 2016).

       , CTV_{nodal} (all patients, excluding cystectomy bed for negative margins): obturator, external iliac, internal iliac, distal common iliac, and presacral.

       , $CTV_{cystectomy\ bed}$ included only for +margins.

       , PTV includes 0.5–0.7 cm expansion.

DOSE PRESCRIPTIONS

    , T1 high-risk.

       , PTV_{pelvis} to 45 Gy, boost up to 61.2 Gy, with concurrent chemo.

, Bladder preservation.
  , Treat PTV_{pelvis} to 40–45 Gy, then cone down to $PTV_{bladder}$ to 54 Gy, then cone down $PTV_{tumor\ bed}$ to 64.8 Gy with concurrent chemo.
, Post-op.
  , pT3-4 pN0-2: Pelvic nodes (and cystectomy bed if +margins) to 50.4 Gy.
  , Local recurrence after cystectomy: 45–50 Gy to pelvic nodes, 60–65 Gy to gross local recurrence with cisplatin.

DOSE LIMITATIONS

, Whole bladder 50 Gy = 5–10% late grade 3–4 effects
, Whole bladder 60 Gy = 10–40% late grade 3–4 effects
, Urethra: max dose <70 Gy associated with <5% risk of stricture
, Small bowel: TD 5/5 1/3: 50 Gy, 3/3 40 Gy

VII

COMPLICATIONS

, Irritative urinary symptoms/bladder spasm: Use terazosin or tamsulosin.
, Acute dysuria: Treat with ibuprofen or pyridium.
, If concern for UTI, order urine culture as leukocyte esterase has high false (+) rate during RT due to inflammation.
, Many patients have frequency, dysuria, intermittent hematuria, but these resolve for most patients within 2–3 yrs.
, Urethral stricture usually <5%.
, Late bowel complications up to 5–15%.
, Late toxicity in RTOG chemo-RT protocols (Efstathiou, JCO 2009):
  , GU toxicity: 10% grade 2, 6% grade 3.
  , GI toxicity: 2% grade 2, 2% grade 3.
, Post-op RT: up to 20–40% GI toxicity.
, Quality of life after bladder preservation therapy remains good.
  , Zietman J Urol 2003: At median follow-up of 6.3 yrs >75% patients retained normal bladder function and >85% reported no bothersome urinary symptoms. Reduced bladder compliance in 22%. Bowel symptoms (e.g., rectal urgency) in 22% (Zietman, J Urol 2003).

FOLLOW-UP (SEE NCCN GUIDELINES AT WWW.NCCN.ORG)

, cTa, cT1, and Tis: Cystoscopy every 3–6 mo for 2 yrs, then increasing intervals as appropriate. Consider imaging of upper tract every 1–2 yrs for high-grade tumors.

, T2–T4: Imaging of chest, upper tracts, abdomen, and pelvis every 3–6 mo for 2 yrs, then increasing intervals as appropriate.

, If bladder preservation, cystoscopy and urine cytology ± mapping biopsy every 3–6 mo for 2 yrs, then increasing intervals as appropriate.

Acknowledgment We thank William Foster MD, Brian Lee MD, PhD, and Joycelyn L. Speight MD, PhD, for their work on the prior edition of this chapter.

REFERENCES

American Cancer Society. Bladder cancer. Atlanta: American Cancer Society; 2016.

Amin, MB, Edge, S, Greene, F, Byrd, DR, Brookland, RK, Washington, MK, Gershenwald, JE, Compton, CC, Hess, KR, Sullivan, DC, Jessup, JM, Brierley, JD, Gaspar, LE, Schilsky, RL, Balch, CM, Winchester, DP, Asare, EA, Madera, M, Gress, DM, Meyer, LR (editos). AJCC cancer staging manual, 8th edition. Springer; 2017

Baumann BC, Bosch WR, Bahl A, et al. Development and validation of consensus contouring guidelines for adjuvant radiation therapy for bladder cancer after radical cystectomy. Int J Radiat Oncol Biol Phys. 2016;96(1):78–86.

Christodouleas JP, Hwang W-T, Baumann BC. Adjuvant radiation for locally advanced bladder cancer? A question worth asking. Int J Radiat Oncol Biol Phys. 2016;94(5):1040–2.

Coppin CM, Gospodarowicz MK, James K, et al. Improved local control of invasive bladder cancer by concurrent cisplatin and preoperative or definitive radiation. The National Cancer Institute of Canada Clinical Trials Group. J Clin Oncol. 1996;14:2901–7.

Edge SB, Byrd DR, Compton CC, Fritz AG, Greene FL, Trotti A, (editors). AJCC cancer staging manual, 7th edition. Springer; 2010.

Efstathiou JA, Bae K, Shipley WU, et al. Late pelvic toxicity after bladder-sparing therapy in patients with invasive bladder cancer: RTOG 89-03, 95-06, 97-06, 99-06. J Clin Oncol. 2009;27(25):4055–61.

Efstathiou JA, Spiegel DY, Shipley WU, et al. Long-term outcomes of selective bladder preservation by combined-modality therapy for invasive bladder cancer: the MGH experience. Eur Urol. 2012;61(4):705–11.

Granfors T, Tomic R, Ljungberg B. Downstaging and survival benefits of neoadjuvant radiotherapy before cystectomy for patients with invasive bladder carcinoma. Scand J Urol Nephrol. 2009;43(4):293–9.

Harland SJ, Kynaston H, Grigor K, et al. A randomized trial of radical radiotherapy for the management of pT1G3 NXM0 transitional cell carcinoma of the bladder. J Urol. 2007;178:807–13.

Huddart RA, Hall E, Hussain SA, et al. Randomized noninferiority trial of reduced high-dose volume versus standard volume radiation therapy for muscle-invasive bladder cancer: results of the BC2001 trial (CRUK/01/004). Int J Radiat Oncol Biol Phys. 2013;87(2):261–9.

James ND, Hussain SA, Hall E, et al. Radiotherapy with or without chemotherapy in muscle-invasive bladder cancer. N Engl J Med. 2012;366(16):1477–88.

Mak RH, Hunt D, Shipley WU, et al. Long-term outcomes in patients with muscle-invasive bladder cancer after selective bladder-preserving combined-modality therapy: a pooled analysis of Radiation Therapy Oncology Group protocols 8802, 8903, 9506, 9706, 9906, and 0233. J Clin Oncol. 2014;32(34):3801–9.

National Comprehensive Cancer Network. Clinical practice guidelines in oncology: bladder cancer v.2.2016. Available at: http://www.nccn.org/professionals/physician_gls/PDF/bladder.pdf

Stein JP, Lieskovsky G, Skinner DG, et al. Radical cystectomy in the treatment of invasive bladder cancer: long-term results in 1,054 patients. J Clin Oncol. 2001;19(3):666–75.

Weiss C, Wolze C, Rodel C, et al. Radiochemotherapy after transurethral resection for high-risk T1 bladder cancer: an alternative to intravesical therapy or early cystectomy? J Clin Oncol. 2006;24(15):2318–24.

Yuan H, Qiu J, Liu L, et al. Therapeutic outcome of fluorescence cystoscopy guided transurethral resection in patients with non-muscle invasive bladder cancer: a meta-analysis of randomized controlled trials. Real FX, ed. PLoS One. 2013;8(9):e74142.

Zietman AL, Sacco D, Skowronski U, et al. Organ conservation in invasive bladder cancer by transurethral resection, chemotherapy and radiation: results of a urodynamic and quality of life study on long-term survivors. J Urol. 2003;170:1772–6.

VII

Chapter 26
Prostate Cancer

Michael A. Garcia, Eric K. Hansen, and Mack Roach III

PEARLS

- Prostate cancer epidemiology:
  - No. 1 non-cutaneous cancer in men – 180,890 estimated cases in the USA in 2016:
    - 1 in 7 men diagnosed in their lifetime, median age at diagnosis is 66.
  - No. 2 cause of cancer death (~26,120 deaths in 2016) after lung cancer.
  - 90% of all prostate cancers are adenocarcinoma.
- Prostate anatomy:
  - Anatomic regions:
    - Apex (inferior): site of 50–80% of cancers, capsule not well defined here and true extracapsular (ECE) is difficult to recognize.
    - Mid-gland.
    - Base (superior, adjacent to bladder).
    - ECE most common at posterior lateral prostate (region penetrated by nerves).
  - Zones:
    - Peripheral zone: 70% of glandular prostate and site of nearly all cancers.
    - Central zone: 25% of the glandular prostate.
    - Transition zone: surrounds urethra and the site of BPH.
    - Anterior fibromuscular stroma.

, Lymph node (LN) drainage:
  , Primarily to internal iliac, obturator, external iliac, and presacral nodes.
  , Disease may also spread to perirectal, common iliac, and para-aortic nodes.
  , Standard prostatectomy LN dissection samples only obturator and external iliac nodes, though 40–60% of involved LN are located in the internal iliac and presacral chains.

, Gleason score (GS) – the sum (2–10) of the major + minor glandular patterns:
  , For each pattern, range is from slight disorganization (1) to anaplastic (5).
  , 2014 International Society of Urological Pathology (ISUP) consensus on Grading of Prostatic Carcinoma (Epstein, Am J Surg Pathol 2016a): group 1 (GS < 6), group 2 (GS 3 + 4), group 3 (GS 4 + 3), group 4 (GS 4 + 4, 3 + 5, 5 + 3), and group 5 (GS 9–10).

SCREENING

, American Cancer Society recommendations (2016):
  , When screening is pursued, should consist of PSA and digital exam.
  , Discussion about uncertainties, risks, and benefits should be had with men at:
    , Age 50 for men at average risk and expected to live at least 10 more years.
    , Age 45 for men at high risk: African-Americans and men with first-degree relative (father, brother, son) diagnosed with prostate cancer at age <65.
    , Age 40 for men at even higher risk: >1 first-degree relative diagnosed at age <65.
    , If the patient asks the physician to decide for him, screening is recommended.

, American Urological Association recommendations (2013):
  , Panel recommends *against* PSA screening in men of age <40.
  , Panel does not recommend routine screening in men ages 40–54. For men at high risk (family history or

African-American), decision for screening should be individualized.

- US Preventative Services Task Force (2012):
  - USPSTF recommends against PSA-based screening for prostate cancer.
  - As a result of USPTF guidelines, screening rates have decreased, and the incidence of metastatic disease may have increased (Jemal, JAMA 2016; Weiner, Prostate Cancer Prostatic Dis 2016).

Table 26.1 Screening Trials

Study	Patients	Arms	Follow-up	RR of death from prostate cancer
PLCO trial* (Andriole, JNCI 2012)	76,685 Age 55–74	**Intervention:** PSA ×6 yrs + DRE ×4 yrs **Control**: Usual care. *Note: Very high PSA screening contamination in control arm (Pinsky, Clin Trials 2010, Shoag, NEJM 2016)*	13 yrs	1.09 (95%CI 0.87–1.36)
ERSPC trial* (Schroder, Lancet 2014)	182,160 Age 55–69	Screening: Offered PSA every year Control: Not offered PSA	13 yrs	0.79 decrease in screened arm (95% CI 0.69–0.91, $p < 0.001$).

*Comment: ERSPC trial appears to be better powered and implemented to answer the question of screening. Additionally, PLCO trial patients were prescreened, while ERSPC trial included index cases diagnosed at the time of recruitment.

VII

WORK-UP

- H&P, including American Urology Association (AUA) urinary symptom score, baseline erectile function, bone pain, and DRE.
- Labs (including PSA, testosterone, CBC, and LFTs).
- TRUS-guided (± MRI fusion) biopsy (>8 separate cores recommended):
  - During TRUS, note prostate volume and any pubic arch interference if considering brachytherapy.

, GS upgrading from ≤6 to ≥7 or from 7 to >7 in 25–30% at prostatectomy (Chun, BJU 2006). Downgrading of GS at prostatectomy is uncommon (Manoharan, BJUI Int 2003).

, Imaging:

  , Bone scan if T1 and PSA >20, T2 and PSA >10, GS ≥8, T3–T4, or symptoms (NCCN).

  , Pelvic CT or MRI if T3–T4 or T1–T2 and risk of LN involvement is >10% (NCCN).

  , MR spectroscopy: decreased citrate and increased choline in prostate cancer:

    , Role in routine management remains controversial.

  , A number of PET/CT tracers have been identified with potential role in staging at initial diagnosis and recurrence (Mertan, Future Oncol 2016):

    , ^{68}Ga prostate-specific membrane antigen (PSMA): very promising with pooled sensitivity 63–86%, specificity 95–100%, even at low PSA values; comparative studies may be superior to choline-PET.

    , ^{11}C-choline: variable sensitivity (38–98%) and specificity (50–100%) for detecting local, node, or distant metastasis, especially at low PSA values (<1 ng/ml). Pooled meta-analysis reports 85% sensitivity and 88% specificity, but difficult to control for variables in different studied populations.

    , ^{18}F—NaF: improved sensitivity (87–89%) for osteoblastic mets but lower specificity (80–91%) than traditional bone scan due to false positives (e.g., healing fractures, bone dysplasia).

STAGING: PROSTATE CANCER

Editors' note: All TNM stage and stage groups referred to elsewhere in this chapter reflect the 2010 AJCC staging nomenclature unless otherwise noted as the new system below was published after this chapter was written.

Table 26.2 AJCC 7TH ED., (2010)

Primary tumor (T) – clinical

TX:	Primary tumor cannot be assessed
T0:	No evidence of primary tumor
T1:	Clinically in apparent tumor neither palpable nor visible by imaging:
T1a:	Tumor incidental histologic finding in 5% or less of tissue resected
T1b:	Tumor incidental histologic finding in more than 5% of tissue resected
T1c:	Tumor identified by needle biopsy (e.g., because of elevated PSA)
T2:	Tumor confined within prostate*
T2a:	Tumor involves one-half of one lobe or less
T2b:	Tumor involves more than one-half of one lobe, but not both lobes
T2c:	Tumor involves both lobes
T3:	Tumor extends through the prostate capsule**
T3a:	Extracapsular extension (unilateral or bilateral)
T3b:	Tumor invades seminal vesicle(s)
T4:	Tumor is fixed or invades adjacent structures other than seminal vesicles such as external sphincter, rectum, bladder, levator muscles, and/or pelvic wall

*Note: Tumor found in one or both lobes by needle biopsy, but not palpable or reliably visible by imaging, is classified as T1c

**Note: Invasion into the prostatic apex or into (but not beyond) the prostatic capsule is classified not as T3 but as T2

Pathologic (pT)*

pT2:	Organ confined
pT2a:	Unilateral, one-half of one side or less
pT2b:	Unilateral, involving more than one-half of side but not both sides
pT2c:	Bilateral disease
pT3:	Extraprostatic extension
pT3a:	Extraprostatic extension or microscopic invasion of bladder neck**
pT3b:	Seminal vesicle invasion
pT4:	Invasion of rectum, levator muscles, and /or pelvic wall

*Note: There is no pathologic T1 classification

**Note: Positive surgical margin should be indicated by an R1 descriptor (residual microscopic disease)

Regional lymph nodes (N)

Clinical

NX:	Regional lymph nodes were not assessed
N0:	No regional lymph node metastasis
N1:	Metastasis in regional lymph node(s)

Pathologic

pNX:	Regional nodes not sampled
pN0:	No positive regional nodes
pN1:	Metastases in regional node(s)

Distant metastasis (M)*

M0:	No distant metastasis
M1:	Distant metastasis
M1a:	Nonregional lymph node(s)
M1b:	Bone(s)
M1c:	Other site(s) with or without bone disease

*Note: When more than one site of metastasis is present, the most advanced category is used. pM1c is most advanced

continued

VII

Table 26.2 (continued)

Anatomic stage/prognostic groups*					
Group	T	N	M	PSA	Gleason
I	T1a–c	N0	M0	PSA < 10	Gleason ≤6
	T2a	N0	M0	PSA < 10	Gleason ≤6
	T1–T2a	N0	M0	PSA X	Gleason X
IIA:	T1a–c	N0	M0	PSA < 20	Gleason 7
	T1a–c	N0	M0	PSA ≥ 10 < 20	Gleason ≤6
	T2a	N0	M0	PSA < 20	Gleason ≤7
	T2b	N0	M0	PSA < 20	Gleason ≤7
	T2b	N0	M0	PSA X	Gleason X
IIB:	T2c	N0	M0	Any PSA	Any Gleason
	T1–T2	N0	M0	PSA ≥ 20	Any Gleason
	T1–T2	N0	M0	Any PSA	Gleason ≥8
III:	T3a–b	N0	M0	Any PSA	Any Gleason
IV:	T4	N0	M0	Any PSA	Any Gleason
	Any T	N1	M0	Any PSA	Any Gleason
	Any T	Any N	M1	Any PSA	Any Gleason

*When either PSA or Gleason is not available, grouping should be determined by T stage and/or either PSA or Gleason as available

Used with the permission from the American Joint Committee on Cancer (AJCC), Chicago, Illinois. The original source for this material is the AJCC Cancer Staging Manual, Seventh Edition (2010), published by Springer Science+Business Media

Table 26.3 AJCC 8TH ED., (2017)

Definitions of AJCC TNM	
Definition of Primary Tumor (T)	
Clinical T (cT)	
T category	**T criteria**
TX	Primary tumor cannot be assessed
T0	No evidence of primary tumor
T1	Clinically inapparent tumor that is not palpable
T1a	Tumor incidental histologic finding in 5% or less of tissue resected
T1b	Tumor incidental histologic finding in more than 5% of tissue resected
T1c	Tumor identified by needle biopsy found in one or both sides, but not palpable
T2	Tumor is palpable and confined within prostate
T2a	Tumor involves one-half of one side or less
T2b	Tumor involves more than one-half of one side but not both sides
T2c	Tumor involves both sides
T3	Extraprostatic tumor that is not fixed or does not invade adjacent structures
T3a	Extraprostatic extension (unilateral or bilateral)
T3b	Tumor invades seminal vesicle(s)
T4	Tumor is fixed or invades adjacent structures other than seminal vesicles such as the external sphincter, rectum, bladder, levator muscles, and/or pelvic wall

PATHOLOGICAL T (PT)

T category	T criteria
T2	Organ confined
T3	Extraprostatic extension
T3a	Extraprostatic extension (unilateral or bilateral) or microscopic invasion of the bladder neck
T3b	Tumor invades seminal vesicle(s)
T4	Tumor is fixed or invades adjacent structures other than seminal vesicles such as the external sphincter, rectum, bladder, levator muscles, and/or pelvic wall

Note: There is no pathological Tl classification
Note: Positive surgical margin should be indicated by an Rl descriptor, indicating residual microscopic disease

DEFINITION OF REGIONAL LYMPH NODE (N)

N category	N criteria
NX	Regional nodes were not assessed
N0	No positive regional nodes
N1	Metastases in regional node(s)

DEFINITION OF DISTANT METASTASIS (M)

M category	M criteria
M0	No distant metastasis
M1	Distant metastasis
M1a	Nonregional lymph node(s)
M1b	Bone(s)
M1c	Other site(s) with or without bone disease

Note: When more than one site of metastasis is present, the most advanced category is used. M1c is most advanced

DEFINITION OF PROSTATE-SPECIFIC ANTIGEN (PSA)

PSA values
<10
≥10<20
<20
≥20
Any value

DEFINITION OF HISTOLOGIE GRADE GROUP (G)

Grade group	Gleason score	Gleason pattern
1	≤6	≤3+3
2	7	3+4
3	7	4+3
4	8	4+4
5	9 or 10	4+5, 5+4, or 5+5

VII

AJCC PROGNOSTIC STAGE GROUPS

When T is...	And N is...	And M is...	And PSA is...	And grade group is...	Then the stage group is...
cT1a–c, cT2a	N0	M0	<10	1	I
pT2	N0	M0	<10	1	I
cT1a–c, cT2a	N0	M0	≥10<20	1	IIA
cT2b–c	N0	M0	<20	1	IIA
T1–2	N0	M0	<20	2	IIB
T1–2	N0	M0	<20	3	IIC
T1–2	N0	M0	<20	4	IIC
T1–2	N0	M0	≥20	1–4	IIIA
T3–4	N0	M0	Any	1–4	IIIB
Any T	N0	M0	Any	5	IIIC
Any T	N1	M0	Any	Any	IVA
Any T	N0	M1	Any	Any	IVB

Note: When either the PSA or grade group is not available, grouping should be determined by T category and/or either the PSA or grade group is available

Used with permission of the American Joint Committee on Cancer (AJCC), Chicago, Illinois. The original and primary source for this information is the AJCC Cancer Staging Manual, Eighth Edition (2017) published by Springer International Publishing

Table 26.4 Risk classification schemes

2016 NCCN risk categories

Very low: T1c, GS ≤6, PSA <10, disease in <3 cores, ≤50% involvement in any core, and PSA density < 0.15

Low: T1–T2a, GS ≤6 and PSA <10

Intermediate: T2b–T2c and/or GS 7 and/or PSA 10–20

High: T3a or GS 8–10 or PSA >20

Very high: T3b–T4 and/or primary Gleason pattern 5 and/or >4 cores with GS 8–10

Roach formulas estimate pathologic stage based on original partin data

ECE = 3/2 × PSA + 10 × (GS-3)

Seminal vesicle involvement = PSA + 10 × (GS-6)

LN involvement = 2/3 × PSA + 10 × (GS-6)

Kattan nomograms predict primarily PSA recurrence, PFS, and prostate cancer-specific mortality after RP, 3DCRT, or brachytherapy (http://www.nomograms.org)

Table 26.5 TREATMENT RECOMMENDATIONS

Stage	Recommended treatment	5–10 years bPFS	5–10 years CSS
Low risk	Life expectancy*≤10 yrs → active surveillance (AS) or EBRT or brachytherapy Life expectancy ≥10 yrs → EBRT, brachytherapy, radical prostatectomy (RP) ± pelvic LN dissection (PLND), or AS	85–95%	>97%

Intermediate risk	Life expectancy <10 yrs → AS, EBRT ± short-term androgen deprivation therapy (stADT) or RP + PLND
	For life expectancy ≥10 years → EBRT + stADT (4–6 month) ± brachytherapy boost, brachytherapy monotherapy, or RP ± PLND:
	    Brachytherapy monotherapy may be considered for favorable intermediate risk (e.g., T1c–T2b, GS 3 + 4 vs. 4 + 3, smaller volume disease)
	    RTOG 0924 investigating role of pelvic LN RT for unfavorable intermediate-risk and favorable high-risk men
		70–85%	85–95%

High risk	EBRT ± brachytherapy boost with long-term ADT (2–3 yrs) (ltADT) ± docetaxel. LN irradiation is indicated Consider RP + PLND for select patients with low-volume disease and no fixation	50–80%	T1–T2: 80–85% N+: 60%
Node+	Lifelong or ltADT alone ± EBRT ± brachytherapy boost. RT + ADT preferred over ADT alone when limited LN disease	10-yr OS 35–60% 5-yr PFS 20–50%	

Metastatic	ADT sensitive:
	    ADT (≥2 yrs) ± (docetaxel ± prednisone)
	ADT resistant:
	    Docetaxel or abiraterone or enzalutamide or radium-233 (if no visceral metastases)
	    Palliative RT ± bisphosphonates
		Median survival for newly diagnosed M1 disease: ~ 3 yrs	

Adjuvant RT after RP	Adjuvant EBRT indications:
	    Residual local disease
	    +margin(s), pT3 disease
		Adjuvant RT
		5-yr bPFS <75%
		5–10-yr LF 5–8%	

Salvage RT after RP	Salvage EBRT indicated for initially undetectable PSA that subsequently rises
	Salvage RT most effective for patients with:
	    Low PSA at time of salvage (≪1 ng/mL)
	    PSA velocity < 2 ng/mL in year before diagnosis
	    Time to PSA failure >3 yrs after RP
	    Pathologic GS ≤7, +margin(s), no LN involvement, and no SVI
	Consider adding ADT, particularly for men with high-risk features (RTOG used 2-yrs bicalutamide; GETUG used 6-mo LHRH agonist)
		Salvage RT
		See Trock and Stephenson/ Tendulkar nomograms to estimate prostate cancer-specific mortality (PCSM) and bPFS	

continued

Table 26.5 (continued)

Residual disease or recurrence after RT	Non-metastatic and +biopsy
	Observation often preferred
	Salvage local therapy (RP, brachytherapy, or cryotherapy) may be considered for select patients. Men most likely to benefit have no/minimal comorbidities, long life expectancy, initial low-risk disease, longer interval to PSA failure (>3 yrs), slow PSA doubling time (>12 mo), lower pre-salvage PSA (<10), and pre-salvage GS ≤7
	Risk of complications of salvage local therapy is increased, so recommend careful patient selection and treatment at experienced center
	Metastatic or not a candidate for local therapy: ADT or observation

*Life expectancy can be estimated using the Social Security Administration tables at http://www.ssa.gov

STUDIES

ACTIVE SURVEILLANCE (AS) AND WATCHFUL WAITING (WW)

- AS generally consists of DRE and PSA every 3–6 months with routine repeat biopsy in 1–2 yrs with definitive treatment given if disease progresses.
  - The goal of AS is to avoid or defer therapy (and side effects) until necessary.
    - Disadvantages of AS include risk of missed opportunity for cure, risk of progression, and/or distant metastases (DM); deferred treatment may be more intense with increased morbidity and anxiety with each new PSA/biopsy.
- WW watches for symptoms that may arise from prostate cancer rather than regimented PSA, DRE, and biopsy, typically in men not suitable for aggressive treatment.
  - WW may forgo possibility of curative treatment but symptoms are addressed.

Table 26.6 Active surveillance and watching waiting trials

Study	Patients	Management	Results
ProtecT trial (Hamdy, NEJM 2016)	1,643 men, 77% GS6, 76% T1c Median age 62	Randomized to AS, RP, or EBRT + 3–6-mo ADT	No difference 10-yr PCSS (99%), but increased DM with AS (6%) vs. RP or RT (2–3%) and increased clinical progression with AS (23%) vs. RP or RT (9%). In AS arm, % men having treatment at 2 yrs 20%, 5 yrs 40%, and 10 yrs 56%. No significant differences between RP and RT
SPCG-4 trial (Bill-Axelson, NEJM 2014)	695 men T1b–T2 Mean age 65	Randomized RP vs. WW	At median f/u of 13.4 yrs RP reduced PCSM by 11%, DM by 12%, and use of ADT by 25%. Subgroup analysis: survival benefit limited to men age <65
ERSPC subset analysis(Bul, BJUI 2012)	509 men low/int. risk median age 68	AS after diagnosed on screening arm of ERSPC	At median f/u of 7 yrs, 43% men switched to deferred treatment after a median of 2.6 yrs. 10-yr CSS 99.1% for low risk and 96.1% for int.-risk patients

ADT ALONE OR WITH RT

Study	Patients	Management	Results
SPCG-7 trial (Fosså, Eur Urol 2016)	875 men 90% high risk, 78% T3, median PSA 16	Arm 1: ADT alone (total blockade ×3 mo then flutamide)arm 2: ADT + RT 70 Gy prostate and SV	Adding RT reduced 10-yr PCSM 19 → 9%, 15-yr PCSM 34% → 17%. Number needed to treat to avert 1 prostate cancer death 5.9. *QOL (Fransson, Lancet Oncol 2009)*: RT increased 4-yr mod/severe urinary bother by 6%, dysuria by 2%, bowel bother by 4%, and erectile dysfunction by 13%
MRC trial (Mason, JCO 2015)	1,205 men T3–T4N0M0 or T1–T2+ PSA > 40 or PSA 20–40 + GS 8–10	ADT alone vs. ADT + RT	Adding RT improved 10-yr OS 55% vs. 49%, PCSM 11% vs. 22%. Adding RT increased urinary frequency by 3%, mild to moderate bowel side effects by 12%, severe diarrhea <0.5%

VII

RADICAL PROSTATECTOMY (RP)

, Retropubic prostatectomy is the standard surgical approach and allows for PLND. Perineal approach is reasonable for men with low-risk disease and small prostates in whom PLND is not indicated, though this approach has largely been abandoned.

, NCCN recommends PLND if risk of LN metastases is >2% by the MSKCC Nomogram (Kattan, Urology 2001).

, High-volume surgeons in high-volume centers generally provide better outcomes.

, Results with laparoscopic and robot-assisted RP in experienced hands are comparable to open approaches.

, Erectile recovery is related to degree of preservation of cavernous nerves and baseline function.

, Multiple studies of neoadjuvant ADT + RP vs. RP alone demonstrate decreased margin positivity and tumor volume but no change in biochemical progression-free survival (bPFS).

, Pathologic GS 3 + 4 has better prognosis than 4 + 3: 10-yr bRFS (48 vs. 38%), DM (8 vs. 15%), and CSS (97 vs. 93%) (Tollefson, J Urol 2006).

, Occult LN mets found in 13% of men with pT3 who were pN0 by H&E. Men with occult LN mets have similar PFS and OS to those with pN+ (Pagliarulo, JCO 2006).

, There is no indisputable evidence that RP is more effective than RT ± ADT (Roach, IJROBP 2015; Hamdy, NEJM 2016; Lennernäs, Acta Oncol 2015). The "meta-analysis" published by Wallis (Wallis, Eur Urol 2016) is flawed; it uses inappropriate RT populations for comparison (Eifler, J Urol 2012) and should be ignored (Roach, Clin Oncol 2016).

RADIATION DOSE ESCALATION

, Several randomized trials report 10–20% increase in bPFS with dose escalation, but no survival benefit (so far), with increased toxicity risk (at least in part related to dosimetric factors).

Table 26.7 Dose escalation trials

Study	Patients	Doses	Benefit	Late toxicity
MDACC (Kuban, IJROBP 2008)	301 men T1–T3N0 No ADT	70 vs. 78 Gy to isocenter (initial 4-field box to 46 Gy)	8-yr bPFS/clinical PFS: Low risk: 63 → 88% Int. risk(PSA > 10): 65 → 94% High risk: 26 → 63% No OS difference	Gr ≥2 GI toxicity: 13 → 26% (16% vs. 46% when <25% vs. >25% rectum received >70 Gy) Gr ≥2 GU toxicity: 8 → 13% (NS)
PROG 9509 (Zietman, JCO 2010)	393 men T1b–T2b, PSA <15 58% low, 33% int. risk no ADT	70.2 vs. 79.2 Gy using proton boost after 50.4 Gy to P and SV	10-yr biochem failure (bF): Low risk: 28 → 7% Int. risk: 42 → 30% No OS difference	No difference Gr ≥ 3 GU 2%, GI 1% toxicity
Netherlands (Al-Mamgani, IJROBP 2008)	669 men T1b–T4N0 PSA < 60 18% low, 28% int., 54% high risk, 10% stADT, 11% ltADT	68 vs. 78 Gy to P ± SV	7-yr bPFS: 45 → 56% greatest risk reduction for int. risk and high risk, but not low risk. No OS difference	Gr ≥2 GI toxicity: 25 → 35%. No difference in GU toxicity
MRC RT01 (Dearnaley, Lancet Oncol 2014)	843 men T1b–T3N0, PSA <50. 25% low, 30% int., 45% high. 3–6-month nADT	64 vs. 74 Gy to P and SV	10-yr bPFS: 43 → 57% Benefit in all risk groups. No OS difference	Gr ≥2 GI toxicity: 24 → 33%. Gr ≥2 GU toxicity: 8–11%
GETUG (Beckendorf, IJROBP 2011)	306 men T1b–T3N0, PSA < 50, no ADT	70 vs. 80 Gy to P (after 46 Gy to P and SV)	5-yr bF: 32 → 24%, subgroup benefit if PSA >15	Gr ≥2 GI toxicity: 14 → 19%. Gr ≥2 GU toxicity: 10 → 18%
RTOG 0126 (Michalski, ASCO GU 2015)	1499 men, T1b–T2b GS 2–6 and PSA 10–20 or GS 7 and PSA <15	70.2 vs. 79.2 Gy EBRT	10-yr bF 26% vs.43%, local progression 4% vs. 8%, DM 5% vs. 8%. No OS difference	10 yr Gr ≥ 2 GI/ GU toxicity 16/10% vs. 22/15%

P prostate; *SV* seminal vesicles; *nADT* neoadjuvant ADT

VII

HYPOFRACTIONATION

- Moderate hypofractionation is 2.4–4 Gy/fx.
- Randomized studies of moderate hypofractionation report similar PFS to conventional fractionation (1.8–2 Gy/fx), but often with small increased toxicity risks.

Table 26.8 Moderate hypofractionation

Study	Patients	Arms (Gy/fx)	Results
CHHiP (Dearnaley, Lancet Oncol 2016)	3,216 men 15% low risk, 73% int. risk, 12% high risk	C-RT: 74/37 H-RT: 57–60/19–20	5-yr biochemical clinical PFS H-RT 60 Gy non-inferior to C-RT 74 Gy: low risk 97%, int. risk 87–90%, and high risk 84–87%. More acute toxicity with H-RT but similar late toxicity: 5-yr Gr 2/3 GI 12–14%/<1%, GU 9–12%/<1%
OCOG (Catton, ASCO 2016)	1,206 men int. risk	C-RT: 78/39 H-RT: 60/20	No difference 5-yr bF 21%. H-RT increased late GU/GI toxicity by 1.9%
RTOG 0415(Lee, JCO 2016)	1,115 menT1–T2cPSA <10	C-RT: 73.8/41 H-RT: 70/28	No difference 5-yr DFS 85% C-RT vs. 86% H-RT or bF C-RT 8% vs. 6% H-RT. H-RT increased late grade 2/3 GI (14% vs. 22%) and GU toxicity (23% vs. 30%)
HYPRO (Incrocci; Aluwini, Lancet Oncol 2016)	820 men 26% int. risk, 74% high risk	C-RT: 78/39 H-RT: 64.6/19	No difference 5-yr RFS 77–81%. H-RT increased late Gr 3 GU toxicity. 3-yr Gr 2/3 GU toxicity C-RT 39/13% vs. H-RT 41/19%, Gr 2/3 GI toxicity C-RT 18/3% vs. 22/3%
Pollack (JCO 2013)	303 men int. and high risk	C-RT: 76/38H-RT: 70.2/26	No difference 5-yr bcF 21–23%. Men with compromised urinary function before RT had slightly worse urinary function after H-RT
Hoffman (Am J Clin Oncol 2016)	206 men mostly low to int. risk	IMRT C-RT: 75.6/42 H-RT: 72/30	8-yr recurrence: 10% H-RT vs. 15% C-RT Late Gr 2/3 GI toxicity: 13% H-RT vs. 5% C-RT
Arcangeli (IJROBP 2012)	168 men high risk	C-RT: 80/40H-RT 62/20	No difference in 70-month bF: C-RT 26% vs. H-RT 21%, but subgroup PSA > 20 men had improved bF with H-RT. No difference in toxicity
Lukka(JCO 2005)	936 menT1–T2, PSA <40, no ADT	C-RT: 66/33H-RT: 52.5/20	5-yr bcPFS C-RT 47% vs. H-RT 40% (non-inferiority not met). Gr 3 late toxicity 3.2% both arms

H-RT hypofractionation; *C-RT* conventional fractionation; *bF* biochemical failure; *bcPFS* biochemical and clinical progression-free survival

꙳ Extreme hypofractionation is 6.5–10 Gy/fx for 4–7 fractions, typically using SBRT with intra-fraction motion management.

꙳ Early data for extreme hypofractionation is promising, but long-term follow-up data is limited.

Table 26.9 Extreme hypofractionation

Study	Patients	Treatment	Results
HYPO-RT-PC (Widmark, ASTRO 2016)	1200 int.-risk men randomized	78 Gy/39 fx vs. 42.7 Gy/7 fx	Median f/u 4.2 yr. No difference in 2-yr Gr 2+ toxicity
PCG GU 002(Vargas, Am JCO 2015)	82 low-risk men randomized	Protons: 38 RBE/5 fx vs. 79.2 RBE/44 fx	Median f/u 18 mo. No difference in urinary, bowel, or sexual function scores. AUA score only worse for H-RT at 12 mo, otherwise similar. No Gr 3/4 toxicity
Pooled analysis (King, Radiother Oncol 2013)	1100 men reviewed 58% low, 30% int., 11% high risk	CyberKnife SBRT 36.25 Gy/4–5 fx	Median f/u 36 mo. 5-yr bPFS low risk 95%, int. risk 84%, high risk 81%
Katz (Frontier, Oncol 2016)	515 men reviewed 63% low, 30% int., 7% high risk	CyberKnife SBRT. 35–36.25 Gy/5 fx	Median f/u 84 mo. 8-yr bPFS low risk 94%, int. risk 84%, high risk 65%. 2% late Gr 3 GU toxicity at 7-yr f/u

VII

RT + ADT

꙳ There is a large body of evidence supporting the addition of ADT to EBRT for patients with intermediate- to high-risk prostate cancer.

꙳ Meta-analysis (Nguyen, JAMA 2011). Among 4,141 men on eight randomized trials of unfavorable-risk prostate cancer, ADT use was not associated with increased risk of cardiovascular death but was associated with lower risk of PCSM and all-cause mortality.

RT + SHORT-TERM ADT

꙳ Randomized trials of stADT vs. no ADT report that adding 3–6-mo ADT improves bPFS by 10–25% and CSS by 3–8%.

Table 26.10 Short term androgen deprivation

Study	Patients	Arms	Benefit
RTOG 9408(Jones, NEJM 2011)	1979 men T1b–T2bPSA < 20	66.6 Gy +/– 4-mo ADT	ST-ADT improved 10-yr OS 61% vs. 54% and PCSM 3% vs. 10% for int.-risk men
RTOG 8610 (Roach, JCO 2008)	456 men Palpable T2–4	66–70 Gy ± 4-mo ADT	10-yr CSS: 64 → 77% DM: 47 → 35% OS: 34 → 43% (GS2–6 subset 52 → 70%)
(D'Amico, JAMA 2015)	206 men T1–T2b + G7–10 or PSA 10–40 or ECE or SVI on MRI)	70 Gy ± 6-mo ADT	Among men with no or minimal comorbidity, RT + ADT improved 15-yr OS (44% vs. 31%), but not men with moderate to severe comorbidity
TTROG 96.01 (Denham, Lancet Oncol 2011)	818 men T2b–T4N0M0 15% int. risk 85% high risk	66 Gy + 0- vs. 3- vs. 6-mo ADT	Compared to no ADT, 3 mo & 6 mo ADT improved bF, LF, and PFS. 6-mo ADT improved DM, PCSM, and OS
Laverdiere (J Urol 2004) Two successive trials reported (L101 and L200)	481 men in L101, 325 in L200 T2–T3N0 70% int. risk	64 Gy. L101: 0- vs. 3-mo vs. 10-mo ADT L200: 5-mo vs. 10-mo ADT	L101: 7-yr bPFS: 42 → 67% with 3–10-mo ADT vs. no ADT. L200: No difference in bPFS with 5- vs. 10-mo ADT
EORTC 22991 (Bolla, JCO 2016)	819 men, 75% int. risk, 25% high risk	70–78 Gy ± 6-mo ADT	ADT improved 5 yr bPFS 70%–83%, DFS 81%–89% and reduced LF 7%–2% and DM 8%–4%, with no difference by RT dose level
RTOG 9910 (Pisansky, JCO 2015)	1579 int.-risk men	70.2 Gy + 4 mo vs. 9-mo ADT	No difference in 10-yr OS, DSS, DM, and bF. Trend for 2% reduced 10-yr LRF (4% vs. 6%) with 9-mo ADT
GETUG-14 (Dubray, ASCO 2016)	377 int.-risk men	80 Gy ± 4 mo ADT	Adding ADT reduced 5-yr bF 10% vs. 21% and improved EFS 84%–76%
PCS III (Nabid, ASCO 2015)	600 int.-risk men	76 Gy alone vs. 70 Gy or 76 Gy + 6 mo ADT	Adding ADT reduced 5-yr bF (76 Gy 14%, 76 Gy + ADT 2%, 70 Gy + ADT 7%) and improved DFS (76 Gy 86%, 76 Gy + ADT 97%, 70 Gy + ADT 93%). Increasing dose to 76 Gy increased late GI toxicity (16% vs. 5%), but did not improve bF or DFS

RT + LONG-TERM ADT

, For high-risk men, long-term ADT improves DFS, CSS, and OS vs. no ADT or 4–6-mo ADT.

, Current standard for most high-risk men is 2–3 yrs ADT, but 18 months may be reasonable for those with limited high-risk features or comorbidity.

Table 26.11 Long term androgen deprivation

Study	Patients	Arms	Benefit
DART01/05 GICOR trial(Zapatero, Lancet Oncol 2015)	355 men, 46% int. risk, 54% high risk	78 Gy + 4-mo ADT vs. 28-mo ADT	28-mo ADT improved 5-yr bPFS (88% vs. 76%), DMFS (94% vs. 79%), and OS (96% vs. 82%) for high-risk men, but no significant benefit for int. risk
RTOG 8531 (Efstathiou, JCO 2009)	977 men cT3, pT3, or N+	65–70 Gy ± indefinite goserelin starting the last week of RT	ADT improved 10-yr OS (49% vs. 39%), CSS (84 vs. 78%), and DM (24 vs. 39%). Subset analysis: OS benefit only for G7–10
EORTC 22863 (Bolla, Lancet 2010)	415 men T3–T4 (92%) or T1–T2 GS ≥ 7 (8%)	70 Gy ±3-yr goserelin starting on first day of RT	Adding ADT improved 10-yr OS (40 → 58%), CSS (70% → 90%)
RTOG 9202 (Horwitz, JCO 2008)	1,554 men T2c–T4 PSA <150	65–70 Gy + 4 mo vs. 28-mo ADT	Long-term ADT improved 10-yr CSS 84 → 89%, DM 23 → 15%, bF 68 → 52%, LF 22 → 12%. Improved 10-yr OS for GS 8–10 32 → 45%.
EORTC 22961 (Bolla, NEJM 2009)	970 men T2c–T4N0/+ or T1c–T2bN+	70 Gy + 6-mo vs. 3-yr ADT	No difference in 5-yr OS, but 3 yrs ADT reduced 5-yr PCSM 3% vs. 5%
PCS IV (Nabid, ASCO GU 2013)	630 high-risk men	70 Gy + 18 mo vs. 36-mo ADT	No difference in 5-yr bF, DM, DSS, or OS
TROG RADAR (Denham, Lancet Oncol 2014)	1071 men, 80% high risk, 20% int. risk	66–74 Gy + 6 mo vs. 18-mo ADT with or without zoledronic acid	Best bPFS with 18-mo ADT for GS 7 and 18-mo ADT + zoledronic acid for GS 8–10

PELVIC NODE RT

, Two contemporary Phase III trials (RTOG 9413 and GETUG-01) reached conflicting results, though smaller field size, ill-defined nADT use, lower nodal risk, and smaller number of men in the GETUG-01 trial make the findings of GETUG-01 difficult to interpret. A number of retrospective studies report improved biochemical control with WPRT (Morikawa, IJROBP 2011).

, RTOG 0924 is comparing high-dose RT to prostate and proximal SV ± WPRT in unfavorable intermediate-risk and favorable high-risk patients.

, *RTOG 9413 field size* (Roach, IJROBP 2006): Compared ncADT arms for WP vs. mini-pelvic vs. prostate-only fields. WP improved 7-yr PFS (40%) vs. mini-pelvis (35%) or prostate-only RT (27%). No difference in late GU toxicity, small increase in late Gr 3+ GI toxicity (1 → 4%) with WPRT. Findings support the superior border of the WP field being at least at the level of L5–S1.

, *GETUG-01* (Pommier, IJROBP 2016, JCO 2007): Men with T1b–T3N0 were randomized to prostate only or "WP." "WP" field smaller than RTOG 9413 with superior field border being S1/S2. ~55% men had LN risk <15% by Roach formula. No difference in 10-yr OS or EFS overall. Subgroup of men treated without ADT with risk of LN involvement <15% had improved 10-yr EFS with pelvic node RT (83% v 50%).

CHEMOTHERAPY WITH RT

, STAMPEDE (James, Lancet 2016): Multiarm randomized trial of standard of care +/− docetaxel, zoledronic acid, or both. Among 2,962 men, 24% were high-risk N0M0 (with at least 2 factors: T3/4, GS 8–10, PSA >40), and 15% N + M0. RT was encouraged until 2011, then mandated for N0M0, and was optional for LN+ patients. Adding docetaxel improved failure free survival for non-metastatic and metastatic patients (HR 0.6), but increased grade 3–5 toxicity (52% vs. 32%).

, RTOG 0521 (Sandler, ASCO 2015): 562 high-risk localized patients treated with RT 72–75.6 Gy with 28-mo ADT ± 6 cycles of docetaxel and prednisone beginning 28 days after RT for localized high-risk prostate cancer. Docetaxel improved 5-yr PFS 66%–73%.

, GETUG 12 (Fizazi, Lancet Oncol 2015): 207 men with high-risk non-metastatic prostate cancer (71% N0, 29% N1) treated with 3 yrs ADT with local therapy 3 months later (87% RT 70–78 Gy, 6% RP) ± 4 cycles of docetaxel. Docetaxel improved 8-yr RFS 62% vs. 50% (greatest benefit for GS 8–10, T3–4, N+, and PSA >20). No treatment-related deaths or difference in long-term toxicity.

, RTOG 9902 (Rosenthal, IJROBP 2015): 397 high-risk localized prostate cancer patients treated with RT 70.2 Gy + 24-mo ADT ± 4 cycles of paclitaxel, estramustine, and etoposide. Terminated early for chemo-related toxicity. No difference in 10-yr bF, LF, DFS, or OS.

LDR BRACHYTHERAPY

, RTOG 0232 (Prestidge, ASTRO 2016): 588 intermediate-risk men with T1c–T2b and either GS 2–6 PSA 10–20 or GS 7 PSA <10 treated with LDR implant alone or with 45 Gy EBRT. No difference in 5-yr PFS (85–86%). Increased grade ≥3 toxicity with EBRT added (GU 7% vs. 3%, GI 3% vs. 2%).

, ASCENDE-RT (Morris, ASCO GU 2015; Rodda, ASTRO 2015): 276 high-risk and 122 intermediate-risk men treated with 46 Gy whole-pelvic RT and 1-yr ADT randomized to 32 Gy EBRT boost vs. 115 Gy I-125 boost. I-125 boost improved 7-yr RFS 86% vs. 71% but increased 5-yr grade 3 GU toxicity (19% vs. 5%) with trend for increased grade 3 GI toxicity (9% vs. 4%).

, Zelefsky (IJROBP 2007a, b): Reviewed 2,693 men with T1–T2 disease treated with LDR monotherapy (68% I-125, 32% Pd-103). 8-yr bRFS 93% if D90 ≥ 130 Gy vs. 76% if <130 Gy; 92% if PSA nadir <0.5, 86% if PSA nadir 0.5 to <1, 79% if PSA nadir 1 to <2, 67% if PSA nadir >2.

, Kittel (IJROBP 2015): 1,989 men with low risk (61%), intermediate (30%), high-int. (5%), and high risk (4%) treated with I-125 monotherapy. 5-yr bPFS low risk 95%, low-intermediate 90%, high-intermediate 81%, high risk 68%. Late grade 3/4 toxicity GU 7/<1%, GI <1/<1%.

, Stone (J Urol 2014): 1,669 men with localized prostate cancer treated with LDR brachytherapy ± ADT ± EBRT. 15-yr CSS: low risk 96%, int. risk 97%, high risk 85%.

, Potters (J Urol 2008): 1,449 men with localized prostate cancer treated with LDR brachytherapy ± ADT ± EBRT. 12-yr bPFS low risk 89%, int. risk 78%, high risk 63%.

VII

⌒ Overall, biochemical PFS appears to be at least as good with brachytherapy compared to other modalities, perhaps better (Grimm, BJUI 2012).

HDR BRACHYTHERAPY

HDR Monotherapy

⌒ Yoshioka (IJROBP 2016): 190 men (42% int. risk, 58% high risk, 73% got ADT) treated with HDR monotherapy (48 Gy/8, 54 Gy/9, or 45.5 Gy/7). Median f/u 92 mo. 8-yr bPFS intermediate risk 91%, high risk 77%. 8-yr late grade 3 GU toxicity 1%, GI toxicity 2%.

⌒ Hauswald (IJROBP 2016): 448 men (64% low risk, 36% int. risk, 9% got ADT) treated with HDR monotherapy (42–43.5 Gy in 7–7.25 Gy fractions in 2 implants 1 week apart). Median f/u 6.5 yrs. 10-yr bPFS low risk 99%, int. risk 95%. Grade 3–4 GU toxicity 5%, 0% GI.

HDR Boost

⌒ Hoskin (Radioth Oncol 2012): 220 men with T1–T3, PSA < 50 (76% ADT) randomized to EBRT 55 Gy/20 alone vs. 35.75 Gy/13 + HDR boost of 17 Gy/2. Median f/u of 30 mo. Mean bRFS 5.1 yrs HDR arm vs. 4.3 yrs (SS). Acute GI toxicity better with HDR arm. QOL better with HDR arm.

⌒ Sathya (JCO 2005): 104 int.-risk (40%) and high-risk (60%) men randomized to 66 Gy EBRT vs. 40 Gy EBRT + 35 Gy HDR boost. HDR boost improved 5-yr bF 61%–29% with no difference in long-term toxicity.

⌒ RTOG 0231 Phase II (Hsu, IJROBP 2010): 129 men with T1c–T3b treated with EBRT 45 Gy + HDR boost of 19 Gy/2. Median f/u of 30 mo, late grade 3–5 GU/GI toxicities were 3%.

⌒ Deutsch (Brachytherapy 2010). Compared 86.4 Gy IMRT ($n = 470$) vs. 50.4 Gy IMRT +21 Gy HDR boost ($n = 160$). HDR boost improved 5-yr bPFS for int. risk (98% vs. 84%) and high risk (93% vs. 71%).

- Marina (Brachytherapy 2014). Compared int.-risk patients treated with 77.4 Gy 3D/IMRT with IGRT (n = 734) vs. 46 Gy WPRT + 19–21 Gy HDR boost (n = 282). HDR boost improved 5-yr bPFS 96% vs. 87% for T2b-c, PNI, or % positive cores >50%.
- Khor (IJROBP 2013): 344 men with int.-high risk treated with 46 Gy EBRT + 19.5 Gy HDR boost in three fractions compared to matched cohort treated with 74 Gy EBRT. HDR boost improved 5-yr bPFS 80% vs. 71% but increased grade 3 urethral stricture 12% vs. 0.3%.

Comparison of Modalities

- There is limited randomized data comparing AS, RP, and RT in newly diagnosed localized prostate cancer. Retrospective studies comparing modalities should be met with caution as patient populations are fundamentally different in regard to comorbidities, clinical vs. pathologic staging, institutional approaches, and use of adjuvant or salvage therapies (Roach, Clin Oncol 2016).

  - Compared to the general American population, overall death rate is lower in men treated with RP (HR of death 0.47), likely due to differences in cardiovascular disease, diabetes, and chronic lung disease (Eifler J Urol 2012).
- Evaluating observational studies by reliability score (taking into account data source, appropriate ADT use, sample size, risk group disclosure, etc.) demonstrate that studies with higher reliability scores are less likely to report benefit of RP over RT (Roach, IJROBP 2015).

VII

Table 26.12 Comparison of modality trials

Study	Clinical characteristics	Modality: 10-yr PCSS
ProtectT (Hamdy, NEJM 2016)	77% GS 6 76% T1c Median PSA 4.6	AS: 98.8% RP: 99.0% RT: 99.6%
Swedish trial(Lennernäs, Acta Oncol 2015)	T1b–T3aN0 (78% T1–T2) PSA ≤ 50	RP: 93% EBRT + HDR: 95%

ProtecT Patient Reported Outcomes (Donovan, NEJM 2016): 1643 men completed validated questionnaires before diagnosis, at 6 and 12 mo after randomization, then annually. Overall, RP had greatest effect on sexual function and urinary continence, whereas RT had more effect on bowel function. At 3/6 yrs, need for ≥1 pad for urinary incontinence was 3/4% RT, 5/8% surveillance, and 20/17% RP. At baseline 67% of men had erection firm enough for intercourse, which fell at 3/6 yrs to 41/30% surveillance, 34/27% RT, and 21/17% RP. RT had small increases in 6-yr bloody stools (5.6% vs. 1.1–1.3%), fecal incontinence (4.1% vs. 1.9–2.6%), and loose stools (15.5% vs. 12.2–13.1%).

Table 26.13 ADJUVANT RADIOTHERAPY AFTER RP

Study	Patients	Arms	Benefits of adjuvant RT	Toxicity
SWOG 8794 (Thompson, J Urol 2009)	431 men pT2-3N0M0 s/p RP with ECE, +margin, or SVI	Observation vs. 60–64 Gy *(33% observation arm got RT)*	15-yr OS: 37 → 47% 15-yr DMFS: 38 → 46% 10-yr bF: 77 → 55% 10-yr LF 22 → 8% Need for ADT at 12 yrs: 50 → 39%	QOL study in 217 men (JCO 2008): increased urinary and GI symptoms w/ RT, though GI difference gone by 2 yrs. No difference in erectile function. QOL initially worse with RT, but improved with time and favored RT arm in long term
EORTC 22911 (Bolla, Lancet 2012; Van der Kwast, JCO 2007)	1,005 men pT-3N0 with ECE, +margin, or SVI	Observation vs. 60 Gy *(~1/2 observation arm got RT)*	10-yr bPFS:39% → 61.8% 5-yr cPFS: 77 → 85% 10-yr cPFS: 66 → 70% 10-yr LRF: 17 → 7% No difference in 5- or 10-yr OS	10-yr cumulative incidence of Gr 3 toxicity 5.3% in RT group vs. 2.5% in observation. No Gr 4 toxicity
ARO 96-02 (Wiegel, Eur Urol 2014)	388 men pT3N0 margin positive or negative	Observation vs. 60 Gy	10-yr bPFS: 35 → 56%. No difference in 10-yr OS or DM (though trial underpowered)	In RT arm, 2% Gr 2 GU toxicity, 1% Gr 2 GI toxicity. 0.3% late Gr 3 toxicity

SALVAGE RADIOTHERAPY

- ˎ PSA failure occurs in 15–40% of patients after RP.
- ˎ Men with rising PSA after RP have up to 60% risk of developing DM and 20% risk of prostate cancer mortality within 10 yrs if untreated. Median time from PSA failure to DM is 8 yrs but only 3 yrs for high GS or PSA doubling time <3 mo. Median time from DM to death is <5 yrs (Pound, JAMA 1999; Freedland, JAMA 2005).
- ˎ Salvage RT can improve bPFS and CSS. Multiple nomograms exist to predict post-RP.

Table 26.14

Study	Patients	Management	Results
Tendulkar, JCO 2016	2,460 men with bF after RP	Salvage RT (SRT) ± ADT	Predictors of biochemical PFS: pre-SRT PSA, GS, EPE, SVI, margins, ADT use, and RT dose. Predictors of DM: pre-SRT PSA, GS, SVI, margins, and ADT
UCSF-CAPRA (Cooperberg, J Urol 2005)	1,439 men s/p RP	Followed in CaPSURE database	Based on Cox analysis, points assigned by PSA, GS, T stage, age, and % biopsy cores. CAPRA score ranges 0–10. RFS at 5 yrs ranged from 85% for score of 0–1 to 8% for a score of 7–10
Genomic classifier (GC) (Den, JCO 2015)	188 men s/p RP with pT3 or + margins	All treated with post-op RT	5-yr DM after RT: 0%, 9%, and 29% for low, average, and high GC scores. GC and pre-RP PSA were independent predictors of DM. Within low GC score (<0.4), no differences in DM for adjuvant vs. salvage RT. But, for higher GC scores (≥0.4), DM at 5 yrs was 6% for adjuvant RT vs. 23% salvage RT. *Note*: the incidence of DM raises the question whether men should have received ADT as well
PORTOS 24-gene score (Zhao, Lancet Oncol 2016)	196 men s/p RP	All treated with post-op RT	Among men with high score, RT reduced 10-yr DM 4% vs. 35% (validation cohort)

VII

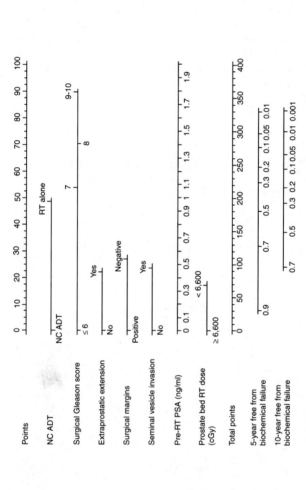

Fig. 26.1 Pretreatment nomogram estimating the 5- and 10-yr rates of biochemical failure after salvage radiotherapy (From: Tendulkar, J Clin Oncol 2016. Reprinted with permission from American Society of Clinical Oncology)

ROLE OF ADT WITH SALVAGE OR ADJUVANT RADIOTHERAPY

- RTOG 9601 (Shipley, NEJM 2017): 760 men post-RP for pT3pN0 or pT2pN0 with +margins who had bF (PSA 0.2–4 ng/ml) randomized to RT ± bicalutamide (24 mo, 150 mg daily). Adding bicalutamide improved 12-yr OS (76% vs. 71%), prostate cancer mortality (6% vs. 13%), DM (15% vs. 23%), and 10-yr bPFS (46% vs. 30%). Greatest DM benefit for GS 8–10, PSA 1.5–4, +margin. Greatest OS benefit for GS 7, PSA 0.7–4, +margin. Bicalutamide 70% gynecomastia, <1% grade 3 liver toxicity.
- GETUG-AFU 16 (Carrie, Lancet Oncol 2016): 743 men with pT2–4a and rising PSA 0.2 to <2 received 66 Gy salvage RT ± 6 months goserelin. Goserelin improved 5-yr bPFS 80% vs. 62%.
- Ramey (ASTRO 2016): Multi-institutional review of 1,861 post-op GS ≥7 patients. For GS 8–10, the combination of WPRT + ADT improved 5-yr bPFS (prostate bed without ADT 34% vs. WPRT without ADT 44% vs. prostate bed with ADT 45% vs. WPRT with ADT 64%); WPRT improved bPFS for GS 7 (67% vs. 53%), but ADT did not.
- RTOG 0534 is randomizing patients with pT2-3N0 and PSA ≥0.1 and <2 to salvage prostate bed RT alone (64.8–70.2 Gy) ± 4–6 months ADT ± 45 Gy pelvic LN RT.

LYMPH NODE INVOLVEMENT

- No prospective evidence for OS benefit with adding local treatment to ADT.
- Messing (Lancet Oncol 2006). 98 pN+ men after RP + PLND were randomized to immediate ADT vs. observation. At 12 yrs, immediate ADT improved MS (11.3 → 13.9 yrs) and MPFS (2.4 → 13.9 yrs). All but three men died of prostate cancer in observation arm.
- NCDB (Lin, JNCI 2015). After propensity score matching among 636 cN+ men, adding RT to ADT was found to 5-yr all-cause mortality by 50%.
- SEER (Tward, Pract Radiat Oncol 2013). 1100 men with cN+ had improved 10-yr CSS with RT 63% vs. no definitive therapy 50%.

VII

- SEER (Rusthoven, IJROBP 2014). 796 cN+ and 2,991 pN+ patients. Adding RT for cN+ improved 10-yr OS (45% vs. 29%). Adding local therapy for pN+ improved 10-yr OS (65% vs. 42%).
- NCDB (Wong, Urol Oncol 2016). 7,225 pN+ patients. On multivariate analysis, ADT and adjuvant RT improved survival vs. no adjuvant therapy, but ADT alone and adjuvant RT alone did not.
- Abdollah (JCO 2014). 1,107 pN1 patients treated with ADT (65%) or ADT + adjuvant RT (35%). Adding adjuvant RT improved 8-yr CSS for pT3b/4 or +margins (93% vs. 84%) and for those with 3–4 involved nodes (97% vs. 79%).
- RTOG 8531 (Lawton, JCO 2005): 173 men biopsy N+ randomized to RT vs. RT + goserelin indefinitely. Goserelin improved 9-yr OS (38 → 62%), bPFS (4 → 10%), and DM (48 → 33%).
- Zagars (Urology 2001): Reviewed 255 pN+ men treated with early ADT ± 70 Gy to prostate. RT improved 10-yr OS (46 → 67%) and PFS.

METASTATIC DISEASE

- Prognosis is best approximated by the absolute level of PSA, PSA-DT, initial stage, and, most importantly, tumor grade.
- Earlier ADT may be better than delayed ADT, although the definitions of early are controversial.
- LHRH agonist (medical castration) and bilateral orchiectomy (surgical castration) appear to be equally effective.
- Antiandrogen therapy should precede or be coadministered with LHRH agonist and be continued in combination for at least 7–14 days to reduce risk of developing symptoms associated with the flare in testosterone with initial LHRH agonist alone.
- Antiandrogen monotherapy appears to be less effective than medical or surgical castration and should not be recommended.
- STAMPEDE (James, NEJM 2017). Adding abiraterone and prednisolone to at least 2 years androgen deprivation for men with locally-advanced (at least 2: T3–4, GS 8–10, PSA >40), node positive, and metastatic disease significantly improves OS (HR 0.63) and failure-free survival (HR 0.29).

, For men with metastatic androgen-sensitive disease, adding chemo appears to have benefit.

  , Sweeny (NEJM 2015): 790 men with metastatic, hormone-sensitive prostate cancer randomized to ADT alone or ADT + docetaxel. MS 44 mo with ADT alone vs. 58 mo with docetaxel.

, For castrate-resistant prostate cancer, options include abiraterone with prednisone, docetaxel with prednisone, enzalutamide, Ra-223 for symptomatic bone metastases, or secondary hormone therapy.

, Expression of androgen-receptor splice variant seven on circulating tumor cell (CTC) may be predictive of response to systemic therapy in castrate-resistant prostate cancer (CRPC) (Scher, JAMA Oncol 2016).

, Retrospective population-based analyses suggest possible survival benefit of local treatment of the prostate (Rusthoven, JCO 2016; Satkunasivam, J Urol 2015). Randomized trials are ongoing to evaluate the impact of local therapy for M1 disease (e.g., NCT01751438 best systemic therapy +/− local therapy).

VII

RADIATION TECHNIQUES

EBRT

, At UCSF, men are treated supine with alpha cradle or knee sponge to align thighs.

, Patients are asked to have full bladder and empty rectum (after enema) for simulation.

, At UCSF, daily image-guided radiation therapy (IGRT) is used to monitor prostate position, using electronic portal imaging device (EPID) or cone-beam CT.

, Gold fiducials are placed in the base and apex of the prostate 7–10 days before simulation.

  , For salvage RT at UCSF, fiducials may be placed at urethral anastomosis by experienced providers to ensure it is consistently in treatment field given high rate of local recurrence in this area (Schiffner, IJROBP 2007; Connolly, Urology 1996).

, Planning is CT-based. The prostate appears larger inferiorly and posteriorly on non-contrast CT images compared to TRUS and MRI.

- Indications for seminal vesicle irradiation include involvement by biopsy, TRUS, or MRI, or estimated risk of involvement >15%.
- Hydrogel spacer may be considered for T1–T2 patients to potentially reduce rectal toxicity (Pieczonka, Urol Pract 2016).
- Indications for WPRT at UCSF include involved LN, seminal vesicle involvement, a calculated risk of LN involvement >15% (by Roach formula), men with T3 GS 6 disease, and men with >50% + biopsy cores or high-risk disease.
- RTOG 0924 is comparing high-dose RT to prostate and proximal SV ± WPRT in unfavorable intermediate- and favorable high-risk patients.
- Traditional WPRT field borders:
  - Superior = L4/L5 interspace (per RTOG 0924); inferior = 0.5–1 cm below the area where the dye narrows on the urethrogram (or 1–1.5 cm below in the post-op setting); lateral = 1.5 cm lateral to the bony margin of the true pelvis.
  - On the AP/PA fields, corners are blocked to decrease dose to the femoral heads, bowel, and bone marrow.
  - On the lateral fields, the anterior border is anterior to the pubic synthesis. The posterior border splits the sacrum to S2/3, and a beam's eye view is generated with CT contours of the rectum present in order to draw the rectal bloc excluding the posterior rectum.
  - "Mini-pelvic" fields are not recommended.
- IMRT may be used for both whole pelvic and boost portions of treatment. For whole pelvic IMRT, careful review of LN mapping is recommended (Shih, IJROBP 2005; Taylor, IJROBP 2005; Harris, IJROBP 2015).
- RTOG GU consensus on pelvic LN CTV volumes:
  - Commence contouring the pelvic CTV LN volumes at the L5/S1 interspace (though RTOG 0924 uses L4/L5 as superior border so entire common iliac nodes are included).

- Use 7 mm margin around the iliac vessels connecting the external and internal iliac contours on each slice, carving out the bowel, bladder, and bone.
- Contour presacral nodes (subaortic only) S1–S3, posterior border being the anterior sacrum, and anterior border approximately 10 mm anterior to the anterior sacral bone carving out the bowel, bladder, and bone.
- Stop external iliac CTV node contours at the top of the femoral heads (bony landmark for the inguinal ligament).
- Stop contours of the obturator CTV nodes at the top of the pubis (Figs. 26.2 and 26.3).
- Proton radiotherapy is an alternative to VMAT/IMRT planning. There is currently no clear evidence supporting benefit or decrement in efficacy or toxicity compared to VMAT/IMRT.
- In the post-op setting, the CTV is based on pre-op imaging, histopathologic size of the prostate, tumor extent, surgical margins, and input from the urologist. RTOG, EORTC, and Australian New Zealand post-prostatectomy contouring guidelines have been published:
  - Inferior border: top of penile bulb or 1.5 cm below urethral beak or 8 mm below vesicourethral anastomosis.
  - Anterior border: posterior edge of pubic symphysis including the entire bladder neck until above the symphysis, then off the bladder.
  - Posterior border: to anterior aspect of the rectum and mesorectal fascia.
  - Lateral borders: to medial edge of obturator internus muscles.
  - Superior border: just above pubic symphysis anteriorly and including surgical clips if limited to the postoperative bed or 5 mm above inferior border of the vas deferens.
  - PTV expansion: 0.6–1.5 cm (Fig. 26.4).

VII

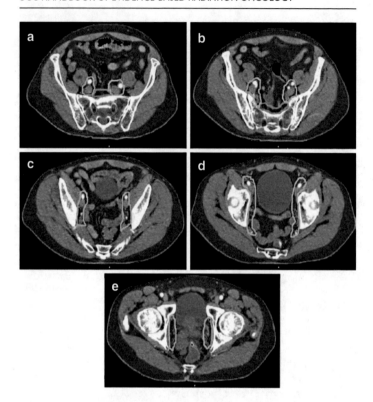

Fig. 26.2 Representative pelvic LN CTV contours: (**a**) Common iliac and presacral (L5/S1). (**b**) External iliac, internal iliac, and presacral (S1–S3). (**c**) External and internal Iliac (below S3). (**d**) End of external iliac (at top of the femoral head, bony landmark for the inguinal ligament). (**e**) Obturator (above the top of the pubic symphysis) (From: Lawton, Int J Radiat Oncol Biol Phys 2009. Reprinted with permission from Elsevier)

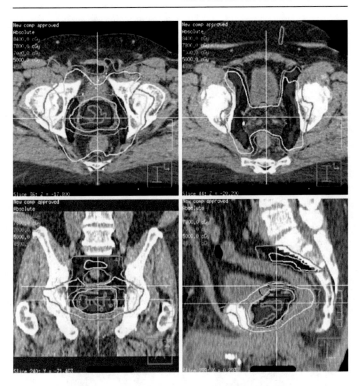

Fig. 26.3 Representative definitive UCSF IMRT plan for a man with cT2b, Gleason 4 + 5 PSA 17.2 adenocarcinoma of the prostate. Purple color wash: prostate and seminal vesicle PTV, blue color wash: lymph node PTV

VII

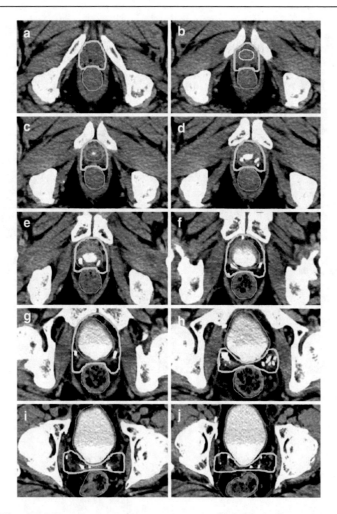

Fig. 26.4 Representative post-op prostate bed CTV, *yellow*; vesico-urethral anastomosis, *white*; rectum, *blue*; bladder, *green*; vas deferens, *red*. (**a**–**c**) Delayed scan following IV contrast so as to ascertain the most inferior slice where urine is last visible (**c**). The anastomosis is one slice below this (**b**), and the most inferior CTV slice 5 mm lower (**a**). (**d**–**g**) The anterior border of the inferior CTV lies behind the symphysis pubis. (**h**–**j**) The most superior slice of the CTV (**j**) encompasses the last slice where the vas deferens is visible and all nonvascular surgical clips (Adapted from Sidhom, Radiother Oncol 2008. Reprinted with permission from Elsevier)

EBRT DOSE

- Prostate dose to 75.6–79.2 Gy at conventional fractionation.
- Prophylactic dose to the seminal vesicles is 54 Gy to the proximal 1 cm. Documented seminal vesicle disease receives full dose.
- Moderately hypofractionated regimens may be considered following published results above with close attention to dose constraints.
- Extreme hypofractionation (>6.5 Gy/fx) may be considered as a cautious alternative at clinics with appropriate technology, physics, and clinical expertise and also with close attention to dose constraints.
- In the post-op setting, the prostate bed is typically treated to 64.8–66.6 Gy at 1.8 Gy/fx for negative margins, 68.4–72 Gy for +margins to gross residual disease.
- Prophylactic dose to the pelvic LN is 45 Gy in 25 fractions. Involved LN goal at least 60 Gy or higher with IMRT, respecting bowel tolerance.

VII

EXAMPLE EBRT DOSE CONSTRAINTS (AT STANDARD FRACTIONATION)

- Bladder: V80 <15%, V75 <25%, V70 <35%, V65 <25–50%, V55 <50%, V40 <50%
- Rectum: V75 <15%, V70 <20–25%, V65 <17–35%, V60 <40–50%, V50 <50%, V40 <35–40%
- Femoral heads: V50 <5%
- Small bowel: V52 0%, <150 cc >45 Gy
- Penile bulb: mean dose <52.5 Gy

LDR BRACHYTHERAPY

- See ABS/ACR guidelines (Bittner, Brachytherapy 2017; Davis, Brachytherapy 2012).
- Traditional indications for monotherapy: T1c–T2a, GS ≤ 6, and PSA ≤ 10.
- Consider adding EBRT if multiple intermediate-risk factors: ≥T2c, GS ≥ 7, PSA >10:
  - RTOG 0232 suggests that favorable intermediate-risk men may receive LDR alone.
- Absolute contraindications: metastases, medically unfit to have general or spinal anesthesia.

- Relative contraindications: high AUA scores (as urinary obstructive symptoms may worsen postoperatively), large prostate size (for >60 cm³, short-course ADT may be considered to shrink prostate), and pubic arch interference; prior TURP is associated with late suburethral necrosis followed by incontinence due to development of a calcified urethra.
- Implants are either preplanned from TRUS images of the prostate taken in the lithotomy position (preferred planning method at UCSF) or by intraoperative TRUS.
- The goal of treatment planning is to cover the prostate with a 3–5 mm margin to cover potential ECE.
- For the procedure, pre-op bowel preparation is necessary, and spinal, epidural, or general anesthesia is generally used.
- In the OR, a catheter or aerated gel is used to visualize the urethra. TRUS frequencies of 5–7 MHz are used. The TRUS is supported on an adjustable 0.5 cm stepping unit mounted to the table. If using a preplan, match the intra-op images to the pre-op images using the seminal vesicles and the base of the gland. Needles are inserted through the template holes until they are viewed in the desired plane. Rotating the needle allows two distinct lines to be seen, corresponding to the bevel. Seeds are deposited from preloaded needles or the Mick applicator. Seeds may be single or suture-mounted. An extended lithotomy position may help reduce pubic arch interference.
- Typically, the patient is discharged after he is able to urinate. Prescriptions are generally provided for tamsulosin, NSAIDs, and antibiotics 3× days. Patients are cautioned to avoid constipation in post-implant period.

LDR DOSE

- Brachytherapy monotherapy doses: I-125 144 Gy; Pd-103 125 Gy.
- After 40–50 Gy EBRT: I-125 110 Gy; Pd-103 90 Gy.
- I-125: source activity 0.2–0.9 mCi, half-life 60 day, photon energy 28 KeV.
- Pd-103: source activity 1.1–2.5 mCi, half-life 17 day, photon energy 21 KeV.

, Review isodose overlays to determine significance of under- and overdosed regions.
, Dosimetric goals:
  , V100 is the percent of the prostate volume covered by 100% of the prescription dose.
  , D90 is the % prescription dose that covers 90% of the prostate volume.
  , Prostate: V100 > 95–99%, D90 > 90–100%, V150 < 70%, V200 < 20%.
  , Urethra: D30% <130%, Dmax <150%, V100 <60%.
  , Rectum: D0.1 mL <200 Gy, D2mL <100%, RV100% <1 mL.

HDR BRACHYTHERAPY

, HDR afterloading catheters are inserted under TRUS guidance using either template or free-hand approach and secured into position.
, With CT planning, CT obtained after implantation of catheters captures catheter positions in treatment planning system.
, With TRUS-based planning, US images are used by treatment planning system instead.
, The treatment planning software determines the optimal loading and duration of the source in a given position in order to accomplish a desired dose distribution. Each catheter is sequentially loaded with Ir-192 by computer-driven stepping motors.
, At UCSF after 45 Gy EBRT, HDR boost is given as 9.5 Gy × 2 fractions in one implant or 15 Gy in a single fraction. Other common HDR boost regimens include 5.5–7.5 Gy × 3 fractions or 4–6 Gy × 4 fractions.
, At UCSF, as monotherapy HDR dose options include 19 Gy in a single fraction, 9.5 Gy BID × 2 day, and 10.5 Gy × 3 fractions with one implant. Another commonly used HDR monotherapy regimen is 13.5 Gy × 2 fractions.
, At UCSF salvage HDR (after EBRT failure): 36 Gy in 2 implants of 3 fractions each separated by 1 week.
, Goals:
  , Prostate: V100 ≥ 90–96%, V150 < 40%, D90 > 90%.

VII

ₐ Rectum and bladder: V75 < 1 mL.
ₐ Urethra: V120 < 0.8 mL.

GYNECOMASTIA DUE TO ANTIANDROGENS

ₐ EBRT 4 Gy × 3 with 9 MeV e – reduces risk of gynecomastia by 70%.

COMPLICATIONS

Table 26.15

Acute EBRT complications	Incidence	Time of onset	Management
Urgency, frequency, nocturia, dysuria	Common	2 weeks	NSAID, alpha-blockers, pyridium
Urinary retention	Rare	>1 week	Catheter
Diarrhea	25–75%	2 weeks	Diet modification, antidiarrheals
Rectal irritation, pain, bleeding	<10–20%	2–6 weeks	Sitz baths, rectal steroids
Fatigue	Common	>3 weeks	Reassurance, light exercise

ₐ Late EBRT complications:
  ₐ Urinary stricture <4%. If prior TURP or prostatectomy, risk is higher (4–9%).
  ₐ Rectal bleeding <5–10% (technique/volume/dose related).
  ₐ Decreased volume of ejaculate is seen with both EBRT and brachytherapy.
  ₐ Absolute excess risk of secondary bladder or rectal cancer risk is <0.5% after RT (SEER, Davis, Cancer 2014).
ₐ Brachytherapy toxicities:
  ₐ Perioperative brachytherapy complications include pain, dysuria, urinary retention, hematuria, and urinary frequency.
  ₐ Obstructive symptoms occur in <1–10% of men and tend to resolve 6–12 mo after the implant. Retention

usually resolves in 1–3 days, but rarely can be chronic requiring a TURP. Urinary retention risk is related to pre-implant AUA score.

- ADT side effects: hot flashes, low libido, fatigue, weight gain, decreased muscle mass, LFT rise, anemia, osteoporosis, and mood changes.
- Prostatectomy toxicities:
  - Penson, J Urol 2005: <1,300 men treated with RP in a population-based cohort. Urinary symptoms: 35% had complete urinary control, 51% had occasional leakage, 11% had frequent leakage, and 3% had no urinary control. Sexual dysfunction: 28% had erections sufficient for intercourse.

FOLLOW-UP

- H&P with DRE (if initially the baseline exam was abnormal) and PSA every 6 mo for 5 yrs and then annually. In the first 1–3 yrs after definitive RT, PSA may be ordered more frequently (every 3–6 mo).
- The "Phoenix Definition" (current ASTRO/RTOG definition) of PSA failure after EBRT, with or without ADT, is defined as a rise by ≥ 2 ng/mL above the nadir PSA (defined as the lowest PSA achieved), with the date of failure "at call" and not backdated. Among men who undergo any salvage therapy, failure is declared at the time of +biopsy or salvage administration (whichever is first).
- The PSA nadir after RP is <3 weeks, after EBRT <2–3 yrs (can be up to 4–5 yrs), and after brachytherapy <3–5 yrs.
- PSA "bounce": About 20% of men have a transient PSA rise (usually <2 ng/mL) after EBRT or brachytherapy with a subsequent fall. <90% occur within 3 yrs (median duration 14 mo). The median time to bounce after EBRT is <9–12 mo. Risk factors for PSA bounce after brachytherapy: age <65, higher implant dose, sexual activity, and larger prostate volume. PSA bounce after brachytherapy or EBRT does not predict PSA failure.

Acknowledgment We thank Siavash Jabbari MD for his work on the prior edition of this chapter.

REFERENCES

Abdollah F, Karnes RJ, Suardi N, et al. Impact of adjuvant radiotherapy on survival of patients with node-positive prostate cancer. J Clin Oncol. 2014;32(35):3939–47.

Al-Mamgani A, van Putten WL, Heemsbergen WD, et al. Update of Dutch multicenter dose-escalation trial of radiotherapy for localized prostate cancer. Int J Radiat Oncol Biol Phys. 2008;72(4):980–8.

Aluwini S, Pos F, Schimmel E, et al. Hypofractionated versus conventionally fractionated radiotherapy for patients with prostate cancer (HYPRO): late toxicity results from a randomised, non-inferiority, phase 3 trial. Lancet Oncol. 2016;17(4):464–74.

American Cancer Society recommendations for prostate cancer early detection: http://www.cancer.org/cancer/prostatecancer/moreinformation/prostatecancerearlydetection/prostate-cancer-early-detection-acs-recommendations. Accessed 9 Aug 2016.

Amin MB, Edge S, Greene F, Byrd DR, Brookland RK, Washington MK, Gershenwald JE, Compton CC, Hess KR, Sullivan DC, Jessup JM, Brierley JD, Gaspar LE, Schilsky RL, Balch CM, Winchester DP, Asare EA, Madera M, Gress DM, Meyer LR. AJCC cancer staging manual. 8th ed: Springer; 2017.

Andriole GL, Crawford ED, Grubb RL, et al. Prostate cancer screening in the randomized prostate, lung, colorectal, and ovarian cancer screening trial: mortality results after 13 years of follow-up. J Natl Cancer Inst. 2012;104(2):125–32.

Arcangeli S, Strigari L, Gomellini S, et al. Updated results and patterns of failure in a randomized hypofractionation trial for high-risk prostate cancer. Int J Radiat Oncol Biol Phys. 2012;84(5):1172–8.

Beckendorf V, Guerif S, Le Prisé E, et al. 70 Gy versus 80 Gy in localized prostate cancer: 5-year results of GETUG 06 randomized trial. Int J Radiat Oncol Biol Phys. 2011;80(4):1056–63.

Bill-Axelson A, Holmberg L, Garmo H, et al. Radical prostatectomy or watchful waiting in early prostate cancer. N Engl J Med. 2014;370(10):932–42.

Bittner HJ, Orio PF, Merrick GS, et al. The American College of Radiology and the American Brachytherapy Society practice parameter for transperineal permanent brachytherapy of prostate cancer. Brachytherapy. 2017;16:59–67.

Bolla M, de Reijke TM, Van Tienhoven G, et al. Duration of androgen suppression in the treatment of prostate cancer. NEJM. 2009;360:2516–27.

Bolla M, van Tienhoven G, Warde P, et al. External irradiation with or without long-term androgen suppression for prostate cancer with high metastatic risk: 10-year results of an EORTC randomised study. Lancet Oncol. 2010;11(11):1066–73.

Bolla M, van Poppel H, Tombal B, et al. Postoperative radiotherapy after radical prostatectomy for high-risk prostate cancer: long-term results of a randomised controlled trial (EORTC trial 22911). Lancet. 2012;380(9858):2018–27.

Bolla M, Maingon P, Carrie C, et al. Short androgen suppression and radiation dose escalation for intermediate- and high-risk localized prostate cancer: results of EORTC trial 22991. JCO. 2016;34(15):1748–56.

Bul M, van den Bergh RCN, Zhu X, et al. Outcomes of initially expectantly managed patients with low or intermediate risk screen-detected localized prostate cancer. BJU Int. 2012;110(11):1672–7.

Carrie C, Hasbini A, de Laroche G, et al. Salvage radiotherapy with or without short-term hormone therapy for rising prostate-specific antigen concentration after radical prostatectomy (GETUG-AFU 16): a randomised, multicentre, open-label phase 3 trial. Lancet Oncol. 2016;17(6):747–56.

Catton CN, Lukka H, Julian JA, et al. A randomized trial of a shorter radiation fractionation schedule for the treatment of localized prostate cancer. ASCO Meeting Abstracts. 2016;34 (suppl; abstr 5003).

Chun FK, Briganti A, Shariat SF, et al. Significant upgrading affects a third of men diagnosed with prostate cancer: predictive nomogram and internal validation. BJU Int. 2006;98(2):329–34.

Connolly JA, Shinohara K, Presti JC, Carroll PR. Local recurrence after radical prostatectomy: characteristics in size, location, and relationship to prostate-specific antigen and surgical margins. Urology. 1996;47(2):225–31.

Cooperberg MR, Pasta DJ, Elkin EP, et al. The University of California, San Francisco cancer of the prostate risk assessment score: a straightforward and reliable preoperative predictor of disease recurrence after radical prostatectomy. J Urol. 2005;173(6):1938–42.

D'Amico AV, Chen M-H, Renshaw A, Loffredo M, Kantoff PW. Long-term follow-up of a randomized trial of radiation with or without androgen deprivation therapy for localized prostate cancer. JAMA. 2015;314(12):1291–3. https://doi.org/10.1001/jama.2015.8577.

D'Amico AV, Renshaw AA, Sussman B, et al. Pretreatment PSA velocity and risk of death from prostate cancer following external beam radiation therapy. JAMA. 2005;294:440–7.

Davis BJ, Horwitz EM, Lee WR, et al. American Brachytherapy Society consensus guidelines for transrectal ultrasound-guided permanent prostate brachytherapy. Brachytherapy. 2012;11(1):6–19.

Davis EJ, Beebe-Dimmer JL, Yee CL, Cooney KA. Risk of second primary tumors in men diagnosed with prostate cancer: a population-based cohort study. Cancer. 2014;120(17):2735–41.

Dearnaley DP, Jovic G, Syndikus I, et al. Escalated-dose versus control-dose conformal radiotherapy for prostate cancer: long-term results from the MRC RT01 randomised controlled trial. Lancet Oncol. 2014;15(4):464–73.

Dearnaley D, Syndikus I, Mossop H, et al. Conventional versus hypofractionated high-dose intensity-modulated radiotherapy for prostate cancer: 5-year outcomes of the randomised, non-inferiority, phase 3 CHHiP trial. Lancet Oncol. 2016;17(8):1047–60.

Den RB, Yousefi K, Trabulsi EJ, et al. Genomic classifier identifies men with adverse pathology after radical prostatectomy who benefit from adjuvant radiation therapy. J Clin Oncol. 2015;33(8):944–51.

Denham JW, Steigler A, Lamb DS, et al. Short-term neoadjuvant androgen deprivation and radiotherapy for locally advanced prostate cancer: 10-year data from the TROG 96.01 randomised trial. Lancet Oncol. 2011;12(5):451–9.

Denham JW, Joseph D, Lamb DS, et al. Short-term androgen suppression and radiotherapy versus intermediate-term androgen suppression and radiotherapy, with or without zoledronic acid, in men with locally advanced prostate cancer (TROG 03.04 RADAR): an open-label, randomised, phase 3 factorial trial. Lancet Oncol. 2014;15(10):1076–89.

Deutsch I, Zelefsky MJ, Zhang Z, et al. Comparison of PSA relapse-free survival in patients treated with ultra-high-dose IMRT versus combination HDR brachytherapy and IMRT. Brachytherapy. 2010;9(4):313–8.

Donovan JL, Hamdy FC, Lane JA, et al. Patient-reported outcomes after monitoring, surgery, or radiotherapy for prostate cancer. N Engl J Med. 2016;375(15):1425–37.

Dubray BM, Beckendorf V, Guerif S, et al. Does short-term androgen depletion add to high dose radiotherapy (80 Gy) in localized intermediate risk prostate cancer? Final analysis of the GETUG 14 randomized trial (EU-20503/NCT00104741). J Clin Oncol. 2016;34(15_suppl):5021.

Edge SB, Byrd DR, Compton CC, Fritz AG, Greene FL, Trotti A. AJCC cancer staging manual. 7th ed: Springer; 2010.

Efstathiou JA, Bae K, Shipley WU, et al. Cardiovascular mortality after androgen deprivation therapy for locally advanced prostate cancer: RTOG 85-31. J Clin Oncol. 2009;27(1):92–9.

Eifler JB, Humphreys EB, Agro M, Partin AW, Trock BJ, Han M. Causes of death after radical prostatectomy at a large tertiary center. J Urol. 2012;188(3):798–802.

Epstein JI, Egevad L, Amin MB, et al. The 2014 International Society of Urological Pathology (ISUP) consensus conference on Gleason grading of prostatic carcinoma: definition of

VII

grading patterns and proposal for a new grading system. Am J Surg Pathol. 2016a;40(2):244.

Fizazi K, Faivre L, Lesaunier F, et al. Androgen deprivation therapy plus docetaxel and estramustine versus androgen deprivation therapy alone for high-risk localised prostate cancer (GETUG 12): a phase 3 randomised controlled trial. Lancet Oncol. 2015;16(7):787–94.

Fosså SD, Wiklund F, Klepp O, et al. Ten- and 15-yr prostate cancer-specific mortality in patients with nonmetastatic locally advanced or aggressive intermediate prostate cancer, randomized to lifelong endocrine treatment alone or combined with radiotherapy: final results of the Scandinavian Prostate Cancer Group-7. Eur Urol. 2016;70(4):684–91.

Fransson P, Lund J-A, Damber J-E, et al. Quality of life in patients with locally advanced prostate cancer given endocrine treatment with or without radiotherapy: 4-year follow-up of SPCG-7/SFUO-3, an open-label, randomised, phase III trial. The Lancet Oncology. 2009;10(4):370–80. https://doi.org/10.1016/S1470-2045(09)70027-0.

Freedland SJ, Humphreys EB, Mangold LA, et al. Risk of prostate cancer-specific mortality following biochemical recurrence after radical prostatectomy. JAMA. 2005;294(4):433–9.

Grimm P, Billiet I, Bostwick D, et al. Comparative analysis of prostate-specific antigen free survival outcomes for patients with low, intermediate and high risk prostate cancer treatment by radical therapy. Results from the Prostate Cancer Results Study Group. BJU Int. 2012;109(Suppl 1):22–9.

Hamdy FC, Donovan JL, Lane JA, et al. 10-year outcomes after monitoring, surgery, or radiotherapy for localized prostate cancer. N Engl J Med. 2016;375(15):1415–24.

Harris VA, Staffurth J, Naismith O, et al. Consensus guidelines and contouring atlas for pelvic node delineation in prostate and pelvic node intensity modulated radiation Harris therapy. Int J Radiat Oncol Biol Phys. 2015;92(4):874–83.

Hauswald H, Kamrava MR, Fallon JM, et al. High-dose-rate monotherapy for localized prostate cancer: 10-year results. Int J Radiat Oncol Biol Phys. 2016;94(4):667–74.

Hoffman KE, Skinner H, Pugh TJ, et al. Patient-reported urinary, bowel, and sexual function after hypofractionated intensity-modulated radiation therapy for prostate cancer: results from a randomized trial. Am J Clin Oncol. 2016. [Epub ahead of print]

Horwitz EM, Bae K, Hanks GE, et al. Ten-year follow-up of radiation therapy oncology group protocol 92-02: a phase III trial of the duration of elective androgen deprivation in locally advanced prostate cancer. J Clin Oncol. 2008;26(15):2497–504.

Hoskin PJ, Rojas AM, Bownes PJ, Lowe GJ, Ostler PJ, Bryant L. Randomised trial of external beam radiotherapy alone or combined with high-dose-rate brachytherapy boost for localised prostate cancer. Radiother Oncol. 2012;103(2):217–22.

Hsu I-C, Bae K, Shinohara K, et al. Phase II trial of combined high-dose-rate brachytherapy and external beam radiotherapy for adenocarcinoma of the prostate: preliminary results of RTOG 0321. Int J Radiat Oncol Biol Phys. 2010;78(3):751–8.

James ND, de Bono JS, Spears MR, et al. Abiraterone for prostate cancer not previously treated with hormone therapy. NEJM. 2017;377(4):338–51.

James ND, Sydes MR, Clarke NW, et al. Addition of docetaxel, zoledronic acid, or both to first-line long-term hormone therapy in prostate cancer (STAMPEDE): survival results from an adaptive, multiarm, multistage, platform randomised controlled trial. Lancet. 2016;387(10024):1163–77.

Jemal A, Ma J, Siegel R, Fedewa S, Brawley O, Ward EM. Prostate cancer incidence rates 2 years after the US preventive services task force recommendations against screening. August: JAMA Oncol; 2016.

Jones CU, Hunt D, McGowan DG, et al. Radiotherapy and short-term androgen deprivation for localized prostate cancer. N Engl J Med. 2011;365(2):107–18.

Kattan MW, Potters L, Blasko JC, et al. Pretreatment nomogram for predicting freedom from recurrence after permanent prostate brachytherapy in prostate cancer. Urology. 2001;58(3):393–9.

Katz SJ. JAMA Surg. 2016 Aug 17; 151(8): e161137.

Khor R, Duchesne G, Tai K-H, et al. Direct 2-arm comparison shows benefit of high-dose-rate brachytherapy boost vs external beam radiation therapy alone for prostate cancer. Int J Radiat Oncol Biol Phys. 2013;85(3):679–85.

King CR, Freeman D, Kaplan I, et al. Stereotactic body radiotherapy for localized prostate cancer: pooled analysis from a multi-institutional consortium of prospective phase II trials. Radiother Oncol. 2013;109(2):217–21.

Kittel JA, Reddy CA, Smith KL, et al. Long-term efficacy and toxicity of low-dose-rate 125I prostate brachytherapy as monotherapy in low-, intermediate-, and high-risk prostate cancer. Int J Radiat Oncol Biol Phys. 2015;92(4):884–93.

Kuban DA, Tucker SL, Dong L, et al. Long-term results of the M. D. Anderson randomized dose-escalation trial for prostate cancer. Int J Radiat Oncol Biol Phys. 2008;70(1):67–74.

Laverdiere J, Nabid A, De Bedoya LD, et al. The efficacy and sequencing of a short course of androgen suppression on freedom from biochemical failure when administered with radiation therapy for T2-T3 prostate cancer. J Urol. 2004;171:1137–40.

Lawton CA, Winter K, Grignon D, et al. Androgen suppression plus radiation versus radiation alone for patients with stage d1/pathologic node-positive adenocarcinoma of the prostate: updated results based on national prospective randomized trial radiation therapy oncology group 85-31. J Clin Oncol. 2005;23:800–7.

Lawton CA, Michalski J, El-Naqa I, et al. RTOG GU radiation oncology specialists reach consensus on pelvic lymph node volumes for high-risk prostate cancer. Int J Radiat Oncol Biol Phys. 2009;74(2):383–7.

Lee WR, Dignam JJ, Amin MB, et al. Randomized phase III noninferiority study comparing two radiotherapy fractionation schedules in patients with low-risk prostate cancer. J Clin Oncol. 2016;34(20):2325–32.

Lennernäs B, Majumder K, Damber J-E, et al. Radical prostatectomy versus high-dose irradiation in localized/locally advanced prostate cancer: a Swedish multicenter randomized trial with patient-reported outcomes. Acta Oncol. 2015;54(6):875–81.

Lin CC, Gray PJ, Jemal A, Efstathiou JA. Androgen deprivation with or without radiation therapy for clinically node-positive prostate cancer. J Natl Cancer Inst. 2015;107(7):1–10.

Lukka H, Hayter C, Julian JA, et al. Randomized trial comparing two fractionation schedules for patients with localized prostate cancer. JCO. 2005;23(25):6132–8.

Manoharan M, Bird VG, Kim SS, Civantos F, Soloway MS. Outcome after radical prostatectomy with a pretreatment prostate biopsy Gleason score of ≥8. BJU Int. 2003;92(6):539–44.

Marina O, Gustafson GS, Kestin LL, et al. Comparison of dose-escalated, image-guided radiotherapy vs. dose-escalated, high-dose-rate brachytherapy boost in a modern cohort of intermediate-risk prostate cancer patients. Brachytherapy. 2014;13(1):59–67.

Mason MD, Parulekar WR, Sydes MR, et al. Final report of the intergroup randomized study of combined androgen-deprivation therapy plus radiotherapy versus androgen-deprivation therapy alone in locally advanced prostate cancer. J Clin Oncol. 2015;33(19):2143–50.

Mertan FV, Lindenberg L, Choyke PL, Turkbey B. PET imaging of recurrent and metastatic prostate cancer with novel tracers. Future Oncol. 2016;12(21):2463–77.

Messing EM, Manola J, Yao J, et al. Immediate versus deferred androgen deprivation treatment in patients with node-positive prostate cancer after radical prostatectomy and pelvic lymphadenectomy. Lancet Oncol. 2006;7(6):472–9.

VII

Michalski JM, Moughan J, Purdy J, et al. A randomized trial of 79.2Gy versus 70.2Gy radiation therapy (RT) for localized prostate cancer. ASCO Meet Abstr. 2015;33(Suppl 7):4.

Morikawa LK, Roach M. Pelvic nodal radiotherapy in patients with unfavorable intermediate and high-risk prostate cancer: evidence, rationale, and future directions. Int J Radiat Oncol Biol Phys. 2011;80(1):6–16.

Morris WJ, Tyldesley S, Pai HH, et al. ASCEND-RT: A multicenter, randomized trial of dose-escalated external beam radiation therapy (EBRT-B) versus low-dose-rate brachytherapy (LDR-B) for men with unfavorable-risk localized prostate cancer. J Clinc Oncol. 2015;33(suppl 7; abstr 3).

Nabid A, Carrier N, Andre-Guy M, et al. High-risk prostate cancer treated with pelvic radiotherapy and 36 versus 18 months of androgen blockade: Results of a phase III randomized study. J Clin Oncol. 2013;31(suppl 6; abstr 3).

Nabid A, Carrier N, Vigneault E, et al. A phase III trial of short-term androgen deprivation therapy in intermediate-risk prostate cancer treated with radiotherapy. J Clin Oncol. 2015;33(suppl; abstr 5019).

Nguyen PL, Je Y, Schutz FAB, et al. Association of androgen deprivation therapy with cardiovascular death in patients with prostate cancer: a meta-analysis of randomized trials. JAMA. 2011;306(21):2359–66.

Pagliarulo V, Hawes D, Brands FH, et al. Detection of occult lymph node metastases in locally advanced node-negative prostate cancer. J Clin Oncol. 2006;24(18):2735–42.

Penson DF, McLerran D, Feng Z, et al. 5-year urinary and sexual outcomes after radical prostatectomy: results from the prostate cancer outcomes study. J Urol. 2005;173(5):1701–5.

Pieczonka CM, Mariados N, Sylvester JE, et al. Hydrogel spacer application technique, patient tolerance and impact on prostate intensity modulated radiation therapy: results from a prospective, multicenter, Pivotal Randomized Controlled Trial. Urol Pract. 2016;3(2):141–6.

Pinsky PF, Blacka A, Kramer BS, Miller A, Prorok PC, Berg C. Assessing contamination and compliance in the prostate component of the prostate, lung, colorectal, and ovarian (PLCO) cancer screening trial. Clin Trials. 2010;7(4):303–11.

Pisansky TM, Hunt D, Gomella LG, et al. Duration of androgen suppression before radiotherapy for localized prostate cancer: radiation therapy oncology group randomized clinical trial 9910. J Clin Oncol. 2015;33(4):332–9.

Pollack A, Walker G, Horwitz EM, et al. Randomized trial of hypofractionated external-beam radiotherapy for prostate cancer. JCO. 2013;31(31):3860–8.

Pommier P, Chabaud S, Lagrange JL, et al. Is there a role for pelvic irradiation in localized prostate adenocarcinoma? Preliminary results of GETUG-01. J Clin Oncol. 2007;25(34):5366–73.

Pommier P, Chabaud S, Lagrange J-L, et al. Is there a role for pelvic irradiation in localized prostate adenocarcinoma? Update of the long-term survival results of the GETUG-01 randomized study. Int J Radiat Oncol Biol Phys. 2016;96(4):759–69.

Potters L, Morgenstern C, Calugaru E, et al. 12-year outcomes following permanent prostate brachytherapy in patients with clinically localized prostate cancer. J Urol. 2008;179(5 Suppl):S20–4.

Pound CR, Partin AW, Eisenberger MA, Chan DW, Pearson JD, Walsh PC. Natural history of progression after PSA elevation following radical prostatectomy. JAMA. 1999;281(1d7):1591–7.

Prestidge BR, Winter K, Sanda MG, et al. Initial report of NRG oncology/RTOG 0232: a phase 3 study comparing combined external beam radiation and transperineal interstitial permanent brachytherapy with brachytherapy alone for selected patients with intermediate-risk prostatic carcinoma. IJROBP. 2016;96(2):S4.

Ramey SJ, Abramowitz MC, Moghanaki D, et al. Benefit of elective nodal irradiation and androgen deprivation therapy with post prostatectomy salvage radiation therapy for prostate cancer. Int J Radiat Oncol Biol Phys. 2016;96(2):S102.

Roach M III. Targeting pelvic lymph nodes in men with intermediate- and high-risk prostate cancer, and confusion about the results of the randomized trials. J Clin Oncol. 2008;26(22):3816–7. author reply 3817-3818

Roach M. Should treatment with radiation and androgen deprivation therapy be considered the "gold standard" for men with unfavourable intermediate- to high-risk and locally advanced prostate cancer? Clin Oncol (R Coll Radiol). 2016;28(8):475–8.

Roach M, Bae K, Speight J, et al. Short-term neoadjuvant androgen deprivation therapy and external-beam radiotherapy for locally advanced prostate cancer: long-term results of RTOG 8610. J Clin Oncol. 2008;26(4):585–91. https://doi.org/10.1200/JCO.2007.13.9881.

Roach M, Ceron Lizarraga TL, Lazar AA. Radical prostatectomy versus radiation and androgen deprivation therapy for clinically localized prostate cancer: how good is the evidence? Int J Radiat Oncol Biol Phys. 2015;93(5):1064–70. https://doi.org/10.1016/j.ijrobp.2015.08.005.

Roach M, DeSilvio M, Lawton C, et al. Phase III trial comparing whole-pelvic versus prostate-only radiotherapy and neoadjuvant versus adjuvant combined androgen suppression: radiation Therapy Oncology Group 9413. JCO. 2003;21(10):1904–11. https://doi.org/10.1200/JCO.2003.05.004.

Roach M, Thomas K. Overview of randomized controlled treatment trials for clinically localized prostate cancer: implications for active surveillance and the United States preventative task force report on screening? J Natl Cancer Inst Monogr. 2012;2012(45):221–9.

Rodda SL, Tyldesley S, Keyes M, et al. Low-dose-rate prostate brachytherapy is superior to dose-escalated EBRT for unfavorable risk prostate cancer: the results of the ASCENDE-RT randomized control trial. Int J Radiat Oncol Biol Phys. 2015;93(3):E191–2.

Rosenthal SA, Hunt D, Sartor AO, et al. A phase 3 trial of 2 years of androgen suppression and radiation therapy with or without adjuvant chemotherapy for high-risk prostate cancer: final results of Radiation Therapy Oncology Group phase 3 randomized trial NRG oncology RTOG 9902. Int J Radiat Oncol Biol Phys. 2015;93(2):294–302.

Rusthoven CG, Carlson JA, Waxweiler TV, et al. The impact of definitive local therapy for lymph node-positive prostate cancer: a population-based study. Int J Radiat Oncol Biol Phys. 2014;88(5):1064–73.

Rusthoven CG, Jones BL, Flaig TW, et al. Improved survival with prostate radiation in addition to androgen deprivation therapy for men with newly diagnosed metastatic prostate cancer. J Clin Oncol. 2016;34(24):2835–42.

Sandler H, Chen H, Seth A, et al. A phase III protocol of androgen suppression (AS) and 3DCRT/IMRT versus AS and 3DCRT/IMRT followed by chemotherapy (CT) with docetaxel and prednisone for localized, high-risk prostate cancer (RTOG 0521). J Clin Oncol. 2015;33(18_suppl); abstr LBA5002.

Sathya JR, Davis IR, Julian JA, et al. Randomized trial comparing iridium implant plus external-beam radiation therapy with external-beam radiation therapy alone in node-negative locally advanced cancer of the prostate. J Clin Oncol. 2005;23:1192–9.

Satkunasivam R, Kim AE, Desai M, et al. Radical prostatectomy or external beam radiation therapy vs no local therapy for survival benefit in metastatic prostate cancer: a SEER-Medicare analysis. J Urol. 2015 Aug;194(2):378–85.

Scher HI, Lu D, Schreiber NA, et al. Association of AR-V7 on circulating tumor cells as a treatment-specific biomarker with outcomes and survival in castration-resistant prostate cancer. June: JAMA Oncol; 2016.

Schiffner DC, Gottschalk AR, Lometti M, et al. Daily electronic portal imaging of implanted gold seed fiducials in patients undergoing radiotherapy after radical prostatectomy. Int J Radiat Oncol Biol Phys. 2007;67(2):610–9.

VII

Schröder FH, Hugosson J, Roobol MJ, et al. Screening and prostate cancer mortality: results of the European randomised study of screening for prostate cancer (ERSPC) at 13 years of follow-up. Lancet. 2014;384(9959):2027–35.

Shih HA, Harisinghani M, Zietman AL, et al. Mapping of nodal disease in locally advanced prostate cancer: rethinking the clinical target volume for pelvic nodal irradiation based on vascular rather than bony anatomy. Int J Radiat Oncol Biol Phys. 2005;63:1262–9.

Shipley WU, Seiferheld W, Lukka H, et al. Radiation with or without antiandrogen therapy in recurrent prostate cancer. NEJM. 2017;376(5):417–28.

Shoag JE, Mittal S, Hu JC. Reevaluating PSA testing rates in the PLCO trial. N Engl J Med. 2016;374(18):1795–6.

Sidhom MA, et al. Post-prostatectomy radiation therapy: consensus guidelines of the Australian and New Zealand Radiation Oncology Genito-Urinary Group. Radiother Oncol. 2008;88(1):10–9.

Stone NN, Stock RG. 15-year cause specific and all-cause survival following brachytherapy for prostate cancer: negative impact of long-term hormonal therapy. J Urol. 2014;192(3):754–9.

Sweeney CJ, Chen Y-H, Carducci M, et al. Chemohormonal therapy in metastatic hormone-sensitive prostate cancer. N Engl J Med. 2015;373(8):737–46.

Taylor A, Rockall AG, Rezneck RH, Powell ME. Mapping pelvic lymph nodes: guidelines for delineation in intensity-modulated radiotherapy. Int J Radiat Oncol Biol Phys. 2005;63:1604–12.

Tendulkar RD, Agrawal S, Gao T, et al. Contemporary update of a multi-institutional predictive nomogram for salvage radiotherapy after radical prostatectomy. J Clin Oncol. 2016;34(30):JCO679647.

Thompson IM, Tangen CM, Paradelo J, et al. Adjuvant radiotherapy for pathological T3N0M0 prostate cancer significantly reduces risk of metastases and improves survival: long-term follow up of a randomized clinical trial. J Urol. 2009;181(3):956–62.

Tollefson MK, Leibovich BC, Slezak JM, Zincke H, Blute ML. Long-term prognostic significance of primary Gleason pattern in patients with Gleason score 7 prostate cancer: impact on prostate cancer specific survival. J Urol. 2006;175(2):547–51.

Tward JD, Kokeny KE, Shrieve DC. Radiation therapy for clinically node-positive prostate adenocarcinoma is correlated with improved overall and prostate cancer-specific survival. Pract Radiat Oncol. 2013;3(3):234–40.

Valicenti RK, Thompson I, Albertsen P, et al. Adjuvant and salvage radiation therapy after prostatectomy: American Society for Radiation Oncology/American Urological Association guidelines. Int J Radiat Oncol Biol Phys. 2013;86(5):822–8.

Van der Kwast TH, Bolla M, Van Poppel H, et al. Identification of patients with prostate cancer who benefit from immediate postoperative radiotherapy: EORTC 22911. J Clin Oncol. 2007;25(27):4178–86.

Vargas CE, Hartsell WF, Dunn M, et al. Hypofractionated versus standard fractionated proton-beam therapy for low-risk prostate cancer: interim results of a randomized trial PCG GU 002. Am J Clin Oncol. 2015;1:1–6.

Wallis CJD, Saskin R, Choo R, et al. Surgery versus radiotherapy for clinically-localized prostate cancer: a systematic review and meta-analysis. Eur Urol. 2016;70(1):21–30.

Weiner AB, Matulewicz RS, Eggener SE, Schaeffer EM. Increasing incidence of metastatic prostate cancer in the United States (2004–2013). July: Prostate Cancer Prostatic Dis; 2016.

Widmark A, Gunnlaugsson A, Beckman L, et al. Extreme hypofractionation vs. conventionally fractionated radiotherapy for intermediate risk prostate cancer: early toxicity results from the scandinavian randomized phase III trial "HYPO-RT-PC." ASTRO Meet Abstr. 2016. Late-breaking abstract 5.

Wiegel T, Bartkowiak D, Bottke D, et al. Adjuvant radiotherapy versus wait-and-see after radical prostatectomy: 10-year follow-up of the ARO 96-02/AUO AP 09/95 trial. Eur Urol. 2014;66(2):243–50.

Wong AT, Schwartz D, Osborn V, Safdieh J, Weiner J, Schreiber D. Adjuvant radiation with hormonal therapy is associated with improved survival in men with pathologically involved lymph nodes after radical surgery for prostate cancer. July: Urol Oncol; 2016.

Yoshioka Y, Suzuki O, Isohashi F, et al. High-dose-rate brachytherapy as monotherapy for intermediate- and high-risk prostate cancer: clinical results for a median 8-year follow-up. Int J Radiat Oncol Biol Phys. 2016;94(4):675–82.

Zagars GK, Pollack A, von Eschenbach AC. Addition of radiation therapy to androgen ablation improves outcome for subclinically node-positive prostate cancer. Urology. 2001;58:233–9.

Zapatero A, Guerrero A, Maldonado X, et al. High-dose radiotherapy with short-term or long-term androgen deprivation in localised prostate cancer (DART01/05 GICOR): a randomised, controlled, phase 3 trial. Lancet Oncol. 2015;16(3):320–7.

Zelefsky MJ, Yamada Y, Cohen GN, et al. Five-year outcome of intraoperative conformal permanent I-125 interstitial implantation for patients with clinically localized prostate cancer. Int J Radiat Oncol Biol Phys. 2007a;67(1):65–70.

Zelefsky MJ, Kuban DA, Levy LB, et al. Multi-institutional analysis of long-term outcome for stages T1-T2 prostate cancer treated with permanent seed implantation. Int J Radiat Oncol Biol Phys. 2007b;67(2):327–33.

Zhao SG, Chang SL, Spratt DE, et al. Development and validation of a 24-gene predictor of response to postoperative radiotherapy in prostate cancer: a matched, retrospective analysis. Lancet Oncol. 2016;17(11):1612–20.

Zietman AL, Bae K, Slater JD, et al. Randomized trial comparing conventional-dose with high-dose conformal radiation therapy in early-stage adenocarcinoma of the prostate: long-term results from proton radiation oncology group/american college of radiology 95-09. J Clin Oncol. 2010;28(7):1106–11.

VII

Chapter 27
Cancer of the Penis

Michael A. Garcia and Alexander R. Gottschalk

PEARLS

- Penile cancer is rare in Western countries (<1% of cancers in men) but accounts for 10–20% of male malignancies in Africa, Asia, and South America.
- Lymph node drainage:
- Skin of penis → bilateral superficial inguinal nodes.
- Glans penis → bilateral inguinal or iliac nodes.
- Penis corporal tissue → bilateral deep inguinal and iliac nodes.
- Up to 25% of non-palpable nodes harbor micrometastases.
- Risk factors: uncircumcised status, phimosis, poor local hygiene, HIV, and HPV.
- Pathology: 95% squamous cell carcinoma; others very rare – melanoma, lymphoma, basal cell carcinoma, and sarcoma.

WORKUP

- H&P, with careful palpation of inguinal nodes and penis.
- Labs: CBC, chemistries, BUN, Cr, and LFTs including alkaline phosphatase.
- Imaging: ultrasound (penis) or MRI for extent of invasion, pelvic/abdominal CT for nodes, CXR for all, and bone scan if advanced/suspicious.
- Biopsy (punch, excisional, or incisional) of primary lesion and needle biopsy for suspicious nodes. If primary lesion is deep, consider cystourethroscopy with biopsy.

VII

STAGING: CANCER OF THE PENIS

Editors' note: All TNM stage and stage groups referred to else-where in this chapter reflect the 2007 AJCC staging nomencla-ture unless otherwise noted as the new system below was published after this chapter was written.

Table 27.1 AJCC 7TH ED., (2010)

Primary tumor (T)

TX: Primary tumor cannot be assessed

T0: No evidence of primary tumor

Tis: Carcinoma in situ

Ta: Noninvasive verrucous carcinoma*

T1a: Tumor invades subepithelial connective tissue without lymph vascular invasion and is not poorly differentiated (i.e., grades 3–4)

T1b: Tumor invades subepithelial connective tissue with lymph vascular invasion or is poorly differentiated

T2: Tumor invades corpus spongiosum or cavernosum

T3: Tumor invades urethra

T4: Tumor invades other adjacent structures

Note: Broad pushing penetration (invasion) is permitted; destructive invasion is against this diagnosis

Regional lymph nodes (N)

*Clinical stage definition**

cNX: Regional lymph nodes cannot be assessed

cN0: No palpable or visibly enlarged inguinal lymph nodes

cN1: Palpable mobile unilateral inguinal lymph node

cN2: Palpable mobile multiple or bilateral inguinal lymph nodes

cN3: Palpable fixed inguinal nodal mass or pelvic lymphadenopathy unilateral or bilateral

Note: Clinical stage definition based on palpation, imaging

*Pathologic stage definition**

pNX: Regional lymph nodes cannot be assessed

pN0: No regional lymph node metastasis

pN1: Metastasis in a single inguinal lymph node

pN2: Metastasis in multiple or bilateral inguinal lymph nodes

pN3: Extranodal extension of lymph node metastasis or pelvic lymph node(s) unilateral or bilateral

Note: Pathologic stage definition based on biopsy or surgical excision

continued

Table 27.1 (continued)

Distant metastasis (M)

M0: No distant metastasis

M1: Distant metastasis*

*Note: Node metastasis outside true pelvis in addition to visceral or bone sites

Anatomic stage/prognostic groups

0:	Tis N0 M0
	Ta N0 M0
I:	T1a N0 M0
II:	T1b N0 M0
	T2 N0 M0
	T3 N0 M0
IIIa:	T1-3 N1 M0
IIIb:	T1-3 N2 M0
IV:	T4 Any N M0
	Any T N3 M0
	Any T Any N M1

Used with the permission from the American Joint Committee on Cancer (AJCC), Chicago, Illinois. The original source for this material is the AJCC Cancer Staging Manual, Seventh Edition (2010), published by Springer Science+Business Media

Table 27.2 AJCC 8TH ED., (2017)

VII

Definitions of AJCC TNM

Definition of Primary Tumor (T)

T category	T criteria
TX	Primary tumor cannot be assessed
T0	No evidence of primary tumor
Tis	Carcinoma in situ (penile intraepithelial neoplasia [PeIN])
Ta	Noninvasive localized squamous cell carcinoma
T1	Glans: tumor invades lamina propria Foreskin: tumor invades the dermis, lamina propria, or dartos fascia Shaft: tumor invades connective tissue between the epidermis and corpora regardless of location. All sites with or without lymphovascular invasion or perineural invasion and is or is not high grade
T1a	Tumor is without lymphovascular invasion or perineural invasion and is not high grade (i.e., grade 3 or sarcomatoid)
T1b	Tumor exhibits lymphovascular invasion and/or perineural invasion or is high grade (i.e., grade 3 or sarcomatoid)
T2	Tumor invades into corpus spongiosum (either glans or ventral shaft) with or without urethral invasion
T3	Tumor invades into the corpora cavernosum (including the tunica albuginea) with or without urethral invasion
T4	Tumor invades into adjacent structures (i.e., the scrotum, prostate, pubic bone)

DEFINITION OF REGIONAL LYMPH NODE (N)
Clinical N (cN)

cN category	cN criteria
cNX	Regional lymph nodes cannot be assessed
cN0	No palpable or visibly enlarged inguinal lymph nodes
cN1	Palpable mobile unilateral inguinal lymph node
cN2	Palpable mobile ≥ 2 unilateral inguinal nodes or bilateral inguinal lymph nodes
cN3	Palpable fixed inguinal nodal mass or pelvic lymphadenopathy unilateral or bilateral

Pathological N (pN)

pN category	pN criteria
pNX	Lymph node metastasis cannot be established
pN0	No lymph node metastasis
pN1	≤2 unilateral inguinal metastases, no ENE
pN2	≥3 unilateral inguinal metastases or bilateral metastases
pN3	ENE of lymph node metastases or pelvic lymph node metastases

DEFINITION OF DISTANT METASTASIS (M)

M category	M criteria
M0	No distant metastasis
M1	Distant metastasis present

AJCC PROGNOSTIC STAGE GROUPS

When T is...	And N is...	And M is...	Then the stage group is...
Tis	N0	M0	0is
Ta	N0	M0	0a
T1a	N0	M0	I
T1b	N0	M0	IIA
T2	N0	M0	IIA
T3	N0	M0	IIB
T1–3	N1	M0	IIIA
T1–3	N2	M0	IIIB
T4	Any N	M0	IV
Any T	N3	M0	IV
Any T	Any N	M1	IV

Used with permission of the American Joint Committee on Cancer (AJCC), Chicago, Illinois. The original and primary source for this information is the AJCC Cancer Staging Manual, Eighth Edition (2017) published by Springer International Publishing

TREATMENT RECOMMENDATIONS

Table 27.3 **TREATMENT RECOMMENDATIONS**

Stage	Recommended treatment
Tis or Ta	Wide local excision with circumcision (Mohs surgery is an option), topical 5-FU or imiquimod, or laser therapy
Early limited lesions (for RT alone, lesions should be T1–T2, <4 cm size)	*Penis preservation*: circumcise first, then brachytherapy alone or EBRT, or chemo-RT. *Brachytherapy alone*: two methods, interstitial implant with Ir-192 (preferred) or radioactive mold – 60 Gy to tumor, 50 Gy to urethra. Contraindicated if >1 cm corpus invasion *EBRT*: 40–50 Gy to whole penile shaft ± lymph nodes (see surgical management below), then boost to primary lesion +2 cm margin (total 65–70 Gy) *Chemo-RT*: based on data extrapolated from anal and cervical cancers Consider prophylactic inguinal node RT based on EUA risk (below) *Surgery* – wide local excision, partial penectomy, or radical penectomy. Ensure 1–2 cm surgical margins For non-palpable inguinal nodes, EAU risks stratify into low (Tis, Ta, T1a), intermediate (T1b, G1–2), and high (T2 or T1b with G3–4) risk. EAU recommends inguinal node dissection for intermediate and high risk. Pelvic node dissection indicated if ≥2 inguinal nodes involved
Advanced lesions	Options: *EBRT*: 45–50.4 Gy to penile shaft and pelvic and inguinal nodes, then boost to primary with 2 cm margin and involved nodes to 60–70 Gy. Consider concurrent chemotherapy *Surgery*: save for salvage partial or radical penectomy; consider inguinal node dissection for tumors extending onto shaft of penis/poorly differentiated; if node positive (biopsy or imaging), need inguinal and pelvic node dissections; post-op RT or chemo-RT for close or positive margins, pN2–3 disease *Neoadjuvant chemo*: consider for bulky nodal disease

VII

STUDIES

There are no randomized trials for primary penile cancers. Studies suggest similar survival rates for early-stage disease between primary RT and surgery when taking into account surgical salvage. Penectomy is associated with higher rates of depression and suicide.

- Penile preservation rates are higher with brachytherapy (about 70% at 5–10 yrs), but brachytherapy patients are more carefully selected with tumors <4 cm diameter with no or minimal shaft involvement.
- Meta-analysis/review (Hasan, Brachytherapy 2015). 1505 surgical patients and 673 brachytherapy patients. 5-yr OS surgery 76% vs. brachytherapy 73%, LC penectomy 84% vs. brachytherapy 79% (84% early-stage), and brachytherapy organ preservation 74%.
- Crook (World J Urol 2009). 67 men treated with LDR brachytherapy to 55–65 Gy. 5-yr CSS 84%, 5-yr LC 87%, and 10-yr LC 72%. Penile preservation rate 5-yr 88%, 10-yr 67%. 5-yr necrosis 12%, and stenosis 9%.
- de Crevoisier (IJROBP 2009). 144 men with glans penis carcinoma treated with LDR to median 65 Gy. 10-yr LC 80%, CSS 92%, and penile preservation 72%. Surgical salvage effective for 86% recurrences. 10-yr painful ulceration 26% and stenosis 29%.
- EBRT series generally include more advanced lesions and report higher rates of LF (about 50%) and need for salvage penectomy.
- Sarin (IJROBP 1997): 101 men treated with primary EBRT (59), brachytherapy (13), penectomy (29). 5-yr OS 57%, CSS 66%, LC 60%, and 50% penile preservation. No difference between surgery and RT in LC after accounting for salvage. Note: 2 attempted suicide after penectomy.
- Ozsahin (IJROBP 2006). 29 men with primary RT (21 EBRT alone, 7 EBRT + brachytherapy, 1 brachytherapy alone) and 22 with post-op RT. LF after organ sparing treatment 56% and 73% of LF salvaged with surgery. Penis preservation rate with definitive RT 52%. No survival difference between surgery and primary RT.

RADIATION TECHNIQUES

SIMULATION AND FIELD DESIGN

- Patients should have circumcision prior to RT to remove portion of tumor involving the prepuce, to expose full extent of the lesion for men with phimosis, and to prevent subsequent contraction or painful necrosis of the irradiated prepuce.

- Interstitial brachytherapy.
- Recommend following ABS guidelines (Crook, Brachytherapy 2013).
- Patient selection: tumor <4 cm diameter, preferably limited to glans or with minor extension across the coronal sulcus. More advanced lesions have higher risk of LF and complications. Combined brachytherapy for primary and surgical evaluation of nodes may be considered. Consider referral to experienced center for penile brachytherapy.
- Implant under general or local anesthesia, takes ~45 min.
- Place Foley catheter during implant and treatment to help identify urethra and avoid transfixing with needles/catheters.
- May use rigid steel needles held in predrilled parallel acrylic templates or parallel flexible nylon catheters, placed 1–1.5 cm apart. Cover gross disease with at least 1 cm margin.
- LDR dose is typically about 60 Gy over 5 days at 0.5 Gy/h.
- HDR with afterloaded Ir-192 may be considered, although there is less published data. ABS reports that 38.4 Gy in 3.2 Gy BID treatments over 6 days with at least 6 h interval between fractions is well tolerated.
- Patients wear supporting Styrofoam collar around penis and may need analgesics and DVT prophylaxis if stay in bed.
- EBRT.
- Simulate patient supine; apply Foley catheter for simulation, and suspend penis in bivalved clear plastic (preferred), such as Lucite or Plexiglas, or wax with central cylindrical chamber custom made to place around the penis.
- If treating inguinal nodes, treat in the frog-leg position. If treating pelvic nodes, may secure penis cranially into pelvic field.
- Volumes.
- GTV: palpable/visible disease (physical exam, CT, MRI).
- CTV:
  - GTV + 2 cm margin or whole shaft of penis.
  - ±Superficial and deep inguinal nodes.
  - ±Pelvic nodes (internal + external iliacs, obturator nodes).
- PTV: depends on technique, 1 cm appropriate.
- Dose: 45–50.4 Gy in 1.8–2 Gy fractions for pelvic fields (up to 54 Gy for extranodal spread). Total dose to primary CTV is 65–70 Gy.
- Plesiobrachytherapy/molds.

VII

꙳ Place penis into cylinder loaded with Ir-192 sources; mold worn for calculated time to give 60 Gy. Limit urethra dose to 50 Gy; requires very compliant patient.

DOSE LIMITATIONS
꙳ Doses >60 Gy increase risk of urethral stenosis and fibrosis.
꙳ For pelvic fields, limit bladder ≤75 Gy, rectum ≤70 Gy, and femoral heads <45 Gy.

COMPLICATIONS
꙳ Dermatitis, dysuria, urethral stricture (10–40%), urethral fistula, erectile dysfunction (10–20%), telangiectasia (nearly universal), penile fibrosis, penile necrosis (3–15%), sterility, and small bowel obstruction (rare)

FOLLOW-UP

(SEE NCCN GUIDELINES AT WWW.NCCN.ORG)
꙳ Need close follow-up, especially if no prophylactic nodal treatment in cN0 patients.
꙳ H&P every 1–2 months for 1st yr, every 3 months for 2nd yr, every 6 months for 3rd to 5th yrs, and then annually.

Acknowledgment We thank Alice Wang-Chesebro MD and William Foster MD for their work on the prior edition of this chapter.

REFERENCES
Amin MB, Edge S, Greene F, Byrd DR, Brookland RK, Washington MK, Gershenwald JE, Compton CC, Hess KR, Sullivan DC, Jessup JM, Brierley JD, Gaspar LE, Schilsky RL, Balch CM, Winchester DP, Asare EA, Madera M, Gress DM, Meyer LR, editors. AJCC cancer staging manual. 8th ed. Springer: Chicago; 2017.
Crook J, Ma C, Grimard L. Radiation therapy in the management of the primary penile tumor: an update. World J Urol. 2009;27(2):189–96.
Crook JM, Haie-Meder C, Demanes DJ, Mazeron JJ, Martinez AA, Rivard MJ. American Brachytherapy Society-Groupe Européen de Curiethérapie-European Society of Therapeutic Radiation Oncology (ABS-GEC-ESTRO) consensus statement for penile brachytherapy. Brachytherapy. 2013;12(3):191–8.

de Crevoisier R, Slimane K, Sanfilippo N, et al. Long-term results of brachytherapy for carcinoma of the penis confined to the glans (N- or NX). Int J Radiat Oncol Biol Phys. 2009;74(4):1150–6.

Edge SB, Byrd DR, Compton CC, Fritz AG, Greene FL, Trotti A, editors. AJCC cancer staging manual. 7th ed. New York: Springer; 2010.

Hasan S, Francis A, Hagenauer A, et al. The role of brachytherapy in organ preservation for penile cancer: a meta-analysis and review of the literature. Brachytherapy. 2015;14(4):517–24.

Ozsahin M, Jichlinski P, Weber DC, et al. Treatment of penile carcinoma: to cut or not to cut? Int J Radiat Oncol Biol Phys. 2006;66(3):674–9.

Sarin R, Norman AR, et al. Treatment results and prognostic factors in 101 men treated for squamous carcinoma of the penis. Int J Radiat Oncol Biol Phys. 1997;38:713–22.

VII

Chapter 28
Testicular Cancer

Michael A. Garcia and Alexander R. Gottschalk

PEARLS

- Spermatogenesis.
  - Spermatogonia → spermatocytes → spermatids → spermatozoa.
- Lymph node (LN) drainage.
  - Left testicle: testicular vein → left renal vein → para-aortic LN.
  - Right testicle: testicular vein → IVC below level of renal vein → paracaval and aortocaval nodes.
  - Prior inguinal surgery may disrupt drainage and redirect through iliac nodes.
- Testicular cancer types:
  - Germ cell tumor (GCT, account for >95% of testicular cancers).
    - Pure seminoma (60% of GCT).
    - Non-seminomatous germ cell tumors (NSGCT, 40% of GCT).
      - Embryonal, yolk sac tumor, choriocarcinoma, teratoma, and mixed.
  - Sex cord-stromal tumors.
    - Sertoli cell, Leydig cell, granulosa cell, and mixed types.
  - Others include lymphoma and embryonal rhabdomyosarcoma.

© Springer International Publishing AG, part of Springer Nature 2018
Eric K. Hansen and M. Roach III (eds.), *Handbook of Evidence-Based Radiation Oncology*, https://doi.org/10.1007/978-3-319-62642-0_28

, Risk factors: cryptorchidism, history of contralateral GCT, family history, and Klinefelter syndrome (47 XXY).
, Estimated 8,700 new testicular cancer cases and 380 deaths in the USA for 2016.

WORKUP

, H&P, bilateral testicular ultrasound, β-hCG, AFP, LDH, chemistry panel, and CXR.
, Radical transinguinal orchiectomy.
, Repeat tumor markers postoperatively if elevated preoperatively.
, β-hCG half-life is 24–36 h; AFP half-life is 3.5–6 days.
, AFP never elevated in pure seminoma; β-hCG may be elevated in pure seminoma.
, Imaging:
  , CT abdomen and pelvis.
  , Seminoma: CT chest if abdominal CT or CXR is abnormal.
  , NSGCT: CT chest.
  , Bone scan and/or MRI brain if clinically indicated.
, Discuss sperm banking prior to initiation of treatment.

Table 28.1 STAGING (AJCC 7TH ED., 2010) TESTICULAR CANCER

Primary tumor (T)*

The extent of primary tumor is usually classified after radical orchiectomy, and for this reason, a pathologic stage is assigned

pTX:	Primary tumor cannot be assessed
pT0:	No evidence of primary tumor (e.g., histologic scar in testis)
pTis:	Intratubular germ cell neoplasia (carcinoma in situ)
pT1:	Tumor limited to the testis and epididymis without vascular/lymphatic invasion; tumor may invade into the tunica albuginea but not the tunica vaginalis
pT2:	Tumor limited to the testis and epididymis with vascular/lymphatic invasion or tumor extending through the tunica albuginea with involvement of the tunica vaginalis
pT3:	Tumor invades the spermatic cord with or without vascular/lymphatic invasion
pT4:	Tumor invades the scrotum with or without vascular/lymphatic invasion

Note: Except for pTis and pT4, the extent of primary tumor is classified by radical orchiectomy. TX may be used for other categories in the absence of radical orchiectomy

Table 28.1 (continued)

Regional lymph nodes (N)
Clinical
NX:	Regional lymph nodes cannot be assessed
N0:	No regional lymph node metastasis
N1:	Metastasis with a lymph node mass 2 cm or less in greatest dimension, or multiple lymph nodes, not more than 2 cm in greatest dimension
N2:	Metastasis with a lymph node mass more than 2 cm but not more than 5 cm in greatest dimension, or multiple lymph nodes, any one mass greater than 2 cm, but not more than 5 cm in greatest dimension
N3:	Metastasis with a lymph node mass more than 5 cm in greatest dimension

Pathologic (pN)
pNX:	Regional lymph nodes cannot be assessed
pN0:	No regional lymph node metastasis
pN1:	Metastasis with a lymph node mass 2 cm or less in greatest dimension and less than or equal to five nodes positive, not more than 2 cm in greatest dimension
pN2:	Metastasis with a lymph node mass more than 2 cm, but not more than 5 cm in greatest dimension; or more than five nodes positive, not more than 5 cm; or evidence of extranodal extension of tumor
pN3:	Metastasis with a lymph node mass more than 5 cm in greatest dimension

Distant metastasis (M)		**Serum markers (S)**
M0:	No distant mets	S0: Markers in normal limits
M1a:	Nonregional LN + or lung mets	S1: LDH < (1.5× normal) and hCG < 5000 and AFP < 1000
		S2: LDH = (1.5–10× normal) or hCG 5000–50,000 or AFP 1000–10,000
M1b:	Mets other than nonregional LN and lung	S3: LDH > (10× normal) or hcG > 50,000 or AFP > 10,000

Anatomic stage/prognostic groups

Group	T	N	M	S (serum tumor markers)
0:	pTis	N0	M0	S0
IA:	pT1	N0	M0	S0
IB:	pT2–4	N0	M0	S0
IS:	Any pT/Tx	N0	M0	S1–S3 (measured post orchiectomy)
IIA:	Any pT/Tx	N1	M0	S0–S1
IIB:	Any pT/Tx	N2	M0	S0–S1
IIC:	Any pT/Tx	N3	M0	S0–S1
IIIA:	Any pT/Tx	Any N	M1a	S0–S1
IIIB:	Any pT/Tx	N1–N3	M0	S2
	Any pT/Tx	Any N	M1a	S2
IIIC:	Any pT/Tx	N1–N3	M0	S3
	Any pT/Tx	Any N	M1a	S3
	Any pT/Tx	Any N	M1b	Any S

Used with the permission from the American Joint Committee on Cancer (AJCC), Chicago, Illinois. The original source for this material is the AJCC Cancer Staging Manual, Seventh Edition (2010), published by Springer Science+Business Media

continued

Table 28.1 (continued)

Royal Marsden staging system	~10-year survival (seminoma)	
I: Limited to testis	I:	RFS 96–98%, CSS 99–100%
IIA: Nodes <2 cm	IIA:	RFS 92%, CSS 96–100%
IIB: Nodes 2–5 cm	IIB:	RFS 86%, CSS 96–100%
IIC: Nodes 5–10 cm	IIC:	RFS 70%, OS 90% (RT alone)
IID: Nodes >10 cm	IID:	RFS 50% (RT alone), 90%
III = Nodes above and below diaphragm		(chemo)
IV = Extralymphatic mets	IIIA/B:	OS 90%
	IIIC:	OS 80%

International Germ Cell Cancer Collaborative Group Risks for NSGCT (JCO 1997)

Good prognosis	*Intermediate prognosis*	*Poor prognosis*
All must be met:	Testis or retroperitoneal	Mediastinal primary or
Testis or retroperitoneal	primary *and* no non-lung	non-lung visceral mets *or* any
primary	visceral mets	of the following:
No non-lung visceral	*and* any of the following:	AFP > 10,000 or hCG > 50,000
mets	AFP < 1,000–10,000 or	or LDH >10× normal
AFP < 1,000,	hCG 5,000–50,000 or LDH	5 yr PFS: 41%
hCG < 5,000, LDH <1.5×	1.5–10× normal	
normal	5 yr PFS: 75%	
5 yr PFS: 89%		

Table 28.2 STAGING (AJCC 8TH ED., 2017)

Definitions of AJCC TNM

Definition of primary tumor (T)

Clinical T (cT)

cT category	cT criteria
cTX	Primary tumor cannot be assessed
cT0	No evidence of primary tumor
cTis	Germ cell neoplasia in situ
cT4	Tumor invades scrotum with or without vascular/ lymphatic invasion

Note: Except for Tis confirmed by biopsy and T4, the extent of the primary tumor is classified by radical orchiectomy. TX may be used for other categories for clinical staging

PATHOLOGICAL T (PT)

pT category	pT criteria
pTX	Primary tumor cannot be assessed
pT0	No evidence of primary tumor
pTis	Germ cell neoplasia in situ
pT1	Tumor limited to testis (including rete testis invasion) without lymphovascular invasion
pT1a*	Tumor smaller than 3 cm in size

pT category	pT criteria
pT1b*	Tumor 3 cm or larger in size
pT2	Tumor limited to testis (including rete testis invasion) with lymphovascular invasion or tumor invading hilar soft tissue or epididymis or penetrating visceral mesothelial layer covering the external surface of tunica albuginea with or without lymphovascular invasion
pT3	Tumor invades spermatic cord with or without lymphovascular invasion
pT4	Tumor invades scrotum with or without lymphovascular invasion

*Subclassification of pT1 applies only to pure seminoma

DEFINITION OF REGIONAL LYMPH NODE (N)

Clinical N (cN)

cN category	cN criteria
cNX	Regional lymph nodes cannot be assessed
cN0	No regional lymph node metastasis
cN1	Metastases with a lymph node mass 2 cm or smaller in the greatest dimension or multiple lymph nodes, not larger than 2 cm in the greatest dimension
cN2	Metastasis with a lymph node mass larger than 2 cm but not larger than 5 cm in the greatest dimension or multiple lymph nodes, any one mass larger than 2 cm but not larger than 5 cm in the greatest dimension
cN3	Metastasis with a lymph node mass larger than 5 cm in the greatest dimension

VII

PATHOLOGICAL N (PN)

pN category	pN criteria
pNX	Regional lymph nodes cannot be assessed
pN0	No regional lymph node metastasis
pN1	Metastasis with a lymph node mass 2 cm or smaller in the greatest dimension and less than or equal to five nodes positive, not larger than 2 cm in the greatest dimension
pN category	**pN criteria**
pN2	Metastasis with a lymph node mass larger than 2 cm but not larger than 5 cm in the greatest dimension or more than five nodes positive, not larger than 5 cm, or evidence of extranodal extension of tumor
pN3	Metastasis with a lymph node mass larger than 5 cm in the greatest dimension

DEFINITION OF DISTANT METASTASIS (M)

M category	M criteria
M0	No distant metastases
M1	Distant metastases
M1a	Non-retroperitoneal nodal or pulmonary metastases
M1b	Non-pulmonary visceral metastases

DEFINITION OF SERUM MARKERS (S)

S category	S criteria
SX	Marker studies not available or not performed
S0	Marker study levels within normal limits
S1	LDH < 1.5 × N* *and* hCG (mIU/mL) < 5,000 *and* AFP (ng/mL) < 1,000
S2	LDH 1.5–10 × N* *or* hCG (mIU/mL) 5,000–50,000 *or* AFP (ng/mL) 1,000–10,000
S3	LDH > 10 × N* *or* hCG (mIU/mL) >50,000 *or* AFP (ng/mL) > 10,000

*N indicates the upper limit of normal for the LDH assay

AJCC PROGNOSTIC STAGE GROUPS

When T is...	And N is...	And M is...	And S is...	Then the stage group is...
pTis	N0	M0	S0	0
pT1–T4	N0	M0	SX	I
pT1	N0	M0	S0	IA
pT2	N0	M0	S0	IB
pT3	N0	M0	S0	IB
pT4	N0	M0	S0	IB
Any pT/TX	N0	M0	S1–3	IS
Any pT/TX	N1–3	M0	SX	II
Any pT/TX	N1	M0	S0	IIA
Any pT/TX	N1	M0	S1	IIA
Any pT/TX	N2	M0	S0	IIB
Any pT/TX	N2	M0	S1	IIB
Any pT/TX	N3	M0	S0	IIC
Any pT/TX	N3	M0	S1	IIC
Any pT/TX	Any N	M1	SX	III
Any pT/TX	Any N	M1a	S0	IIIA
Any pT/TX	Any N	M1a	S1	IIIA

When T is...	And N is...	And M is...	And S is...	Then the stage group is...
Any pT/TX	N1–3	M0	S2	IIIB
Any pT/TX	Any N	M1a	S2	IIIB
Any pT/TX	N1–3	M0	S3	IIIC
Any pT/TX	Any N	M1a	S3	IIIC
Any pT/TX	Any N	M1b	Any S	IIIC

Used with permission of the American Joint Committee on Cancer (AJCC), Chicago, Illinois. The original and primary source for this information is the AJCC Cancer Staging Manual, Eighth Edition (2017) published by Springer International Publishing

TREATMENT RECOMMENDATIONS

Table 28.3 TREATMENT RECOMMENDATIONS FOR SEMINOMA

Stage	Recommended treatment
All patients	Radical inguinal orchiectomy with high ligation of spermatic cord
I seminoma	Post resection: surveillance preferred for pT1–T3 for compliant patients (relapse rate 16%). Alternatively, RT (20 Gy to para-aortic ± pelvic LN) or carboplatinum × 1–2c
IIA/IIB seminoma	RT 20 Gy to pelvic and para-aortic LN with boost to gross disease (30 Gy for IIA, 36 Gy for IIB), or primary chemotherapy with etoposide/cisplatin (EP) chemo × 4c or bleomycin/etoposide/cisplatin (BEP) x 3c
IIC/D and III seminoma	Chemo: EP × 4c or BEP × 3c
NSGCT	IA: open nerve-sparing retroperitoneal LN dissection (nsRPLND) or surveillance in compliant patients IB: nsRPLND or BEP × 1–2c or surveillance if T2 and compliant patient IS: EP × 4c or BEP × 3c IIA: if markers negative, nsRPLND or EP × 4c or BEP × 3c. If persistent tumor marker elevation, EP × 4c or BEP × 3c IIB: if markers negative and LN mets within drainage sites, nsRPLND or EP × 4c or BEP × 3c. If persistent tumor marker elevation or multifocal LN mets with aberrant drainage, EP × 4c or BEP × 3c IIC/IIIA: EP × 4c or BEP × 3c IIIB: BEP × 4c IIIC: BEP × 4c or etoposide/ifosfamide/cisplatin (VIP) × 4

STUDIES

Table 28.4 SURVEILLANCE

Study	Patients	Management after orchiectomy	Findings
Warde et al. (JCO 2002) retrospective	638 patients w/ stage I seminoma	Surveillance Median f/u 7 yrs	Relapses in 19% Risk factors for relapse: tumors >4 cm, and invasion of rete testis (but these risk factors were not validated in subsequent analysis by Chung (ASCO 2010))
Mortenson et al. (Eur Urol 2014) retrospective	1,954 patients w/ stage I seminoma	Surveillance then salvage for relapse Median f/u 15.1 yrs	Relapses in 18.9% pts., 73% within first 2 yrs 62% relapses treated w/ RT, 36% treated w/ chemo. Disease-specific survival (DSS) at 15 yrs: 99.3%. Relapse risk factors: tumor size, vascular invasion, epididymal invasion
Kollmannsberger et al. (JCO 2015) Retrospective	2,483 patients with stage I testis cancer (54% seminoma)	Surveillance, then salvage for relapse Median f/u 5.2 yrs	Relapse in 13% of seminomas, 92% within 3 yrs. relapse in 19% non-seminomas, 90% within 2 yrs. All relapses treated with chemo or RT. 5 yr DSS: 99.7%
SGCCG (Aparicio, Ann Oncol 2014)	744 patients with stage I seminoma	Low risk: surveillance. High risk: carboplatin × 2c. Median f/u 6.7 yrs	Surveillance for low risk: relapse 14.8% overall (8.3% if tumor <4 cm and no rete testis involvement). 5-yr CSS 100% with salvage chemo (95%) or RT (5%)

RT FIELD AND DOSE FOR STAGE I

- MRC Trial TE 10 (Fossa, JCO 1999): 478 patients with stage I seminoma randomized to dogleg vs. para-aortic (PA) RT. No difference in 3-yr RFS/OS with dogleg (97/96%) vs. PA (99/100%). 3-yr pelvic RFS was 100% with dogleg vs. 98% with PA. PA arm had decreased nausea/vomiting, lower azoospermia (11% vs. 35%), and faster recovery of sperm count.

- MRC Trial 18 (Jones, JCO 2005): 625 patients with stage I seminoma randomized to 20 Gy vs. 30 Gy RT (2Gy/fx). RT was PA (dogleg for patients with prior inguinal surgery). No difference in 5-yr RFS (97% 30Gy, 96.4% 20Gy). 30 Gy arm had worse rates of lethargy and inability to carry out normal work at 4 weeks post-RT.

CHEMO FOR STAGE I

- MRC TE19/EORTC 30982 (Oliver, JCO 2011; Lancet 2005): 1,447 patients with stage I seminoma randomized to carboplatin × 1c vs. RT (20–30 Gy, 87% PA, and 13% dogleg). Median f/u 6.5 yrs. 5-yrs RFS: RT 96.0% vs. carbo 94.7% (p = 0.36). Relapse sites: carboplatin 74% PA, 0% pelvic vs. RT 9% PA, 28% pelvic. Fewer contralateral GCTs in AUC arm (HR 0.22, p = 0.03).

SECOND CANCER RISK

- Travis (JNCI 2005). Review of 40,576 patients with testicular cancer in 14 registries in Europe and North America. If diagnosed by age 35, cumulative risk of second solid cancer 40 yrs after treatment was 36% for seminoma and 31% for non-seminoma vs. 23% for the general population. Increased relative risk of solid cancers was noted for RT (RR = 2.0), chemo (RR = 1.8), and both (RR = 2.9).
- Horwich (Br J Cancer 2014). Review of 2629 patients with stage I seminoma treated with RT in the UK or Norway 1960–1992. RT was 91% abdominal + pelvic, 6% PA only, 1% included the mediastinum or neck. Standardized incidence ratio for 2nd cancer was 1.62 for pelvic or abdominal sites with no significant elevated risk of cancers elsewhere. Absolute excess risk of 29 cancers per 10,000 person years.

RADIATION TECHNIQUES

SIMULATION AND FIELD DESIGN

- ، Simulate supine. Place clamshell on uninvolved testicle. Position penis out of field.
- ، Non-contrast CT simulation.
- ، AP/PA field borders:
  - ، Superior: T11/T12.
  - ، Inferior:
- ، Stage I: L5/S1 for PA field.
- ، Stage II: Top of acetabulum for dogleg to cover ipsilateral common, external, and proximal internal iliac nodes.
  - ، Lateral: traditionally, tips of transverse processes of vertebra, but with 3D planning, may contour aorta and inferior vena cava and add 1.2–1.9 cm CTV (plus 2 cm block margin on all nodes), 0.5 cm PTV, and 7 mm margin from PTV to block edge for beam penumbra.
  - ، For left-sided tumors, widen field to include left renal hilar nodes.
- ، If prior inguinal surgery, treat ipsilateral inguinal and iliac regions.
- ، For IIA/IIB, boost nodal mass with 2 cm block margin.

DOSE PRESCRIPTIONS

- ، Stage I: 20 Gy at 2.0 Gy/fx. Alternatively, 25.5 Gy at 1.5 Gy/fx.
- ، Stage II: Boost IIA nodes to 30 Gy and IIB nodes to 36 Gy.

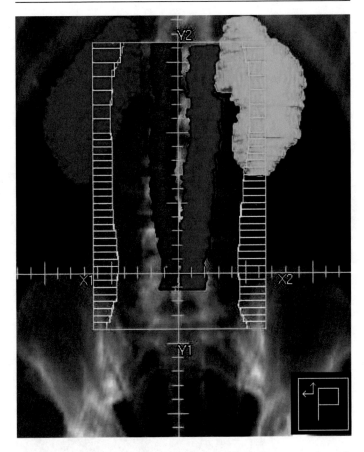

VII

Fig. 28.1 DRR of a para-aortic field used to treat a stage I semi-noma (Reprinted from Wilder et al., Int J Radiat Oncol Biol Phys 2012 with permission from Elsevier)

Fig. 28.2 DRR of a **(a)** dogleg field and **(b)** boost field used to treat a stage IIB seminoma (Reprinted from Wilder et al., Int J Radiat Oncol Biol Phys 2012 with permission from Elsevier)

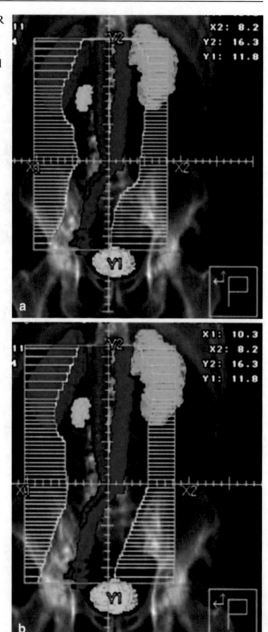

DOSE LIMITATIONS

- RT doses of 0.2–0.5 Gy cause temporary azoospermia, 0.5–1.0 Gy can cause long-term azoospermia, and 2 Gy can cause sterilization.
  - Clamshell reduces testicle dose by 2–3×.
- For dogleg field ~4 cGy/fx → ~1.5 cGy/fx.
- For PA field ~2 cGy/fx → ~0.7 cGy/fx.
- Kidneys: Total kidney V20Gy <30% acceptable, but aim for D50% <8 Gy for each kidney. If solitary kidney, D15% <20 Gy.
  - Rule out horseshoe kidney prior to treatment with IVP or CT.

COMPLICATIONS

- Acute: nausea, vomiting, and diarrhea. Antiemetic prophylaxis recommended 2 h before each treatment.
- Late: small bowel obstruction, chronic diarrhea, and peptic ulcer disease (<2% if <35 Gy).
- With clamshell, most patients will have oligospermia at 4 months to ~1 year.
- Infertility: 50% patients have subfertile counts at presentation or post-op. After RT, 30% able to have children.
- BEP causes immediate azoospermia, but >50% recover sperm count.

FOLLOW-UP (SEE NCCN GUIDELINES AT WWW.NCCN. ORG)

- After RT for stage I seminoma.
- H&P every 6–12 months for the first 2 yrs, then annually. Abdominal +/− pelvic CT annually for 3 yrs. CXR as clinically indicated, consider CT chest if symptomatic.
- Stage I surveillance.
- H&P every 3–6 months for year 1, then every 6–12 months for yrs 2 and 3, and then annually. CT abdomen and pelvis at each visit. CXR as clinically indicated, consider CT chest if symptomatic.
- PET/CT valuable in evaluating postchemotherapy residual disease.

Acknowledgment We thank Brian Missett MD for his work on the prior edition of this chapter.

REFERENCES

Amin MB, Edge S, Greene F, Byrd DR, Brookland RK, Washington MK, Gershenwald JE, Compton CC, Hess KR, Sullivan DC, Jessup JM, Brierley JD, Gaspar LE, Schilsky RL, Balch CM, Winchester DP, Asare EA, Madera M, Gress DM, Meyer LR, editors. AJCC cancer staging manual. 8th ed. New York: Springer; 2017.

Aparicio J, Maroto P, García del Muro X, et al. Prognostic factors for relapse in stage I seminoma: a new nomogram derived from three consecutive, risk-adapted studies from the Spanish Germ Cell Cancer Group (SGCCG). Ann Oncol. 2014;25(11):2173–8.

Chung PW, Daugaard G, Tyldesley S, et al. Prognostic factors for relapse in stage I seminoma managed with surveillance: A validation study. J Clin Oncol. 2010;28:15s. (suppl; abstr 4535)

Edge SB, Byrd DR, Compton CC, Fritz AG, Greene FL, Trotti A, editors. AJCC cancer staging manual. 7th ed. New York: Springer; 2010.

Fossa SD, Horwich A, Russell JM, et al. Optimal planning target volume for stage I testicular seminoma: a Medical Research Council randomized trial. Medical Research Council Testicular Tumor Working Group. J Clin Oncol. 1999;17:1146.

Horwich A, Fosså SD, Huddart R, et al. Second cancer risk and mortality in men treated with radiotherapy for stage I seminoma. Br J Cancer. 2014;110(1):256–63.

International Germ Cell Cancer Collaborative Group. International germ cell consensus classification: a prognostic factor-based staging system for metastatic germ cell cancers. JCO. 1997;15(2):594–603.

Jones WG, Fossa SD, Mead GM, et al. Randomized trial of 30 versus 20 Gy in the adjuvant treatment of stage I Testicular Seminoma: a report on Medical Research Council Trial TE18, European Organisation for the Research and Treatment of Cancer Trial 30942 (ISRCTN18525328). J Clin Oncol. 2005;23:1200–8.

Kollmannsberger C, Tandstad T, Bedard PL, et al. Patterns of relapse in patients with clinical stage I testicular cancer managed with active surveillance. J Clin Oncol. 2015;33(1):51–7.

Mortensen MS, Lauritsen J, Gundgaard MG, et al. A nationwide cohort study of stage I seminoma patients followed on a surveillance program. Eur Urol. 2014;66(6):1172–8.

National Comprehensive Cancer Network. Clinical practice guidelines in oncology: Testicular cancer. Available at: https://www.nccn.org/professionals/physician_gls/PDF/testicular.pdf. Accessed 10 Jan 2017.

Oliver RTD, Mason MD, Mead GM, et al. Radiotherapy versus single-dose carboplatin in adjuvant treatment of stage I seminoma: a randomized trial. Lancet. 2005;266:293–300.

Oliver RT, Mead GM, Fogarty PJ, et al. Radiotherapy vs carboplatin for stage I seminoma: updated analysis of the MRC/EORTC randomized trial. J Clin Oncol. 2008;26:abstr 1.

Oliver RTD, Mead GM, Rustin GJS, et al. Randomized trial of carboplatin versus radiotherapy for stage I seminoma: mature results on relapse and contralateral testis cancer rates in MRC TE19/EORTC 30982 study (ISRCTN27163214). J Clin Oncol. 2011;29(8):957–62.

Travis LB, Fossa SD, Schonfeld SJ, et al. Second cancers among 40,576 testicular cancer patients: focus on long-term survivors. J Natl Cancer Inst. 2005;97:1354–65.

Warde P, Specht L, Horwich A, et al. Prognostic factors for relapse in stage I seminoma managed by surveillance: a pooled analysis. J Clin Oncol. 2002;20:4448–52.

Wilder RB, Buyyounouski MK, Efstathiou JA, Beard CJ. Radiotherapy treatment planning for testicular seminoma. Int J Radiat Oncol Biol Phys. 2012;83(4):e445–52.

PART VIII
Gynecologic Sites

Chapter 29
Cervical Cancer

Serah Choi and I-Chow J. Hsu

PEARLS

- In the United States, cervical cancer incidence was ~12,990 (decreasing ~0.9%/yr over the last 10 yrs) and ~4120 deaths in 2016.
- Worldwide, it is the fourth most common cancer in women and seventh most common cancer overall, with ~528,000 new cases and ~266,000 deaths in 2012.
- Clinical presentation includes: irregular and/or heavy vaginal bleeding, postcoital bleeding and/or abnormal vaginal discharge or asymptomatic (detected on exam or by screening). Advanced disease: pelvic pain, lower back pain, bowel symptoms and/or urinary symptoms.
- Regular Pap screening decreases incidence and mortality by at least 80%.
- ACS guidelines: start Pap screening at age 21 and test q3 yrs. At 30 yo, can do Pap smear combined with an human papillomavirus (HPV) test q5 yrs (co-testing) until 65 yo; and it is also ok to do just Pap smear q3 yrs. Women >65 yo can stop if normal Pap tests in previous 10 yrs and no history of CIN2 or CIN3 in last 20 yrs.
- Risk factors include early first intercourse, multiple partners, history of other STDs, high parity, smoking, immunosuppression, and prenatal diethylstilbestrol (DES) exposure (clear-cell carcinoma).
- ~64% of invasive tumors are squamous cell and ~28% are adenocarcinomas.

VIII

- HPV types 16 and 18 cause ~70% of invasive cervical cancers. HPV 31, 33, 45, 52, and 58 cause ~19%.
- HPV vaccines in the United States: the quadrivalent vaccine (Gardasil) includes HPV6, 11, 16, and 18; the 9-valent vaccine (Gardasil 9) includes HPV6, 11, 16, 18, 31, 33, 45, 52, and 58; and the bivalent vaccine (Cervarix) includes HPV 16 and 18.
- HPV18+ and HPV58+ genotypes predictive for response to chemoradiation treatment (chemo-RT).
- Preinvasive disease: atypical squamous cells of uncertain significance (ASCUS), low-grade squamous intraepithelial lesion (LGSIL), and high-grade squamous intraepithelial lesion (HGSIL).
- ASCUS: 2/3 resolve spontaneously. Perform HPV test and if + for high-risk (HR) strain, do colposcopy. Alternatively, repeat Pap in 1 yr and if abnormal, perform colposcopy.
- LGSIL = Mild dysplasia/CIN 1. Half resolve spontaneously. Repeat Pap in 1 yr (ages 21–24) and, if abnormal, perform colposcopy. If >24 yo, HPV testing and if + for high risk strain, colposcopy.
- HGSIL = Severe dysplasia/CIN 2 or 3/CIS. 1/3 resolves spontaneously. Perform colposcopy with biopsy.
- Anatomy: cylindrical, fibrous organ ~3–4 cm in length. The cervical os is at the inferior aspect of the endocervical canal and the internal os is at the superior aspect. The cervix is lined by squamous cells at the outer aspect, and columnar, glandular cells along the inner canal. The transition between squamous cells and columnar cells is the squamo-columnar junction, where most precancerous/cancerous changes arise.
- Lymphatics of cervix: course laterally along uterine artery to external iliac nodes and eventually to the paraaortic nodes (PAN); posterolaterally behind ureters to internal iliac nodes and eventually to the PAN; posteriorly to common iliac nodes and lateral sacral nodal groups.
- Prognostic factors include lymph node (LN) metastases, tumor size, stage, uterine extension, and hemoglobin level <10.
- Risk of pelvic LN involvement for stage I, II, and III disease is ~15%, 30%, and 45%, respectively.
- Cervical cancer can spread by direct extension, lymphatics or hematogenous dissemination (most often to lungs, liver, and bones).
- Most common site for metastases is pelvic LNs followed by lungs and para-aortic nodes.

WORKUP

- History and physical examination (H&P) including gynecologic history, abnormal vaginal bleeding or discharge and pelvic pain. Examine abdomen, supraclavicular (SCV) LNs and inguinal LNs. Perform pelvic exam under anesthesia, including bimanual palpation, jointly with a Gynecologic Oncologist.
- Pap smear if not bleeding.
- Colposcopy with 15× magnification, cold conization if no gross lesion noted and cannot visualize entire lesion with colposcope. Alternatively, four quadrant punch biopsies or dilation and curettage for pathology.
- Cystoscopy, sigmoidoscopy and/or barium enema for IIB, III, or IVA disease or for symptoms.
- Labs: CBC (including platelets), renal function tests and LFTs. Consider HIV testing.
- Imaging: PET/CT or CT chest/abdomen/pelvis. Can consider chest X-ray (CXR) for chest imaging for stage 1. pelvic MRI for stage IB-IV to assess local disease extent.
  - PET scans are sensitive (~85–90%) and specific (~95–100%).
  - MRI is ~90% accurate for parametrial/vaginal involvement.
  - Because access to imaging may be limited in developing countries, FIGO clinical staging does not include CT, MRI, bone scan, PET, lymphangiography or laparotomy, and intravenous pyelogram is the only imaging allowed to affect FIGO stage. However, FIGO acknowledges the benefits of modern imaging in staging and encourages its use when available.
- If stage IIIB, place renal stent prior to starting chemo.

VIII

STAGING: CERVICAL CANCER

Editors' note: All TNM stage and stage groups referred elsewhere in this chapter reflect the 2007 AJCC staging nomenclature unless otherwise noted as the new system below was published after this chapter was written.

Table 29.1 (AJCC 7TH ED., 2010/FIGO 2008)

Primary tumor (T)

TNM categories	FIGO stages	
TX		Primary tumor cannot be assessed
T0		No evidence of primary tumor
Tis*		Carcinoma in situ (preinvasive carcinoma)
T1	I	Cervical carcinoma confined to uterus (extension to corpus should be disregarded)
T1a**	IA	Invasive carcinoma diagnosed only by microscopy. Stromal invasion with a maximum depth of 5.0 mm measured from the base of the epithelium and a horizontal spread of 7.0 mm or less. Vascular space involvement, venous or lymphatic, does not affect classification
T1a1	IA1	Measured stromal invasion 3.0 mm or less in depth and 7.0 mm or less in horizontal spread
T1a2	IA2	Measured stromal invasion more than 3.0 mm and not more than 5.0 mm with a horizontal spread 7.0 mm or less
T1b	IB	Clinically visible lesion confined to the cervix or microscopic lesion greater than T1a/IA2
T1b1	IB1	Clinically visible lesion 4.0 cm or less in greatest dimension
T1b2	IB2	Clinically visible lesion more than 4.0 cm in greatest dimension
T2	II	Cervical carcinoma invades beyond uterus, but not to pelvic wall or to lower third of vagina
T2a	IIA	Tumor without parametrial invasion
T2a1	IIA1	Clinically visible lesion 4.0 cm or less in greatest dimension
T2a2	IIA2	Clinically visible lesion more than 4.0 cm in greatest dimension
T2b	IIB	Tumor with parametrial invasion
T3	III	Tumor extends to pelvic wall and/or involves lower third of vagina, and/or causes hydronephrosis or nonfunctioning kidney
T3a	IIIA	Tumor involves lower third of vagina, no extension to pelvic wall
T3b	IIIB	Tumor extends to pelvic wall and/or causes hydronephrosis or nonfunctioning kidney
T4	IVA	Tumor invades mucosa of bladder or rectum, and/or extends beyond true pelvis (bullous edema is not sufficient to classify a tumor as T4)

* *Note*: FIGO no longer includes Stage 0 (Tis)

** *Note*: All macroscopically visible lesions – even with superficial invasion – are T1b/IB

Regional lymph nodes (N)

TNM categories	FIGO stages	
NX		Regional lymph nodes cannot be assessed
N0		No regional lymph node metastasis
N1	IIIB	Regional lymph node metastasis

Distant metastasis (M)

TNM categories	FIGO stages	
M0		No distant metastasis
M1	IVB	Distant metastasis (including peritoneal spread, involvement of supraclavicular, mediastinal, or para-aortic LNs, lung, liver, or bone)

Anatomic stage/prognostic groups (FIGO 2008)

0:	Tis N0 M0
I:	T1 N0 M0
IA:	T1a N0 M0
IA1:	T1a1 N0 M0
IA2:	T1a2 N0 M0
IB:	T1b N0 M0
IB1:	T1b1 N0 M0
IB2:	T1b2 N0 M0
II:	T2 N0 M0
IIA:	T2a N0 M0
IIA1:	T2a1 N0 M0
IIA2:	T2a2 N0 M0
IIB:	T2b N0 M0
III:	T3 N0 M0
IIIA:	T3a N0 M0
IIIB:	T3b any N M0
	T1-3 N1 M0
IVA:	T4 any N M0
IVB:	any T any N M1

[a]*Note*: FIGO no longer includes Stage 0 (Tis)

Used with the permission from the American Joint Committee on Cancer (AJCC), Chicago, Illinios. The original source for this material is the AJCC Cancer Staging Manual, Seventh Edition (2010), published by Springer Science + Business Media

Table 29.2 (AJCC 8TH ED., 2017)

Definitions of AJCC TNM

Definition of primary tumor (T)

T category	FIGO stage	T criteria
TX		Primary tumor cannot be assessed
T0		No evidence of primary tumor
T1	I	Cervical carcinoma confned to the uterus (extension to corpus should be disregarded)

continued

Table 29.2 (continued)

T1a	IA	Invasive carcinoma diagnosed only by microscopy. Stromal invasion with a maximum depth of 5.0 mm measured from the base of the epithelium and a horizontal spread of 7.0 mm or less. Vascular space involvement, venous or lymphatic, does not affect classifcation.
T1a1	IA1	Measured stromal invasion of 3.0 mm or less in depth and 7.0 mm or less in horizontal spread
T1a2	IA2	Measured stromal invasion of more than 3.0 mm and not more than 5.0 mm, with a horizontal spread of 7.0 mm or less
T1b	IB	Clinically visible lesion confned to the cervix or microscopic lesion greater than T1a/IA2. Includes all macroscopically visible lesions, even those with superfcial invasion.
T1b1	IB1	Clinically visible lesion 4.0 cm or less in greatest dimension
T1b2	IB2	Clinically visible lesion more than 4.0 cm in greatest dimension
T2	II	Cervical carcinoma invading beyond the uterus but not to the pelvic wall or to lower third of the vagina
T2a	IIA	Tumor without parametrial invasion
T2a1	IIA1	Clinically visible lesion 4.0 cm or less in greatest dimension
T2a2	IIA2	Clinically visible lesion more than 4.0 cm in greatest dimension
T2b	IIB	Tumor with parametrial invasion
T3	III	Tumor extending to the pelvic sidewall* and/or involving the lower third of the vagina and/or causing hydronephrosis or nonfunctioning kidney
T3a	IIIA	Tumor involving the lower third of the vagina but not extending to the pelvic wall
T3b	IIIB	Tumor extending to the pelvic wall and/ or causing hydronephrosis or nonfunctioning kidney
T4	IVA	Tumor invading the mucosa of the bladder or rectum and/or extending beyond the true pelvis (bullous edema is not suffcient to classify a tumor as T4)

*The pelvic sidewall is defined as the muscle, fascia, neurovascular structures, and skel-etal portions of the bony pelvis. On rectal examination, there is no cancer-free space between the tumor and pelvic sidewall.

DEFINITION OF REGIONAL LYMPH NODE (N)

N category	FIGO stage	N criteria
NX		Regional lymph nodes cannot be assessed
N0		No regional lymph node metastasis
N0(i+)		Isolated tumor cells in regional lymph node(s) no greater than 0.2 mm
N1		Regional lymph node metastasis

DEFINITION OF DISTANT METASTASIS (M)

M category	FIGO stage	M criteria
M0		No distant metastasis
M1	IVB	Distant metastasis (including peritoneal spread or involvement of the supraclavicular, mediastinal, or distant lymph nodes; lung; liver; or bone)

AJCC PROGNOSTIC STAGE GROUPS

When T is...	And N is...	And M is...	Then the stage group is...
T1	Any N	M0	I
T1a	Any N	M0	IA
When T is...	And N is...	And M is...	Then the stage group is...
T1a1	Any N	M0	IA1
T1a2	Any N	M0	IA2
T1b	Any N	M0	IB
T1b1	Any N	M0	IB1
T1b2	Any N	M0	IB2
T2	Any N	M0	II
T2a	Any N	M0	IIA
T2a1	Any N	M0	IIA1
T2a2	Any N	M0	IIA2
T2b	Any N	M0	IIB
T3	Any N	M0	III
T3a	Any N	M0	IIIA
T3b	Any N	M0	IIIB
T4	Any N	M0	IVA
Any T	Any N	M1	IVB

Used with permission of the American Joint Committee on Cancer (AJCC), Chicago, Illinois. The original and primary source for this information is the AJCC Cancer Staging Manual, Eighth Edition (2017) published by Springer International Publishing

VIII

Table 29.3 Local control and survival by stage	~LC (%)	~Survival (%)
	IA: 95–100	IA: 95–100
	IB1: 90–95	IB1: 85–90
	IB2: 60–80	IB2: 60–70
	IIA: 80–85	IIA: 75
	IIB: 60–80	IIB: 60–65
	IIIA: 60	IIIA: 25–50
	IIIB: 50–60	IIIB: 25–50
	IVA: 30	IVA: 15–30
		IVB: <10

SURGICAL TECHNIQUES

- Class I: total abdominal hysterectomy (extrafascial). Removal of cervix, small rim of vaginal cuff and outside of the pubocervical fascia.
- Class II: modified radical hysterectomy (extended). Unroofing of ureters to resect parametrial and paracervical tissue medial to ureters (cardinal and uterosacral ligaments) and vaginal cuff (1–2 cm).
- Class III: radical abdominal hysterectomy (Wertheim-Meigs). Mobilization of ureters, bladder, and rectum to remove parametrial tissue to pelvic sidewall and vaginal cuff (upper 1/3–1/2) and lymphadenectomy.
- Class IV: extended radical hysterectomy. Removal of superior vesicular artery, part of ureter and bladder and more vaginal cuff.
- Radical vaginal trachelectomy: fertility sparing surgery for select stage IA2 or stage IB1 lesions (≤2 cm diameter) which involves removal of the cervix, upper vagina, and supporting ligaments, but preservation of the uterine corpus. Abdominal radical trachelectomy involves a larger resection of parametria (compared to vaginal) for select stage IB1 cases and used for lesions up to 4 cm in diameter.
- Indications for postoperative RT or chemo-RT:
  - Postoperative pelvic RT: lymphovascular space invasion (LVSI), >1/3 stromal invasion, or >4 cm tumor.
  - Postoperative chemo-RT: +margin, +LN, or parametrial or greater extension.

TREATMENT RECOMMENDATIONS

Table 29.4 **TREATMENT RECOMMENDATIONS**

Stage	Recommended treatment
Preinvasive	Conization or loop electrosurgical excisional procedure (LEEP) or laser or cryotherapy ablation or simple hysterectomy
IA	Total abdominal hysterectomy or trachelectomy or large cone biopsy with negative margins and close follow-up (if fertility preservation desired). Radical hysterectomy preferred for IA2 lesions OR Brachytherapy alone (LDR 65–75 Gy or HDR 7 Gy × 5–6 fx). If HR pathologic features, treat as IB

continued

Table 29.4 (continued)

Stage	Recommended treatment
IB1	Radical hysterectomy with pelvic LN dissection OR Definitive RT: External beam radiation therapy (EBRT) to WP (45 Gy) and brachytherapy (HDR 6 Gy × 5 fx, 7 Gy × 4 fx or LDR 15–20 Gy × 2 fx)
IB2–IIA	Concurrent chemo-RT with cisplatin. WP RT (45 Gy). Brachytherapy = HDR 6 Gy × 5 fx, 7 Gy × 4 fx or LDR 15–20 Gy × 2 fx
IIB	Concurrent chemo-RT with cisplatin. WP RT (45, nodal boost 50–50.4 Gy). Brachytherapy = HDR 6 Gy × 5 fx, 7 Gy × 4 fx or LDR 15–20 Gy × 2 fx
IIIA	Concurrent chemo-RT with cisplatin. RT to WP, vagina, and inguinal LN (45, nodal boost 50–50.4 Gy). Brachytherapy = HDR 6 Gy × 5 fx, 7 Gy × 4 fx or LDR 17–20 Gy × 2 fx
IIIB–IVA	Concurrent chemo-RT with cisplatin. WP RT (45, nodal boost 50–60 Gy). Brachytherapy = HDR 6 Gy × 5, 7 Gy × 4 fx or LDR 20 Gy × 2. If para-aortic LN+, add paraaortic LN IMRT (45–60 Gy)
IVB	Combination chemotherapy

STUDIES

SURGERY VERSUS RADIATION

- Landoni (Lancet 1997): 343 pts with IB–IIA randomized to RT vs. surgery ± RT. Surgery was radical hysterectomy + pelvic LND with optional adjuvant RT to 50.4 Gy for stage > IIA, <3 mm uninvolved cervix, +margin or LN+. 45 Gy given to + PAN. 63% of pts in surgery arm received adjuvant RT, including 83% with tumors >4 cm. RT alone arm was 47 Gy EBRT + LDR 76 Gy point A dose. No significant differences in 5-yr overall survival (OS) (83%), DFS (74%), or recurrence (25%). Morbidity worse with surgery ± RT arm vs. RT alone arm (28% vs. 12%).

EXTENDED-FIELD RT (EFRT)

- *RTOG 79–20* (Rotman, JAMA 1995): 337 pts with IIB without clinical or radiographically involved PAN randomized to WP 45 Gy or EFRT 45 Gy. EFRT improved 10-yr OS (55 vs. 44%), but no difference on LRC (65%) or DM (25–30%). Toxicity increased with EFRT (8 vs. 4%).
- Vargo (IJROBP 2014): retrospective, 61 pts, IBI-IVA, with PET-avid pelvic LNs treated with EF-IMRT (45 Gy/25 fx,

VIII

with concomitant boost to involved nodes to 55 Gy/25 fx) with concurrent cisplatin and HDR brachy. PET/CT at 12–16 wks. Mean f/u 29 mo. Sites of persistent/recurrent disease: cervix (16.3%), regional nodes (4.9%), and distant (23%). PAN failure in pts with pelvic only LN+ was 2.5%. Rate of late grade 3 adverse events was 4%. EF-IMRT was well tolerated with low regional recurrence.

CHEMO-RT

- *RTOG 90–01* (Morris, NEJM 1999; Eifel, JCO 2004): 386 pts with surgically staged IIB–IVA, IB–IIA ≥ 5 cm, or LN + randomized to EFRT + brachy (total 85 Gy point A dose) or to WP RT + brachy (total 85 Gy point A dose) + cisplatin/5FU. Chemo-RT improved 8-yr OS (67 vs. 41%), DFS (61 vs. 46%), and decreased LRF (18 vs. 35%) and DM (20 vs. 35%).

- *GOG 120* (Rose, NEJM 1999, JCO 2007): 526 pts with IIB–IVA (surgically staged PAN) randomized to WP + LDR brachy (total 81 Gy point A dose) + three different chemo regimens: weekly cisplatin vs. cisplatin/5FU/hydroxyurea vs. hydroxyurea alone. Cisplatin arms decreased stage IIB and III 10-yr LR (21–22 vs. 34%) and improved PFS (43–46 vs. 26%), OS (53 vs. 34%). No difference in grade 3–4 late toxicities among the 3 regimens.

- *GOG 85 / SWOG 8695 Intergroup* (Whitney and Sause, JCO 1999): 368 pts, IIB-IVA with negative cytologic washings and PAN randomized to WP RT with concurrent 5-FU + cisplatin vs. WP RT plus oral hydroxyurea (HU). IIB pts received 40.8 Gy/24 fx WP EBRT then 40 Gy IC brachy boost to point A and, if necessary, point B boost to 55 Gy; III-IVA pts received 51 Gy/30 fx EBRT +30 Gy brachy boost, point B 60 Gy. If no implant, then 61.2 Gy EBRT. Grade ≥ 3 toxicities: 4% in 5-FU/cis vs. 24% in HU group. PFS 5-FU/cis 57% vs. HU 47%; OS 5-FU/cis 55% vs. HU 43%. 5-FU/cisplatin greater PFS, OS, and less toxicity than hydroxyurea.

- *GOG 123* (Keys, NEJM 1999; Stehman, Am J Obstet Gynecol 2007): 369 pts with IB2 randomized to WP + LDR RT (total 75 Gy to point A) followed by adjuvant simple hysterectomy vs. same RT + concurrent weekly cisplatin (40 mg/m^2) × 6 cycles followed by same surgery. Chemo-RT improved 5-yr PFS (71 vs. 60%) and OS (78 vs. 64%), without increasing serious late adverse effects.

ˌ *NCIC* (Pearcey, JCO 2002): 353 pts with IA, IIA >5 cm, or IIB randomized to WP45 Gy + LDR 35 Gy × 1 or HDR 8 Gy × 3 vs. same RT + weekly cisplatin 40 mg/m² x 6 cycles. No difference in 5-yr OS (62% vs. 58%).

ˌ *GOG 165* (Lanciano, JCO 2005): 316 pts with IIB, IIIB, and IVA randomized to WP 45 Gy + parametrial boost + IC brachytherapy with standard weekly cisplatin (40 mg/m²) vs. same RT with 6 cycles protracted venous infusion (PVI) 5-FU. Study closed prematurely when planned interim analysis demonstrated a 35% higher distant failure rate with RT + PVI 5-FU.

ˌ *B9E-MC-JHQS* (Duenas-Gonzalez, JCO 2011): 515 pts with IIB-IVA randomized to arm A (cisplatin and gemcitabine weekly x 6 wks with concurrent EBRT (50.4 Gy/28 fx) followed by brachy (30 to 35 Gy in 96 h), and then 2 adjuvant cycles cisplatin + gemcitabine) or to arm B (cisplatin chemo-RT followed by brachy only; dosing same as for arm A). 3-yr PFS better in arm A vs. arm B (74.4% vs. 65.0%) and overall PFS and OS. Grade ≥ 3 toxicities greater in arm A vs. arm B (86.5% vs. 46.3%), with two deaths related to study treatment in arm A. Readers encouraged to review accompanying editorial with this publication.

ˌ *Korea Cancer Center Hospital* (Ryu, IJROBP 2011): 104 pts with IIB–IVA randomized to weekly cisplatin (40 mg/m² × 6 cycles) or triweekly cisplatin (cisplatin 75 mg/m² q3 wks × 3 cycles). All pts got concurrent EBRT and IC brachy. Less grade 3–4 neutropenia in triweekly arm vs. weekly arm (22.6% vs. 39.2%). Higher 5-yr OS in triweekly arm (88.7% vs. 66.5%).

ˌ *NRG/GOG Nomograms* (Rose, JCO 2015). 2,042 pts with locally advanced cervical cancer treated with cisplatin-based chemo-RT. Nomograms generated to predict 2-yr PFS, 5-yr OS, and pelvic recurrence.

VIII

ADJUVANT HYSTERECTOMY AFTER RT

ˌ *GOG 71* (Keys, Gynecol Oncol 2003): 256 pts with ≥4 cm tumors randomized to EBRT + brachy (80 Gy point A dose) vs. same RT (except 75 Gy point A dose) followed by extrafascial hysterectomy. No difference in OS (61 vs. 64%), but trend for higher LR without surgery (26 vs. 14%, p = 0.08).

POST-OP RT

- *GOG 92 / RTOG 87–06* (Sedlis, Gynecol Onc 1999; Rotman, IJROBP 2006): 277 pts with bulky IB treated with radical hysterectomy with negative margins and LNs, but with ≥2 risk factors (LVSI, >1/3 stromal invasion, or ≥4 cm tumors) randomized to observation vs. post-op WP RT (46–50.4 Gy). Median f/u 9.6 yrs. No difference in OS. Trend toward 5-yr PFS 53% (RT) vs. 62% (RT + surgery) (p = 0.09). No difference in severe toxicity.

POST-OP CHEMO-RT

- *GOG 109/SWOG 8797/RTOG 91–12* (Peters, JCO 2000; Monk, Gynecol Onc 2005): 243 pts s/p radical hysterectomy with IA2, IB, IIA, and + LN or + margin or + parametrium randomized to WP RT (49.3 Gy with 45 Gy to PAN if common iliac LN+) vs. WP RT + cisplatin/5FU q3 wks x 4 cycles. Post-op chemo-RT improved 4-yr PFS (80% vs. 63%) and OS (81% vs. 71%) [30]. Unplanned exploratory analysis showed that the absolute improvement on 5-yr survival for adjuvant chemo-RT (vs. RT alone) was 5% in pts with tumors ≤2 cm (82% vs. 77%), 19% in tumors >2 cm (77% vs. 58%), 4% in pts with one LN+ (83% vs. 79%) and 20% in pts with ≥2 LN+ (75% vs. 55%).

BRACHYTHERAPY

- Several retrospective and population-based studies report better LC and survival with EBRT + brachy boost vs. EBRT alone.
- *French STIC study* (Charra-Brunaud, Radiother Oncol 2012): Prospective study demonstrated that image-guided three-dimensional (3D) brachy dosimetry improved LC with half the toxicity observed with conventional 2D dosimetry.

⌖ *National Cancer database* (Gil, IJROBP 2014): 7,654 pts, stage IIB-IVA in the NCDB. 90.3% received brachy. From 2004 to 2011, brachy use decreased from 96.7% to 86.1%, and IMRT and SBRT use increased from 3.3% to 13.9% in the same period. IMRT or SBRT boost resulted in inferior OS vs. brachy boost.

⌖ American Brachytherapy Society (ABS) review (Mayadev, Brachy 2017). Literature review of cervix HDR brachy. Pts treated with chemo-RT and image-based HDR brachy technique had improved pelvic control and DFS compared to pts treated to traditional Point A dose specification.

RADIATION TECHNIQUES

EBRT SIMULATION AND FIELD DESIGN

⌖ Consider placing radiopaque marker(s) in cervix or at distal margin of any vaginal disease.

⌖ There is no standard pelvic EBRT field. Blocking should be individualized based on 3D imaging when treating with four field technique.

⌖ Simulate patient supine with CT planning. Borders: superior = L4/5; inferior = 3 cm below most inferior vaginal involvement as marked by seeds (often at inferior obturator foramen); lateral = 2 cm lateral to pelvic brim; posterior = include entire sacrum and cover the parametrial tissue lateral to the rectum; anterior = splitting the pubic symphysis.

⌖ Treat inguinal nodes if stage IIIA (lower 1/3 vagina). Inferior border should flash the perineum.

⌖ If common iliac nodes involved, raise superior border to allow for at least a 4 cm margin (~L3/4 level).

⌖ EFRT for para-aortic nodes: superior border = T12/L1, lateral = encompass tips of transverse processes. Block kidneys as determined by CT planning. Use IMRT to minimize dose to kidneys and small bowel. Use IMRT contouring atlas for IMRT CTV.

⌖ When used, midline block reduces dose to bladder and rectum, but may underdose sacrum. Since T&O has 100% dose through point A, which is ~2 cm from midline, a 4 cm midline block would be at the 100% IDL. Superior border of midline block = midsacroiliac

VIII

joint. If concerned about toxicity, use a wider midline block (6 cm, ~50% IDL), or if concerned about tumor dose, use a narrower block. Midline blocks narrower than 5 cm may include the ureters which are ~2–2.5 cm from midline.

- At some institutions, it is preferred to deliver higher EBRT doses with a midline block for advanced lesions. After 45 Gy to the WP, the superior border may be lowered to the midsacroiliac joint and EBRT continued to 50 Gy. At 50 Gy, the superior border is further lowered to the bottom of the sacroiliac joint and treated to 54 Gy. If parametrial tumor persists after 50–54 Gy, it may boost parametria to 60 Gy.
- IMRT is encouraged to treat involved nodes and/or for EFRT with chemotherapy to boost to higher dose to 54–60 Gy.
- IMRT contouring guidelines for intact cervix (Lim, IJROBP 2011):
  - GTV = entire GTV; intermediate/high signal seen on T2-weighted MRI.
  - CTV includes:
    - GTV.
    - Entire cervix (if not already encompassed by the GTV).
    - Entire uterus.
    - Entire parametria (including ovaries and include entire mesorectum if uterosacral ligament is involved). Anterior border = posterior wall of bladder or posterior border of external iliac vessel. Posterior border = uterosacral ligaments and mesorectal fascia. Lateral border = medial edge of internal obturator muscle/ischial ramus bilaterally. Superior border = top of fallopian tube/ broad ligament; depending on degree of uterus flexion, this may also form the anterior boundary of parametrial tissue. Inferior border = urogenital diaphragm.
    - Vagina: if minimal or no vaginal extension, include upper 1/2 of the vagina; if upper vaginal involved, include upper 2/3 of the vagina; if extensive vaginal involvement, include entire vagina.

, Nodal CTV: involved nodes and relevant draining nodal groups (common, internal, and external iliac and obturator and presacral LNs). Inclusion of PANs depends on the extent of disease and staging.

, PTV margin: Add 1.5 to 2 cm on primary CTV and 0.7 cm on nodal CTV.

, Use of generous margins is encouraged to compensate for internal target motion. Consider target movement due to bladder and rectal filling.

BRACHYTHERAPY

, See ABS cervix LDR and HDR guidelines (Viswanathan, Brachytherapy 2012; Viswanathan, Brachytherapy 2012; Lee, Brachytherapy 2012; Suneja, Brachytherapy 2017).

, First intracavitary application should be performed within 4–6 weeks of the initiation of EBRT. The second application should be performed 1–2 weeks later to complete all therapy within 8 weeks.

, Tandem and ovoid or tandem and ring applicators may be used with or without interstitial catheters. Optimal positioning is essential for best dose distribution.

, LDR uses manual after loading Cs-137. PDR uses remote after loading Ir-192 with source strength ~4 kU (1 Ci) [vs ~42 kU (10 Ci) as in HDR]. Dose rate with LDR and PDR is about 0.4–0.6 Gy/h.

, ABS endorses GEC-ESTRO guidelines for contouring, image-based treatment planning, and dose reporting (Haie-Meder, Radiother Oncol 2005; Pötter, Radiother Oncol 2006).

GTV-D = GTV at diagnosis.

GTV-B = GTV at at time of brachy.

HR-CTV-B = HR-CTV includes GTV-B, entire cervix, and presumed extracervical tumor extension at time of brachy (taking into account disease extent at diagnosis and suspected pathological residual tissue defined by clinical exam and MRI findings).

IR-CTV = Intermediate-risk CTV includes 5–15 mm around HR-CTV as indicated to cover initial macroscopic extent of disease with concern for at most residual microscopic disease.

VIII

HDR BRACHYTHERAPY TECHNIQUE AT UCSF

- Unless greater tumor shrinkage is needed, the first implant can occur after 20 Gy EBRT and the second implant 1–2 weeks later (e.g. 7 Gy × 4 fx over 2 implants).
- If small lesion and narrow vagina, treat first with IC brachytherapy before EBRT, which can cause vaginal narrowing.
- If large lesion and narrow vagina, use EBRT first to shrink the tumor.
- An MRI with T2-weighted images should be obtained ~1 week prior to brachy to determine the extent of residual disease and to help guide applicator selection.
- Placement of tandem, applicator, and interstitial catheters are performed in the OR. After induction of sedation or anesthesia, the patient is placed in dorsal lithotomy position and an EUA using TRUS is performed to visualize tumor extent. The patient's perineum is prepped and draped in a sterile fashion.
- Using a speculum, a countertraction suture is always placed on the cervix or on the left and right upper lateral vaginal walls. The suture is used to secure the tandem to the uterus.
- A Foley catheter is placed and the balloon is inflated with 7 cc of diluted contrast (1:10) and the bladder is filled with 200 cc of saline. The Foley is plugged to keep the bladder full to decrease the anteversion of the uterus to improve TRUS imaging.
- The cervix is then sounded with TRUS guidance. The cervical os is dilated using Hanks/Hegar dilators of progressively larger sizes.
- An intrauterine tandem is custom bent to fit the curvature and length of the uterine canal. Once the cervical os is dilated to at least 6 mm in diameter, the tandem is inserted into the uterine canal. TRUS is used to verify the placement of the tandem in the uterus. Tandem length is ~6–8 cm (~4 cm for postmenopausal women).
- A minimum of 2, 30-cm Flexi-Guide interstitial catheters are inserted transvaginally into the vagina at the 3 o'clock and 9 o'clock positions and advanced superiorly into the cervix under TRUS guidance (freehand), keeping parallel to the tandem and keeping the tips of the catheters inside the uterus. Additional interstitial catheters can be added to improve coverage if needed.

, The tandem and catheters are then passed through the center of a ring applicator. The ring and tandem are secured using the counter traction suture(s) placed previously.

, For cervical tumors with extensive vaginal extension, a tandem and cylinder applicator is used in addition to the TRUS-guided interstitial catheters.

   , A vaginal cylinder applicator is introduced into the vagina without dislodging the interstitial catheters and placed flush against the vagina apex.

   , Additional Flex-Guide vaginal surface catheters are inserted along the grooves on the surface of the cylinder and secured using a rubber O-ring; these catheters remain on the surface of the cylinder and do not enter the cervix.

   , The cylinder is then secured to the vaginal using the two counter traction sutures placed previously.

, Vaginal packing imbedded with radiopaque wire and lubricated with K-Y jelly is used to stabilize the implant apparatus and to minimize bladder neck, urethral and vaginal mucosa doses (anterior vagina packing), and rectal dose (posterior vagina packing).

, The position of friction collars on the Flexi-Guide catheters are adjusted so dental putty can be applied around them to secure them together to the tandem and ring (or to the tandem and cylinder).

, The patient is then transferred to the recovery room before HDR treatment.

, After recovery, a pelvic noncontrast CT scan is obtained for treatment planning.

, Target volumes and organs at risk (OARs) (bladder, bowel, vagina, rectum) are contoured:

   , HR-CTV encompasses the cervix and any residual tumor extension into the parametrium, vagina, or uterus at the time of brachy.

   , At UCSF, all treatment optimization are done by Inverse Planning Simulated Annealing (IPSA). Dose is optimized to HR-CTV.

   , Intermediate-risk CTV is the disease extent at diagnosis. IR-CTV is not used for prescribing dose at UCSF.

   , IR-CTV = HR-CTV plus 1–1.5 cm margin, but not into bladder or bowel.

VIII

- After contouring and optimization using IPSA, the HR-CTV V100 is usually 85–95%. V75 of OARs is almost always < 1 cc.
- HDR brachy uses a high-activity Ir-192 (<10 Ci) source with dose rate ~ 12 Gy/h.
- Image-guided brachy requires modification of dwell time based on 3D images. Treatment delivery is accomplished by HDR afterloaders.
- No chemotherapy or EBRT is administered on HDR treatment days.
- Overall treatment, including EBRT and brachy, should be completed within 8 weeks from initiation of treatment.

DOSE PRESCRIPTIONS

- EBRT: 1.8 Gy/fx with concurrent cisplatin-based chemotherapy
  - Whole pelvis = 45 Gy
  - Sidewall boost cumulative doses: IB–IIA = 45–50 Gy, IIB = 45–54 Gy, III–IVA = 54–60 Gy
  - Persistent or bulky parametrial tumor = 60 Gy
  - Para-aortic Elective PANs (if treated) = 45 Gy
  - Bulky LN = 54–60 Gy
  - Post-op = 45–50.4 Gy covering upper 3–4 cm of vaginal cuff, parametria, and pelvic nodes
- At UCSF, simultaneously integrated boost (SIB) IMRT is used for involved LNs to reduce overall treatment duration:
  - PTV nodes: 45 Gy/25 fx
  - SIB to CTV nodes: 50 Gy/25 fx (cumulative)
  - SIB to the GTV nodes: 54 Gy/25 fx (cumulative)
- Brachy boost to HR-CTV
  - Cumulative dose 80–90 Gy is recommended; 85–90 Gy for nonresponders or for tumors >4 cm at the time of brachy
  - LDR = 35–45 Gy at dose rate of 0.4–0.6 Gy/h
  - HDR = 7 Gy x 4 fx over 2 implants (UCSF) or 6 Gy x 5 fx

DOSE LIMITATIONS

- HDR: D2cc to the sigmoid <75 Gy, D2cc to the rectum <75 Gy, D2cc <90 Gy to the bladder (MRI/CT based planning).
- Ovarian failure with 5–10 Gy and sterilization with 2–3 Gy.

- Limit upper vaginal mucosa <120 Gy, midvaginal mucosa <80–90 Gy, and lower vaginal mucosa <60–70 Gy. Vaginal doses >50–60 Gy cause significant fibrosis and stenosis.
- Limit uterus <100 Gy, ureters <75 Gy.
- Femoral heads: max dose <52 Gy, V35 <10%.
- Rectum: V40 <40–60%, V50 <50%, V60 <35%, V65 <25%.
- Bladder: V40 <40–60%, V45 <35%, V65 <50%.
- Bowel bag: V40 <30%. Small bowel: V35 <35%; max pt. dose <56 Gy; V45 <195 cc.
- Bone marrow: V20 <75%, V10 <90%, V40 <37%.
- Bilateral kidneys: V16 <25%; mean total kidney <15 Gy.
- Liver: mean dose <30 Gy.

COMPLICATIONS

- Acute: pruritus, dry/moist desquamation, nausea, colitis, cystitis and vaginitis
- HDR and LDR morbidity are equivalent: uterine perforation (<3%), vaginal laceration (<1%), deep vein thrombosis (<1%).
- Late: vaginal stenosis, ureteral stricture (1–3%), vesicovaginal or rectovaginal fistula (<2%), intestinal obstruction or perforation (<5%), and femoral neck fracture (<5%).
- Recommend vaginal dilation as needed to maintain vaginal vault size and sexual function.
- Standard post-op complications. Surgical mortality is 1%.

VIII

FOLLOW-UP

- See NCCN guidelines.
- H&P every 3–6 mo for 2 yrs, then every 6–12 mos for 3–5 yrs, then annually based on the risk of disease recurrence.
- Cervical/vaginal cytology annually as indicated for detection of lower genital tract lesions.
- Imaging (chest X-ray, CT, PET-CT, and MRI) and labs as indicated based on exam, symptoms and risk of recurrence.
- Patient education on sexual health, vaginal dilator use, and vaginal lubricants.

Acknowledgment We thank R. Scott Bermudez MD and Kim Huang MD for their work on the prior edition of this chapter.

REFERENCES

Charra-Brunaud C, Harter V, Delannes M, et al. Impact of 3D image-based PDR brachytherapy on outcome of pts treated for cervix carcinoma in France: results of the French STIC prospective study. Radiother Oncol. 2012;103(3):305–13.

Dueñas-González A, Zarbá JJ, Patel F, et al. Phase III, open-label, randomized study comparing concurrent gemcitabine plus cisplatin and radiation followed by adjuvant gemcitabine and cisplatin versus concurrent cisplatin and radiation in patients with stage IIB to IVA carcinoma of the cervix. J Clin Oncol. 2011;29(13):1678–85.

Edge S, Byrd DR, Compton CC, Fritz AG, Greene FL, Trotti A. AJCC cancer staging handbook. New York: Springer; 2011.

Eifel PJ, Winter K, Morris M, et al. Pelvic irradiation with concurrent chemotherapy versus pelvic and para-aortic irradiation for high-risk cervical cancer: an update of radiation therapy oncology group trial (RTOG) 90-01. J Clin Oncol. 2004;22:872–80.

Garland SM, Steben M, Sings HL, et al. Natural history of genital warts: analysis of the placebo arm of 2 randomized phase III trials of a quadrivalent human papillomavirus (types 6, 11, 16, and 18) vaccine. J Infect Dis. 2009;199(6):805–14.

Gill BS, Lin JF, Krivak TC, et al. National Cancer Data Base analysis of radiation therapy consolidation modality for cervical cancer: the impact of new technological advancements. Int J Radiat Oncol Biol Phys. 2014;90(5):1083–90.

Haie-Meder C, Pötter R, Van Limbergen E, et al. Recommendations from Gynaecological (GYN) GEC-ESTRO Working Group (I): concepts and terms in 3D image based 3D treatment planning in cervix cancer brachytherapy with emphasis on MRI assessment of GTV and CTV. Radiother Oncol. 2005;74(3):235–45.

Han K, Milosevic M, Fyles A, Pintilie M, Viswanathan AN. Trends in the utilization of brachytherapy in cervical cancer in the United States. Int J Radiat Oncol Biol Phys. 2013;87(1):111–9.

Hanks GE, Herring DF, Kramer S. Patterns of care outcome studies. Results of the national practice in cancer of the cervix. Cancer. 1983;51(5):959–67.

Hsu IJ, Swift PS. Cancer of the uterine cervix. In: Leibel SA, Phillips TL, editors. Textbook of radiation oncology. 3rd ed. Philadelphia: Saunders; 2010. p. 1002–25.

Keys HM, Bundy BN, Stehman FB, et al. Cisplatin, radiation, and adjuvant hysterectomy compared with radiation and adjuvant hysterectomy for bulky stage IB cervical carcinoma. N Engl J Med. 1999;340:1154–61.

Keys HM, Bundy BN, Stehman FB, et al. Radiation therapy with and without extrafascial hysterectomy for bulky stage IB cervical carcinoma: a randomized trial of the gynecologic oncology group. Gynecol Oncol. 2003;89:343–53.

Lanciano RM, Martz K, Coia LR, Hanks GE. Tumor and treatment factors improving outcome in stage III-B cervix cancer. Radiat Oncol Biol. 1991;20(1):95–100.

Lanciano R, Calkins A, Bundy BN, et al. Randomized comparison of weekly cisplatin or protracted venous infusion of fluorouracil in combination with pelvic radiation in advanced cervix cancer: a gynecologic oncology group study. J Clin Oncol. 2005;23:8289–95.

Landoni F, Maneo A, Colombo A, et al. Randomised study of radical surgery versus radiotherapy for stage Ib-IIa cervical cancer. Lancet. 1997;350:535–40.

Lee LJ, Das IJ, Higgins SA, et al. American Brachytherapy Society consensus guidelines for locally advanced carcinoma of the cervix. Part III: low-dose-rate and pulsed-dose-rate brachytherapy. Brachytherapy. 2012;11:53–7.

Lim K, Small W Jr, Portelance L, et al. Consensus guidelines for delineation of clinical target volume for intensity-modulated pelvic radiotherapy for the definitive treatment of cervix cancer. Int J Radiat Oncol Biol Phys. 2011;79:348–55.

Logsdon MD, Eifel PJ. Figo IIIB squamous cell carcinoma of the cervix: an analysis of prognostic factors emphasizing the balance between external beam and intracavitary radiation therapy. Radiat Oncol Biol. 1999;43(4):763–75.

Mayadev J, Viswanathan A, Liu Y, et al. American Brachytherapy Task Group Report: a pooled analysis of clinical outcomes for high-dose-rate brachytherapy for cervical cancer. Brachytherapy. 2017;16:22–43.

Monk BJ, Wang J, Im S, et al. Rethinking the use of radiation and chemotherapy after radical hysterectomy: a clinical-pathologic analysis of a Gynecologic Oncology Group/Southwest Oncology Group/Radiation Therapy Oncology Group trial. Gynecol Oncol. 2005;96(3):721–8.

Montana GS, Fowler WC, Varia MA, Walton LA, Mack Y, Shemanski L. Carcinoma of the cervix, stage III. Results of radiation therapy. Cancer. 1986;57(1):148–54.

Morris M, Eifel PJ, Lu J, et al. Pelvic radiation with concurrent chemotherapy compared with pelvic and para-aortic radiation for high-risk cervical cancer. N Engl J Med. 1999;340:1137–43.

National Cancer Institute Surveillance. Epidemiology, and End Results Program (SEER). 2016. http://seer.cancer.gov/statfacts/html/corp.html. Accessed 22 Aug 2016.

National Comprehensive Cancer Network. Clinical Practice Guidelines in Oncology: Cervical Cancer (Version 1.2016). 2016. https://www.nccn.org/professionals/physician_gls/pdf/cervical.pdf. Accessed 27 Aug 2016.

PDQ Screening and Prevention Editorial Board. Cervical Cancer Screening (PDQ®): Health Professional Version. 4 Mar 2016.

Pearcey R, Brundage M, Drouin P, et al. Phase III trial comparing radical radiotherapy with and without cisplatin chemotherapy in pts with advanced squamous cell cancer of the cervix. J Clin Oncol. 2002;20:966–72.

Peters WA III, Liu PY, Barrett RJ II, et al. Concurrent chemotherapy and pelvic radiation therapy compared with pelvic radiation therapy alone as adjuvant therapy after radical surgery in high-risk early-stage cancer of the cervix. J Clin Oncol. 2000;18:1606–13.

Pötter R, Haie-Meder C, Van Limbergen E, et al. Recommendations from gynaecological (GYN) GEC ESTRO working group (II): concepts and terms in 3D image-based treatment planning in cervix cancer brachytherapy-3D dose volume parameters and aspects of 3D image-based anatomy, radiation physics, radiobiology. Radiother Oncol. 2006;78(1):67–77.

Rose PG, Bundy BN, Watkins EB, et al. Concurrent cisplatin-based radiotherapy and chemotherapy for locally advanced cervical cancer. N Engl J Med. 1999;340:1144–53.

Rose PG, Ali S, Watkins E, et al. Long-term follow-up of a randomized trial comparing concurrent single agent cisplatin, cisplatin-based combination chemotherapy, or hydroxyurea during pelvic irradiation for locally advanced cervical cancer: a gynecologic oncology group study. J Clin Oncol. 2007;25:2804–10.

Rose PG, Java J, Whitney CW, et al. Nomograms Predicting Progression-Free Survival, Overall Survival, and Pelvic Recurrence in Locally Advanced Cervical Cancer Developed From an Analysis of Identifiable Prognostic Factorsin Patients From NRG Oncology/Gynecologic Oncology Group Randomized Trials of Chemoradiotherapy. J Clin Oncol. 2015;33:2136–42.

Rotman M, Pajak TF, Choi K, et al. Prophylactic extended-field irradiation of para-aortic lymph nodes in stages IIB and bulky IB and IIA cervical carcinomas. Ten-yr treatment results of RTOG 79-20. JAMA. 1995;274:387–93.

Rotman M, Sedlis A, Piedmonte MR, et al. A phase III randomized trial of postoperative pelvic irradiation in stage IB cervical carcinoma with poor prognostic features: follow-up of a gynecologic oncology group study. Int J Radiat Oncol Biol Phys. 2006;65:169–76.

Ryu S-Y, Lee W-M, Kim K, et al. Randomized clinical trial of weekly vs. triweekly cisplatin-based chemotherapy concurrent with radiotherapy in the treatment of locally advanced cervical cancer. Int J Radiat Oncol Biol Phys. 2011;81(4):e577–81.

Sedlis A, Bundy BN, Rotman MZ, et al. A randomized trial of pelvic radiation therapy versus no further therapy in selected pts with stage IB carcinoma of the cervix after radical hysterectomy and pelvic lymphadenectomy: a gynecologic oncology group study. Gynecol Oncol. 1999;73:177–83.

SEER Cancer Statistics Review, 1975–2012. National Cancer Institute. 2016. http://seer.cancer.gov/archive/csr/1975_2012/results_merged/sect_05_cervix_uteri.pdf. Accessed 26 Aug 2016.

VIII

Serrano B, Alemany L, Tous S, et al. Potential impact of a nine-valent vaccine in human papillomavirus related cervical disease. Infect Agent Cancer. 2012;7(1):38.

Stehman FB, Ali S, Keys HM, et al. Radiation therapy with or without weekly cisplatin for bulky stage 1B cervical carcinoma: follow-up of a gynecologic oncology group trial. Am J Obstet Gynecol. 2007;197(5):503.e1–6.

Suneja G, Brown D, Chang A, et al. American Brachytherapy Society: brachytherapy treatment recommendations for locally advanced cervix cancer for low-income and middle-income countries. Brachytherapy. 2017;16:85–94.

The American Cancer Society guidelines for the prevention and early detection of cervical cancer. 2016. http://www.cancer.org/cancer/cervicalcancer/moreinformation/cervical-cancerpreventionandearlydetection/cervical-cancer-prevention-and-early-detection-cervical-cancer-screening-guidelines. Accessed 26 Aug 2016.

Vargo JA, Kim H, CHOI S, et al. Extended field intensity modulated radiation therapy with concomitant boost for lymph node-positive cervical cancer: analysis of regional control and recurrence patterns in the positron emission tomography/computed tomography era. Int J Radiat Oncol Biol Phys. 2014;90(5):1091–8.

Viswanathan AN and Thomadsen B. American Brachytherapy Society consensus guidelines for locally advanced carcinoma of the cervix. Part I: general principles. Brachytherapy. 2012;11:33–46.

Viswanathan AN, Beriwal S, De Los Santos JF, et al. American Brachytherapy Society consensus guidelines for locally advanced carcinoma of the cervix. Part II: high-dose-rate brachytherapy. Brachytherapy. 2012;11:47–52.

Viswanathan AN. Uterine cervix. In: Halperin CE, Wazer DE, Perez CA, Brady LW, editors. Principles and practice of radiation oncology. 6th ed. Philadelphia: Lippincott Williams & Wilkins; 2013. p. 1355–425.

Viswanathan AN, Erickson B, Gaffney DK, et al. Comparison and consensus guidelines for delineation of clinical target volume for CT- and MR-based brachytherapy in locally advanced cervical cancer. Int J Radiat Oncol Biol Phys. 2014;90(2):320–8.

Viswanathan AN, Dizon DS, Gien LT, Koh W. Cervical cancer. In: Gunderson LL, Tepper JE, editors. Clinical radiation oncology. 4th ed. Philadelphia: Churchill Livingstone; 2015. p. 1173–1202.e6.

Wang C-C, Lai C-H, Huang Y-T, Chao A, Chou H-H, Hong J-H. HPV genotypes predict survival benefits from concurrent chemotherapy and radiation therapy in advanced squamous cell carcinoma of the cervix. Int J Radiat Oncol Biol Phys. 2012;84(4):e499–506.

Whitney CW, Sause W. Randomized comparison of fluorouracil plus Cisplatin versus Hydroxyurea as an adjunct to radiation therapy in stage IIB-IVA carcinoma of the cervix with negative para-aortic lymph nodes: a gynecologic oncology group and southwest oncology group study. 1999:1137-1143. J Clin Oncol. 1999;17(5):1339–48.

Chapter 30
Endometrial Cancer

Serah Choi and I-Chow J. Hsu

PEARLS

- 60,050 estimated new cases and 10,470 deaths in 2016.
- Most common gynecological cancer in the USA; fourth most common malignancy in women after breast, lung, and colorectal.
- Patients can present with abnormal uterine bleeding (~90% cases, early stage), nonbloody vaginal discharge (~10%), pelvic pain, and/or palpable pelvic mass.
- Risk factors: unopposed estrogen, postmenopausal (median age at diagnosis is 61), nulliparity, early menarche, late menopause, obesity, tamoxifen (7.5×), oral contraceptives use.
- Patients with Lynch Syndrome (HPNCC) have 16–54% cumulative risk of endometrial cancer by age 70 (Bonadona, 2011).
- Grade is determined by percentage of dedifferentiated solid growth pattern. Grade 1: ≤5%, Grade 2: 5–50%, Grade 3: >50%.
- 75–80% of tumors are endometrioid endometrial adenocarcinomas that arise from endometrial hyperplasia.
- Rate of progression to invasive cancer from simple hyperplasia is rare (<2%) with progression to carcinoma in patients with simple and complex hyperplasia, with atypia being more common (30–40%).
- 20% of endometrial carcinomas are nonendometrioid, including papillary serous (UPSC), clear cell, and mucinous.

VIII

© Springer International Publishing AG, part of Springer Nature 2018   **653**
Eric K. Hansen and M. Roach III (eds.), *Handbook of Evidence-Based Radiation Oncology*, https://doi.org/10.1007/978-3-319-62642-0_30

- Up to 5% of uterine cancers are sarcomas, including carcinosarcoma (most common), leiomyosarcoma, and endometrial stromal sarcomas.
- Type 1: estrogen related, endometrioid histology, associated with prolonged unopposed estrogen and have better prognosis (Bokhman, 1983).
- Type 2: more often nonendometrioid (serous, clear cell, and carcinosarcomas), not stimulated by estrogen, arise from atrophic endometrium or from an endometrial polyp in older pts., not associated with obesity, worse prognosis (Brinton, 2013).
- TCGA identified four genomic subgroups: *POLE*-mutant tumors (ultrahypermutated), which have significantly better PFS; MSI (hypermutated) and copy-number low (endometrioid), which have relatively intermediate PFS; copy-number high tumors (serous-like), which have the poorest outcomes (Cancer Genome Atlas Research Network, 2013).
- Prognostic factors: stage, cell type, grade, LVSI, depth of invasion, cervical extension, and age.
- Primary lymphatic drainage of the uterine body is to pelvic LN (internal and external iliac, obturator, common iliac, presacral, parametrial); direct spread may occur to paraaortic LN. There are few lymphatics in endometrium, but myometrium and subserosa have a rich lymphatic network.
- ~1/3 of patients with + pelvic LN have + paraaortic LN.

WORKUP

- H&P with attention to uterine size, cervical and vaginal involvement, ascites, nodes.
- Labs: CBC, blood chemistries, LFTs, CA-125 (elevated in 60%), UA.
- Endometrial biopsy is diagnostic gold standard with >90% sensitivity and 85% specificity, thereby largely obviating need for D&C.
- D&C if endometrial biopsy is nondiagnostic.
- Pap smear has limited sensitivity (as low as 40%).
- Imaging: CXR, CT, or MRI of abdomen and pelvis or transvaginal ultrasound to evaluate symptomatic disease.
- Cystoscopy and/or sigmoidoscopy as clinically indicated.

STAGING (AJCC 7TH ED., 2010/ FIGO 2008)

Editors' note: All TNM stage and stage groups referred to elsewhere in this chapter reflect the 7th Ed AJCC staging nomenclature unless otherwise noted, as the new system was published after this chapter was written.

Table 30.1 Uterine carcinomas

Primary tumor (T) (surgical–pathologic findings)		
TNM categories	*FIGO stages*	
TX		Primary tumor cannot be assessed
T0		No evidence of primary tumor
Tis*		Carcinoma in situ (preinvasive carcinoma)
T1	I	Tumor confined to corpus uteri
T1a	IA	Tumor limited to endometrium or invades less than one-half of the myometrium
T1b	IB	Tumor invades one-half or more of the myometrium
T2	II	Tumor invades stromal connective tissue of the cervix, but does not extend beyond uterus**
T3a	IIIA	Tumor involves serosa and/or adnexa (direct extension or metastasis)
T3b	IIIB	Vaginal involvement (direct extension or metastasis) or parametrial involvement
T4	IVA	Tumor invades bladder mucosa and/or bowel mucosa (bullous edema is not sufficient to classify a tumor as T4)

Note: FIGO no longer includes Stage 0 (Tis)
*Endocervical glandular involvement only should be considered Stage I and not Stage II

Regional lymph nodes (N)		
TNM categories	*FIGO stages*	
NX		Regional lymph nodes cannot be assessed
N0		No regional lymph node metastasis
N1	IIIC1	Regional lymph node metastasis to pelvic lymph nodes
N2	IIIC2	Regional lymph node metastasis to paraaortic lymph nodes, with or without positive pelvic lymph nodes

continued

Table 30.1 (continued)

Distant metastasis (M)		
TNM categories	*FIGO stages*	
M0		No distant metastasis
M1	IVB	Distant metastasis (includes metastasis to inguinal lymph nodes intraperitoneal disease, or lung, liver, or bone. Excludes metastasis to paraaortic lymph nodes, vagina, pelvic serosa, or adnexa)

Anatomic stage/prognostic groups

Carcinomas[*]

0[**]:	Tis N0 M0
I:	T1 N0 M0
IA:	T1a N0 M0
IB:	T1b N0 M0
II:	T2 N0 M0
III:	T3 N0 M0
IIIA:	T3a N0 M0
IIIB:	T3b N0 M0
IIIC1:	T1-T3 N1 M0
IIIC2:	T1-T3 N2 M0
IVA:	T4 any N M0
IVB:	any T any N M1

[*]Carcinosarcomas should be staged as carcinoma
[**]*Note*: FIGO no longer includes Stage 0 (Tis)
Used with permission from the American Joint Committee on Cancer (AJCC), Chicago, Illinois. The original source for this material is the AJCC Cancer Staging Manual, Seventh Edition (2010), published by Springer Science + Business Media

Table 30.2 Leiomyosarcoma, endometrial stromal sarcoma

Primary tumor (T)		
TNM categories	*FIGO stages*	
TX		Primary tumor cannot be assessed
T0		No evidence of primary tumor
T1	I	Tumor limited to the uterus
T1a	IA	Tumor 5 cm or less in greatest dimension
T1b	IB	Tumor more than 5 cm
T2	II	Tumor extends beyond the uterus, within the pelvis
T2a	IIA	Tumor involves adnexa
T2b	IIB	Tumor involves other pelvic tissues
T3	III[*]	Tumor infiltrates abdominal tissues
T3a	IIIA	One site
T3b	IIIB	More than one site
T4	IVA	Tumor invades bladder or rectum

Note: Simultaneous tumors of the uterine corpus and ovary/pelvis in association with ovarian/pelvic endometriosis should be classified as independent primary tumors
[*]Lesions must infiltrate abdominal tissues and not just protrude into the abdominal cavity

Table 30.2 (continued)

Regional lymph nodes (N)		
TNM Categories	*FIGO Stages*	
NX		Regional lymph nodes cannot be assessed
N0		No regional lymph node metastasis
N1	IIIC	Regional lymph node metastasis

Distant metastasis (M)		
TNM categories	*FIGO stages*	
M0		No distant metastasis
M1	IVB	Distant metastasis (excluding adnexa, pelvic, and abdominal tissues)

Used with permission from the American Joint Committee on Cancer (AJCC), Chicago, Illinois. The original source for this material is the AJCC Cancer Staging Manual, Seventh Edition (2010), published by Springer Science + Business Media

Table 30.3 Adenosarcoma

Primary tumor (T)		
TNM Categories	*FIGO Stages*	
TX		Primary tumor cannot be assessed
T0		No evidence of primary tumor
T1	I	Tumor limited to the uterus
T1a	IA	Tumor limited to the endometrium/endocervix
T1b	IB	Tumor invades to less than half of the myometrium
T1c	IC	Tumor invades more than half of the myometrium
T2	II	Tumor extends beyond the uterus, within the pelvis
T2a	IIA	Tumor involves adnexa
T2b	IIB	Tumor involves other pelvic tissues
T3	III*	Tumor involves abdominal tissues
T3a	IIIA	One site
T3b	IIIB	More than one site
T4	IVA	Tumor invades bladder or rectum

Note: Simultaneous tumors of the uterine corpus and ovary/pelvis in association with ovarian/pelvic endometriosis should be classified as independent primary tumors
*In this stage, lesions must infiltrate abdominal tissues and not just protrude into the abdominal cavity

Table 30.3 (continued)

Regional lymph nodes (N)		
TNM Categories	*FIGO Stages*	
NX		Regional lymph nodes cannot be assessed
N0		No regional lymph node metastasis
N1	IIIC	Regional lymph node metastasis

Distant metastasis (M)		
TNM Categories	*FIGO Stages*	
M0		No distant metastasis
M1	IVB	Distant metastasis (excluding adnexa, pelvic, and abdominal tissues)

Used with permission from the American Joint Committee on Cancer (AJCC), Chicago, Illinois. The original source for this material is the AJCC Cancer Staging Manual, Seventh Edition (2010), published by Springer Science + Business Media

Table 30.4 Uterine sarcoma

Anatomic stage/prognostic groups	
I:	T1 N0 M0
IA*:	T1a N0 M0
IB*:	T1b N0 M0
IC**:	T1c N0 M0
II:	T2 N0 M0
IIIA:	T3a N0 M0
IIIB:	T3b N0 M0
IIIC:	T1, T2, T3 N1 M0
IVA:	T4 any N M0
IVB:	any T any N M1

*Note: Stages IA and IB differ from those applied for leiomyosarcoma and endometrial stromal sarcoma
**Note: Stage IC does not apply for leiomyosarcoma and endometrial stromal sarcoma
Used with the permission of the American Joint Committee on Cancer (AJCC), Chicago, Illinois. The original source for this material is the AJCC Cancer Staging Manual, Seventh Edition (2010) published by Springer Science + Business Media

STAGING (AJCC 8TH ED., 2017)

Table 30.5 Uterine carcinomas

T category	FIGO stage	T criteria
Definitions of AJCC TNM		
Definition of primary tumor (T)		
TX		Primary tumor cannot be assessed
T0		No evidence of primary tumor
T1	I	Tumor confined to the corpus uteri, including endocervical glandular involvement
T1a	IA	Tumor limited to the endometrium or invading less than half the myometrium
T1b	IB	Tumor invading one half or more of the myometrium
T2	II	Tumor invading the stromal connective tissue of the cervix but not extending beyond the uterus. Does *not* include endocervical glandular involvement
T3	III	Tumor involving serosa, adnexa, vagina, or parametrium
T3a	IIIA	Tumor involving the serosa and/or adnexa (direct extension or metastasis)
T3b	IIIB	Vaginal involvement (direct extension or metastasis) or parametrial involvement
T4	IVA	Tumor invading the bladder mucosa and/or bowel mucosa (bullous edema is not sufficient to classify a tumor as T4)

DEFINITION OF REGIONAL LYMPH NODE (N)

N category	FIGO stage	N criteria
NX		Regional lymph nodes cannot be assessed
N0		No regional lymph node metastasis
N0(i+)		Isolated tumor cells in regional lymph node(s) not greater than 0.2 mm
N1	IIIC1	Regional lymph node metastasis to pelvic lymph nodes
N1mi	IIIC1	Regional lymph node metastasis (greater than 0.2 mm but not greater than 2.0 mm in diameter) to pelvic lymph nodes
N1a	IIIC1	Regional lymph node metastasis (greater than 2.0 mm in diameter) to pelvic lymph nodes
N2	IIIC2	Regional lymph node metastasis to para-aortic lymph nodes, with or without positive pelvic lymph nodes

continued

| N2mi | IIIC2 | Regional lymph node metastasis (greater than 0.2 mm but not greater than 2.0 mm in diameter) to para-aortic lymph nodes, with or without positive pelvic lymph nodes |
| N2a | IIIC2 | Regional lymph node metastasis (greater than 2.0 mm in diameter) to para-aortic lymph nodes, with or without positive pelvic lymph nodes |

DEFINITION OF DISTANT METASTASIS (M)

M category	FIGO stage	M criteria
M0		No distant metastasis
M1	IVB	Distant metastasis (includes metastasis to inguinal lymph nodes, intraperitoneal disease, lung, liver, or bone) (it excludes metastasis to pelvic or para-aortic lymph nodes, vagina, uterine serosa, or adnexa)

AJCC PROGNOSTIC STAGE GROUPS

When T is...	And N is...	And M is...	Then the stage group is...
T1	N0	M0	I
T1a	N0	M0	IA
T1b	N0	M0	IB
T2	N0	M0	II
T3	N0	M0	III
T3a	N0	M0	IIIA
T3b	N0	M0	IIIB
T1-T3	N1/N1mi/N1a	M0	IIIC1
T1-T3	N2/N2mi/N2a	M0	IIIC2
T4	Any N	M0	IVA
Any T	Any N	M1	IVB

Table 30.6 Leiomyosarcoma, endometrial stromal sarcoma

Definitions of AJCC TNM		
Definition of primary tumor (T)		
Leiomyosarcoma and endometrial stromal sarcoma		
T category	**FIGO stage**	**T criteria**
TX		Primary tumor cannot be assessed
T0		No evidence of primary tumor
T1	I	Tumor limited to the uterus
T1a	IA	Tumor 5 cm or less in the greatest dimension
T1b	IB	Tumor more than 5 cm
T2	II	Tumor extends beyond the uterus, within the pelvis
T2a	IIA	Tumor involves adnexa
T2b	IIB	Tumor involves other pelvic tissues
T3	III	Tumor infiltrates abdominal tissues
T3a	IIIA	One site
T3b	IIIB	More than one site
T4	IVA	Tumor invades bladder or rectum

AJCC PROGNOSTIC STAGE GROUPS
Leiomyosarcoma and Endometrial Stromal Sarcoma

When T is...	And N is...	And M is...	Then the stage group is...
T1	N0	M0	I
T1a	N0	M0	IA
T1b	N0	M0	IB
T1c	N0	M0	IC
T2	N0	M0	II
T3a	N0	M0	IIIA
T3b	N0	M0	IIIB
T1–3	N1	M0	IIIC
T4	Any N	M0	IVA
Any T	Any N	M1	IVB

VIII

Table 30.7 Adenosarcoma

Definitions of AJCC TNM
Definition of primary tumor (T)
Adenosarcoma

T category	FIGO stage	T criteria
TX		Primary tumor cannot be assessed
T0		No evidence of primary tumor
T1	I	Tumor limited to the uterus
T1a	IA	Tumor limited to the endometrium/endocervix
T1b	IB	Tumor invades to less than half of the myometrium
T1c	IC	Tumor invades more than half of the myometrium
T2	II	Tumor extends beyond the uterus, within the pelvis
T2a	IIA	Tumor involves adnexa
T2b	IIB	Tumor involves other pelvic tissues
T3	III	Tumor infiltrates abdominal tissues
T3a	IIIA	One site
T3b	IIIB	More than one site
T4	IVA	Tumor invades bladder or rectum

AJCC PROGNOSTIC STAGE GROUPS
Adenosarcoma

When T is...	And N is...	And M is...	Then the stage group is...
T1	N0	M0	I
T1a	N0	M0	IA
T1b	N0	M0	IB
T2	N0	M0	II
T3a	N0	M0	IIIA
T3b	N0	M0	IIIB
T1–3	N1	M0	IIIC
T4	Any N	M0	IVA
Any T	Any N	M1	IVB

Table 30.8 Uterine sarcoma

Definitions of AJCC TNM
Definition of regional lymph node (N)
All uterine sarcomas

N category	FIGO stage	N criteria
NX		Regional lymph nodes cannot be assessed
N0		No regional lymph node metastasis
N0(i+)		Isolated tumor cells in regional lymph node(s) not greater than 0.2 mm
N1	IIIC	Regional lymph node metastasis

DEFINITION OF DISTANT METASTASIS (M)
All Uterine Sarcomas

M category	FIGO stage	M criteria
M0		No distant metastasis
M1	IVB	Distant metastasis (excluding adnexa, pelvic, and abdominal tissues)

Used with permission of the American Joint Committee on Cancer (AJCC), Chicago, Illinois. The original and primary source for this information is the AJCC Cancer Staging Manual, Eighth Edition (2017) published by Springer International Publishing

TREATMENT RECOMMENDATIONS

Table 30.9 TREATMENT RECOMMENDATIONS

Stage	Recommended treatment
All patients	The primary treatment for all medically operable patients is TAH/BSO and lymph node assessment, unless patients want (and are candidates for) fertility-sparing options. Patients with metastatic disease are also candidates for surgery, in select cases. Lymph node assessment includes pelvic nodal dissection (external iliac, internal iliac, obturator and common iliac nodes) with or without aortic nodal dissection. Visual inspection and biopsies (if indicated) of the liver, omentum, peritoneal, diaphragmatic, serosal and mucosal surfaces are often done. Peritoneal cytology does not affect staging but is often obtained
IA, IB	IA Grade 1 without adverse risk factors*: observation IA Grade 2–3 without adverse risk factors, 1A Grade 1 with adverse features, 1B Grade 1–2 without adverse risk factors: observation or vaginal brachy 1A Grade 2 with adverse risk factors, 1B Grade 1–2 with adverse risk factors: observation or vaginal brachy and/or EBRT 1A Grade 3 with adverse risk factors, 1B Grade 3 without adverse risk factors: vaginal brachy and/or EBRT +/– systemic therapy 1B Grade 3 with adverse risk factors: EBRT and/or vaginal brachy +/– systemic therapy

continued

Table 30.9 (continued)

Stage	Recommended treatment
II	Pelvic RT +/– VC brachytherapy boost. Consider VC brachytherapy alone only if Grade 1–2, surgical nodal staging, no LVSI Consider chemotherapy for Grade 3
III-IVB	Chemotherapy + tumor-directed RT to reduce pelvic recurrences and improve PFS
Medically inoperable	Stage I minimal myometrial invasion by MRI, Grade 1–2: Intracavitary brachy alone Stage I deep myometrial invasion by MRI, or Stage I MRI not available: Tumor-directed EBRT to uterus, cervix, upper vagina, pelvic LN, and other involved areas (~45–50.4 Gy), followed by intracavitary brachytherapy boost Stage II: EBRT 45-50 Gy + brachy boost to uterus and cervix Stage III confined to pelvis: EBRT with dose-escalation to extrauterine gross disease up to 65 Gy using image-guided IMRT + brachy boost
Recurrence	If no prior RT → EBRT and IC or IS brachytherapy boost to total dose 60–70 Gy. Consider IS salvage brachytherapy for select previously irradiated patients
Serous carcinoma, clear cell carcinoma, carcinosarcoma, undifferentiated/ dedifferentiated carcinoma	Surgery. For IA: observe, chemo +/– vaginal brachy, or EBRT +/– vaginal brachy. For stage IB-IV: chemo +/– EBRT +/– vaginal brachy
Low-grade endometrial stromal sarcoma	Surgery. For stage I, observe or estrogen blockade. For stage II-IVA, estrogen blockade +/– EBRT. For stage IVB, estrogen blockade +/– palliative EBRT
High-grade endometrial stromal sarcoma, undifferentiated uterine sarcoma, uterine leiomyosarcoma	Surgery. If stage I, observe or consider systemic therapy. If stage II or III, consider systemic therapy and/or consider EBRT. If stage IVA, systemic therapy and/or EBRT. If stage IVB, systemic therapy +/– palliative EBRT

*Adverse risk factors include: older age, LVSI, tumor size, lower uterine segment or surface cervical glandular involvement

STUDIES

LYMPHADENECTOMY

   MRC ASTEC (Kitchener, Lancet 2009): 1,408 women thought preoperatively to have corpus-confined disease randomized to surgery (TAH/BSO/washings/PALN palpation) ± lymphadenectomy. With adjustment for baseline characteristics and pathology, lymphadenectomy provided no significant OS or RFS benefit.

ADJUVANT RADIOTHERAPY

   GOG 99 (Keys, Gyn Onc 2004): 392 pts with IB (60%), IC (30%), and occult II (10%) treated with TAH/BSO, pelvic and PALN sampling, and peritoneal cytology with media f/u 69 mos. Randomized to no additional therapy vs. post-op WP RT (50.4 Gy). 2/3 of patients had low–intermediate risk (LIR) disease and 1/3 of patients were high intermediate risk (HIR) (G2-3, outer 1/3 involvement, and LVSI or age >50 years +2 factors, or age >70 yo + 1 factor). WP RT improved LRR (12 → 3%), mostly among HIR pts (26 → 6%) vs. LIR pts (6 → 2%). No difference in OS (86 → 92%), but not powered to detect OS change. 4-yr severe complication rate was 13% with EBRT. Majority of pelvic recurrences in vaginal cuff.

   PORTEC-1 (Creutzberg, Lancet 2000): 714 pts with IB G2–3 or IC G1–2 treated with TAH/BSO randomized to observation vs. WP RT (46 Gy). No LN dissection (only sampling of suspicious LN). 90% of pts had G1–2 and 40% were IB. WP RT decreased LRR (14 → 4%), with 75% of failures occurring in the vaginal vault. No difference in OS (81 vs. 85%) or DM (8 vs. 7%). Update with 10-yr f/u and central pathology review for 80% of pts (Scholten, IJROBP 2005): confirmed WP RT reduces LRR (14 → 5%) without OS benefit (66 vs. 73%, p = 0.09), even after excluding IB grade 1 patients. Pts with two or more risk factors (age ≥60 years, Grade 3, and ≥50% myometrial invasion) had greatest LRR benefit with RT (23 → 5%). Update with 13-yr median f/u (Nout, JCO 2011; Creutzberg, IJROBP

VIII

2011): 15-yr LRR 5.8% vs.15.5% (mostly vaginal recurrences 11%) and OS 52% vs. 60% (*P* = 0.14) for RT vs. observation, respectively. Long-term urinary and bowel symptoms and lower physical and role-physical functioning even 15 yrs after treatment with EBRT.

- *ASTEC EN.5* (Blake, Lancet 2009): 905 pts with IA/B Grade 3, IC any grade, or I-II papillary serous or clear cell histology randomized after surgery to observation or WP RT (40–46 Gy). However, vaginal cuff brachytherapy was used in 51% of patients randomized to the observation arm. No difference in 5-yr OS (84%) or DSS (89–90%). WP RT reduced isolated pelvic or vaginal recurrences (6.1 → 3.2%), and increased acute toxicity (27 → 57%) and late severe toxicity (3 → 7%).

- *Norwegian Radium Hospital* (Aalders, Obstet Gynecol 1980; Onsrud, JCO 2013): 500 pts with IB-IC any grade treated with TAH/BSO without LN sampling. 65% of pts had IB G1-2. Randomized to VC vs. VC → WP RT. VC = LDR 60 Gy to surface. WP RT = 40 Gy with central shielding at 20 Gy. Addition of WP RT decreased pelvic and vaginal recurrences (7 → 2%), but did not change OS (90%) because more DM in WP RT arm. On subset analysis, most improvement in LRR with IC G3 (20 → 5%). Poor prognostic factors = IC, G3, LVSI, age >60 years. With 20-yr f/u, women age <60 years had worse OS and increased risk of secondary cancer with EBRT.

- *PORTEC 2* (Nout, Lancet 2010): 427 pts with HIR (age >60 years and IC Grade 1–2 or IB Grade 3; any age and IIA Grade 1–2 or Grade 3 with <50% invasion) randomized to WP RT (46 Gy) vs. VC (21 Gy HDR in 3 fx or 30 Gy LDR). Median f/u 45 mos. No significant difference in 5-yr LR relapse (5.1 vs. 2.1%), isolated pelvic recurrence (1.5 vs. 0.5%) or DM (8.3 vs. 5.7%) for VC vs. EBRT, respectively. Acute Grade 1–2 GI toxicity rate significantly lower with VC (12.6 vs 53.8%). Patient-reported QoL significantly better with VC (Nout, JCO 2009).

- *Swedish low-risk trial* (Sorbe, Int J Gynecol Cancer 2009): RCT, 645 pts, FIGO Stage IA–IB, endometrioid, FIGO (2009) Grade 1–2, randomized to VC (3–8 Gy x 3–6 fx) vs. observation. Vaginal recurrences 1.2% with VBT, 3.1% with observation (*p* = 0.114). G1-2 toxicity 2.8% with VC, 0.6% with observation. Safe to omit VC if low risk.

, *Swedish intermediate risk trial* (Sorbe, IJROBP 2012): 527 pts, Stage I, endometrioid, with one of the following risk factors (Grade 3, >50% myometrial infiltration or DNA aneuploidy) randomized after surgery to VC brachytherapy +/– 46 Gy pelvic RT. Adding pelvic RT reduced 5-yr LRR 5% to 1.5% without OS difference and increased intestinal, urinary, and vaginal toxicity.

, *SEER* (Chino, Int J Radiat Oncol Biol Phys 2012) 56,360 pts, FIGO Stage I, 70% low risk, 26% intermediate risk, and 3% high risk. 41.6% had LND and 18% adjuvant RT. Increased survival associated with WPRT or VC alone in the intermediate-risk group. In the high-risk group, in the absence of LND, only WPRT is associated with increased survival.

RADIATION VERSUS CHEMOTHERAPY

, *GOG 122* (Randall, JCO 2006): 396 pts with III/IV disease treated with surgery with maximal residual disease ≤2 cm randomized to WART (30 Gy + 15 Gy pelvic boost +15 Gy PA boost if pelvic LN+ or no sampling of pelvic and PA LN) vs. chemo (doxorubicin + cisplatin every 3 weeks × 7c → cisplatin × 1c). 21% of patients had UPSC in each arm. Chemo improved 5-yr OS (42 → 55%) and DFS (38 → 50%), but increased Grade 3–4 hematologic, GI, and cardiac toxicity.

, *Italian* (Maggi, Br J Cancer 2006): 345 pts with IC G3, II G3 with >50% myometrial invasion, and IIIA-IIIC randomized to pelvic RT 45–50 Gy vs. CAP chemo (cyclophosphamide/doxorubicin/cisplatin) monthly x 5c. Note 64% of the patient had Stage III disease. No difference in 7-yr OS 62% or PFS 56–60%. RT delayed LF (11 → 7%) and chemo delayed DM (21 → 16%).

, *JGOG 2033* (Susumu, Gynecol Oncol 2008): 385 pts, Stage IC–III, >50% myometrial invasion s/p surgery and PLND randomized to pelvic RT (45–50 Gy) vs. CAP chemo (cyclophosphamide, doxorubicin, cisplatin) q4 wks for 3 cycles. Only 3% received brachy. No difference in 5 yr PFS (82–84%) or OS (85–87%). On subset analysis, no difference for ICG1-2<70 years (low–intermediate risk), but chemo improved PFS (66 → 84%) and OS (74 → 90%) for

VIII

higher-risk group (ICG3 or IC >70 yrs or Stage II or IIIA (+cytology)). 7% pelvic failures in each arm, but fewer vaginal recurrences in RT arm. No differences in extrapelvic recurrences (~15%).

COMBINED MODALITY TREATMENT

- *GOG 34* (Morrow, Gynecol Oncol 1990): 181 pts, clinically Stage I or II (occult) found to have one 1 or more risk factors for recurrence: greater than 50% myometrial invasion, pelvic or aortic node metastasis, cervical involvement, or adnexal metastases. After surgery + RT (WP 50 Gy; if PA LN+ then PA field to top of T12 45/30) randomized to observation vs. doxorubicin. No difference in 5-yr PFS or OS. Toxicity: 6.9% SBO in RT arm; treatment-related deaths 25% (chemo) vs. RT 2%. Study underpowered. 25/92 pts in doxorubicin group received no chemo.

- *RTOG 9708* (Greven, Gynecol Oncol 2006): Phase II trial of 46 patients with Grade 2–3 disease with either >50% myometrial invasion and cervical stromal invasion or pelvic-confined extrauterine disease treated with WP RT (45 Gy) and cisplatin on days 1 and 28. 4-yr pelvic, regional, and distant recurrence rates were 2%, 2%, and 19%, respectively. 4-yr OS and DFS were 85% and 81%, respectively. No recurrences for Stages IC, IIA, or IIB.

- *Ontario Canada group* (Lupe, IJROBP 2007): 33 pts with III/IV disease treated with carboplatin/paclitaxel every 3 weeks × 4c, then pelvic RT 45 Gy, then 2 more cycles chemo. PA RT and/or VC HDR were optional. 2-yr DFS and OS 55%, with only 3% pelvic relapse.

- *Finland* (Kuoppala, Gynecol Oncol 2008): 156 pts, Stage IA–B, Grade 3 or Stage IC–IIIA, Grade 1–3 postoperatively randomized to RT alone (56 Gy, 3 wk split after 28 Gy) vs. RT+ 3 cycles of cisplatin/epirubicin/cyclophosphamide. No difference in disease-specific 5-yr OS: 84.7% (RT) vs. 82.1% chemoRT. No difference in median disease-free survival: 18 mos (RT) vs. 25 mos (chemoRT).

- *NSGO-EC-9501/EORTC-55991 and MaNGO ILIADE-III pooled data* (Hogberg, Eur J Cancer. 2010): 534 pts, Stages I–III, no residual tumor and prognostic factors implying high risk. Randomly allocated to adjuvant RT alone vs. RT + sequential chemo (various regimens). Neither study alone showed differences in the overall survival. Combined analysis showed 5-yr OS 75% RT vs. 82% chemoRT (P = 0.07) and cancer-specific survival 75% RT vs. 82% chemoRT (P = 0.01). 5-yr PFS: 78% RT vs. 69% chemoRT (p = 0.009).

- *GOG 249* (McMeekin, Gynecol Oncol 2014): RCT, 601 pts, randomly assigned to pelvic EBRT vs. VC followed by paclitaxel/carboplatin chemotherapy (VC/C). At median f/u 24 mos, no difference in RFS: 82% vs. 84% for EBRT and VC/C. No difference in OS: 93% vs. 92% for EBRT and VC/C. Acute toxicity more common with VC/C.

- *PORTEC-3* (de Boer, Lancet Oncol 2016): 686 high-risk pts randomized to RT alone (48.6 Gy) vs. chemoRT (2 cycles concurrent cisplatin and 4 adjuvant cycles of carboplatin + paclitaxel). 570 pts evaluated for 2-yr toxicity and health-related QoL as secondary outcomes. ChemoRT increased 2-yr severe tingling or numbness (25% vs. 6%), acute grade ≥3 toxicity (61% vs. 13%) mostly hematological.

- *GOG 258*: Randomized phase III trial of cisplatin + tumor volume directed irradiation followed by carboplatin + paclitaxel vs. chemo alone (carboplatin + paclitaxel) for optimally debulked, advanced endometrial carcinoma. Awaiting results.

VIII

UTERINE CARCINOSARCOMA

- *EORTC 55874* (Reed, Eur J Cancer 2008): 224 pts, Stage I/II of all uterine sarcoma subtypes after TAH/BSO/washings with optional nodal sampling randomized to observation vs. post-op WP RT (50.4 Gy). RT reduced LRR (22% vs. 40%), but had no effect on OS, PFS, or DM. In subset analysis, WP RT increased LC for carcinosarcomas, but not leiomyosracomas.

- *GOG 150* (Wolfson, Gynecol Oncol 2007): 232 pts with Stages I–IV uterine carcinosarcoma ≤1 cm residual and/or no extraabdominal spread randomized to WART (whole abdomen 30 Gy/pelvis 49.8-50 Gy at 1 Gy bid or 1.5 Gy QD) vs. chemotherapy (cisplatin/ifosfamide/mesna × 3c). No significant difference in recurrence rate or survival between the two arms.

⸏ *Sampath* et al. (IJROBP 2010): Retrospective study of 3,650 uterine sarcoma pts from the National Oncology Database. 5-yr OS 37%. Adjuvant RT (post-op EBRT to pelvis ± brachy) not predictive for OS. RT provided 53% reduction in the risk of LRF at 5 yrs.

⸏ *GOG 261:* Randomized phase III, paclitaxel + carboplatin vs. ifosfamide + paclitaxel in chemo-naive pts with newly diagnosed Stage I–IV, persistent or recurrent carcinosarcoma of the uterus or ovary. Awaiting results.

IMRT

⸏ *RTOG 0418 (*Klopp, IJROBP 2013): Phase II study. 43 pts with adenocarcinoma of endometrium treated with pelvic IMRT (no chemo), 50.4 Gy/28 fx to the vaginal and nodal PTVs. 7% had Grade 2, 16% Grade 3 hematologic toxicity.

⸏ *French multicenter trial (*Barillot, Radiother Oncol 2014*)*: Phase II study. 46 pts with postoperative Stage Ib G3, Ic or II endometrial carcinomas received post-op IMRT. Vaginal and nodal PTV dose: 45 Gy/25 fx. 75% got additional vaginal vault HDR boost. Low rate (<30%) of acute GI Grade 2 toxicity.

⸏ *RTOG 0921* (Viswanathan, Cancer 2015): Phase II study. 30 pts s/p hysterectomy and PLND with: Grade 3 with >50% myometrial invasion; Grade 2 or 3 with any cervical stromal invasion; or extrauterine extension confined to the pelvis. Treated with IMRT and concurrent cisplatin + bevacizumab followed by optional VC boost then adjuvant carboplatin + paclitaxel for 4 cycles. 45 Gy/25 fx to the vaginal and nodal PTVs; 14.4 Gy/8 fx boost (total 59.4 Gy) to enlarged/involved LNs. 7 pts had Grade 3 nonhematologic toxicities within 90 days; 6 pts had Grade 3 toxicities between 90 and 365 days post-treatment. At follow-up of 3.92 yrs (Viswanathan, IJROP 2016): 5 pts with Grade 3 or 4 AEs >1 yr from treatment start. 4-yr OS 86.7%, DFS 73.2%, paraaortic failure 6.7%, and DF 23.5%. No pts with recurrent disease in the pelvis.

⸏ *RTOG 1203*: Randomized phase III, standard vs. IMRT pelvic radiation for post-op endometrial and cervical cancer. Closed to accrual, awaiting results.

RADIATION TECHNIQUES

SIMULATION AND FIELD DESIGN

- Tumor-directed RT refers to RT directed to sites of known or suspected tumor and may include EBRT and/or brachytherapy.

EBRT

- Simulate patient supine with CT planning; administer presimulation enema.
- WP borders: superior = L5-S1; inferior = below obturator canal and including upper 1/2–2/3 of vagina; lateral = 2 cm lateral to pelvic brim; posterior = split sacrum to S3; anterior = pubic symphysis. Consider using IMRT (Fig. 30.1).
- EFRT borders: Extend superior border to top of L1 with CT planning to avoid kidneys. Recommend IMRT.
- If IMRT is used, careful attention to target delineation is necessary, and consider using internal target volume (ITV) or volume of vagina that is in both the empty and full bladder CT. Refer to RTOG CTV consensus guidelines (Small, IJROBP 2008). Fig. 30.1.

Vaginal Brachytherapy

- Place two marker seeds in vaginal cuff at both ends of hysterectomy scars. Use largest vaginal cylinder possible (2.5–3.5 cm). Target upper 2/3 of vaginal cuff. Consider CT planning. We recommend prescribing dose to vaginal surface because it represents the Dmax of normal tissue. However, some institutions prescribe to 0.5 cm, and dose and fractionation should be modified based on institutional experience.

Brachytherapy for Intact Uterus

- Use Martinez-Y applicator or combination of tandem and cylinder +/− interstitial catheters. Consider US guidance and 3D image-guided brachytherapy. Use tandem with ring or ovoids for pre-op stage II.

VIII

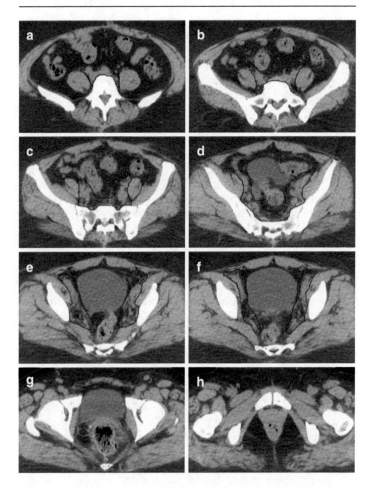

Fig. 30.1 Example pelvic nodal IMRT clinical tumor volumes on representative axial CT slices: (**a**) upper common iliacs, (**b**) mid-common iliacs and presacral area, (**c**) lower common iliacs and presacral area, (**d**) upper internal and external iliacs and presacral area, (**e** and **f**) internal and external iliacs, (**g**) vagina and parametrium, (**h**) vagina

DOSE PRESCRIPTIONS

- Post-op (see ASTRO guideline, Klopp, PRO 2014; ABS guideline, Small, Brachytherapy 2012).
    - VC alone:
        HDR: 10.5 Gy x 3 (UCSF), 6 Gy x 5, 4 Gy x 6 at vaginal surface.
        LDR: 50–60 Gy at vaginal surface.
    - Pelvic LN: 1.8 Gy/fx to 45–50.4 Gy.
    - VC brachytherapy boost:
        HDR: 6 Gy x 3 at vaginal surface.
        LDR: 20 Gy at vaginal surface.
    - Paraaortic LN+: EFRT to 45-50 Gy and boost enlarged unresectable nodes up to 65 Gy (sequential) or 54 Gy/25 fx with simultaneous integrated boost (SIB) using IMRT/IGRT."
- Inoperable: Follow ABS guidelines (Schwarz, Brachytherapy 2015).
    - HDR alone for selected MRI Stage I Grade 1–2 with limited myometrial invasion: 6 Gy × 6, 8.5 Gy × 4, 5 Gy × 9–10.
    - Tumor-directed EBRT 45-50 Gy and boost involved nodes up to 65 Gy (sequential) or 54 Gy/25 fx (SIB) with IMRT/IGRT.
    - HDR boost examples: 6.5 Gy × 3, 5 Gy × 5, 8.5 Gy × 2.

VIII

DOSE LIMITATIONS

- Upper vaginal mucosa 150 Gy, midvaginal mucosa 80–90 Gy, lower vaginal mucosa 60–70 Gy.
- Ovarian failure with 5–10 Gy. Sterilization with 2–3 Gy.
- Small bowel <45–50.4 Gy, rectal point dose <70 Gy, bladder point <75 Gy based on 2D planning.
- For IMRT: small bowel <30% to receive 40 Gy; rectum <60% to receive 30 Gy; bladder <35% to receive 45 Gy; femoral head ≤15% to receive 30 Gy, bone marrow ≤37% to receive 40 Gy (RTOG 0418, Jhingran, IJROBP 2012; Klopp, IJROBP 2013).

COMPLICATIONS

- TAH/BSO complications – mortality (<1%), infection, wound dehiscence, fistula, bleeding
- Frequency and urgency of urine and/or stool
- Vaginal stenosis – use dilators

FOLLOW-UP

- H&P exam every 3 mos × 2 yrs, then every 6 mos × 3 yrs, then annually. Vaginal cytology every 6 mos for 2 yrs, then annually. CA-125 optional. Annual chest X-ray. CT imaging (chest/abdomen/pelvis) every 3–6 mo for 2–3 yrs, then every 6 mo for next 2 yrs, then annually for high-grade sarcomas. Other imaging (MRI/PET) as clinically indicated.

Acknowledgment We thank R. Scott Bermudez MD and Kim Huang MD for their work on the prior edition of this chapter.

REFERENCES

Aalders JG, Abeler V, Kolstad P, et al. Postoperative external irradiation and prognostic parameters in stage I endometrial carcinoma: clinical and histopathologic study of 540 patients. Gynecol Oncol. 1980;56:419.

Amant F, Coosemans A, Debiec-Rychter M, Timmerman D, Vergote I. Clinical management of uterine sarcomas. Lancet Oncol. 2009;10(12):1188–98.

ASTEC study group, Kitchener H, Swart AM, et al. Efficacy of systematic pelvic lymphadenectomy in endometrial cancer (MRC ASTEC trial): a randomized study. Lancet. 2009;373:125–36.

ASTEC/EN.5 study group, Blake P, Swart AM, Orton J, et al. Adjuvant external beam radiotherapy in the treatment of endometrial cancer (MRC ASTEC and NCIC CTG EN.5 randomised trials): pooled trial results, systematic review, and meta-analysis. Lancet. 2009;373:137–46.

Barillot I, Tavernier E, Peignaux K, et al. Impact of post operative intensity modulated radiotherapy on acute gastro-intestinal toxicity for patients with endometrial cancer: results of the phase II RTCMIENDOMETRE French multicentre trial. Radiother Oncol. 2014;111(1):138–43.

de Boer SM, Powell ME, Mileshkin L, et al. Toxicity and quality of life after adjuvant chemoradiotherapy versus radiotherapy alone for women with high-risk endometrial cancer (PORTEC-3): an open-label, multicentre, randomised, phase 3 trial. Lancet Oncol. 2016;17(8):1114–26.

Bokhman JV. Two pathogenetic types of endometrial carcinoma. Gynecol Oncol. 1983;15(1):10–7.

Bonadona V, Bonaïti B, Olschwang S, et al. Cancer risks associated with germline mutations in MLH1, MSH2, and MSH6 genes in lynch syndrome. JAMA. 2011;305(22):2304–10.

Brinton LA, Felix AS, McMeekin DS, et al. Etiologic heterogeneity in endometrial cancer: evidence from a gynecologic oncology group trial. Gynecol Oncol. 2013;129(2):277–84.

Cancer Genome Atlas Research Network, et al. Integrated genomic characterization of endometrial carcinoma. Nature. 2013;497:67–73.

Chino JP, Jones E, Berchuck A, et al. The influence of radiation modality and lymph node dissection on survival in early-stage endometrial cancer. Int J Radiat Oncol Biol Phys. 2012;82:1872–9.

Cardenes HR, Look K, Michael H, et al. Endometrium. In: Halperin CE, Perez CA, Brady LW, et al., editors. Principles and practice of radiation oncology. 5th ed. Philadelphia: Lippincott Williams & Wilkins; 2008. p. 1610–28.

Creutzberg CL, Fleming GF. Endometrial Cancer. In: Gunderson LL, Tepper JE, editors. Clinical radiation oncology. 4th ed. Philadelphia: Churchill Livingstone; 2015. p. 1203–1229.e7.

Creutzberg CL, van Putten WL, Koper PC, et al. Surgery and postoperative radiotherapy versus surgery alone for patients with stage-1 endometrial carcinoma: multicentre randomised trial. PORTEC study group. Post operative radiation therapy in endometrial carcinoma. Lancet. 2000;355:1404–11.

Creutzberg CL, Nout RA, Lybeert ML, et al. Fifteen-year radiotherapy outcomes of the randomized PORTEC-1 trial for endometrial carcinoma. Int J Radiat Oncol Biol Phys. 2011;81:e631–8.

FIGO Committee. On gynecologic oncology. FIGO staging for uterine sarcomas. Int J Gynaecol Obstet. 2009;104:179.

Greven K, Winter K, Underhill K, et al. Final analysis of RTOG 9708: adjuvant postoperative irradiation combined with cisplatin/paclitaxel chemotherapy following surgery for patients with high risk endometrial cancer. Gynecol Oncol. 2006;103:155–9.

Hogberg T, Signorelli M, de Oliveira CF, et al. Sequential adjuvant chemotherapy and radiotherapy in endometrial cancer--results from two randomised studies. Eur J Cancer. 2010;46(13):2422–31.

Hsu IJ, Alektiar KM, Nori D. Cancer of the endometrium. In: Leibel SA, Phillips TL, editors. Textbook of radiation oncology. 3rd ed. Philadelphia: Saunders; 2010. p. 1026–51.

Jhingran A, Winter K, Portelance L, et al. A phase II study of intensity modulated radiation therapy to the pelvis for postoperative patients with endometrial carcinoma: radiation therapy oncology group trial 0418. Int J Radiat Oncol Biol Phys. 2012;84(1):e23–8.

Johnson N, Cornes P. Survival and recurrent disease after postoperative radiotherapy for early endometrial cancer: systematic review and meta-analysis. BJOG. 2007; 114(11):1313–20.

Keys HM, Roberts JA, Brunetto VL, et al. A phase III trial of surgery with or without adjunctive external pelvic radiation therapy in intermediate risk endometrial adenocarcinoma: a gynecologic oncology group study. Gynecol Oncol. 2004;92:744–51.

Klopp AH, Moughan J, Portelance L, et al. Hematologic toxicity in RTOG 0418: a phase 2 study of postoperative IMRT for gynecologic cancer. Int J Radiat Oncol Biol Phys. 2013;86(1):83–90.

Klopp A, Smith BD, Alektiar K, et al. The role of postoperative radiation therapy for endometrial cancer: executive summary of an American Society for Radiation Oncology evidence-based guide- line. Pract Radiat Oncol. 2014;4:137–44.

VIII

Kong A, Simera I, Collingwood M, et al. Adjuvant radiotherapy for stage I endometrial cancer: systematic review and meta-analysis. Ann Oncol. 2007;18(10):1595–604.

Kuoppala T, Mäenpää J, Tomas E, et al. Surgically staged high-risk endometrial cancer: randomized study of adjuvant radiotherapy alone vs. sequential chemo-radiotherapy. Gynecol Oncol. 2008;110:190–5.

Lee CM, Szabo A, Shrieve DC, et al. Frequency and effect of adjuvant radiation therapy among women with stage I endometrial adenocarcinoma. JAMA. 2006;295:389–97.

Lupe K, Kwon J, D'Souza D, et al. Adjuvant paclitaxel and carboplatin chemotherapy with involved field radiation in advanced endometrial cancer: a sequential approach. Int J Radiat Oncol Biol Phys. 2007;67(1):110–6.

Maggi R, Lissoni A, Spina F, et al. Adjuvant chemotherapy vs radiotherapy in high-risk endometrial carcinoma: results of a randomised trial. Br J Cancer. 2006;95(3):266–71.

McMeekin DS, Filiaci VL, Aghajanian C, et al. A randomized phase III trial of pelvic radiation therapy (PXRT) versus vaginal cuff brachytherapy followed by paclitaxel/carboplatin chemotherapy (VCB/C) in patients with high risk (HR), early stage endometrial cancer (EC): a gynecologic oncology group trial. Gynecol Oncol. 2014;134(2):438.

Meyer LA, Bohlke K, Powell MA, et al. Postoperative radiation therapy for endometrial cancer: American Society of Clinical Oncology clinical practice guideline endorsement of the American Society for Radiation Oncology evidence-based guideline. J Clin Oncol. 2015;33(26):2908–13.

Morrow CP, Bundy BN, Homesley HD. Doxorubicin as an adjuvant following surgery and radiation therapy in patients with high-risk endometrial carcinoma, stage I and occult stage II: a gynecologic oncology group study. Gynecol Oncol. 1990;36(2):166–71.

National Cancer Institute Surveillance, Epidemiology, and End Results Program (SEER) (2016). http://seer.cancer.gov/statfacts/html/corp.html. Accessed 22 Aug 2016. National Comprehensive Cancer Network. Clinical Practice Guidelines in Oncology: Endometrial cancers (Version 2.2016). 2016. https://www.nccn.org/professionals/physician_gls/pdf/uterine.pdf. Accessed on 22 Aug 2016.

Nout RA, Putter H, Jürgenliemk-Schulz IM, et al. Quality of life after pelvic radiotherapy or vaginal brachytherapy for endometrial cancer: first results of the randomized PORTEC-2 trial. J Clin Oncol. 2009;27(21):3547–56.

Nout RA, Smit V, Putter H, et al. Vaginal brachytherapy versus pelvic external beam radiotherapy for patients with endometrial cancer of high-intermediate risk (PORTEC-2): an open-label, non-inferiority, randomised trial. Lancet. 2010;375(9717):816–23.

Nout RA, van de Poll-Franse LV, Lybeert MLM, et al. Long-term outcome and quality of life of patients with endometrial carcinoma treated with or without pelvic radiotherapy in the post operative radiation therapy in endometrial carcinoma 1 (PORTEC-1) trial. J Clin Oncol. 2011;29(13):1692–700.

Onsrud M, Cvancarova M, Hellebust TP, et al. Long-term outcomes after pelvic radiation for early-stage endometrial cancer. J Clin Oncol. 2013;31:3951–6.

Pecorelli S. Revised FIGO staging for carcinoma of the vulva, cervix, and endometrium. Int J Gynaecol Obstet. 2009;105(2):103–4.

Randall ME, Filiaci VL, Muss H, et al. Randomized phase III trial of whole-abdominal irradiation versus doxorubicin and cisplatin chemotherapy in advanced endometrial carcinoma: a gynecologic oncology group study. J Clin Oncol. 2006;24:36–44.

Reed NS, Mangioni C, Malstrom H, et al. Phase III randomized study to evaluate the role of adjuvant pelvic radiotherapy in the treatment of uterine sarcomas stages I and II:

an European organization for research and treatment of cancer gynaecological cancer group study (protocol 55874). Eur J Cancer. 2008;44:808–18.

Sampath S, Schultheiss TE, Ryu JK. The role of adjuvant radiation in uterine sarcomas. Int J Radiat Oncol Biol Phys. 2010;76(3):728–34.

Scholten AN, van Putten WLJ, Beerman H, et al. Postoperative radiotherapy for stage 1 endometrial carcinoma: long-term outcome of the randomized PORTEC trial with central pathology review. Int J Radiat Oncol Biol Phys. 2005;63:834–8.

Schwarz JK, Beriwal S, Esthappan J, et al. Consensus statement for brachytherapy for the treatment of medically inoperable endometrial cancer. Brachytherapy. 2015;14:587–99.

Small W, Mell LK, Anderson P, et al. Consensus guidelines for delineation of clinical target volume for intensity-modulated pelvic radiotherapy in postoperative treatment of endometrial and cervical cancer. Int J Radiat Oncol Biol Phys. 2008;71(2):428–34.

Small W Jr, Beriwal S, Demanes DJ, et al. American brachytherapy Society consensus guidelines for adjuvant vaginal cuff brachyther- apy after hysterectomy. Brachytherapy. 2012;11:58–67.

Sorbe B, Nordström B, Mäenpää J, et al. Intravaginal brachytherapy in FIGO stage I low-risk endometrial cancer: a controlled randomized study. Int J Gynecol Cancer. 2009;19(5):873–8.

Sorbe B, Horvath G, Andersson H, et al. External pelvic and vaginal irradiation versus vaginal irradiation alone as postoperative therapy in medium-risk endometrial carcinomaDOUBLEHYPHENa prospective randomized study. Int J Radiat Oncol Biol Phys. 2012;82:1249–55.

Susumu N, Sagae S, Udagawa Y, et al. Randomized phase III trial of pelvic radiotherapy versus cisplatin-based combined chemotherapy in patients with intermediate- and high-risk endometrial cancer: a Japanese gynecologic oncology group study. Gynecol Oncol. 2008;108(1):226–33.

Viswanathan AN, Moughan J, Miller BE, et al. NRG oncology/RTOG 0921: a phase 2 study of postoperative intensity-modulated radiotherapy with concurrent cisplatin and bevacizumab followed by carboplatin and paclitaxel for patients with endometrial cancer. Cancer. 2015;121(13):2156–63.

Viswanathan AN, Winter K, Miller BE, et al. Updated 4-year results for NRG oncology/ RTOG 0921: a phase 2 study of postoperative intensity modulated radiation therapy with concurrent Cisplatin and Bevacizumab followed by carboplatin and paclitaxel for patients with endometrial cancer. Int J Radiat Oncol Biol Phys. 2016;96(2S):S49–50.

Wolfson A, Brady M, Rocereto T, et al. Gynecologic oncology group. Randomized phase III trial of whole abdominal irradiation (WAI) vs. cisplatin-ifosfamide and mesna (CIM) as post-surgical therapy in stage I-IV carcinosarcoma (CS) of the uterus. Gynecol Oncol. 2007;107(2):177–85.

VIII

Chapter 31
Ovarian Cancer

Serah Choi and I-Chow J. Hsu

PEARLS

- 22,280 estimated new cases and 14,240 deaths in 2016.
- 5th leading cause of cancer death in women; leading cause of gynecologic cancer death.
- Average lifetime risk is 1 in 70 with median age at diagnosis of 63 years.
- Highly curable if diagnosed at an early stage, but 75% present with Stage III or IV disease.
- Symptoms rare in early stages. Abdominal pain/bloating/pressure, irregular vaginal bleeding/discharge, adnexal mass, GI symptoms (gas, bloating, constipation) are usually associated with advanced stages. There are no good screening tests.
- Risk factors: family history, nulliparity, first parity >35 years, infertility, early menarche, late menopause, ovulation-inducing drugs, hormone replacement therapy, obesity, endometriosis, smoking.
- Strongest risk factor is a family history of ovarian cancer (20% are familial), yet only 5–10% of tumors result from a known genetic disposition. Lifetime risk: general population 1.8%, one first-degree relative: 5%, two first-degree relatives: 25–50%.
- Consider genetic testing and/or prophylactic salpingo-oophorectomy for a strong family history.

VIII

Eric K. Hansen and M. Roach III (eds.), *Handbook of Evidence-Based Radiation Oncology*, https://doi.org/10.1007/978-3-319-62642-0_31

» Familial syndromes tend to occur earlier and have a more indolent course than sporadic variants:
  » BRCA1 (lifetime risk 45%), BRCA2 (lifetime risk 25%), HNPCC.
» Anatomy: paired ovaries, each ~4 cm × 3 cm × 2 cm in size, beneath the external iliac artery, anterior to the ureter and internal iliac artery, attached on either side of the uterus by the ovarian ligament and attached to the body wall via the suspensory ligament of the ovary. Surface is covered by ovarian epithelium.
» Pathology: epithelial 85%, germ cell 10%, sex cord stromal 5%
  » Epithelial types: serous 40–50%, endometrioid 15–25%, mucinous 6–16%, clear cell 5–11%; transitional, mixed epithelial, and undifferentiated are less frequent.
» Patterns of spread: exfoliation into peritoneal cavity (most common), lymphatic (mainly pelvic/paraaortic, but inguinals also at risk via round ligament), direct extension (most common to fallopian tubes) and hematogenous (<5%).
» 90% recurrences occur within 5 years; 85% of relapses are intraabdominal.
» "Platinum resistant" if disease progresses during platinum therapy or relapse <6 mos from completion of treatment; associated with worse prognosis.
» Most patients die from local disease (small bowel obstruction, ascites, abdominal organ infiltration, etc.).
» Most important negative prognostic factors: stage, grade, residual volume of disease.
  » Other negative factors: age >65, pre-op ascites, CA125 elevated after 3 cycles of chemo or nadir >20 U/mL after first-line therapy.

WORKUP

» H&P with family history, complete gynecologic exam and Pap smear.
» Signs/symptoms: abdominal discomfort/pain, increasing girth, change in bowel habits, early satiety, dyspepsia, nausea, ascites, adnexal mass, pleural effusion, Sister Mary Joseph's nodule, Blumer's shelf, Leser–Trélat sign

(sudden appearance of seborrheic keratoses), hypercalcemia with clear cell, subacute cerebellar degeneration and/or precocious puberty (germ cell).

- Labs: CBC, LFT, BUN/Cr, serum tumor markers as follows:
  - CA125: elevated in 80% of epithelial ovarian tumors; may serve as an early marker for disease recurrence. False positives possible, especially in premenopausal women.
  - CA 19–9: low sensitivity but may be positive in GI or Müllerian tumors.
  - CEA: elevated in 58% with Stage III disease.
  - AFP and βHCG: measure if <30 years old to help rule out germ cell tumors.
- Imaging:
  - Transvaginal US (more useful than transabdominal US for adnexal masses).
    Ovarian enlargement during reproductive years usually benign.
    Simple cyst <3 cm can be followed by serial US.
    Complex ovarian cyst or postmenopausal women with simple cyst and CA-125 > 65 U/mL suggestive of cancer → surgery indicated.
  - CT/MRI abdomen/pelvis: especially helpful preoperatively if advanced disease.
  - Chest X-ray or chest CT as clinically indicated.
- Cystoscopy, sigmoidoscopy, barium enema, upper GI series, or endoscopy as clinically indicated.
- Endometrial biopsy preoperatively in women with abnormal vaginal bleeding.
- Pre-op percutaneous assessment of ascites or mass not recommended as it may lead to tumor seeding along tract or peritoneum and delay surgical staging/management.
- Surgical exploration: EUA, excise intact suspicious mass, frozen sections → if malignant, proceed to complete surgical staging.
- Surgical staging: vertical incision, collect ascites/washings, TAH/BSO, complete abdominal exploration, omentectomy, random peritoneal biopsies (including diaphragm), aortic/pelvic lymph node sampling, optimal debulking, ±appendectomy. If proven Stage IA, may preserve fertility with unilateral salpingo-oophrectomy (USO).

VIII

Table 31.1 STAGING (AJCC 7TH ED., 2010/FIGO 2008): OVARIAN CANCER

Primary tumor (T)		
TNM Categories	*FIGO Stages*	
TX		Primary tumor cannot be assessed
T0		No evidence of primary tumor
T1	I	Tumor limited to ovaries (one or both)
T1a	IA	Tumor limited to one ovary; capsule No malignant cells in ascites or peritoneal washings
T1b	IB	Tumor limited to both ovaries; capsules intact, no tumor on ovarian surface. No malignant cells in ascites or peritoneal washings
T1c	IC	Tumor limited to one or both ovaries with any of the following: Capsule ruptured, tumor on ovarian surface, malignant cells in ascites or peritoneal washings
T2	II	Tumor involves one or both ovaries with pelvic extension
T2a	IIA	Extension and/or implants on uterus and/or tube(s). No malignant cells in ascites or peritoneal washings
T2b	IIB	Extension to and/or implants on other pelvic tissues. No malignant cells in ascites or peritoneal washings
T2c	IIC	Pelvic extension and/or implants (T2a or T2b) with malignant cells in ascites or peritoneal washings
T3	III	Tumor involves one or both ovaries with microscopically confirmed peritoneal metastasis outside the pelvis
T3a	IIIA	Microscopic peritoneal metastasis beyond pelvis (no macroscopic tumor)
T3b	IIIB	Macroscopic peritoneal metastasis beyond pelvis 2 cm or less in greatest dimension
T3c	IIIC	Peritoneal metastasis beyond pelvis more than 2 cm in greatest dimension and/or regional lymph node metastasis

Note: Liver capsule metastasis T3/Stage III; liver parenchymal metastasis M1/Stage IV. Pleural effusion must have positive cytology for M1/Stage IV

Table 31.2   (continued)

Regional lymph nodes (N)		
TNM	*FIGO*	
Categories	*Stages*	
NX		Regional lymph nodes cannot be assessed
N0		No regional lymph node metastasis
N1	IIIC	Regional lymph node metastasis

Distant metastasis (M)		
TNM	*FIGO*	
Categories	*Stages*	
M0		No distant metastasis
M1	IV	Distant metastasis (excludes peritoneal metastasis)

Anatomic stage/prognostic groups	
I	T1 N0 M0
IA	T1a N0 M0
IB	T1b N0 M0
IC	T1c N0 M0
II	T2 N0 M0
IIA	T2a N0 M0
IIB	T2b N0 M0
IIC	T2c N0 M0
III	T3 N0 M0
IIIA	T3a N0 M0
IIIB	T3b N0 M0
IIIC	T3c N0 M0
IV	Any T N1 M0
	Any T any N M1

VIII

Used with the permission from the American Joint Committee on Cancer (AJCC), Chicago, Illinois. The original source for this material is the AJCC Cancer Staging Manual, 7th ed. (2010), published by Springer Science + Business Media

Table 31.2 STAGING (AJCC 8TH ED., 2017)

Definitions of AJCC TNM

T category	FIGO stage	T criteria
TX		Primary tumor cannot be assessed
T0		No evidence of primary tumor
T1	I	Tumor limited to ovaries (one or both) or fallopian tube(s)
T1a	IA	Tumor limited to one ovary (capsule intact) or fallopian tube surface; no malignant cells in ascites or peritoneal washings
T1b	IB	Tumor limited to one or both ovaries (capsules intact) or fallopian tubes; no tumor on ovarian or fallopian tube surface; no malignant cells in ascites or peritoneal washings
T1c	IC	Tumor limited to one or both ovaries or fallopian tubes, with any of the following
T1c1	IC1	Surgical spill
T1c2	IC2	Capsule ruptured before surgery or tumor on ovarian or fallopian tube surface
T1c3	IC3	Malignant cells in ascites or peritoneal washings
T2	II	Tumor involves one or both ovaries or fallopian tubes with pelvic extension below pelvic brim or primary peritoneal cancer
T2a	IIA	Extension and/or implants on the uterus and/or fallopian tube(s) and/or ovaries
T2b	IIB	Extension to and/or implants on other pelvic tissues
T3	III	Tumor involves one or both ovaries or fallopian tubes, or primary peritoneal cancer, with microscopically confirmed peritoneal metastasis outside the pelvis and/or metastasis to the retroperitoneal (pelvic and/ or para-aortic) lymph nodes
T3a	IIIA2	Microscopic extrapelvic (above the pelvic brim) peritoneal involvement with or without positive retroperitoneal lymph nodes
T3b	IIIB	Macroscopic peritoneal metastasis beyond pelvis 2 cm or less in the greatest dimension with or without metastasis to the retroperitoneal lymph nodes
T3c	IIIC	Macroscopic peritoneal metastasis beyond the pelvis more than 2 cm in the greatest dimension with or without metastasis to the retroperitoneal lymph nodes (includes extension of tumor to capsule of liver and spleen without parenchymal involvement of either organ)

DEFINITION OF REGIONAL LYMPH NODE (N)

N category	FIGO stage	N criteria
NX		Regional lymph nodes cannot be assessed
N0		No regional lymph node metastasis
N0(i+)		Isolated tumor cells in regional lymph node(s) not greater than 0.2 mm
N1	IIIA1	Positive retroperitoneal lymph nodes only (histologically confirmed)
N1a	III A1i	Metastasis up to 10 mm in the greatest dimension
N1b	III A1ii	Metastasis more than 10 mm in the greatest dimension

DEFINITION OF DISTANT METASTASIS (M)

M category	FIGO stage	M criteria
M0		No distant metastasis
M1	IV	Distant metastasis, including pleural effusion with positive cytology, liver or splenic parenchymal metastasis, metastasis to extra-abdominal organs (including inguinal lymph nodes and lymph nodes outside the abdominal cavity), and transmural involvement of intestine
M1a	IVA	Pleural effusion with positive cytology
M1b	IVB	Liver or splenic parenchymal metastases; metastases to extra-abdominal organs (including inguinal lymph nodes and lymph nodes outside the abdominal cavity); transmural involvement of intestine

VIII

AJCC PROGNOSTIC STAGE GROUPS

When T is...	And N is...	And M is...	Then the stage group is...
T1	N0	M0	I
T1a	N0	M0	IA
T1b	N0	M0	IB
T1c	N0	M0	IC
T2	N0	M0	II
T2a	N0	M0	IIA
T2b	N0	M0	IIB
T1/T2	N1	M0	IIIA1
T3a	N0/N1	M0	IIIA2
T3b	N0/N1	M0	IIIB
T3c	N0/N1	M0	IIIC
Any T	Any N	M1	IV
Any T	Any N	M1a	IVA
Any T	Any N	M1b	IVB

Used with permission of the American Joint Committee on Cancer (AJCC), Chicago, Illinois. The original and primary source for this information is the AJCC Cancer Staging Manual, Eighth Edition (2017) published by Springer International Publishing

TREATMENT RECOMMENDATIONS

Table 31.3 TREATMENT RECOMMENDATIONS

Stage	Recommended treatment
IA/B gr 1	Surgery → observation
IA/B gr 2	Surgery → observation or Surgery → intravenous (IV) taxane/carboplatin × 3–6 cycles
IA/B gr 3 or IC	Surgery → IV taxane/carboplatin × 3–6 cycles
II, III or IV	IV taxane/carboplatin × 6 cycles or intraperitoneal chemo (IP) in <1 cm optimally debulked stage II and III patients → completion surgery as indicated by tumor response and potential resectability in select patients.

STUDIES

ADJUVANT CHEMO: EARLY STAGE

- *ICON and EORTC-ACTION* (JNCI 2003): 925 pts, ICON included mainly Stages I–II, ACTION included IA/BG2–3, IC, IIA randomized to observation vs. 4–6 cycles immediate adjuvant platinum-based chemo (57% single agent carboplatin, 27% combo cisplatin). Immediate chemo improved 5-year OS 8% (82 vs. 74%) and 5-year RFS 11% (76 vs. 65%).
- *GOG 157* (Bell, Gyn Oncol 2006): 457 pts, included IA/BG2–3, IC, II randomized to 3 cycles (considered standard arm) vs. 6 cycles adjuvant paclitaxel/carboplatin. No significant difference in 5-year recurrence between 3 cycles and 6 cycles chemo (25.4 vs. 20.1%), but 6 cycles associated with greater toxicity.

ADJUVANT CHEMO: ADVANCED STAGE

- *GOG 111* (McGuire, NEJM 1996): 410 pts, Stage III/IV with <1 cm residual randomized to cisplatin with either cyclophosphamide or paclitaxel. Paclitaxel improved PFS (18 vs. 13 mo), and MS (38 vs. 24 mo). Results confirmed in large European/Canadian Intergroup trial (Piccart et al. 2000).
- *GOG 158* (Ozols, JCO 2003): 792 pts, advanced stage with <1 cm residual randomized to paclitaxel with either

cisplatin or carboplatin. Carboplatin regimen was less toxic, easier to administer, and equally effective.

˒ Dose-dense weekly paclitaxel with carboplatin may improve PFS vs. every 3 week, but dose-dense regimen is more toxic (JGOG 3016, Katsumata, Lancet Oncol 2013; GOG 262, Chan, NEJM 2016).

˒ Adding bevacizumab to every 3 week carboplatin paclitaxel may improve PFS and OS for pts with ascites (*GOG 218*, Burger, NEJM 2011) or high-risk pts with poor prognosis (ICON7, Perren, NEJM 2011).

˒ 3 GOG randomized trials have reported improved OS with IP chemo vs. IV chemo in pts with advanced ovarian carcinoma (GOG 104, GOG 114, GOG 172) with best results using the GOG 172 regimen (Armstrong 2006, NEJM 2006), median PFS 24 vs. 18 mo, MS 66 vs. 50 mo. However, IP chemo increases toxicity, only 42% of pts treated with GOG 172 regimen completed all 6 cycles.

ADJUVANT WHOLE ABDOMINAL RADIATION THERAPY (WART)

˒ In general, WART is now rarely used and is included here for historical reference. The role of radiation in ovarian cancer is mainly palliative localized radiation for symptom control.

˒ No randomized trials have evaluated best modern chemo and WART techniques.

˒ Dembo (Am J Obstet Gynecol 1979; Cancer 1985; IJROBP 1992): 190 pts with IB, II, asymptomatic III randomized to pelvic RT vs. pelvic RT + chlorambucil vs. WART. In pts with no residual or <2 cm residual, WART improved 10-year OS vs. pelvic RT ± chlorambucil (10 year 64 vs. 40%) with 30% decrease in abdominal recurrences with WART.

˒ Kojs (Cancer Radiother 2001). 150 pts with IA, IB grade 2–3, and IC/IIA without residual after surgery randomized to cisplatin, doxorubicin, and cyclophosphamide x 6c vs WART (30 Gy in 24 fx + pelvic boost to 50 Gy). 5-yr RFS 81% both groups, 3 late Grade 3 intestinal complications in WART arm.

˒ NOCGI (Chiara, Am J Clin Oncol 1994): 70 pts with high-risk, Stage I or II randomized to cisplatin + cyclophosphamide vs. WART (43.2 Gy/24 fx to the pelvis, 30.2 Gy to the upper

VIII

abdomen). Closed prematurely due to protocol violations and low accrual. 5-yr OS 71% for chemo vs. 53% for WART (p = 0.16). Relapse-free survival 74% for chemo and 50% for WART (p = 0.07). Chemo toxicities mild and tolerable, whereas 28% of patients in WAI arm had Gr 3–4 acute diarrhea, 2 pts hospitalized for severe enteritis, 1 pt had late bowel obstruction requiring surgery.

- Chemo-resistant non-serous histologies, such as clear cell and mucinous, may benefit from adjuvant WART (Hoskins, JCO 2012; Swenerton, Ann Oncol 2011), but have not yet been prospectively studied.

CONSOLIDATIVE RADIATION

- *North Thames Ovary Group Study* (Lambert, JCO 1993): 254 pts locally advanced, Stage IIB-IV who received surgery followed by 5 cycles of carboplatin. If residual disease <2 cm at second look surgery, then randomized to Arm (1) carboplatin 400 mg/m^2 × 5 courses or Arm (2) WART (24 Gy/20 fx). Median OS 2 yrs, no difference in OS or DFS. Chemo well tolerated. WART well tolerated, but one treatment-related death from fecal fistula. No advantage to consolidative WART over further chemo.
- *Swedish-Norgewian Ovarian Cancer Study Group* (Sorbe, *Int J Gynecol Cancer* 2003): RCT, 172 pts, FIGO Stage III, epithelial ovarian cancer status post complete surgical remission after primary cytoreductive surgery and induction chemo (cisplatin + doxorubicin/epirubicin) randomized to: WART (20 Gy/20 fx + pelvic boost to L3/L4 20.4 Gy/12 fx), chemo (6 courses of cis + doxorubicin/epirubicin), or observation. In pts with complete surgical and pathologic remission, 5-yr PFS was better in the RT group 56% vs. 36% for chemo and 35% for observation. Treatment-related toxicity greatest with RT, with 10% Grade 3 late GI toxicity.

PALLIATIVE RADIOTHERAPY

- A number of series report palliative response in up to 50–80% of pts for bleeding or pain.

RADIATION TECHNIQUES

WART SIMULATION AND FIELD DESIGN

- Supine, alpha cradle or knee sponge, planning CT scan.
- Include entire peritoneal cavity; pelvic RT alone is never adequate as primary adjuvant therapy (Dembo 1985).
- Treat AP/PA. Borders: superior = above diaphragm; inferior = below obturator foramen; lateral = outside peritoneal reflection.
- Shield kidneys at 15 Gy and liver at 25 Gy (UCSF does not use liver blocks).
- Consider IMRT to reduce dose to bone marrow, kidneys, and liver (Rochet, BMC Cancer 2011; Strahlenther Onkol 2015).

DOSE PRESCRIPTIONS

- 30 Gy at 1.2–1.5 Gy/fx whole field; kidney blocks at 15 Gy, liver blocks at 25 Gy.
- Paraaortic boost to 45 Gy.
- Pelvis boost to 45–50.4 Gy.
- Palliation: 30 Gy in 10 fx, 14.8 Gy at 3.7 Gy BID, repeat up to 44.4 Gy with 2–4-week intervals.

VIII

DOSE LIMITATIONS (TD 5/5)

- Kidney <20 Gy
- Liver <25 Gy
- Lung: limit volume receiving ≥20 Gy (V20) <20%
- Spinal cord <45 Gy
- Bone marrow <30 Gy
- Stomach <45 Gy
- Small bowel <45–50 Gy
- Rectum <60 Gy
- Bladder <60 Gy

WART COMPLICATIONS

- Fyles et al. (1992): 598 pts received WART 1971–1985.
  - Acute: diarrhea (~70%), nausea/vomiting (60%), leukopenia (11%), thrombocytopenia (11%); 23% required treatment breaks, primarily for hematologic toxicity.

› Late: transient LFT elevation (44%), chronic diarrhea (14%), basal pneumonitis (4%), serious bowel obstruction (4.2%).

FOLLOW-UP

› H&P, including pelvic exam, every 2–4 months for 2 years, then every 3–6 months for 3 years, then annually.
› CBC annually, CA-125 at each visit if initially elevated, other labs and imaging as indicated.
› US as indicated in patients who underwent USO.
› Referral to genetic risk evaluation.

Acknowledgment We thank R. Scott Bermudez MD, James Rembert MD for their work on the prior edition of this chapter.

REFERENCES

Alektiar KM, Chi DS, Kauff ND, Fuks ZY. Cancer of the ovary. In: Leibel SA, Phillips TL, editors. Textbook of radiation oncology. 3rd ed. Philadelphia: Saunders; 2010. p. 1052–66.

Armstrong DK, Bundy B, Wenzel L, et al. Intraperitoneal cisplatin and paclitaxel in ovarian cancer. N Engl J Med.2006;354:34–43.

Bell J, Brady MF, Young RC, et al. Randomized phase III trial of three versus six cycle of adjuvant carboplatin and paclitaxel in early stage epithelial ovarian carcinoma: a gynecologic oncology group study. Gyn Oncol. 2006;102:432–9.

Bundy B, Alberts DS, et al. Phase III trial of standard-dose intravenous Cisplatin plus paclitaxel versus moderately high-dose carboplatin followed by intravenous paclitaxel and Intraperitoneal Cisplatin in Small-Volume Stage III Ovarian Carcinoma: An Intergroup Study of the Gynecologic Oncology Group, Southwestern Oncology Group, and Eastern Cooperative Group. J Clin Oncol. 2001;19:1001–7.

Burger RA, Brady MF, Bookman MA, et al. Incorporation of bevacizumab in the primary treatment of ovarian cancer. N Engl J Med. 2011;365(26):2473–83.

Chan JK, Brady MF, Penson RT, et al. Weekly vs. every-3-week paclitaxel and carboplatin for ovarian cancer. N Engl J Med. 2016;374(8):738–48.

Chiara S, Conte P, Franzone P, et al. High-risk early-stage ovarian cancer. Randomized clinical trial comparing cisplatin plus cyclophosphamide versus whole abdominal radiotherapy. Am J Clin Oncol. 1994;17(1):72–6.

Dembo AJ. Abdominopelvic radiotherapy in ovarian cancer. A 10-year experience. Cancer. 1985;55(9 Suppl):2285–90.

Edge SB, American Joint Committee on Cancer. American Cancer Society. AJCC cancer staging manual. 7th ed. New York: Springer Science+Business Media; 2010.

Ferriss JS, Java JJ, Bookman MA, et al. Ascites predicts treatment benefit of bevacizumab in front-line therapy of advanced epithelial ovarian, fallopian tube and peritoneal cancers: an NRG oncology/GOG study. Gynecol Oncol. 2015;139(1):17–22.

Fyles AW, Dembo AJ, Bush RS, et al. Analysis of complications in patients treated with abdomino-pelvic radiation therapy for ovarian carcinoma. Int J Radiat Oncol Biol Phys. 1992;22(5):847–51.

Hoskins PJ, Le N, Gilks B, et al. Low-stage ovarian clear cell carcinoma: population-based outcomes in British Columbia, Canada, with evidence for a survival benefit as a result of irradiation. J Clin Oncol. 2012;30(14):1656–62.

ICON and EORTC-ACTION investigators. International collaboration on ovarian neoplasm trial 1 and adjuvant chemotherapy in ovarian neoplasm trial: two parallel randomized phase III trials of adjuvant chemotherapy in patients with early stage ovarian cancer. J Natl Cancer Inst. 2003;95:105–12.

Katsumata N, Yasuda M, Isonishi S, et al. Long-term results of dose-dense paclitaxel and carboplatin versus conventional paclitaxel and carboplatin for treatment of advanced epithelial ovarian, fallopian tube, or primary peritoneal cancer (JGOG 3016): a randomised, controlled, open-label trial. Lancet Oncol. 2013;14(10):1020–6.

Kojs Z, Glinski B, Reinfuss M, et al. Results of a randomized prospective trial comparing postoperative abdominopelvic radiotherapy with postoperative chemotherapy in early ovarian cancer. Cancer Radiother. 2001;5:5–11.

Lambert HE, Rustin GJ, Gregory WM, Nelstrop AE. A randomized trial comparing single-agent carboplatin with carboplatin followed by radiotherapy for advanced ovarian cancer: a North Thames Ovary Group study. J Clin Oncol. 1993;11(3):440–8.

Lee L, Berkowitz R, Matulonis U. Ovarian and fallopian tube cancer. In: Halperin CE, Wazer DE, Perez CA, Brady LW, editors. Principles and practice of radiation oncology. 6th ed. Philadelphia: Lippincott Williams & Wilkins; 2013. p. 1446–64.

McGuire WP, Hosking WJ, Brady MF, et al. Taxol and cisplatin improves outcome in patients with advanced ovarian cancer as compared to cytoxan/cisplatin. N Engl J Med. 1996;334(1):1–6.

National Cancer Institute Surveillance, Epidemiology, and End Results Program (SEER). 2016. http://seer.cancer.gov/statfacts/html/ovary.html. Accessed 20 Aug 2016.

National Comprehensive Cancer Network. Clinical Practice Guidelines in Oncology: Ovarian Cancer (Version 1.2016). 2016. Available at: https://www.nccn.org/professionals/physician_gls/pdf/ovarian.pdf. Accessed on 21 Aug 2016.

Oza AM, Cook AD, Pfisterer J, et al. Standard chemotherapy with or without bevacizumab for women with newly diagnosed ovarian cancer (ICON7): overall survival results of a phase 3 randomised trial. Lancet Oncol. 2015;16(8):928–36.

Ozols RF, Bundy BN, Greer E, et al. Phase III trials of carboplatin and paclitaxel compared with cisplatin and paclitaxel in patients with optimally resected stage III ovarian cancer: a Gynecology Oncology Group study. J Clin Oncol. 2003;21:3194–200.

Perren TJ, Swart AM, Pfisterer J, et al. A phase 3 trial of bevacizumab in ovarian cancer. N Engl J Med. 2011;365(26):2484–96.

Piccart M, Bertelsen K, James K, et al. Randomized intergroup trial of cisplatin-paclitaxel versus cisplatin-cyclophosphamide in women with advanced epithelial ovarian cancer: three-year results. J Natl Cancer Inst. 2000;92:699–708.

Rochet N, Kieser M, Sterzing F, et al. Phase II study evaluating consolidation whole abdominal intensity-modulated radiotherapy (IMRT) in patients with advanced ovarian cancer stage FIGO III--the OVAR-IMRT-02 Study. BMC Cancer. 2011;11:41.

Rochet N, Lindel K, Katayama S, et al. Intensity-modulated whole abdomen irradiation following adjuvant carboplatin/taxane chemotherapy for FIGO stage III ovarian cancer: four-year outcomes. Strahlenther Onkol. 2015;191:582-9.

Sorbe B. Consolidation treatment of advanced (FIGO stage III) ovarian carcinoma in complete surgical remission after induction chemotherapy: a randomized, controlled, clinical trial comparing whole abdominal radiotherapy, chemotherapy, and no further treatment. Int J Gynecol Cancer. 2003;13(3):278–86.

Swenerton KD, Santos JL, Gilks CB, et al. Histotype predicts the curative potential of radiotherapy: the example of ovarian cancers. Ann Oncol. 2011;22:341–7.

Vicus D, Small W Jr, Covens A. Ovarian cancer. In: Gunderson LL, Tepper JE, editors. Clinical radiation oncology. 4th ed. Philadelphia: Churchill Livingstone; 2015. p. 1264–1283.e5.

VIII

Chapter 32
Vaginal Cancer

Serah Choi and Tracy Sherertz

PEARLS

- Primary vaginal cancers are rare (only 1–2% of all gynecologic malignancies).
- The most common tumors of the vagina are metastatic lesions (endometrial, ovarian, colorectal, breast, uterus, bladder, kidney).
- Presenting symptoms include: vaginal bleeding, discharge, pruritus, dyspareunia and/or pain or alterations of urinary or anorectal functions.
- 20% of vaginal tumors are detected incidentally as a result of Pap smear for cervical cancer screening.
- Tumors that involve the cervix or vulva are classified as cervical or vulvar primaries, not vaginal cancer primaries.
- ~ 50% of women diagnosed with primary vaginal carcinomas have had a prior hysterectomy for benign, premalignant, or malignant disease.
- A cancer-free period of at least 5 years distinguishes a recurrent cervical or vulvar carcinoma from a newly diagnosed primary vaginal cancer.
- ~80% of primary vaginal carcinomas are squamous cell carcinomas, which are frequently associated with HPV infection.
- HPV infection and p16 expression are associated with better prognosis in squamous cell vaginal cancers.

VIII

© Springer International Publishing AG, part of Springer Nature 2018
Eric K. Hansen and M. Roach III (eds.), *Handbook of Evidence-Based Radiation Oncology*, https://doi.org/10.1007/978-3-319-62642-0_32

- The vagina is a 3–4 in. fibromuscular tube extending from the lower aspect of the cervix to the vulva. The lower 1/3 is below the bladder base with the urethra anteriorly, the middle 1/3 is adjacent to bladder base, and the upper 1/3 at the level of the vaginal fornices.

- The most common location of primary vaginal cancer is the upper 1/3 of the vagina (~50%).

- Lymph node drainage: upper 1/3 of the vagina drains into the external iliac and paraaortic chain, the middle third into the common and internal iliac chains and the lower third into the superficial inguinal, femoral, and perirectal chains.

- Vaginal intraepithelial neoplasia (VAIN) is associated with HPV infection; frequently multifocal, and can progress to invasive disease.

- Melanoma comprises 5% and most frequently occurs in the lower 1/3 of the vagina. Verrucous carcinomas tend to recur locally, but rarely metastasize. Rare histologies include papillary serous adenocarcinoma, small cell carcinoma, botryoid variant of embryonal rhabdomyosarcoma, lymphoma, and clear cell adenocarcinoma.

- Clear cell carcinoma is associated with in utero exposure to diethylstilbestrol (DES), with a peak incidence at <30 years; adenocarcinomas not associated with DES exposure usually occur during postmenopausal years.

- Risk factors: carcinoma in situ, HPV, chronic vaginal irritation, previous abnormal Pap smears, early hysterectomy, multiple lifetime sex partners, early age at first intercourse, current smoker, in utero exposure to DES.

- For squamous cancers, the most significant prognostic factor is FIGO stage.

- Other adverse prognostic factors: age >60 years, middle or lower 1/3 location, poorly differentiated, tumor size, and anemia.

- Pelvic disease control is worse in primary non-DES–associated adenocarcinoma compared to squamous cell carcinoma (31% vs. 81%) (Frank, Gynecol Oncol 2007).

- Brachytherapy in combination with EBRT improves survival compared to EBRT alone.

, The role for chemotherapy (usually cisplatin-based) is based on small phase I and II studies and extrapolated from the cervical cancer literature.

, Combined analysis of three randomized clinical trials of the FDA-approved human papillomavirus quadrivalent (Types 6, 11, 16, 18) vaccine shows 50% efficacy (95% CI) for HPV18-related VAIN2/3 in the intention-to-treat population (Joura, Lancet 2007).

WORKUP

, H&P with bimanual and rectal exam, speculum examination, and Pap smear. On speculum exam, rotate the speculum while withdrawing to visualize the posterior wall. Examination under anesthesia, preferably with the Gynecologic Oncologist, and with biopsy if not previously performed or definitive diagnosis not yet established.

, Colposcopy with Schiller's test and multiple directed biopsies including the cervix and vulva to rule out primary cervical and/or vulvar cancer.

, Fine needle aspiration or excision of clinically or radiographically suspicious inguinal nodes.

, Cystoscopy and sigmoidoscopy for stage $\geq$ II or symptoms.

, Labs: CBC, electrolytes, BUN, Cr, LFTs including alkaline phosphatase.

, Imaging: CXR, CT $\pm$ PET (for nodal and distant metastasis), and/or MRI (to define local disease extent and assist in brachytherapy planning). On MRI, tumors are best visualized on T2-weighted imaging and appear hyperintense.

, Risk of nodal involvement generally increases with stage: I = 5%, II = 25%, III = 75%, IV = 85%. Consider biopsy of enlarged LN to confirm involvement as may be inflammatory. Conversely, normal size LN may be pathologically involved.

VIII

Table 32.1 STAGING (AJCC 7TH ED., 2010/FIGO 2008):VAGINAL CANCER

Primary tumor (T)		
TNM Categories	*FIGO* Stages*	
TX		Primary tumor cannot be assessed
T0		No evidence of primary tumor
Tis*		Carcinoma in situ (preinvasive carcinoma)
T1	I	Tumor confined to vagina
T2	II	Tumor invades paravaginal tissues, but not to pelvic wall
T3	III	Tumor extends to pelvic wall**
T4	IVA	Tumor invades mucosa of the bladder or rectum and/or extends beyond the true pelvis (bullous edema is not sufficient evidence to classify a tumor as T4)

*Note: FIGO no longer includes Stage 0 (Tis)
**Note: Pelvic wall is defined as muscle, fascia, neurovascular structures, or skeletal portions of the bony pelvis. On rectal examination, there is no cancer-free space between the tumor and pelvic wall

Regional lymph nodes (N)		
TNM Categories	*FIGO Stages*	
NX		Regional lymph nodes cannot be assessed
N0		No regional lymph node metastasis
N1	III	Pelvic or inguinal lymph node metastasis

Distant metastasis (M)		
TNM Categories	*FIGO Stages*	
M0		No distant metastasis
M1	IVB	Distant metastasis

Anatomic stage/prognostic groups

0*:	Ti N0 M0
I:	T1N0M0
IIi:	T2N0M0
III:	T1–T3N1M0
	T3N0M0
IVA:	T4 Any N M0
IVB:	Any T Any N M1

*Note: FIGO no longer includes Stage 0 (Tis)
Used with the permission from the American Joint Committee on Cancer (AJCC), Chicago, Illinois. The original source for this material is the AJCC Cancer Staging Manual, Seventh Edition (2010), published by Springer Science + Business Media

Table 32.2 STAGING (AJCC 8TH ED., 2017)

Definitions of AJCC TNM

Definition of primary tumor (T)

T category	FIGO stage	T criteria
TX		Primary tumor cannot be assessed
T0		No evidence of primary tumor
T1	I	Tumor confined to the vagina
T1a	I	Tumor confined to the vagina, measuring ≤2.0 cm
T1b	I	Tumor confined to the vagina, measuring >2.0 cm
T2	II	Tumor invading paravaginal tissues but not to the pelvic sidewall
T2a	II	Tumor invading paravaginal tissues but not to the pelvic wall, measuring ≤2.0 cm
T2b	II	Tumor invading paravaginal tissues but not to the pelvic wall, measuring >2.0 cm
T3	III	Tumor extending to the pelvic sidewall* and/or involving the lower third of the vagina and/or causing hydronephrosis or nonfunctioning kidney
T4	IVA	Tumor invading the mucosa of the bladder or rectum and/or extending beyond the true pelvis (bullous edema is not sufficient evidence to classify a tumor as T4)

Pelvic sidewall is defined as the muscle, fascia, neurovascular structures, or skeletal portions of the bony pelvis. On rectal examination, there is no cancer-free space between the tumor and the pelvic sidewall

VIII

DEFINITION OF REGIONAL LYMPH NODE (N)

N category	FIGO stage	N criteria
NX		Regional lymph nodes cannot be assessed
N0		No regional lymph node metastasis
N0(i+)		Isolated tumor cells in regional lymph node(s) not greater than 0.2 mm
N1	III	Pelvic or inguinal lymph node metastasis

DEFINITION OF DISTANT METASTASIS (M)

M category	FIGO stage	M criteria
M0		No distant metastasis
M1	IVB	Distant metastasis

AJCC PROGNOSTIC STAGE GROUPS

When T is...	And N is...	And M is...	Then the stage group is...
T1a	N0	M0	IA
Tib	N0	M0	IB
T2a	N0	M0	IIA
T2b	N0	M0	IIB
T1–T3	N1	M0	III
T3	N0	M0	III
T4	Any N	M0	IVA
Any T	Any N	M1	IVB

Used with permission of the American Joint Committee on Cancer (AJCC), Chicago, Illinois. The original and primary source for this information is the AJCC Cancer Staging Manual, Eighth Edition (2017) published by Springer International Publishing

TREATMENT RECOMMENDATIONS

Table 32.3 TREATMENT RECOMMENDATIONS

Stage	Recommended treatment	~Outcomes (5 year)
CIS	CO_2 laser or topical 5-FU or wide local excision. Close follow-up required because of multifocality and frequent progression. For recurrent cases, intracavitary (IC) brachytherapy 60–70 Gy to the entire vaginal mucosa	LC: >90% DSS: >90%
I (<0.5 cm thick, <2 cm, and low-grade)	*Surgery* (wide local excision or total vaginectomy with vaginal reconstruction). Preserves ovarian function. Post-op RT for close/+ margins *Alternative*: IC ± IS RT. treat entire vaginal mucosa to surface dose 65 Gy (60–70 Gy). Tumor with 2 cm radial margin boosted to 90 Gy mucosal dose (corresponding to ~67 Gy at 0.5 cm depth)	LC: 90% DSS: 80–85% Pelvic control: 80% DM: 10–20%
I (>0.5 cm thick, >2 cm, or high-grade)	*Surgery*: Radical vaginectomy and pelvic lymphadenectomy (for upper 2/3) or inguinal lymphadenectomy (for lower 1/3). Post-op RT for close/+ margins *Alternative*: RT. EBRT to whole pelvis ± inguinal LN to 45 Gy. IS ± IC boost to tumor with 2 cm radial margin to 75–80 Gy (corresponding to ~100–105 Gy tumor mucosal dose)	

Table 32.3 (continued)

II	EBRT to whole pelvis ± inguinal LN to 45 Gy. IS ± IC boost to tumor with 2 cm radial margin to 75–80 Gy (corresponding to ~100–105 tumor mucosal dose)	LC: 65–90% Pelvic: 65–85% DM: 20% DSS: 75–80%
III, IVA	EBRT to whole pelvis to 45–50 Gy. If lower 1/3 involvement, treat inguinal nodes to 45–50 Gy IS ± IC boost tumor with 2 cm radial margin to 75–85 Gy (corresponding to 100–110 Gy tumor mucosal dose)	*III* LC: 50–75% Pelvic: 65–70% DM: 25% DSS: 30–60%
	For lesions involving >50% of vagina, rectovaginal (RV) septum, and/or bladder, use of brachytherapy tailored to the individual patient due to risk of fistula formation	*IVA* LC: 20–40% Pelvic: 40% DM: >30% DSS: <10–20%
	For parametrial and paravaginal extension, EBRT or IS boost to 65–70 Gy For +LN, boost to 60 Gy with EBRT Consider concomitant cisplatin-based chemo (based on cervix and vulvar literature) for tumors >4 cm and III–IVA	
	If fistula or high risk of fistula, options include total vaginectomy, exenteration, and repair of fistula, if possible. LND generally performed. Avoid primary RT, especially brachytherapy	
Clear cell adeno-carcinoma	Surgery may preserve ovarian function, but it is morbid because it includes radical hysterectomy, vaginectomy, pelvic lymphadenectomy, and paraaortic lymph node sampling. If elected, definitive radiation techniques are the same as those described for Stages II, III, IV	
Metastasis	Tumor-directed palliative RT ± chemo	
Recurrence	Pelvic exenteration if no extension to side wall (removes vulva, vagina, uterus, anorectum, bladder, urethra, and pelvic and groin lymph node dissections). Interstitial brachytherapy with or without external beam radiotherapy can effectively salvage vaginal recurrence (Nag et al. 2002) in previously unradiated patients. Isolated vaginal recurrences can be salvaged with radiation therapy (Huh et al. 2007). HDR interstitial brachytherapy may be effective means of dose escalation, and HDR brachytherapy is efficacious for primary or recurrent vaginal cancer (Beriwal et al. 2008).	

VIII

STUDIES

, Most trials are retrospective and have small pt numbers. Data concerning chemotherapy are limited, and their use is extrapolated from the cervix and vulvar literature.

, There are no prospective trials comparing HDR to LDR brachytherapy.

, In general, RT is preferred over surgery, except for early or posterior Stage I lesions, distal lesions, or in the presence of a fistula.

, *Univ of Alberta experience* (Lian, Gynecol Oncol 2008): Retrospective review of 68 pts. Vaginal morbidity low if BT alone (0%), and highest in the EBRT and BT group (82.1%). Five-year DSS by stage: I 90%, II 87%, III 32%, IV 26%.

, *Gustave-Roussy Instit experience* (de Crevoisier, Radiother Oncol 2007): Retrospective review of 91 pts Five-year DSS by stage: I 83%, II 76%, III 52%. Pelvic control by stage: I 79%, II 62%, III 62%.

, *MDACC experience* (Frank, IJROBP 2005): Retrospective review of 193 pts. Tumors >4 cm did worse. Most relapse was LR (68–83%). Major complications increased with stage (4–21%). Five-year DSS by stage: I 85%, II 78%, III–IVA 58%. Vaginal control by stage: I–II 91%, III–IVA 83%. Pelvic control by stage: I 86%, II 84%, III–IVA 71%.

, Platta et al. (*J Contemp Brachytherapy*, 2013): Retrospective review of 63 pts, 1983–2009. Median f/u 44.2 mo. 5-year survival: Stages I and II, 73.3%, Stages III and IVA, 34.4%. Worse prognosis if >1/3 vaginal involvement vs. <1/3: 5-year DFS (84.0 vs. 52.4%), 5-year LC (86.9 vs. 60.4%). 5-year grade 3+ toxicity rate 23.1%. Concurrent chemo no impact on outcomes or toxicity.

, Miyamoto et al. (*PloS One*, 2013): Retrospective review of 71 pts treated between 1972 and 2009. 3-yr OS was 56% (RT) vs. 79% (chemoRT). 3-yr DFS was 43% (RT) vs. 73% (chemoRT). Relapse at any site: 23 pts. (45%) in the RT group vs. 3 (15%) in the CCRT group.

, Rajagopalan et al. (*Gynecology Oncology*, 2014): Retrospective review of 13,689 pts from the National Cancer Data Base (1998 to 2011). 8222 (60.1%) received RT and 3932 (47.8%) received CCRT. CCRT use increased from 20.8% (in 1998) to 59.1% (in 2011). Median survival for CCRT vs. RT alone: 56.2 vs. 41.2 mo. 5.9% increase in 5- yr OS with CCRT.

, Orten et al. (*Gynecology Oncology*, 2016): retrospective study of 2517 pts from the SEER database with primary vaginal cancer diagnosed from 1988 to 2011. Median OS: 3.6 yr (EBRT alone) vs. 6.1 yr (any brachy). Brachy reduced risk of death in all stage groups and tumors >5 cm had greatest benefit (HR 0.68).

RADIATION TECHNIQUES

SIMULATION AND FIELD DESIGN
EBRT

, Simulate the pt supine with tumor and introitus markers. Bolus on inguinal nodes may be needed (correlate with CT scan). If treating the inguinal nodes, treat pt in the frog-leg position. If IMRT will be used, simulate with a full and empty bladder.

, Traditional AP/PA field borders: *superior* = L5/S1 interspace (node negative pts); *inferior* = cover entire vagina and 3 cm below lowest extent of disease as marked with a radiopaque marker; *lateral* = 2 cm lateral to the pelvic brim.

, If distal 1/3 vaginal involvement, lateral borders widened to include the inguinofemoral nodes (*lateral* = greater trochanter; *inferior* = inguinal crease or 2.5 cm below ischium; *superolateral* = anterior superior iliac spine).

, If treating inguinal nodes, techniques such as IMRT may be used to protect the femoral heads as described for vulvar and anal cancer.

, A midline block/central sparing is optional in effort to decrease dose to the bladder and rectum. If a midline block is not used, the brachytherapy dose must be reduced, depending on the total cumulative EQD2 dose.

, If 4-field technique is used, care must be taken to avoid underdosing the presacral, perirectal, and anterior external iliac LN. On the lateral fields: *anterior border* = pubic symphysis and *posterior border* = S2/S3 or behind sacrum, depending on stage. Contour nodal volumes to ensure coverage.

VIII

- IMRT techniques require great care in treatment planning and careful attention to primary tumor and LN mapping (Frumovitz, Gynecol Oncol 2008). The vaginal apex can be displaced by 1.5–2 cm in the AP direction with organ filling.
- External beam RT CTV generally includes GTV + 1–2 cm margin; entire vagina; paravaginal area up to pelvic side-walls; and bilateral pelvic nodes (common iliac, external iliac, internal iliac, obturator, presacral). Treat to 45–50.4 Gy in 25–28 fx.
- Prior to brachy boost, consider restaging with MRI of the pelvis with IV contrast and intravaginal contrast for brachy planning.
- Consider concurrent chemotherapy for high-risk pts. (tumors >4 cm or Stage III–IVA) with good performance status.

Brachytherapy

- Brachytherapy monotherapy may be used for early-stage, well-defined lesions involving <50% vagina and not involving rectovaginal septum.
- IC brachytherapy uses largest possible vaginal cylinder to improve the ratio of mucosa to tumor dose.
- Dome cylinders are used for homogenous irradiation of the vaginal cuff.
- Upper 1/3 lesions may be treated with an intrauterine tandem and vaginal colpostats, followed by treatment of the middle and lower 1/3 of the vagina with a vaginal cylinder with a blank source at the top of the cylinder if full dose has already been reached at the apex. Careful attention to cumulative doses to the bladder and rectum are critical.
- IS brachytherapy is preferred for lesions >0.5 cm to improve coverage. Use CT or MRI-based planning. Follow ABS recommendations (Beriwal, Brachytherapy 2012).
- HDR dose is ~60% of LDR dose.
- Typical HDR boost dose after 45 Gy EBRT = 6–7 Gy × 3 (~30 Gy LDR equivalent).

DOSE LIMITATIONS

- Upper vaginal mucosa tolerance is 120 Gy, mid-vaginal mucosal tolerance is 80–90 Gy, and lower-vaginal mucosa

tolerance is 60–70 Gy. Vaginal doses >50–60 Gy increase risk of significant vaginal fibrosis and stenosis.
, Ovarian failure is age-dependent, usually occurs with 5–10 Gy. Sterilization occurs with 2–3 Gy.
, Limit bladder D2cc <90 Gy and rectum D2cc <65 Gy (EQD2).

COMPLICATIONS

, Complications are dose-related and include vaginal dryness and atrophy, pubic hair loss, vaginal stenosis and fibrosis (~50%), cystitis (~50%), proctitis (~40%), rectovaginal or vesicovaginal fistula (<5%), vaginal necrosis (<5–15%), lymphedema (increased risk in post-op setting), urethral stricture (rare), and small bowel obstruction (rare in the absence of prior abdominal surgery).
, Vaginal dilators and topical estrogen used to minimize stenosis.
, Radiation-induced menopause; consider ovarian transposition prior to pelvic radiation for premenopausal patients.
, Smoking cessation should be encouraged to reduce risk of late radiation toxicity.

VIII

FOLLOW-UP

, H&P (with pelvic exam and Pap smear) every 3 months for 1 year, every 4 months for second year, every 6 months for third and fourth years, then annually. CXR annually for 5 years.

Acknowledgment We thank Thomas T. Bui MD, Eric K. Hansen MD, and Joycelyn L. Speight MD, PhD for their work on the prior edition of this chapter.

REFERENCES

Alonso I, Felix A, Torné A, et al. Human papillomavirus as a favorable prognostic biomarker in squamous cell carcinomas of the vagina. Gynecol Oncol. 2012;125(1):194–9.

Beriwal S, Demanes DJ, Erickson B, et al. American Brachytherapy Society consensus guidelines for interstitial brachytherapy for vaginal cancer. Brachytherapy. 2012;11(1):68–75.

Beriwal S, Heron DE, Mogus R, et al. High-dose rate brachytherapy (HDRB) for primary or recurrent cancer in the vagina. Radiat Oncol. 2008;3:7.

Chyle V, Zagars GK, Wheeler JA, et al. Definitive radiotherapy for carcinoma of the vagina: outcome and prognostic factors. Int J Radiat Oncol Biol Phys. 1996;35:891–905.

de Crevoisier R, Sanfilippo N, et al. Exclusive radiotherapy for primary squamous cell carcinoma of the vagina. Radiother Oncol. 2007;85(3):362–70.

Edge SB, American Joint Committee on Cancer. American Cancer Society. AJCC cancer staging manual. 7th ed. New York: Springer Science+Business Media; 2010.

Feldbaum VM, Flowers LC, Oprea-Ilies GM. Improved survival in p16-positive vaginal cancers across all tumor stages but no correlation with MIB-1. Am J Clin Pathol. 2014;142(5):664–9.

Frank SJ, Deaver MT, Jhingran A, et al. Primary adenocarcinoma of the vagina not associated with diethylstilbestrol (DES) exposure. Gynecol Oncol. 2007;105(2):470–4.

Frank SJ, Jhingran A, Levenback C, et al. Definitive radiation therapy for squamous cell carcinoma of the vagina. Int J Radiat Oncol Biol Phys. 2005;62:138–47.

Frumovitz M, Gayed IW, Jhingran A, et al. Lymphatic mapping and sentinel lymph node detection in women with vaginal cancer. Gynecol Oncol. 2008;108(3):478–81.

Gardner CS, Sunil J, Klopp AH, et al. Primary vaginal cancer: role of MRI in diagnosis, staging and treatment. BJR. 2015;88(1052):20150033–11.

Green S, Stock RG. Cancer of the vagina. In: Leibel SA, Phillips TL, editors. Textbook of radiation oncology. 3rd ed. Philadelphia: Saunders; 2010. p. 1067–84.

Harris EE, Latifi K, Rusthoven C, Javedan K, Forster K. Assessment of organ motion in postoperative endometrial and cervical cancer pts treated with intensity-modulated radiation therapy. Int J Radiat Oncol Biol Phys. 2011;81(4):e645–50.

Huh WK, Straughn JM Jr, Mariani A, et al. Salvage of isolated vaginal recurrences in women with surgical stage I endometrial cancer: a multiinstitutional experience. Int J Gynecol Cancer. 2007;17(4):886–9.

Jhingran A, Salehpour M, Sam M, Levy L, Eifel PJ. Vaginal motion and bladder and rectal volumes during pelvic intensity-modulated radiation therapy after hysterectomy. Int J Radiat Oncol Biol Phys. 2012;82(1):256–62.

Joura EA, Leodolter S, Hernandez-Avila M, et al. Efficacy of a quadrivalent prophylactic human papillomavirus (types 6, 11, 16, and 18) L1 virus-like-particle vaccine against high-grade vulval and vaginal lesions: a combined analysis of three randomised clinical trials. Lancet. 2007;369(9574):1693–702.

Kang J, Viswanathan AN. Vaginal Cancer. In: Perez CA, Brady LW, Halperin EC, et al., editors. Principles and practice of radiation oncology. 6th ed. Philadelphia: Lippincott Williams & Wilkins; 2013. p. 1465–501.

Klopp AH, Eifel PJ, Berek JS, Konstantinopoulous PA. Cancer of the cervix, vagina, and vulva. In: DeVita Jr VT, Lawrence TS, Rosenberg SA, editors. DeVita, Hellman, and Rosenberg's cancer principles & practice of oncology. 10th ed. Philadelphia: Wolters Kluwer Health; 2015. p. 1013–47.

Lian J, Dundas G, Carlone M, Ghosh S, Pearcey R. Twenty-year review of radiotherapy for vaginal cancer: an institutional experience. Gynecol Oncol. 2008;111(2):298–306.

Miyamoto DT, Viswanathan AN. Concurrent chemoradiation for vaginal cancer. PLoS One. 2013;8(6):e65048.

Morris M, Blessing JA, Monk BJ, et al. Phase II study of cisplatin and vinorelbine in squamous cell carcinoma of the cervix: a Gynecologic Oncology Group Study. J Clin Oncol. 2004;22(16):3340–4.

Nag S, Yacoub S, Copeland LJ, Fowler JM. Interstitial brachytherapy for salvage treatment of vaginal recurrences in previously unirradiated endometrial cancer pts. Int J Radiat Oncol Biol Phys. 2002;54:1153–9.

National Cancer Institute. Vaginal Cancer (PDQ): Treatment. 2016. Available at: http://www.cancer.gov/types/vaginal/hp/vaginal-treatment-pdq. Accessed on 15 Aug 2016.

Orton A, Boothe D, Williams N, et al. Brachytherapy improves survival in primary vaginal cancer. Gynecol Oncol. 2016;141(3):501–6.

Platta CS, Anderson B, Geye H, Das R, Straub M, Bradley K. Adjuvant and definitive radiation therapy for primary carcinoma of the vagina using brachytherapy and external beam radiation therapy. J Contemp Brachytherapy. 2013;2:76–82.

Perez CA, Grigsby PW, Garipagaoglu M, et al. Factors affecting long-term outcome of irradiation in carcinoma of the vagina. Int J Radiat Oncol Biol Phys. 1999;44:37–45.

Rajagopalan MS, Xu KM, Lin JF, Sukumvanich P, Krivak TC, Beriwal S. Adoption and impact of concurrent chemoradiation therapy for vaginal cancer: a National Cancer Data Base (NCDB) study. Gynecol Oncol. 2014;135(3):495–502.

Russell AH, Horowitz NS. Vulvar and vaginal carcinoma. In: Gunderson LL, Tepper JE, editors. Clinical radiation oncology. 4th ed. Philadelphia: Churchill Livingstone; 2015. p. 1230–63.

Samant R, Lau B, Choan E, et al. Primary vaginal cancer treated with concurrent chemoradiation using cis-platinum. Int J Radiat Oncol Biol Phys. 2007;69:746–50.

Stock RG, Chen AS, Seski J. A 30-year experience in the management of primary carcinoma of the vagina: analysis of prognostic factors and treatment modalities. Gynecol Oncol. 1995;56(1):45–52.

Tran PT, Su Z, Lee P, et al. Prognostic factors for outcomes and complications for primary squamous cell carcinoma of the vagina treated with radiation. Int J Radiat Oncol Biol Phys. 2006;S66:1052.

VIII

Chapter 33
Vulvar Cancer

Serah Choi and Tracy Sherertz

PEARLS

- ~5% of all gynecologic malignancies in the United States.
- Anatomy: mons pubis, clitoris, labia majora, labia minora, vaginal vestibule, Bartholin's glands (at posterior labia majora), prepuce over clitoris, posterior fourchette, perineal body.
- Approximately 70% arise in the labia and ~15% arise in the clitoris or perineal body.
- Common presenting symptoms: pruritus, pain, and/or palpable vulvar mass or ulcer.
- Risk factors: HPV, vulvar intraepithelial neoplasia (2–5% progress to vaginal cancer), history of genital warts, multiple sexual partners, history of abnormal Pap smears, immunosuppression, smoking, increasing age, Bowen's disease, Paget's disease, leukoplakia.
- ~80–90% are squamous cell carcinomas. Bartholin's tumors can be adenocarcinomas, adenoid cystic carcinomas, or squamous if they arise in the ductal squamous epithelium. Other histologies: melanoma, sarcoma, basal cell carcinoma, Merkel cell tumors, carcinoid, transitional cell carcinoma, apocrine gland cancer, Paget's disease, and metastatic lesions.

VIII

© Springer International Publishing AG, part of Springer Nature 2018   **707**
Eric K. Hansen and M. Roach III (eds.), *Handbook of Evidence-Based Radiation Oncology*, https://doi.org/10.1007/978-3-319-62642-0_33

- Melanomas <10% of primary tumors, but are the second most common malignancy of the vulva.
- LN involvement is the most important prognostic factor for survival. 5-yr OS: 86% if limited to vulva, 54% if regional nodes involved, 16% if metastatic disease. ~23% of pts have a local recurrence at 5 years.
- LN spread is to inguinofemoral nodes (superficial and deep). Most superior deep femoral node = Cloquet's node.
- Clitoris can theoretically drain directly to pelvic LN, but rare without inguinofemoral LN involvement.
- Risk of nodal involvement correlates with stage and depth of tumor invasion:
  - IA <1 mm deep <5%, 1–3 mm deep 8–10%, 3–5 mm deep 20%.
  - 5 mm deep or >2 cm size 40%.
  - III 30–80%.
  - IV 80–100%.
- Approximately 20–25% of cN0 pts are pN+.
- Overall incidence of pelvic LN+ is 5%. If inguinal LN+, ~30% risk of pelvic LN+.
- HPV or p16 positivity is associated with better PFS and fewer in-field relapses after RT in vulvar SCC

WORKUP

- H&P with examination under anesthesia (EUA).
- Colposcopy and biopsy of primary and FNA or excisional biopsy of clinically positive inguinal nodes.
- Pap smear of cervix and vagina.
- Cystoscopy, urethroscopy, and/or sigmoidoscopy may be indicated for advanced stages and/or bladder/bowel symptoms.
- CBC, UA, LFT/renal function studies.
- CXR. CT/PET/MRI as needed for evaluating extent of tumor, nodal involvement, and/or for treatment planning.
- Smoking cessation and counseling, if indicated.

STAGING: VULVAR CANCER

Editors' note: All TNM stage and stage groups referred to elsewhere in this chapter reflect the 2010 AJCC staging nomenclature unless otherwise noted as the new system below was published after this chapter was written.

Table 33.1   (AJCC 7TH ED., 2010/FIGO 2008)

Primary tumor (T)		
TNM *Categories*	FIGO *Stages*	
TX		Primary tumor cannot be assessed
T0		No evidence of primary tumor
Tis*		Carcinoma in situ (preinvasive carcinoma)
T1a	IA	Lesions 2 cm or less in size, confined to the vulva or perineum and with stromal invasion 1.0 mm or less**
T1b	IB	Lesions more than 2 cm in size *or* any size with stromal invasion more than 1.0 mm, confined to the vulva or perineum
T2***	II	Tumor of any size with extension to adjacent perineal structures (lower/distal 1/3 urethra, lower/distal 1/3 vagina, anal involvement)
T3****	IVA	Tumor of any size with extension to any of the following: upper/proximal 2/3 of urethra, upper/proximal 2/3 vagina, bladder mucosa, rectal mucosa, or fixed to pelvic bone

Note: FIGO no longer includes stage 0 (Tis)
**Note*: The depth of invasion is defined as the measurement of the tumor from the epithelial–stromal junction of the adjacent most superficial dermal papilla to the deepest point of invasion
****FIGO uses the classification T2/T3. This is defined as T2 in TNM
*****FIGO uses the classification T4. This is defined as T3 in TNM

VIII

Table 33.1 (CONTINUED)

Regional lymph nodes (N)

TNM Categories	FIGO Stages	
NX		Regional lymph nodes cannot be assessed
N0		No regional lymph node metastasis
N1		One or two regional lymph nodes with the following features
N1a	IIIA	One lymph node metastasis each 5 mm or less
N1b	IIIA	One lymph node metastasis 5 mm or greater
N2	IIIB	Regional lymph node metastasis with the following features
N2a	IIIB	Three or more lymph node metastases each less than 5 mm
N2b	IIIB	Two or more lymph node metastases 5 mm or greater
N2c	IIIC	Lymph node metastasis with extracapsular spread
N3	IVA	Fixed or ulcerated regional lymph node metastasis

Distant metastasis (M)

TNM Categories	FIGO Stages	
M0		No distant metastasis
M1	IVB	Distant metastasis (including pelvic lymph node metastasis)

Anatomic stage/prognostic groups

0*:	Tis N0 M0
I:	T1 N0 M0
IA:	T1a N0 M0
IB:	T1b N0 M0
II:	T2 N0 M0
IIIA:	T1, T2 N1a, N1b M0
IIIB:	T1, T2 N2a, N2b M0
IIIC:	T1, T2 N2c M0
IVA:	T1, T2 N3 M0
	T3 Any N M0
IVB:	Any T Any N M1

Used with the permission from the American Joint Committee on Cancer (AJCC), Chicago, Illinois. The original source for this material is the AJCC Cancer Staging Manual, Seventh Edition (2010), published by Springer Science + Business Media

FIGO staging: Pecorelli 2009, Copyright 2009, with permission from Elsevier

*Note: FIGO no longer includes stage 0 (Tis)

Table 33.2 (AJCC 8TH ED., 2017)

Definitions of AJCC TNM

Definition of primary tumor (T)

T category	FIGO stage	T criteria
TX		Primary tumor cannot be assessed
T0		No evidence of primary tumor
T1	I	Tumor confined to the vulva and/or perineum Multifocal lesions should be designated as such. The largest lesion or the lesion with the greatest depth of invasion will be the target lesion identified to address the highest pT stage The depth of invasion is defined as the measurement of the tumor from the epithelial-stromal junction of the adjacent most superficial dermal papilla to the deepest point of invasion
T1a	IA	Lesions 2 cm or less, confined to the vulva and/or perineum, and with stromal invasion of 1.0 mm or less
T1b	IB	Lesions more than 2 cm, or any size with stromal invasion of more than 1.0 mm, confined to the vulva and/or perineum
T2	II	Tumor of any size with extension to adjacent perineal structures (lower/distal third of the urethra, lower/distal third of the vagina, anal involvement)
T3	IVA	Tumor of any size with extension to any of the following—upper/proximal two thirds of the urethra, upper/proximal two thirds of the vagina, bladder mucosa, or rectal mucosa—or fixed to the pelvic bone

VIII

DEFINITION OF REGIONAL LYMPH NODE (N)

N category	FIGO stage	N criteria
NX		Regional lymph nodes cannot be assessed
N0		No regional lymph node metastasis
N0(i+)		Isolated tumor cells in regional lymph node(s) not greater than 0.2 mm
N1	III	Regional lymph node metastasis with one or two lymph node metastases each less than 5 mm, or one lymph node metastasis =5 mm
N1a*	IIIA	One or two lymph node metastases each less than 5 mm
N1b	IIIA	One lymph node metastasis =5 mm
N2		Regional lymph node metastasis with three or more lymph node metastases each less than 5 mm, or two or more lymph node metastases =5 mm, or lymph node(s) with extranodal extension
N2a*	IIIB	Three or more lymph node metastases each less than 5 mm
N2b	IIIB	Two or more lymph node metastases =5 mm
N2c	IIIC	Lymph node(s) with extranodal extension
N3	IVA	Fixed or ulcerated regional lymph node metastasis

*Includes micrometastasis, N1mi, and N2mi

Note: The site, size, and laterality of the lymph node metastases should be recorded

DEFINITION OF DISTANT METASTASIS (M)

M category	FIGO stage	M criteria
M0		No distant metastasis (no pathological M0; use clinical M to complete stage group)
M1	IVB	Distant metastasis (including pelvic lymph node metastasis)

AJCC PROGNOSTIC STAGE GROUPS

When T is...	And N is...	And M is...	Then the stage group is...
T1	N0	M0	I
T1a	N0	M0	IA
T1b	N0	M0	IB
T2	N0	M0	II
T1–T2	N1–N2c	M0	III
T1–T2	N1	M0	IIIA
T1–T2	N2a, N2b	M0	IIIB
T1–T2	N2c	M0	IIIC
T1–T3	N3	M0–M1	IV
T1–T2	N3	M0	IVA
T3	Any N	M0	IVA
Any T	Any N	M1	IVB

Used with permission of the American Joint Committee on Cancer (AJCC), Chicago, Illinois. The original and primary source for this information is the AJCC Cancer Staging Manual, eighth edition (2017), published by Springer International Publishing

TREATMENT RECOMMENDATIONS

Table 33.3 TREATMENT RECOMMENDATIONS

Stage	Recommended treatment
CIS	Local excision or CO_2 laser
IA	Wide local excision (WLE). Post-op RT (50 Gy) to vulva for + margin, margin<8 mm, LVSI, or depth > 5 mm. [Sample lymph nodes for lesion with >1 mm depth of invasion]
IB/II	WLE with ipsilateral (superficial) LN dissection or sentinel lymph node biopsy for lateralized lesions. Bilateral (superficial) LN dissection for central lesions, lesions>5 mm deep, LVSI, or poorly differentiated lesions. If LN+, add deep inguinal dissection. Post-op RT to vulva for + margin, margin<8 mm, LVSI, or lesions >5 mm deep. Post-op RT to inguinal and pelvic nodes for >1 LN+, or nodal ECE
	Alternatively, consider pre-op chemo-RT (50 Gy for cN- or 54 Gy for cN+) for lesions close to urethra, clitoris, or rectum because margin may be difficult to obtain. Either elective chemo-RT to groins or planned LN dissection (before or after chemo-RT). If bilateral LN dissection performed initially, pathologic LN findings dictate whether or not RT needed to groins. However, chemo-RT to primary lesion could be delayed. If primary lesion has CR to chemo-RT, consider biopsy, and if negative observation. If <CR or biopsy demonstrates persistent disease, resect with functional preservation if possible, or boost primary to 65–70 Gy or consider radical vulvectomy

Table 33.3 (CONTINUED)

Stage	Recommended treatment
III/IVA	If cN0, perform bilateral LN dissection first followed by chemo-RT to vulva or vulva and inguinal/pelvic nodes (for ECE, >1 LN+)
	If cN+ fixed or ulcerated, pre-op chemo-RT (45–50 Gy with cisplatin, 5-FU, and/or mitomycin C) provides about 50% CR. Follow with bilateral LN dissection. Surgical salvage for persistent or recurrent disease. If nodal ECE boost to 60 Gy; if gross residual take to 65–70 Gy

STUDIES

INDICATIONS FOR ADJUVANT POST-OP VULVAR RT

- Heaps (Gynecol Oncol 1990): review of surgical-pathologic factors predictive of LR for 135 pts with vulvar CA. Increased LR with + margin, margin <8 mm pathologically or <1 cm clinically, LVSI, and depth > 5 mm.

INDICATIONS FOR PELVIC/INGUINAL RT

- GOG 37 (Homesley, Obstet Gynecol 1986): 114 pts treated with radical vulvectomy and b/l inguinal LND and found to have any inguinal LN+ were randomized to pelvic LN dissection (n = 55) vs. post-op RT (n = 59) with 45–50 Gy to pelvic and b/l inguinal LN (but not to vulva). RT decreased groin recurrence (5% vs. 24%) and improved 2-yr OS (68% vs. 54%). Subset analysis showed benefit only in cN+, pts with >1 pN+ or +LN with ECE. No difference in pelvic recurrence.
- GOG 37 update (Kunos, Obstet Gynecol 2009): 74 mo median survivor f/u. 6-yr OS: 51% post-op RT vs. 41% PLND (p = 0.18). 6-yr cancer-related deaths: 51% post-op RT vs. 29% PLND (SS). >20% ratio of positive ipsilateral LN (# positive LN/# resected) associated with contralateral LN met, relapse, and cancer-related death. Similar late toxicities rates between post-op RT and PLND.

VIII

NODAL EVALUATION AND MANAGEMENT

- GOG 88 (Stehman, IJROBP 1992): 121 pts with IB–III cN0 treated with radical vulvectomy randomized to b/l inguinal RT (50 Gy to D3, without pelvic RT) vs. b/l radical LN dissection. If pLN+, then received RT (50 Gy) to b/l groin and pelvis. Interim analysis of only 58 pts demonstrated improved 2-yr OS (90% vs. 70%) with surgery and decreased inguinal recurrences.
  - Criticisms: RT addressed only inguinal nodes, whereas surgery included pelvic LN dissection if inguinal LN+; arms biased since no CT used for staging; poor technique of RT (prescribed to D3, all inguinal recurrences received < prescribed dose); 50 Gy should sterilize microscopic disease as evidenced by University of Wisconsin retrospective review with good technique (Petereit, *IJROBP* 1993).
- Kirby (Gynecol Oncol 2005): retrospective review of 65 pts with stage I/II vulvar cancer treated with vulvectomy and superficial inguinal lymphadenectomy (SupIL). Pts with pathologically negative SupIL had 4.6% recurrence rate in the inguinal region and 16.9% recurrence on the vulva. 5-yr DFS and OS were 66% and 97%, respectively.
- Van der Zee (JCO 2008): observational study looking at 623 groins in 403 pts. 259 pts with unifocal vulvar disease and negative sentinel node (SN). 3-yr groin recurrence rate was 2.3% and OS 97%. Short-term and long-term morbidity was decreased with sentinel node removal vs. sentinel node removal + inguino-femoral lymphadenectomy. Basis for GOG 173.
- GOG 173 (Levenbach, JCO 2012): 452 pts with SCC vulva, depth of invasion at least 1 mm, tumor limited to the vulva, primary tumor size 2–6 cm, no inguinal LN on exam, had SLNB followed by lymphadenectomy. SLN identified in 92% of pts, of which 32% were positive, but 8% false-negative SLN rate (positive LN found with complete dissection). For pts with tumors <4 cm, if SLN negative, the risk of a false-negative SLN is <3%.

CHEMO-RT

- GOG 101 (Moore, IJROBP 1998): phase II trial of 41 pts with unresectable T3 or T4, any LN status treated with pre-op chemo-RT with 1.7 Gy b.i.d. d1–4, 1.7 Gy qd d5–12 to 23.8 Gy with cisplatin on d1 and 5-FU on d1–4 → 2 week break → repeat to total dose 47.6 Gy. For cN0, RT was to vulvar area only and for cN+ included inguinal and pelvic LN. Surgery 4–8 wks after chemo-RT. Pre-op chemo-RT had 47% cCR and 55% 4-yr OS (expect 20–50%). 54% had gross residual disease, but only 3% were unresectable.

- GOG 101 (Montana, IJROBP 2000): 46 pts with advanced disease in the inguino-femoral nodes (stage IVA) N2/N3 received a split course of RT (47.6 Gy) to the primary and LN with concurrent cisplatin/5-FU followed by surgery. 95% were deemed resectable after chemo-RT. LC of primary and lymph nodes was 76% and 97%, respectively.

- Landrum (Gynecol Oncol 2008): 63 pts with stage III/IV disease treated with primary surgery vs. primary chemo-RT (weekly cis or 2 cycles of cisplatin plus 5-FU with RT). Primary chemo-RT pts were younger (61 vs. 72 yo), had fewer nodal metastasis (54% vs. 83%), and larger tumors (6 vs. 3.5 cm). No difference in OS, PFS, or recurrence rates between surgery and chemo-RT groups.

- GOG 205 (Moore, Gynecol Oncol 2012): phase II, 58 pts, unresectable T3 or T4, any N. RT (1.8 × 32 daily fx = 57.6 Gy) with weekly cisplatin (no 5-FU) followed by resection of residual disease. cCR in 37 pts (64%), of which 29 had pCR (50% of total).

VIII

IMRT

- Beriwal (IJROBP, 2006): retrospective study, 15 pts treated with IMRT; 7 pts with pre-op chemo-RT (cis + 5FU) and 8 pts with post-op RT. Median dose: 46 Gy in the pre-op, 50.4 Gy post-op groups. Mean volume > 30 Gy was reduced with IMRT vs. 3D CRT: small bowel (44% vs. 71%); rectum (45% vs. 87%); bladder (62% vs. 88%). Grade 3 small-bowel toxicity in 1 pt. At median f/u 12 mos, 5 pts (71%) had cCR and 3 pts (42.8%) had pCR in pre-op group. In the adjuvant group, 2 pts had recurrences in the treatment field. No late Grade 3 toxicities.

- Beriwal (IJROBP, 2013): retrospective study, 42 pts, stage I-IVA treated twice-daily IMRT and with 5-FU/cisplatin during the first and last weeks of treatment or weekly cisplatin with daily RT. Median dose 46.4 Gy. 33 pts (78.6%) had resection of vulva, 13 of which had inguinal LND. pCR in 48.5%, of which 15 had no recurrence within a median time of 26.5 mos. 17 pts had partial CR, 8 of which (47.1%) developed recurrence in the vulvar surgical site within a median follow-up of 8 mos. No grade 3 chronic GI/GU toxicities.

MIDLINE BLOCK
- Dusenberry (IJROBP 1994): 27 pts with stage III/IV disease with pLN+ treated with post-op RT with a midline block. 48% central recurrence rate with the use of the midline block. Authors recommended including tumor bed (no midline block) post-op RT for pts with LN+.

RADIATION TECHNIQUES

SIMULATION AND FIELD DESIGN
- Simulate supine, frog-leg position with custom immobilization.
- Wire vulva, anus, scars. Simulate with and without bolus or use virtual bolus in planning. If rectum distended >3.5 cm, repeat simulation after further bowel prep.
- Traditional borders: superior = L5/S1 or mid SI if clinically no involved pelvic LN (L4/5 if pelvic LN+); inferior = flash vulva and 3 cm inferior to bottom of ischium; lateral = 2 cm beyond pelvic brim and greater trochanter (anterior superior iliac spine) to include inguinal LN.
- Bolus vulva +/- groin(s) prn. Confirm dose received under bolus with TLDs early in treatment course.
- CT plan depth of groin nodes. May need to boost groins with en face electrons.
- MRI may identify satellite lesions, muscle invasion, and/or dermal involvement not easily identified on CT.

- Follow consensus recommendations for contouring vulva and regional nodes (Gaffney, IJROBP 2016). Consider IMRT to reduce dose to normal structures.
- GTV = gross disease on exam, CT, MRI.
- Primary CTV:
  - Always include at least 1 cm margin on GTV and entire vulva.
  - If GTV invades vagina, include 3 cm CTV margin on GTV or entire vaginal canal.
  - If GTV invades anus, bladder, or rectum, include 2 cm CTV margin on anorectum or bladder.
  - If GTV invades urethral meatus, include 2 cm CTV margin.
  - If GTV invades mid or proximal urethra, include entire urethra and bladder neck in CTV.
  - If GTV invades clitoris, include 2 cm CTV margin.
  - If post-op, negative margins, include entire operative bed. If close/+ margin, add 2 cm margin.
- LN CTV:
  - In general, include entire nodal bed plus echelon above grossly involved LN. If groin node grossly involved, include contralateral groin in CTV too.
  - For lesions involving only vulva or vulva and distal vagina, include bilateral inguino-femoral, obturator, internal and external iliac LN.
  - If proximal half of posterior vagina involved, also include presacral S1–S3 nodes.
  - If anus/anal canal involved, include bilateral inguino-femoral, obturator, internal and external iliac, peri-rectal, and presacral nodes.
- PTV = CTV + 0.7–1 cm depending on body habitus, stability.

VIII

DOSE PRESCRIPTIONS
- 1.8 Gy/fx.
- Post-op: 45-50.4 Gy to vulva tumor bed and regional LN. Boost primary up to 60–70 Gy for close or involved margins. Boost nodal extracapsular extension to 54–60 Gy.

- Definitive: primary and involved nodes 60–70 Gy; 45–50.4 Gy for elective nodes.
  - Boost may require brachytherapy.

DOSE LIMITATIONS
- Small bowel <45–55 Gy, prefer V40 Gy to V45 Gy <30%
- Femoral heads <45 Gy, prefer V30 Gy <50%, V40 Gy < 35%, V44 Gy <5%
- Bladder <60 Gy, prefer V45 Gy to V50 Gy <35%
- Rectum <60 Gy, prefer V45 Gy <60%
- Lower vagina <75–80 Gy

COMPLICATIONS
- Acute: epilation of pubic hair, hyperpigmentation, skin reaction, moist desquamation, diarrhea, cystitis.
- Late: atrophy of skin and telangiectasia, shortening and narrowing of vagina, vaginal dryness. Femoral neck fracture <5%, associated with osteoporosis and smoking.

FOLLOW-UP

- H&P q3–6 mo × 2 yrs, every 6–12 mo × 3–5 yrs, then annually based on risk of disease recurrence.

Acknowledgment We thank Stephen Shiao MD, PhD, Brian Missett MD, and Joycelyn L. Speight MD, PhD for their work on the prior edition of this chapter.

REFERENCES

Beriwal S, Heron DE, Kim H, et al. Intensity-modulated radiotherapy for the treatment of vulvar carcinoma: a comparative dosimetric study with early clinical outcome. Int J Radiat OncolBiolPhys. 2006;64(5):1395–400.

Beriwal S, Shukla G, Shinde A, et al. Preoperative intensity modulated radiation therapy and chemotherapy for locally advanced vulvar carcinoma: analysis of pattern of relapse. Radiat Oncol Biol. 2013;85(5):1269–74.

Burger MP, Hollema H, Emanuels AG, Krans M, Pras E, Bouma J. The importance of the groin node status for the survival of T1 and T2 vulval carcinoma patients. Gynecol Oncol. 1995;57(3):327–34.

Dusenbery KE, Carlson JW, LaPorte RM, et al. Radical vulvectomy with postoperative irradiation for vulvar cancer: therapeutic implications of a central block. Int J Radiat Oncol Biol Phys. 1994;29:989–98.

Gaffney DK, King B, Viswanathan AN, et al. Consensus recommendations for radiation therapy contouring and treatment of vulvar carcinoma. Int J Radiat Oncol Biol Phys. 2016;95(4):1191–200.

Gill BS, Bernard ME, Lin JF, et al. Impact of adjuvant chemotherapy with radiation for node-positive vulvar cancer: a National Cancer Data Base (NCDB) analysis. Gynecol Oncol. 2015;137(3):365–72.

Heaps JM, Fu YS, Montz FJ, et al. Surgical–pathologic variables predictive of local recurrence in squamous cell carcinoma of the vulva. Gynecol Oncol. 1990;38:309–14.

Homesley HD, Bundy BN, Sedlis A, et al. Radiation therapy versus pelvic node resection for carcinoma of the vulva with positive groin nodes. Obstet Gynecol. 1986;68:733–40.

Kirby TO, Rocconi RP, Numnum TM, et al. Outcomes of stage I/II vulvar cancer patients after negative superficial inguinal lymphadenectomy. Gynecol Oncol. 2005;98:309–12.

Klopp AH, Eifel PJ, Berek JS, Konstantinopoulous PA. Cancer of the cervix, vagina, and vulva. In: DeVita Jr VT, Lawrence TS, Rosenberg SA, editors. DeVita, Hellman, and Rosenberg's cancer principles & practice of oncology. 10th ed. Philadelphia: Wolters Kluwer Health; 2015. p. 1013–47.

Kunos C, Simpkins F, Gibbons H, et al. Radiation therapy compared with pelvic node resection for node-positive vulvar cancer: a randomized controlled trial. Obstet Gynecol. 2009;114:537–46.

Landrum LM, Grainger SL, Skaggs VJ, et al. Gynecologic Oncology Group risk groups for vulvar carcinoma: improvement in survival in the modern era. Gynecol Oncol. 2007;106:521–5.

Landrum LM, Skaggs V, Gould N. Comparison of outcome measures in patients with advanced squamous cell carcinoma of the vulva treated with surgery or primary chemoradiation. Gynecol Oncol. 2008;108(3):584–90.

Lee LJ, Howitt B, Catalano P, et al. Prognostic importance of human papillomavirus (HPV) and p16 positivity in squamous cell carcinoma of the vulva treated with radiotherapy. Gynecol Oncol. 2016;142(2):293–8.

Levenback CF, Ali S, Coleman RL, et al. Lymphatic mapping and sentinel lymph node biopsy in women with squamous cell carcinoma of the vulva: a gynecologic oncology group study. J Clin Oncol. 2012;30(31):3786–91.

Montana GS, Kang S. Carcinoma of the vulva. In: Perez CA, Brady LW, Halperin EC, et al., editors. Principles and practice of radiation oncology. 5th ed. Philadelphia: Lippincott Williams & Wilkins; 2008. p. 1692–707.

Montana GS, Thomas GM, Moore DH, et al. Preoperative chemo-radiation for carcinoma of the vulve with N2/N3 nodes: a gynecologic oncology group study. Int J Radiat Oncol Biol Phys. 2000;48:1007–13.

Moore DH, Ali S, Koh W-J, et al. A phase II trial of radiation therapy and weekly cisplatin chemotherapy for the treatment of locally-advanced squamous cell carcinoma of the vulva: a gynecologic oncology group study. Gynecol Oncol. 2012;124(3):529–33.

Moore DH, Thomas GM, Montana GS, et al. Preoperative chemoradiation for advanced vulvar cancer: a phase II study of the Gynecologic Oncology Group. Int J Radiat Oncol Biol Phys. 1998;42:79–85.

National Cancer Institute.Surveillance, epidemiology, and end results program (SEER). 2016. http://seer.cancer.gov/statfacts/html/vulva.html. Accessed 17 Aug 2016.

National Comprehensive Cancer Network.Vulvar cancer (version 1.2016). 2016. https://www.nccn.org/professionals/physician_gls/pdf/vulvar.pdf. Accessed 17 Aug 2016.

Pecorelli S. Revised FIGO staging for carcinoma of the vulva, cervix, and endometrium. Int J Gynaecol Obstet. 2009;105(2):103–4.

Petereit DG, Mehta MP, Buchler DA, et al. Inguinofemoral radiation of N0, N1 vulvar cancer may be equivalent to lymphadenectomy if proper radiation technique is used. Int J Radiat Oncol Biol Phys. 1993;27(4):963–7.

VIII

Russell AH, Horowitz NS. Vulvar and vaginal carcinoma. In: Gunderson LL, Tepper JE, editors. Clinical radiation oncology. 4th ed. Philadelphia: Churchill Livingstone; 2015. p. 1230–63.

Stehman FB, Bundy BN, Thomas G, et al. Groin dissection versus groin radiation in carcinoma of the vulva: a Gynecologic Oncology Group study. Int J Radiat Oncol Biol Phys. 1992;24:389–96.

Van der Zee AG, Oonk MH, DeHullu JA, et al. Sentinel node dissection is safe in the treatment of early-stage vulvar cancer. J Clin Oncol. 2008;26(6):884–9.

Chapter 34
Urethral Cancer

Serah Choi and Tracy Sherertz

PEARLS

- Primary urethral cancer is rare: <1% of all malignancies and 0.1% of gynecologic malignancies.
- Risk factors in females: chronic irritation from UTIs or STDs, HPV infection, urethral diverticulum, urethral caruncle.
- Average age is 60 (50–80) years, with increasing incidence with age (greatest in >75 age group), more common among African Americans.
- Ratio of female to male incidence for urethral cancer (1:3).
- Among females:
  - 30% = TCC.
  - 29% = adenocarcinoma.
  - 28% = squamous cell.
  - Rare = melanoma, lymphomas, mets, adenoid cystic, anaplastic tumors, Kaposi's sarcoma, clear-cell adenocarcinoma.
- Female urethra is ~3–4 cm long, 0.6 cm in resting diameter. Located in the anterior vaginal wall, posterior to the pubic symphysis, extends inferiorly and anteriorly from the bladder through the urogenital diaphragm to the vestibule, to form the urethral meatus. Lower distal half = anterior urethra, upper proximal half = posterior urethra.

VIII

© Springer International Publishing AG, part of Springer Nature 2018   **721**
Eric K. Hansen and M. Roach III (eds.), *Handbook of Evidence-Based Radiation Oncology*, https://doi.org/10.1007/978-3-319-62642-0_34

- Three layers: muscular layer (continuous with that of the bladder), erectile, and mucous.
- Two sphincters: internal at bladder neck and voluntary sphincter at plane of urogenital diaphragm.
- Proximal 1/3 epithelium = transitional cells.
- Distal 2/3 epithelium = non-keratinizing squamous cells.
- Periurethral Skene's glands secrete mucous near meatus (and extend along distal urethra).
- LN spread is to inguinal and pelvic LNs (including presacral and obturators).
  - T1 lesions = uncommon.
  - T2–T3 lesions = 35–50% of cases.
  - For urethra, clinically involved LN are almost always pathologically involved (vs. penile carcinoma only ~50% are pathologically involved).
- At presentation, ~10% of patients have DM.
- Most important prognostic factors = tumor size, local invasion, and location (distal more favorable).

WORKUP

- H&P: symptoms include bleeding, pain, dysuria, urinary frequency. Less common: mass, inguinal LN, perineal pain, dyspareunia.
- Detailed pelvic EUA.
- Urethroscopy and cystoscopy.
- CT/MRI of pelvis, Chest X-Ray (CXR).
- Biopsy.

Table 34.1 STAGING (AJCC 7TH ED., 2010): URETHRAL CANCER

Primary tumor (T): male and female	
TX:	Primary tumor cannot be assessed
T0:	No evidence of primary tumor
Ta:	Noninvasive papillary, polypoid, or verrucous carcinoma
Tis:	Carcinoma in situ
T1:	Tumor invades subepithelial connective tissue
T2:	Tumor invades any of the following: corpus spongiosum, prostate, periurethral muscle
T3:	Tumor invades any of the following: corpus cavernosum, beyond prostatic capsule, anterior vagina, bladder neck
T4:	Tumor invades other adjacent organs

Table 34.1 (continued)

Regional lymph nodes (N)

NX: Regional lymph nodes cannot be assessed

N0:   No regional lymph node metastasis

N1:   Metastasis in a single lymph node 2 cm or less in greatest dimension

N2:   Metastasis in a single node more than 2 cm in greatest dimension, or in multiple nodes

Distant metastasis (M)

M0:   No distant metastasis

M1:   Distant metastasis

Anatomic stage/prognostic groups

0a:	Ta N0 M0
0is:	Tis N0 M0
	Tis pu N0 M0
	Tis pd N0 M0
I:	T1 N0 M0
II:	T2 N0 M0
III:	T1 N1 M0
	T2 N1 M0
	T3 N0 M0
	T3 N1 M0
IV:	T4 N0 M0
	T4 N1 M0
	Any T N2 M0
	Any T Any N M1

Used with the permission from the American Joint Committee on Cancer (AJCC), Chicago, Illinois. The original source for this material is the AJCC Cancer Staging Manual, Seventh Edition (2010), published by Springer Science + Business Media

VIII

Table 34.2 STAGING (AJCC 8TH ED., 2017)

Definitions of AJCC TNM

Definition of Primary Tumor (T)

Male Penile Urethra and Female Urethra

T Category	T Criteria
TX	Primary tumor cannot be assessed
T0	No evidence of primary tumor
Ta	Non-invasive papillary carcinoma
Tis	Carcinoma *in situ*
T1	Tumor invades subepithelial connective tissue
T2	Tumor invades any of the following: corpus spongiosum, periurethral muscle
T3	Tumor invades any of the following: corpus cavernosum, anterior vagina
T4	Tumor invades other adjacent organs (e.g., invasion of the bladder wall)

PROSTATIC URETHRA

T Category	T Definition
Tis	Carcinoma *in situ* involving the prostatic urethra or periurethral or prostatic ducts without stromal invasion
T1	Tumor invades urethral subepithelial connective tissue immediately underlying the urothehum
T2	Tumor invades the prostatic stroma surrounding ducts either by direct extension from the urothelial surface or by invasion from prostatic ducts
T3	Tumor invades the periprostatic fat
T4	Tumor invades other adjacent organs (e.g., extraprostatic invasion of the bladder wall, rectal wall)

DEFINITION OF REGIONAL LYMPH NODE (N)

N Category	N Criteria
NX	Regional lymph nodes cannot be assessed
N0	No regional lymph node metastasis
N1	Single regional lymph node metastasis in the inguinal region or true pelvis [perivesical, obturator, internal (hypogastric) and external iliac], or presacral lymph node
N2	Multiple regional lymph node metastasis in the inguinal region or true pelvis [perivesical, obturator, internal (hypogastric) and external iliac], or presacral lymph node

DEFINITION OF DISTANT METASTASIS (M)

M Category	M Criteria
M0	No distant metastasis
M1	Distant metastasis

AJCC PROGNOSTIC STAGE GROUPS

When T is...	And N is...	And M is...	Then the stage group is...
Tis	N0	M0	0is
Ta	N0	M0	0a
T1	N0	M0	I
T1	N1	M0	III
T2	N0	M0	II
T2	N1	M0	III
T3	N0	M0	III
T3	N1	M0	III
T4	N0	M0	IV
T4	N1	M0	IV
Any T	N2	M0	IV
Any T	Any N	M1	IV

HISTOLOGIC GRADE (G)
Urothelial Carcinoma

G	G Definition
LG	Low grade
HG	High grade

SQUAMOUS CELL CARCINOMA AND ADENOCARCINOMA

G	G Definition
GX	Grade cannot be assessed
G1	Well differentiated
G2	Moderately differentiated
G3	Poorly differentiated

Used with permission of the American Joint Committee on Cancer (AJCC), Chicago, Illinois. The original and primary source for this information is the AJCC Cancer Staging Manual, Eighth Edition (2017) published by Springer International Publishing

Table 34.3 Local control and survival by stage

~LC	~5-year OS
I–II: 70–90%	I–II: 70–90%
III: 20–60%	III: 20–40%
IV: 10–20%	IV: 10–20%

TREATMENT RECOMMENDATIONS

VIII

Table 34.4 TREATMENT RECOMMENDATIONS

2002 stage	Recommended treatment
CIS	Surgical options: laser coagulation, open excision, or partial or total urethrectomy
I–II	Distal lesions Surgical resection of primary ± regional LN dissection (LND) Interstitial (IS) brachytherapy alone EBRT (including prophylactic regional LN) + IS brachy boost (± concurrent chemotherapy for squamous cell histology) Proximal lesions or those of entire urethra Pre-op RT → surgery with urinary diversion
III, IV	Distal lesions Surgical resection of primary + inguinal LND EBRT (including prophylactic regional LN) + IS brachy boost (± concurrent chemotherapy for squamous cell histology) Proximal lesions or those of entire urethra Pre-op RT → surgery (radical cystourethrectomy or female anterior exenteration with the removal of gynecologic organs too) with pelvic LND and urinary diversion. May require exenteration, if extensive

continued

Table 34.4 (continued)

Mets	Investigational chemo protocols, palliative symptom-directed radiotherapy
Recurrence	After RT, surgical excision or exenteration
	After surgery, RT + further surgery

STUDIES

- Because of its rarity, most studies are retrospective with small patient numbers.
- Data concerning chemotherapy are limited. Some use cisplatin or 5-FU/MMC-based concurrent chemo with EBRT for squamous-cell histology, with extrapolation from the cervix and anal cancer literature.
- Weghaupt (Gynecol Oncol 1984): 62 female patients treated high-dose intracavitary vaginal radium and EBRT, with tumor dose 55–70 Gy. 42 patients (68%) had tumors of the anterior urethra, and in 20 patients (32%) the posterior urethra was involved. 19 patients (31%) LN+. 5-year overall survival (OS) 64.5%. 5-year OS for anterior lesions 71% vs. 50% for posterior lesions.
- Garden (Cancer 1993): Of 97 patients, 86 received RT only after excision or biopsy of primary, 35 EBRT + brachy, 21 EBRT only, 30 brachy only, and 11 preop RT. RT doses 40–106 Gy (median, 65 Gy). The median f/u 105 months (range, 20–337 months). 5-year OS 41%, 10-year OS 31%, 64% LC at 5 year with RT alone. 49% of patients with LC had symptomatic complications (urethral stenosis, fistula, necrosis).
- Grisby (IJROBP 1998): 44 patients, T1-T4, median f/u 8.25 years. 7 patients treated with surgery, 25 patients with RT, and 12 patients with surgery + RT. 5-year OS 42%, 5-year cause-specific survival (CSS) 40%. Tumor size (>4 cm) and histology (adenocarcinoma) were poor prognostic factors on multivariate analysis.
- Milosevic (Radiother Oncol 2000): 34 patients, stage I–IV. 15 patients RT only to primary and 19 patients RT to primary and regional LNs. 20 patients got brachy to primary. 7-year OS 41%, 7-year CSS 45%. Benefit of brachy greatest in patients with bulky primary tumor. Brachy improves local control. Large tumor size was the only independent predictor of recurrence and death from cancer.

- Gakis (Ann Oncol 2015): 124 patients (86 men, 38 women) with primary urethral cancer; neoadjuvant chemo and neoadjuvant chemoRT associated with improved 3-year relapse-free survival and overall survival for cT3/T4 and/ or cN+ lesions, versus surgery +/– adjuvant chemo.

RADIATION TECHNIQUES

SIMULATION AND FIELD DESIGN
- Interstitial implant most often used for distal or meatus lesions.
- CT or MRI are used to verify needle placement.
- Larger, more invasive, or proximal tumors should be treated with a combination of EBRT and IS brachy.
- Consider IMRT for bowel sparing.
- Bolus may be required to ensure adequate dose for superficial tumors and/or inguinal LN.
- Traditional EBRT borders = whole pelvis and inguinal LN.
  - Superior = L5/S1.
  - Inferior = flash perineum.
  - Lateral = cover inguinal LN.
- EBRT dose.
  - WP = 50 Gy.
  - Involved LN = boost to 60–66 Gy.
- Brachy dose.
  - With implant alone for early lesions = 60–70 Gy (LDR equivalent).
  - As boost after 50 Gy WP = 10–30 Gy boost to 60–80 Gy (LDR equivalent).

DOSE LIMITATIONS
- Perineal skin reaction is a limiting factor for EBRT and thus limit to ~50–66 Gy.
- Upper vaginal mucosa tolerance is 120 Gy, midvaginal mucosal tolerance is 80–90 Gy, and lower vaginal mucosa tolerance is 60–70 Gy.
- Vaginal doses >50–60 Gy cause significant vaginal fibrosis and stenosis.
- Ovarian failure occurs with 5–10 Gy. Sterilization occurs with 2–3 Gy.

VIII

- Limit total bladder dose to <90 Gy and total rectum and sigmoid doses to <75 Gy (equivalent doses in 2 Gy per fraction).

COMPLICATIONS

- Complications are dose related and include skin reaction, urethral stricture (that could necessitate dilatation or urinary diversion), urinary incontinence, cystitis, vaginal dryness and atrophy, vaginal stenosis and fibrosis, vaginal necrosis, vesicovaginal fistula, proctitis, pubic hair loss, small bowel obstruction (rare).
- Vaginal dilators should be used to minimize stenosis.

FOLLOW-UP

- H&P with careful pelvic examination every 3 months for 1 year, every 4 months for second year, every 6 months for third and fourth years, then annually. CXR annually for 5 years.

Acknowledgments We thank Siavash Jabbari MD, Eric K. Hansen MD, and Alexander R. Gottschalk MD for their work on the prior edition of this chapter.

REFERENCES

Eng TY. Cancer of the female urethra. In: Perez CA, Brady LW, Halperin EC, et al., editors. Principles and practice of radiation oncology. 6th ed. Philadelphia: Lippincott Williams & Wilkins; 2013. p. 1491–502.

Foens CS, Hussey DH, Staples JJ, Doornbos JF, Wen BC, Vigliotti AP. A comparison of the roles of surgery and radiation therapy in the management of carcinoma of the female urethra. Int J Radiat Oncol Biol Phys. 1991;21(4):961–8.

Forman JD, Lichter AS. The role of radiation therapy in the management of carcinoma of the male and female urethra. Urol Clin North Am. 1992;19(2):383–9.

Gakis G, Morgan TM, Daneshmand S, et al. Impact of perioperative chemotherapy on survival in patients with advanced primary urethral cancer: results of the international collaboration on primary urethral carcinoma. Ann Oncol. 2015;26(8):1754–9.

Garden AS, Zagars GK, Delclos L. Primary carcinoma of the female urethra. Results of radiation therapy. Cancer. 1993;71(10):3102–8.

Grigsby PW. Carcinoma of the urethra in women. Int J Radiat Oncol Biol. 1998;41(3):535–41.

Jemal A, Siegel R, Ward E, et al. Cancer statistics, 2008. CA Cancer J Clin. 2008;58(2):71–96.

Kuettel MR, Parda DS, Harter KW, Rodgers JE, Lynch JH. Treatment of female urethral carcinoma in medically inoperable patients using external beam irradiation and high dose rate intracavitary brachytherapy. J Urol. 1997;157(5):1669–71.

Micaily B, Dzeda MF, Miyamoto CT, Brady LW. Brachytherapy for cancer of the female urethra. Semin Surg Oncol. 1997;13(3):208–14.

Milosevic MF, Warde PR, Banerjee D, et al. Urethral carcinoma in women: results of treatment with primary radiotherapy. Radiother Oncol. 2000;56(1):29–35.

Mostofi FK, Davis CJ Jr, Sesterhenn IA. Carcinoma of the male and female urethra. Urol Clin North Am. 1992;19(2):347–58.

Swartz MA, Porter MP, Lin DW, Weiss NS. Incidence of primary urethral carcinoma in the United States. Urology. 2006;68(6):1164–8.

VanderMolen LA, Sheehy PF, Dillman RO. Successful treatment of transitional cell carcinoma of the urethra with chemotherapy. Cancer Investig. 2002;20(2):206–7.

Weghaupt K, Gerstner GJ, Kucera H. Radiation therapy for primary carcinoma of the female urethra: a survey over 25 years. Gynecol Oncol. 1984;17(1):58–63.

VIII

PART IX

Lymphomas and Myeloma

Chapter 35
Hodgkin's Lymphoma

Jason Chan and Steve E. Braunstein

EPIDEMIOLOGY

- 10% of all lymphomas.
- Incidence/mortality in the USA for 2015 is 9050/1150 (Advani JCO 2007).
- Males slightly greater incidence than females (1.3:1).
- Bimodal age distribution at presentation: ages 25–30 and >55.
- First-degree relatives of patients have 5× risk for HL.
- Epstein–Barr virus associated with mixed cellularity HL.
- HIV associated with mixed cellularity and lymphocyte depleted.

HISTOLOGY

- HL falls into two general histologic categories:
  - Classic type (95%): four subtypes, characteristic Reed–Sternberg cells (binucleate B cells, CD15+, CD30+).
  - Nodular lymphocyte predominant (5%): characteristic "popcorn" cells (CD19/20/79a/Oct2+), best prognosis.

IX

Table 35.1 Characteristics of Hodgkin's lymphoma subtypes

WHO classification	Nodular lymphocyte predominant (NLPHL)	Classic HL (CHL) Nodular sclerosis (NSCHL)	Mixed cellularity (MCCHL)	Lymphocyte rich (LRCHL)	Lymphocyte depleted (LDCHL)
CD15	–	+	+	+	+
CD30	–	+	+	+	+
CD20	+	+/–	+/–	+/–	+/–
CD45	+	–	–	–	–
Incidence/epidemiology	5% all HL More common age > 40	70% CHL More common in adolescents and young adults	20% CHL More common in young children	15% CHL	≤ 5% CHL
Presentation	Often stage I–II, B symptoms <10%	Mediastinum often involved. One-third have B symptoms	Often advanced disease, often subclinical subdiaphragmatic disease in patients with clinically staged I–II above diaphragm	Usually early stage	Rare, mostly advanced with B symptoms in older patients, associated with HIV
Prognosis	Best, occasional late relapse	Intermediate between LRCHL and LDCHL	Intermediate between LRCHL and LDCHL	Good, infrequent relapses	Worst
30 month EFS	94%	89%	86%	97%	55%
30 month OS	97%	97%	94%	97%	87%

Treatment outcomes of 2715 HL patients within trials HD7 to HD12 of the German Hodgkin's Study Group (Advani JCO 2011)
EFS event-free survival, *OS* overall survival

WORK-UP

Table 35.2 Workup

H&P	B symptoms (fever ≥38 C, >10% weight loss in ≤6 mo, drenching sweats) occur in 15–20% of stage I–II, 33% overall. Complete lymph node exam. Most common presentation is painless lymphadenopathy (cervical 80%, mediastinal 50%)
Labs	CBC with differential, LFTs, BUN/Cr, ESR, chemistries, alkaline phosphatase, LDH, albumin. Pregnancy test. HIV test (if risk factors)
Pathology	Excisional LN biopsy. Bone marrow biopsy for B symptoms, stage III–IV, bulky disease, recurrent disease
Imaging	CXR; CT chest, abdomen and pelvis; PETCT scan
Pre-chemo	MUGA (adriamycin); PFTs (bleomycin); fertility preservation

STAGING

Table 35.3 Staging (AJCC 7th ed., 2010): Hodgkin's lymphoma

Anatomic stage/prognostic groups

I	Involvement of a single lymphatic site (i.e., nodal region, Waldeyer's ring, thymus, or spleen) (I) or localized involvement of a single extralymphatic organ or site in the absence of any lymph node involvement (IE) (rare in Hodgkin's lymphoma)
II	Involvement of two or more lymph node regions on the same side of the diaphragm (II) or localized involvement of a single extralymphatic organ or site in association with regional lymph node involvement with or without involvement of other lymph node regions on the same side of the diaphragm (IIE). The number of regions involved may be indicated by a subscript, as in, for example, II 3
III	Involvement of lymph node regions on both sides of the diaphragm (III), which also may be accompanied by extralymphatic extension in association with adjacent lymph node involvement (IIIE) or by involvement of the spleen (IIIS) or both (IIIE,S). Splenic involvement is designated by the letter S
IV	Diffuse or disseminated involvement of one or more extralymphatic organs, with or without associated lymph node involvement or isolated extralymphatic organ involvement in the absence of adjacent regional lymph node involvement but in conjunction with disease in distant site(s). Stage IV includes any involvement of the liver or bone marrow, lungs (other than by direct extension from another site), or cerebrospinal fluid

Used with the permission from the American Joint Committee on Cancer (AJCC), Chicago, Illinois. The original source for this material is the *AJCC Cancer Staging Manual, Seventh Edition* (2010), published by Springer Science + Business Media
Lymph node groups: Waldeyer's ring; occipital/cervical/preauricular/supraclavicular; infraclavicular; axillary; epitrochlear; mediastinal; right and left hilar (separate); para-aortic; splenic; mesenteric; iliac; inguinal/femoral; popliteal
A no B symptoms, *B* B symptoms, *X* bulky disease

IX

Table 35.4 Staging (AJCC 8th ed., 2017)

AJCC prognostic stage groups

Lugano classification for Hodgkin and Non-Hodgkin lymphoma

Stage	Stage description
Limited stage	
I	Involvement of a single lymphatic site (i.e., nodal region, Waldeyer's ring, thymus, or spleen)
IE	Single extralymphatic site in the absence of nodal involvement (rare in Hodgkin lymphoma)
II	Involvement of two or more lymph node regions on the same side of the diaphragm
IIE	Contiguous extralymphatic extension from a nodal site with or without involvement of other lymph node regions on the same side of the diaphragm
II bulky[a]	*Stage II with disease bulk*[b]
Advanced stage	
III	Involvement of lymph node regions on both sides of the diaphragm; nodes above the diaphragm with spleen involvement
IV	Diffuse or disseminated involvement of one or more extralymphatic organs, with or without associated lymph node involvement
	or *noncontiguous* extralymphatic organ involvement in conjunction with nodal Stage II disease
	or *any* extralymphatic organ involvement in nodal Stage III disease
	Stage IV includes *any* involvement of the CSF, bone marrow, liver, or lungs (other than by direct extension in Stage IIE disease)

[a]Stage II bulky may be considered either early or advanced stage based on lymphoma histology and prognostic factors (see discussion of Hodgkin lymphoma prognostic factors)

[b]The definition of disease bulk varies according to lymphoma histology. In the Lugano classification, bulk in Hodgkin lymphoma is defined as a mass greater than one third of the thoracic diameter on CT of the chest or a mass >10 cm. For NHL, the recommended definitions of bulk vary by lymphoma histology. In follicular lymphoma, 6 cm has been suggested based on the Follicular Lymphoma International Prognostic Index-2 (FLIPI-2) and its validation. In DLBCL, cutoffs ranging from 5 to 10 cm have been used, although 10 cm is recommended

Note: Hodgkin lymphoma uses A or B designation with stage group. A/B is no longer used in NHL

CHRONIC LYMPHOCYTIC LEUKEMIA/SMALL LYMPHOCYTIC LYMPHOMA

Modified Rai staging system (mainly used in North America)

Stage	Risk	Findings	Survival (months)
0	Low	Lymphocytosis only	>120
I	Intermediate	+ adenopathy	95
II	Intermediate	+ enlarged spleen and/or liver	72
III	High	Lymphocytosis + Hgb <11 g/dL	30
IV	High	Lymphocytosis + Plt <100,000/µL	30

Binet staging system

Stage	Findings	Survival (months)
A	Lymphocytosis only	>120
B	+ adenopathy	95
C	+ enlarged spleen and/or liver	72

Used with permission of the American Joint Committee on Cancer (AJCC), Chicago, Illinois. The original and primary source for this information is the *AJCC Cancer Staging Manual, Eighth Edition* (2017) published by Springer International Publishing

RISK CLASSIFICATION

- Early stage HL (Stage I–II)
  - Favorable (no risk factors)
  - Unfavorable (≥1 risk factor)

IX

Table 35.5 Unfavorable risk factors for stage I–II HL

Risk factor	GHSB	EORTC	NCIC	NCCN
Age	–	≥50	≥40	–
Histology	–	MC or LD	–	–
ESR or B sx	>50 if A or >30 if B	>50 if A or >30 if B	>50 or any B sx	>50 or any B sx
Large mediastinal adenopathy	MMR > 0.33	MMR > 0.35	MMR > 0.33 or > 10 cm	MMR > 0.33
# nodal sites	>2	>3	>3	>3
Extranodal lesions	Any	–	–	–
Bulky	–	–	–	>10 cm

Mediastinal mass measured on CXR by the mediastinal mass ratio (MMR) maximum width of mass/maximum intrathoracic diameter
Early stage treated with chemo-RT, 5-year FFF 95% and OS >95%
ESR erythrocyte sedimentation rate, *LD* lymphocyte depletion, *MC* mixed cellularity

, Advanced stage HL (Stage IIB, III, and IV)

Table 35.6 International prognostic score (IPS-7) 1 point per factor for advanced stage HL

Gender	Male	Albumin	<4 g/dL
Age	≥45	Hgb	<10.5 g/dL
Stage	IV	WBC	>15,000/uL
–	–	Lymphocyte	<8% or <600 uL

Table 35.7 IPS-7 risk group for advanced stage HL (Hasenclever et al. 1998)

	IPS score	5-year PFS (%)	5-year OS (%)
Good	0	84	89
	1	77	90
Fair	2	67	81
	3	60	78
Poor	4	51	61
	>5	42	56

Table 35.8 IPS-3 risk group for advanced stage HL (Aleman IJROBP 2007)

	IPS score	5-year PFS (%)	5-year OS (%)
1 point per factor	0	83	95
Age ≥ 45	1	74	85
Stage IV	2	68	75
Hgb < 10.5 g/dL	3	63	52

TREATMENT

CHEMOTHERAPY

, Chemo regimens

Table 35.9 Chemotherapy Regimens

Combination	Drug	Days	Cycle (days)	Comment
ABVD	Adriamycin (doxorubicin)	1, 15	28	Decreased sterility and second malignancies vs. MOPP
	Bleomycin	1, 15		
	Vinblastine	1, 15		
	Dacarbazine	8–14		
Stanford V	Mechlorethamine	1	28	Decreased bleomycin and doxorubicin toxicity vs. ABVD
	Doxorubicin	1, 15		
	Vinblastine	1, 15		
	Vincristine	8, 22		
	Bleomycin	8, 22		
	Etoposide	15, 16		
	Prednisone	Qod		
BEACOPP	Bleomycin	8	21	Eight cycles total. Filgrastim from day 8 of each cycle until leukocyte count normalizes. RT given for disease >5 cm
	Etoposide	1–3		
	Adriamycin (doxorubicin)	1		
	Cyclophosphamide	1		
	Oncovin (vincristine)	8		
	Procarbazine	1–7		
	Prednisone	1–14		
EPOCH	Etoposide [why underlined?]	1–4	21	DA-EPOCH = dose adjustment each cycle based on neutropenia and thrombocytopenia
	Prednisone	1–5		
	Oncovin (vincristine)	1–4		
	Cyclophosphamide	5		
	Hydroxydaunorubicin (doxorubicin)	1–4		
Other	Rituximab (anti-CD20)	NLPHL expresses CD20		
	Brentuximab (anti-CD30)	CHL expresses CD30		
	Nivolumab (anti-PD1)	HL has a high immune cell infiltrate		

IX

ROLE OF PET/CT

, PET/CT is valuable for initial, interim, and posttreatment staging. Interim PET may stratify patients that may be treated with chemo alone vs. the benefit from additional chemotherapy and/or involved site radiotherapy. The prognostic significance of interim PET is well established for advanced disease, less so for early-stage disease.

, End-of-treatment PET positivity is a negative prognostic factor for both early- and advanced-stage disease.

, Biopsy is recommended for Deauville 5 classification (below), and if positive, treat as refractory disease.

Table 35.10 PET 5-point scale (Deauville criteria)

Score	PET/CT scan result
1	No uptake
2	Uptake ≤ mediastinum
3	Uptake ≥ mediastinum but ≤ liver
4	Uptake moderately higher than liver
5	Uptake markedly higher than liver and/or new lesions
X	New areas of uptake unlikely to be related to lymphoma

TREATMENT RECOMMENDATIONS

TABLE 35.11 TREATMENT OF CLASSICAL HL

Stage	Recommended treatment
IA/IIA favorable (no bulky mediastinal disease, <10 cm adenopathy, ≤3 sites, ESR < 50, no B sx)	**ABVD × 4 cycles → PETCT → ISRT 20 Gy (CR) or 30 Gy (PR)** **ABVD × 2 cycles → PETCT → ISRT 20 Gy (CR) or 30 Gy (PR)** Stanford V × 8 weeks → PETCT → ISRT 30 Gy ABVD × 2 cycles → CT → ABVD × 2 (CR) or 4 (PR) (total 4–6) → PETCT Deauville 1–3 → observe Deauville 4 or 5 (with negative biopsy) → ISRT ABVD × 3 cycles → PETCT Deauville 1–2 → observe Deauville 3–4 → ABVD × 1 (4 total) → ISRT Deauville 5 (with negative biopsy) → ISRT
I–II unfavorable (bulky mediastinal disease or >10 cm adenopathy)	**ABVD × 4 cycles → PETCT** **Deauville 1–3 → ± ABVD × 2 cycles (4–6 total) → ISRT** **Deauville 4 or 5 (negative biopsy) → ABVD × 2 cycles (6 total) → ISRT** Stanford V × 12 weeks → PETCT → ISRT 30 Gy – 36 Gy to initial sites >5 cm Escalated BEACOPP × 2 + ABVD × 2 → PETCT → ISRT
I–II unfavorable (non-bulky)	ABVD × 4 cycles → PETCT Deauville 1–3 ABVD × 2 cycles (6 total) ISRT Deauville 4 or 5 (negative biopsy) ABVD × 2 cycles (6 total) → PETCT → ISRT Stanford V × 12 weeks → PETCT → ISRT 30 Gy – 36 Gy to initial sites >5 cm Escalated BEACOPP × 2 + ABVD × 2 → PETCT → ISRT

Stage	Recommended treatment
III–IV	ABVD × 2 cycles → PETCT
	Deauville 1–3
	ABVD × 4 cycles (6 total)
	Observe
	ISRT
	Deauville 4–5
	ABVD (6 total) or escalated BEACOPP × 4 cycles → PETCT
	Deauville 1–3 or Deauville 4–5 (with negative biopsy)
	observe
	ISRT
	Stanford V × 12 weeks → PETCT → ISRT 30–36 Gy to initial >5 cm
	sites, involved spleen
	Escalated BEACOPP × 6 → PETCT
	Deauville 1–2 → observe
	Deauville 2–3 → ISRT to residual >2.5 cm PET+
	Deauville 5 (biopsy negative)
	Observe
	ISRT

NCCN category 1 recommendations are bolded

TABLE 35.12 TREATMENT OF NODULAR LYMPHOCYTE-PREDOMINANT HL

Stage	Recommended treatment
IA/IIA favorable (no bulky disease, ≤3 sites, ESR < 50)	Observe (completely excised solitary lymph node) ISRT (preferred)
I–II unfavorable (bulky disease, >3 sites, or ESR > 50)	Chemotherapy → ISRT ±rituximab
IIIA–IVA	Chemotherapy → ± ISRT ± rituximab Local RT (palliation only) Rituximab alone
IIIB–IVB	Chemotherapy → ± ISRT ± rituximab

IX

TABLE 35.13 TREATMENT OF REFRACTORY / RELAPSED HL

Stage	Recommended treatment

Primary refractory disease (no clear superior approach, individualized treatment is recommended)	**Second-line systemic therapy → PETCT**
	Deauville 1–3
	  High-dose therapy (HDT) + autologous stem cell rescue (ASCR) → brentuximab 1 year
	  Observe ± ISRT (if ASCR contraindicated)
	Deauville 4
	  HDT/ASCR ± ISRT → brentuximab 1 year
	  Additional second-line systemic therapy ± ISRT
	Deauville 5
	  ISRT
	  Additional second-line systemic therapy ± ISRT

Relapse	Most chemo-alone failures occur in sites of initial disease IFRT or extended-field RT alone as salvage only in highly selected cases Otherwise same algorithm as primary refractory

NCCN category 1 recommendations are bolded

, General Primary Treatment Algorithm with ABVD (most common chemo in the USA)

Stage	Primary treatment	PFS (%)	OS (%)
I–II favorable CHL	ABVD × 2–4 cycles → restage → ISRT	90	95
I–II favorable NLPHL	RT alone	90	90
I–II unfavorable bulky	ABVD × 4 cycles → restage → ±ABVD × 2 cycles (4–6 total) → ISRT	85	90
I–II unfavorable non-bulky	ABVD × 4 cycles → restage → ABVD × 2 cycles (6 total) → ±ISRT		
III–IV	ABVD × 6–8 cycles	60	70

RADIOTHERAPY STUDIES

EARLY-STAGE CLASSICAL HL

- Randomized trials report improved PFS with chemotherapy added to radiotherapy vs. radiotherapy alone:
  - *GHSG HD7* (Engert, JCO 2007), *SWOG 9133/CALGB 9391* (Press, JCO 2001), *EORTC-GELA H8F/U* (Ferme, NEJM 2007), and *EORTC H7F* (Noordijk, JCO 2006).
- When chemotherapy is used, smaller radiotherapy field sizes can replace extended-field or subtotal nodal irradiation (STNI) fields:
  - *EORTC-GELA H8F/U* (Ferme, NEJM 2007); *EORTC H7F* (Noordijk, JCO 2006); Milan (Bonadonna, JCO 2004), and *GHSG HD8* (Engert JCO 2003).
- A number of studies have investigated chemotherapy +/– RT for early-stage HL. Omitting radiotherapy reduces PFS but not OS. Representative studies include:
  - *EORTC H9F* (ASCO 2005 abstr, Haematologica abstr 2007): 783 patients with favorable IA–IIB randomized to no IFRT, IFRT (20 Gy), or IFRT (36 Gy), after attaining CR with EBVP ×6c (79% of patients had CR and were randomized). 4-year EFS decreased without IFRT (70%) vs. 84% (20 Gy) and 87% (36 Gy). No RT arm stopped because of unacceptable failure rate (>20%). No difference in OS (98% all three arms).
  - *NCIC/ECOG HD.6* (Meyer, NEJM 2012): 405 patients CS IA or IIA non-bulky stratified into favorable or unfavorable groups, randomized to ABVD ×4c vs. STNI alone (favorable) or STNI + ABVD ×2c (unfavorable). In favorable group, no difference in OS or EFS at 12 years. In unfavorable group, ABVD + STNI improved 12-year freedom from disease progression (94% vs. 86%) but worse 12-year OS (81% vs. 92%) compared to ABVD alone due to more non-cancer deaths. More secondary cancers (23 vs. 10) and cardiac events (26 vs. 16) with STNI.
  - *EORTC 20051/GELA H10* (Raemaekers, JCO 2014): 444 I–II randomized to ABVD × 3 + INRT vs. ABVD × 2 → FDG-PET, if PET positive, then escalated BEACOPP × 2 + INRT; if PET negative then ABVD × 2. Interim analysis showed worse PFS for PET-negative pts who did not receive INRT in favorable (94.9% vs. 100%) and unfavorable (94.7% vs. 97.3%) subgroups.

IX

- *Hay* (Ann Oncol 2013). 588 pts with non-bulky IA–IIA treated on GHSG HD10/HD11 or NCIC HD.6. Adding IFRT improved 8-year PFS particularly for 162 pts not achieving complete response after 2c ABVD (88% vs. 74%).
- Picardi (Leukemia & Lymphoma 2007): 166 pts with bulky >5 cm who became PET negative after VEBEP chemo with residual CT mass > 1.3 cm randomized to observation vs. IFRT 32 Gy. 65% stage I–II. Median follow-up 40 months. IFRT reduced failures 14 → 4%, and all chemo-alone failures were in initial site and contiguous nodal regions.
- *RAPID* (Radford, NEJM 2015): 602 CS I–IIA treated with ABVD ×3c followed by PET. 426 PET-negative (Deauville 1 or 2) patients randomized to IFRT 30 Gy or no further treatment. 3-year PFS 94.6% in RT group vs. 90.8% in ABVD alone arm. Did not meet non-inferiority criteria.
- *NCDB* (Olszewski, JCO 2015). 20,600 pts with early stage HL treated with chemotherapy with or without radiotherapy. In adjusted population, adding RT improved 5-yr OS (95% vs. 91%) and relative survival (98% vs. 94%).
- *Meta-analysis* (Sickinger, Critical Reviews in Hem Onc 2016): In three RCTs involving 1480 early-stage patients, PFS inferior in PET-adapted arms that omitted radiotherapy compared to standard treatment. No data on long-term sequelae of treatment or quality of life.
- Reduced early-stage IFRT dose:
  - *EORTC H9F*: see description above. No difference at 4 years between IFRT dose 36 Gy and 20 Gy after CR to 6 cycles chemo for favorable early-stage disease.
  - *GHSG HD10* (Engert, NEJM 2010): 1370 patients with favorable I–II with no risk factors randomized to ABVD ×2c vs. ×4c, followed by IFRT 20 vs. 30 Gy. At medium follow-up 7.5 years, no statistically significant difference between any of the arms.
  - *GHSG HD11* (Eich, JCO 2010): 1395 patients with clinical stage I–II randomized to ABVD × 4 + IFRT (30 Gy) vs. ABVD × 4 + IFRT (20 Gy) vs. BEACOPP × 4 IFRT (30 Gy) vs. BEACOPP × 4 + IFRT (20 Gy). Median FU 82 months. No difference in overall freedom from treatment failure (FFTF) or OS between ABVD vs. BEACOPP or 20 Gy vs. 30 Gy, though there was more toxicity with BEACOPP and more relapses in the 20 Gy arm requiring salvage.

ADVANCED STAGE

 A number of studies have investigated consolidative radio-therapy after chemotherapy for an advance-stage disease. It appears to improve PFS particularly for patients with bulky disease or poor responders to chemotherapy.

 SWOG 7808 (Ann Int Med 1994). CS III–IV MOP-BAP × 6 months. If CR, randomized to observation vs. 20 Gy IFRT. Improved FFP for NSHD (60–82%), bulky >6 cm (57–75%) and patients who actually completed assigned treatment (67–85%). No difference in OS.

 GHSG HD3 (Ann Oncol 1995). CS IIIB/IV COPP/ABVD × 6 months. If CR, randomized to 2 months COPP/ABVD or 20 Gy IFRT. No diff RFS (77%) or OS (90%).

 GELA H89 (Blood 2000): 418 patients CS IIIB/IV who achieved CR/PR after six cycles of MOPP/ABV or ABVPP were randomized to STLI or two more cycles of chemo. Five-year DFS (79 vs. 74%) and OS (88 vs. 85%) were not different.

 EORTC 20884/GPMC H34 (NEJM 2003; IJROBP 2007). CS III/IV MOPP-ABV × 6–8c. If CR, randomized to observation vs. consolidative IFRT (24 Gy). IFRT did not improve RFS or OS and had higher rate of myelodysplastic syndrome and leukemia. For those in PR (33%, all received RT), 8-year EFS 76% and OS 84% not significantly different from those with CR ± RT (75 and 82%), therefore the role for RT in patients with PR.India (Laskar, JCO 2004). 179 (71%) of 251 pts with stage I–IV achieved CR after ABVD × 6 and then were randomized to no RT or consolidation RT. IFRT was given in 84%. 47% were <15 years, and 68% had MC histology. RT improved 8-year EFS (76 vs. 88%) and OS (89 vs. 100%).

 UKLG LYO9 (Johnson, JCO 2010): 702 pts treated with at least 6c ABVD with two other multidrug regimens. IFRT recommended for incomplete response to chemo or bulky disease at presentation. IFRT improved 5-year PFS (86% vs. 71%) and OS (93% vs. 87%).

 GHSG HD12 (Borchmann, JCO 2011): 1670 patients with CS IIB/IIIA and risk factors or stage IIIB/IV randomized to escalated BEACOPP × 8 vs. escalated BEACOPP × 4 + and std BEACOPP × 4 with IFRT to residual vs. no RT to residual for both arms. Second randomization of IFRT (30 Gy) vs. no IFRT to initial bulky or residual enlarged nodes. At 5 years, no statistical difference between any of the four arms. RT improved FFTF (87 → 90.4%), but no difference

IX

Table 35.14 Active trials

Trial	Clinical stage	Standard arm	Experimental arm(s)	Favorable interim PET
HD16	Early favorable (resembling H10F)	ABVD × 2c + IFRT 20 Gy irrespective of interim PET	ABVD × 2c → interim PET	IFRT 20 Gy vs. observation
HD17	Early unfavorable (resembling H10U)	BEACOPP × 2c + ABVD × 2c + IFRT 30 Gy irrespective of interim PET	BEACOPP × 2c + ABVD × 2c → interim PET	INRT 30 Gy vs. observation
HD18	Advanced	escBEACOPP × 8c irrespective of interim PET. RT to PET+ residual disease ≥2.5 cm	escBEACOPP × 2c → interim PET	escBEACOPP × 2c (4 total) if PET-positive, escBEACOPP × 6c (8 total) + rituximab

in survival. Because RT was given to 11% of patients in "non-RT" arms, equivalency of a non-RT strategy cannot be proved. *GHSG HD15* (Engert, Lancet 2012). 2182 pts with advanced HL treated with 6–8c BEACOPP and PET-guided RT (30 Gy) restricted to pts in PR with PET+ residual disease ≥2.5 cm. PET-negative pts received no additional RT. Negative predictive value of PET was 94%. 4-year PFS was 92% for PET-negative CT-persistent residual disease not irradiated suggesting consolidative RT may be omitted. 4-year PFS for PET+ PR pts irradiated was 86% suggesting consolidative RT effective.

NODULAR LYMPHOCYTE PREDOMINANT HL

꜒ GHSG (Eichenauer, JCO 2015). 256 pts with stage IA NLPHL treated on GHSG protocols. 8-year PFS/OS was IFRT 92/99%, EFRT 84/96%, and combined modality treatment 89/99%. IFRT is considered the standard of care due to the lowest risk of toxic effects. Rituximab alone had poorer 4-year PFS 81%.

PRIMARY REFRACTORY OR RELAPSED HD

꜒ Kahn (IJROBP 2011). 92 pts with relapsed/refractory HL treated with high-dose chemo and stem cell transplant. Median FU 5 years 50% received IFRT (median dose 30 Gy) and had trend for improved disease control: 22% vs. 37% relapse/progression.

꜒ Levis (Clin Lymphoma Myeloma Leuk 2017). 73 pts with relapsed/refractory HL treated with autologous stem cell transplant. Median FU 41 mo. 29% received IFRT (median dose 30 Gy). For pts with limited stage disease at relapse and PET+, IFRT had trend for improved 3-year PFS (68% vs. 50%) and OS (92% vs. 62%). IFRT appeared to compensate for worse prognostic factors.

꜒ Poen (IJROBP 1996). 100 pts with relapsed/refractory HL treated with high-dose chemo and autologous bone marrow transplant. Median FU 40 mo. 24% received RT (median dose 30 Gy). IFRT improved 3-year freedom from relapse for stage I–III disease (100% vs. 67%) and trend for improved OS (85% vs. 60%).

IX

RADIATION TECHNIQUES

SIMULATION AND FIELD DESIGN

, Contemporary treatment for HD involves small field RT with chemotherapy:

, INRT/ISRT has replaced IFRT and EFRT/STNI (Fig. 35.1).

, Recommend following ILROG working group guidelines (Specht, IJROBP 2014):

, In both involved-node RT (INRT) and involved-site RT (ISRT), the pre-chemo GTV determines CTV. When optimal pre-chemo PET/CT imaging is not available, ISRT is used with clinical judgment used to contour a larger CTV to accommodate uncertainties in defining the pre-chemo GTV.

, 3D simulation (CT, PET/CT, or MRI) is always recommended, when possible in the same position as in pre-chemo imaging, with appropriate immobilization.

, Fuse pre- and post-chemotherapy imaging studies when available. Contour pre-chemo GTV on pre-chemo CT and/or PET/CT. When image fusion is not available, contour the target volumes on the planning CT scan with

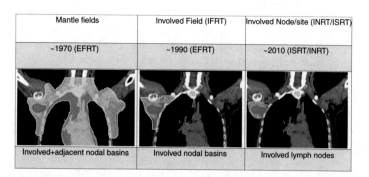

Mantle fields	Involved Field (IFRT)	Involved Node/site (INRT/ISRT)
~1970 (EFRT)	~1990 (EFRT)	~2010 (ISRT/INRT)
Involved+adjacent nodal basins	Involved nodal basins	Involved lymph nodes

Fig. 35.1 Evolution of RT field design. Large fields such as with extended field radiation therapy (EFRT) have been replaced by smaller fields with involved-field radiation therapy (IFRT) followed by involved node/site radiation therapy (INRT/ISRT)

larger CTV to account for uncertainties and differences of patient positioning.

- CTV encompasses all pre-chemotherapy lymphoma involvement, modified for normal tissue boundaries, tumor shrinkage, and other anatomic changes.
- More generous margins should be used for early-stage NLPHL when RT is used as the sole treatment modality, including as a minimum adjacent lymph nodes to the originally involved GTV.
- 4DCT and breath hold/respiratory gating may be considered with ITV for situations where internal organ movement is of concern.
- Irradiation of residual mass after chemotherapy for advanced disease.
  - GTV is the residual mass after chemotherapy.
  - CTV encompasses all pre-chemotherapy lymphoma involvement.
  - Usually 1 cm margin is sufficient, but in the chest and upper abdomen, a larger margin in the superior-inferior direction may be needed to compensate for respiratory motion.
- IMRT, image guidance, proton therapy, and other advanced techniques may be considered to reduce normal tissue toxicity while achieving local control.
- PTV expansion for setup uncertainty should be determined on a case-by-case and institutional basis.
- Start radiation 3–4 weeks after completion of chemotherapy.
- Larger field RT is now limited to salvage treatment for pts unable to have effective systemic therapy.
- IFRT is no longer routinely used but may be considered on a case-by-case basis if imaging is suboptimal or for salvage treatment:
  - IFRT encompasses a region, not an individual LN.
  - Traditionally involved field regions are the neck (unilateral), mediastinum (including bilateral hilum), axilla (including supraclavicular and infraclavicular LN), spleen, para-aortic, and inguinal (femoral and iliac nodes).
  - Shield testes for men and consider oophoropexy for women.

IX

DOSE PRESCRIPTIONS

- See treatment algorithms above.
- Early stage classic HL, CR to chemotherapy.
  - 20 Gy if favorable (I–IIA, ESR <50, no extralymphatic disease, <1–2 regions involved) treated with ABVD.
  - 30 Gy if unfavorable or treated with Stanford V.
- Early stage NLPHL: 30–35 Gy.
- Residual lymphoma after chemotherapy: 36–40 Gy.

DOSE LIMITATIONS

- Radiation dose to all normal structures should be ALARA to minimize long-term complications.
- At a minimum attempt to meet well-documented QUANTEC dose constraints (Marks, IJROBP 2010).

COMPLICATIONS

- Acute and late complications are site dependent (see other chapters for different regions).
- Late risks of particular concern include coronary artery disease, hypothyroidism, gastric ulcer, pulmonary toxicity, second malignancies, and infertility.
- Heart disease (van Nimwegen, JCO 2015): Excess relative risk of 7.4% per Gy that increases linearly with no threshold. Twofold relative risk for CHD following a mean heart dose of 12 Gy.
- Second cancer (Schaapveld, NEJM 2015): 3905 patients from the Netherlands with ≥5 yr survival since treatment between 1965 and 2000. At median FU 19.1 years, standardized incidence ratio (SIR) of 4.6 compared to general population (1055 second cancers in 908 patients). Secondary leukemia declined due to reduced use of alkylating agents. Secondary solid cancer risk overall was unchanged in the most recent study period (1989–2000) as compared to earlier periods.

FOLLOW-UP

- Every 3–6 months for 1–2 years, then every 6–12 months until year 3, and then annually with H&P, labs as indicated.
- CT at 6, 12, and 24 months after treatment. Or, PET/CT if last PET was Deauville 4–5.
- Follow thyroid function if in RT field.

, Annual breast screening initiated 8–10 years after therapy or at age 40, whichever first, for women treated with chest or axillary RT.
, Consider referral to survivorship clinic.
, Recommend following NCCN follow-up guidelines.

Acknowledgment We thank Hans T. Chung MD, Stephen L. Shiao MD, PhD, and Naomi R. Schechter MD for their work on the prior edition of this chapter.

REFERENCES

Advani R, Maeda L, Lavori P, et al. Impact of positive positron emission tomography on prediction of freedom from progression after Stanford V chemotherapy in Hodgkin's disease. J Clin Oncol. 2007;25(25):3902–7.

Advani R, Horning SJ, Jonathan E, et al. Abbreviated 8-week chemotherapy (CT) plus involved node radiotherapy (INRT) for nonbulky stage I-II Hodgkin lymphoma: preliminary results of the Stanford G5 Study. J Clin Oncol (Meeting abstracts). 2011;29:8064.

Aleman BM, Raemaekers JM, Tomasic R, et al. Involved field radiotherapy for patients in partial remission after chemotherapy for advanced Hodgkin's lymphoma. Int J Radiat Oncol Biol Phys. 2007;67(1):19–30.

Aleman BMP, Raemaekers JMM, Tirelli U, et al. Involved-field radiotherapy for advanced Hodgkin's lymphoma. N Engl J Med. 2003;348:2396–406.

Bonadonna G, Bonfante V, Viviani S, Di Russo A, Villani F, Valagussa P. ABVD plus subtotal nodal versus involved-field radiotherapy in early-stage Hodgkin's disease: long-term results. J Clin Oncol. 2004;22(14):2835–41.

Borchmann P, Haverkamp H, Diehl V, et al. Eight cycles of escalated-dose BEACOPP compared with four cycles of escalated-dose BEACOPP followed by four cycles of baseline-dose BEACOPP with or without radiotherapy in patients with advanced-stage Hodgkin's lymphoma: final analysis of the HD12 trial of the German Hodgkin Study Group. J Clin Oncol. 2011;29:4234–42.

Borchmann P, Haverkamp H, Diehl V, et al. Eight cycles of escalated-dose BEACOPP compared with four cycles of escalated-dose BEACOPP followed by four cycles of baseline-dose BEACOPP with or without radiotherapy in patients with advanced-stage Hodgkin's lymphoma: final analysis of the HD12 trial of the German Hodgkin Study Group. J Clin Oncol. 2011;29:4234–42.

Borchmann P, Haverkamp H, Lohri A, et al. Addition of rituximab to BEACOPP escalated to improve the outcome of early interim PET positive advanced stage Hodgkin lymphoma patients: second planned interim analysis of the HD18 study. Blood (Meeting abstracts). 2014;124:500.

Canellos GP, Anderson JR, Propert KJ, et al. Chemotherapy of advanced Hodgkin's disease with MOPP, ABVD, or MOPP alternating with ABVD. N Engl J Med. 1992;327:1478–84.

Canellos GP, Niedzwiecki D. Long-term follow-up of Hodgkin's disease trial. N Engl J Med. 2002;346:1417–8.

Diefenbach CS, Li H, Hong F, et al. Evaluation of the International Prognostic Score (IPS-7) and a Simpler Prognostic Score (IPS-3) for advanced Hodgkin lymphoma in the modern era. Br J Haematol. 2015;171:530–8.

Diehl V, Brillant C, Engert A, et al. HD10: investigating reduction of combined modality treatment intensity in early stage Hodgkin's lymphoma. Interim analysis of a randomized trial of the German Hodgkin Study Group (GHSG). J Clin Oncol (Meeting abstracts). 2005a;23:6506.

IX

Diehl V, Brillant C, Engert A, et al. Recent interim analysis of the HD11 trial of the GHSG: intensification of chemotherapy and reduction of radiation dose in early unfavorable stage Hodgkin's lymphoma. Blood. 2005b;106:abstract no. 816.

Diehl V, Franklin J, Pfistner B, et al. Ten-year results of a German Hodgkin Study Group randomized trial of standard and increased dose BEACOPP chemotherapy for advanced Hodgkin lymphoma (HD9). J Clin Oncol (Meeting abstracts). 2007a;25:LBA8015.

Diehl V, Franklin J, Pfreundschuh M, et al. Standard and increased-dose BEACOPP chemotherapy compared with COPP-ABVD for advanced Hodgkin's disease. NEJM. 2003;348:2386–95.

Diehl V, Franklin J, Tesch H, et al. Dose escalation of BEACOPP chemotherapy for advanced Hodgkin's disease in the HD9 trial of the German Hodgkin's Lymphoma Study Group (GHSG). Proc ASCO. 2007;8544:(abstract no. 7).

Diehl V, Haverkamp H, Mueller R, et al. Eight cycles of BEACOPP escalated compared with 4 cycles of BEACOPP baseline with or without radiotherapy in patients in advanced stage Hodgkin lymphoma (HL): final analysis of the HD12 trial of the Germa Hodgkin Study Group (GHSG). J Clin Oncol. 2009;27:15s (Suppl; abstr 8544)

Diehl V, Loeffler M, Pfreundschuh M, et al. Further chemotherapy versus low-dose involved-field radiotherapy as consolidation of complete remission after six cycles of alternating chemotherapy in patients with advance Hodgkin's disease. German Hodgkins' Study Group (GHSG). Ann Oncol. 1995;6(9):901–10.

Eich H, Gossmann A, Engert A, et al. A contribution to solve the problem of the need for consolidative radiotherapy after intensive chemotherapy in advanced stages of Hodgkin's lymphoma – analysis of a quality control program initiated by the radiotherapy reference Center of the German Hodgkin Study Group (GHSG). Int J Radiat Oncol Biol Phys. 2007;69:1187–92.

Eich HT, Diehl V, Gorgen H, et al. Intensified chemotherapy and dose-reduced involved-field radiotherapy in patients with early unfavorable Hodgkin's lymphoma: final analysis of the German Hodgkin Study Group HD11 trial. J Clin Oncol. 2010;28:4199–206.

Eichenauer DA, Plütschow A, Fuchs M, von Tresckow B, Böll B, Behringer K, Diehl V, Eich HT, Borchmann P, Engert A. Long-term course of patients with stage IA nodular lymphocyte-predominant Hodgkin lymphoma: a report from the German Hodgkin Study Group. J Clin Oncol. 2015;33(26):2857–62.

Engert A, Haverkamp H, Kobe C, Markova J, Renner C, Ho A, Zijlstra J, Král Z, Fuchs M, Hallek M, Kanz L. Reduced-intensity chemotherapy and PET-guided radiotherapy in patients with advanced stage Hodgkin's lymphoma (HD15 trial): a randomised, open-label, phase 3 non-inferiority trial. Lancet. 2012;379(9828):1791–9.

Engert A, Diehl V, Franklin J, et al. Escalated-dose BEACOPP in the treatment of patients with advanced-stage Hodgkin's lymphoma: 10 years of follow-up of the GHSG HD9 study. J Clin Oncol. 2009;27(27):4548–54.

Engert A, Franklin J, Eich HT, et al. Two cycles of doxorubicin, bleomycin, vinblastine, and dacarbazine plus extended-field radiotherapy is superior to radiotherapy alone in early favorable Hodgkin's lymphoma: final results of the GHSG HD7 trial. J Clin Oncol. 2007;25(23):3495–502.

Engert A, Plütschow A, Eich HT, et al. Reduced treatment intensity in patients with early-stage Hodgkin's lymphoma. N Engl J Med. 2010;363:640–52.

Engert A, Schiller P, Josting A, Herrmann R, Koch P, Sieber M, Boissevain F, de Wit M, Mezger J, Dühmke E, Willich N. Involved-field radiotherapy is equally effective and less toxic compared with extended-field radiotherapy after four cycles of chemotherapy in patients with early-stage unfavorable Hodgkin's lymphoma: results of the HD8 trial of the German Hodgkin's Lymphoma Study Group. J Clin Oncol. 2003;21 (19):3601–8.

Fabian CJ, Mansfield CM, Dahlberg S, et al. Low-dose involved field radiation after chemotherapy in advanced Hodgkin disease. A Southwest Oncology Group randomized study. Ann Intern Med. 1994;120(11):903–12.

Ferme C, Eghbali H, Meerwaldt JH, et al. Chemotherapy plus involved-field radiation in early-stage Hodgkin's disease. N Engl J Med. 2007;357(19):1916–27.

Firme C, Sebban C, Hennequin C, et al. Comparison of chemotherapy to radiotherapy as consolidation of complete or good partial response after six cycles of chemotherapy for patients with advanced Hodgkin's disease: results of the Groupe d'etudes des Lymphomes de l'Adulte H89 trial. Blood. 2000;95:2246–52.

Gallmini A, Hutchings M, Rigacci L, et al. Early interim 2-[18F]fluoro-2-deoxy-D-glucose positron emission tomography is prognostically superior to international prognostic score in advanced-stage Hodgkin's lymphoma: a report from a joint Italian-Danish study. J Clin Oncol. 2007;25:3746–52.

Girinsky T, Specht L, Ghalibafian M, et al. The conundrum of Hodgkin lymphoma nodes: to be or not to be included in the involved node radiation fields. The EORTC-GELA lymphoma group guidelines. Radiother Oncol. 2008;88:202–10.

Gobbi PG, Levis A, Chisesi T, et al. ABVD versus modified Stanford V versus MOPPEBVCAD with optional and limited radiotherapy in intermediate- and advanced stage Hodgkin's lymphoma. Final results of a multicenter randomized trial by the Intergruppo Italiano Linfomi. J Clin Oncol. 2005;23:9198–207.

Hasenclever D, Diehl V, Armitage JO, et al. A prognostic score for advanced Hodgkin's disease. N Engl J Med. 1998;339:1506–14.

Hay AE, Klimm B, Chen BE, Goergen H, Shepherd LE, Fuchs M, Gospodarowicz MK, Borchmann P, Connors JM, Markova J, Crump M. An individual patient-data comparison of combined modality therapy and ABVD alone for patients with limited-stage Hodgkin lymphoma. Ann Oncol. 2013;24(12):3065–9.

Horning SJ, Hoppe RT, Advani R, et al. Efficacy and late effects of Stanford V chemotherapy and radiotherapy in untreated Hodgkin's disease: mature data in early and advanced stage patients. Blood. 2004;104:308 (abstr 308).

Johnson PW, Sydes MR, Hancock BW, Cullen M, Radford JA, Stenning SP. Consolidation radiotherapy in patients with advanced Hodgkin's lymphoma: survival data from the UKLG LY09 randomized controlled trial (ISRCTN97144519). J Clin Oncol. 2010;28(20):3352–9.

Juweid ME, Stroobants S, Hoekstra OS, et al. Use of positron emission tomography for response assessment of lymphoma: consensus of the imaging subcommittee on International Harmonization Project in Lymphoma. J Clin Oncol. 2007;25(5):571–8.

Khan N, Khan MK, Almasan A, Singh AD, Macklis R. The evolving role of radiation therapy in the management of malignant melanoma. Int J Radiat Oncol Biol Phys. 2011;80(3):645–54.

Kobe C, Dietlein M, Franklin J, et al. FDG-PET for assessment of residual tissue after completion of chemotherapy in Hodgkin lymphoma – report on the second interim analysis of the PET investigation in the trial HD15 of the GHSG. Haematol. 2007;92(Suppl 5):CO21.

Laskar S, Gupta T, Vimal S, et al. Consolidation radiation after complete remission in Hodgkin's disease following six cycles of doxorubicin, bleomycin, vinblastine, and dacarbazine chemotherapy: is there a need? J Clin Oncol. 2004;22:62–8.

Lavoie JC, Connors JM, Phillips GL, et al. High-dose chemotherapy and autologous stem cell transplantation for primary refractory or relapsed Hodgkin lymphoma: long-term outcome in the first 100 patients treated in Vancouver. Blood. 2005;106(4):1473–8.

Levis M, Piva C, Filippi AR, Botto B, Gavarotti P, Pregno P, Nicolosi M, Freilone R, Parvis G, Gottardi D, Vitolo U. Potential benefit of involved-field radiotherapy for patients with relapsed-refractory hodgkin's lymphoma with incomplete response before autologous stem cell transplantation. Clin Lymphoma Myeloma Leuk. 2017;17(1):14–22.

Macdonald DA, Ding K, Gospodarowicz MK, et al. Patterns of disease progression and outcomes in a randomized trial testing ABVD alone for patients with limited-stage Hodgkin lymphoma. Ann Oncol. 2007;18(10):1680–4.

IX

Marks LB, Yorke ED, Jackson A, et al. Use of normal tissue complication probability models in the clinic. Int J Radiat Oncol Biol Phys. 2010;76:S10–9.

Meyer RM, Gospodarowicz MK, Connors JM, et al. ABVD alone versus radiation-based therapy in limited-stage Hodgkin's lymphoma. N Engl J Med. 2012;366:399–408.

Noordijk E, Carde P, Hagenbeek A. Combination of radiotherapy and chemotherapy is advisable in all patients with clinical stage I-II Hodgkin's disease. Six-year results of the EORTC-GPMC controlled clinical trials "H7-VF", "H7-F" and "H7-U". Presented at ASTRO 1997.

Noordijk EM, Thomas J, Ferme C, et al. First results of the EORTC-GELA H9 random-ized trials: the H9-F trial (comparing 3 radiation dose levels) and H9-U trial (com-paring 3 chemotherapy schemes) in patients with favorable or unfavorable early stage Hodgkin's lymphoma (HL). J Clin Oncol (Meeting abstracts). 2005;23:6505.

Noordijk EM, Carde P, Dupouy N, et al. Combined-modality therapy for clinical stage I or II Hodgkin's lymphoma: long-term results of the European Organization for Research and Treatment of Cancer (EORTC) H7 randomized controlled trials. J Clin Oncol. 2006;24:3128–35.

Olszewski AJ, Shrestha R, Castillo JJ. Treatment selection and outcomes in early-stage classical Hodgkin lymphoma: analysis of the National Cancer Data Base. J Clin Oncol. 2015;33(6):625–33.

Pavlovsky S, Maschio M, Santarelli MT, et al. Randomized trial of chemotherapy versus chemotherapy plus radiotherapy for stage I–II Hodgkin's disease. J Natl Cancer Inst. 1988;80(18):1466–73.

Picardi M, De Renzo A, Pane F, et al. Randomized comparison of consolidation radiation versus observation in bulky Hodgkin's lymphoma with post-chemotherapy negative positron emission tomography scans. Leuk Lymphoma. 2007;48(9):1721–7.

Poen JC, Hoppe RT, Horning SJ. High-dose therapy and autologous bone marrow trans-plantation for relapsed/refractory Hodgkin's disease: the impact of involved field radiotherapy on patterns of failure and survival. Int J Radiat Oncol Biol Phys. 1996;36(1):3–12.

Press OW, LeBlanc M, Lichter AS, et al. Phase III randomized intergroup trial of subtotal lymphoid irradiation versus doxorubicin, vinblastine, and subtotal lymphoid irradi-ation for stage IA to IIA Hodgkin's disease. J Clin Oncol. 2001;19:4238–44.

Radford J, Illidge T, Counsell N, et al. Results of a trial of PET-directed therapy for early-stage Hodgkin's lymphoma. N Engl J Med. 2015;372:1598–607.

Raemaekers JMM, Andre MPE, Federico M, et al. Omitting radiotherapy in early posi-tron emission tomography-negative stage I/II Hodgkin lymphoma is associated with an increased risk of early relapse: clinical results of the preplanned interim analysis of the randomized EORTC/LYSA/FIL H10 trial. J Clin Oncol. 2014;32:1188–94.

Rigacci L, Vitolo U, Nassi L, et al. Positron emission tomography in the staging of patients with Hodgkin's lymphoma. Ann Hematol. 2007;86:897–903.

Schaapveld M, Aleman BMP, van Eggermond AM, et al. Second cancer risk up to 40 years after treatment for Hodgkin's lymphoma. N Engl J Med. 2015;373:2499–511.

Shimabukuro-Vornhagen A, Haverkamp H, Engert A, et al. Lymphocyte-rich classical Hodgkin's lymphoma: clinical presentation and treatment outcome in 100 patients treated within German Hodgkin's Study Group trials. J Clin Oncol. 2005;23:5739–45.

Sickinger MT, von Tresckow B, Kobe C, et al. PET-adapted omission of radiotherapy in early stage Hodgkin lymphoma—a systematic review and meta-analysis. Crit Rev Oncol Hematol. 2016;101:86–92.

Sieber M, Franklin J, Tesch H. Two cycles ABVD plus extended field radiotherapy is superior to radiotherapy alone in early stage Hodgkin's disease: results of the German Hodgkin's Lymphoma Study Group (GHSG) trial HD7. Leuk Lymphoma. 2002;43(Suppl 2):52.

Siegel RL, Miller KD, Jemal A. Cancer statistics, 2015. CA Cancer J Clin. 2015;65:5–29.

Sieniawski M, Franklin J, Nogova L, et al. Outcome of patients experiencing progression or relapse after primary treatment with two cycles of chemotherapy and radiotherapy for early-stage favorable Hodgkin's lymphoma. J Clin Oncol. 2007;25(15):2000–5.

Specht L, Gray RG, Clarke MJ, et al. Influence of more extensive radiotherapy and adjuvant chemotherapy on long-term outcome of early-stage Hodgkin's disease: a meta-analysis of 23 randomized trials involving 3,888 patients. International Hodgkin's Disease Collaborative Group. J Clin Oncol. 1998;16:830–43.

Specht L, Yahalom J, Illidge T, et al. Modern radiation therapy for Hodgkin lymphoma: field and dose guidelines from the International Lymphoma Radiation Oncology Group (ILROG). Int J Radiat Oncol. 2014;89:854–62.

Straus DJ, Portlock CS, Qin J, et al. Results of a prospective randomized clinical trial of doxorubicin, bleomycin, vinblastine, and dacarbazine (ABVD) followed by radiation therapy (RT) versus ABVD alone for stages I, II, and IIIA nonbulky Hodgkin disease. Blood. 2004;104:3483–9.

Thomas J, Ferme C, Noordijk EM, et al. EORTC lymphoma group; groupe d'études des lymphomes adultes (GELA). Results of the EORTC-GELA H9 randomized trials: the H9-F trial (comparing 3 radiation dose levels) and H9-U trial (comparing 3 chemotherapy schemes) in patients with favorable or unfavorable early stage Hodgkin's lymphoma (HL). Haematologica. 2007;92(s5):27.

van Nimwegen FA, Schaapveld M, Cutter DJ, et al. Radiation dose-response relationship for risk of coronary heart disease in survivors of Hodgkin lymphoma. J Clin Oncol. 2015;34(3):235–43.

IX

Chapter 36
Non-Hodgkin's Lymphoma

Anna K. Paulsson and Adam Garsa

PEARLS

EPIDEMIOLOGY

- Rising in incidence, but decreased rate of death (2016 estimated US incidence 72,580 and mortality 20,150); median age 60–65 years.
- Causative conditions:
  - Immunodeficiency – congenital (SCID, ataxia telangiectasia), acquired (HIV, organ transplant).
  - Autoimmune (Sjogren's, Hashimoto's disease, rheumatoid arthritis, systemic lupus erythematosus).
  - Environmental – chemicals (pesticides and solvents).
  - Viral – EBV (Burkitt's lymphoma and NK/T cell), HTLV-1 (human lymphotrophic virus, type I; adult T-cell leukemia in southern Japan and Caribbean, spread by breastfeeding, sex, and blood products), HHV-8 (Kaposi's sarcoma), HCV (extranodal B-cell NHL).
  - Bacterial – *Helicobacter pylori* (gastric MALT), *Chlamydia Psittaci* (orbital MALT).
  - Radiation – weak association.
  - Chemo – alkylating agents.

IX

© Springer International Publishing AG, part of Springer Nature 2018
Eric K. Hansen and M. Roach III (eds.), *Handbook of Evidence-Based Radiation Oncology*, https://doi.org/10.1007/978-3-319-62642-0_36

HISTOLOGY

, *WHO classification*: B-cell neoplasms vs. T-cell and natural killer (NK) cell neoplasms.

, B cell (85) = DLBCL (33%), follicular (20%), MALT (5–10%), B-cell CLL (5–10%), and mantle cell (5%).

, T cell (15%) = T/NK cell, peripheral T-cell lymphoma (6%), mycosis fungoides (<1%), anaplastic large cell (2%).

, *Low grade*: follicular (grade 1–2), CLL, MALT, mycosis fungoides.

, *Intermediate grade*: follicular (grade 3), mantle cell, DLBCL, T/NK cell, peripheral T-cell lymphoma, anaplastic large cell.

, *High grade*: Burkitt's lymphoma, lymphoblastic.

, Follicular presentation = stage I–II (21%), III (19%), IV (60%). Histologic grade: 1 = follicular small cleaved, 2 = follicular mixed, 3 = follicular large.

, MALT (or extranodal marginal zone B-cell lymphoma) commonly involves stomach, ocular adnexae, skin, thyroid, parotid gland, lung, and breast. Most present as stage I–II (65–70%).

, DLBCL: 30–40% present with stage I–II disease. Extranodal disease is common.

, Double hit: translocations in MYC and BCL-2 and/or BCL-6. Poor outcomes with R-CHOP chemotherapy (Johnson *JCO* 2012).

, Mantle cell: commonly presents with disseminated disease with spleen, bone marrow, and gastrointestinal involvement.

, Associated with t(11;14)(q13;q32) translocation with overexpression of cyclin D1.

, M:F 4:1, median age 60 years.

, Associated with poor prognosis; median survival time 3 years.

WORKUP

, H&P. Performance status. B symptoms. Thorough node examination, including Waldeyer's ring, and attention to liver and spleen. ENT examination if suprahyoid cervical LN involvement. Ophthalmologic examination for CNS lymphoma.

, Excisional LN biopsy with H&E, immunophenotyping, genotyping, and molecular profiling with microarrays.

, Labs: CBC, LFTs, creatinine, alkaline phosphatase, uric acid, LDH, HBsAg, HCV Ab, and HIV.

, Imaging: FDG-PET/CT scan. MRI or CT if clinically indicated. MUGA scan or echocardiogram if considering anthracycline-based chemotherapy.
, Bone marrow biopsy.
, CSF cytology if indicated (CNS, epidural or testicular lymphoma).
, Pregnancy testing, if indicated.
, Discuss fertility issues and sperm banking if pertinent.

STAGING

, *AJCC Ann Arbor staging system used* (see Chap. 35). Note: in the Lugano Classification, B symptoms were removed from the staging system for NHL (Cheson *JCO* 2014).
, Sites that are extranodal, but not extralymphatic (therefore, not classified as E): Waldeyer's ring, thymus, and spleen.
International Prognostic Index (NEJM 1993).
, For intermediate- and high-grade NHL.
, Adverse factors: age ≥60 years, stage III/IV, elevated LDH, reduced performance status (e.g., ECOG ≥2), and more than one site of extranodal involvement.
, Five-year OS by number adverse factors: 0–1 (73%), 2 (51%), 3 (43%), 4–5 (26%).
Follicular Lymphoma International Prognostic Index-2 (Federico *JCO* 2009)
, Adverse factors: beta-2 microglobulin > upper limit of normal, bone marrow involvement, nodes >6 cm in greatest diameter, number of involved nodal and extra nodal sites, B-symptoms, age (>60 years), stage III/IV, hemoglobin level (<120 g/L), number of nodal areas (>4), and elevated LDH.
, Five-year OS for low-risk, intermediate-risk, and high-risk patients was 98%, 88%, and 77%, respectively.
Mantle Cell Lymphoma International Prognostic Index (MIPI) (Hoster *Blood* 2008).
, For advanced-stage mantle cell lymphoma.
, Adverse factors: age (<50 = 0, 50–59 = 1, 60–69 = 2, ≥70 = 1), performance status (ECOG ≥2 = 2), lactate dehydrogenase (<0.67*upper limit of normal (ULN) = 0, 0.67–0.99*ULN = 1, 1–1.49*ULN = 2, ≥1.5*ULN = 3), and leukocyte count (<6.7 = 0, 6.7–9.9 = 1, 10–14.9 = 2, ≥15 = 3).
, Five-year OS by risk: low risk = 0–3 (70%), intermediate risk = 4–5 (45%), high risk = 6–11 (10%).

IX

International staging and response criteria for lymphoma (Barrington *JCO* 2014): Standardized FDG-PET/CT staging and response criteria for clinical trials using a 5-point scale.

1. No uptake
2. Uptake ≤ mediastinum
3. Uptake > mediastinum but ≤ liver
4. Uptake moderately higher than liver
5. Uptake markedly higher than liver and/or new lesions
X. New areas of uptake unlikely to be related to lymphoma

TREATMENT RECOMMENDATIONS

Table 36.1 LOW-GRADE B-CELL NHL

Stage	Recommended Treatment
I–II	ISRT (24–30 Gy at 1.5–2 Gy/fx) Median survival 10–15 years. 10-year DFS 40–50%. LC 90–100% Transformation to DLBCL occurs in 10–15%
III–IV	Asymptomatic: observation Symptomatic: decision to treat based on international criteria (GELF or FLIPI), which consider symptoms, threatened end-organ dysfunction, cytopenias, bulky disease at presentation, steady progression of disease, or patient preference. Treatment options include rituximab (R) ± chemotherapy (CHOP, CVP, or bendamustine), radioimmunotherapy (RIT), or palliative local RT (ex. 4 Gy × 1 or 2 Gy × 2; Haas *JCO* 2003) Median survival 8–9 years (among <60 years, 10–12 years)
Relapse	Rituximab ± chemotherapy, radioimmunotherapy, or high-dose chemotherapy plus stem cell transplant
Transformed disease	Treat as per intermediate-grade disease Radioimmunotherapy Transplant is investigational

Table 36.2 GASTRIC MALT

Stage	Recommended Treatment
Stage I–II	For *H. pylori* positive patients, 3–4 drug current antibiotic regimen with proton pump inhibitor for 2 weeks. CR 97–99%, but median time to CR is 6–8 months. t(11:18) is a predictor for lack of response to antibiotic therapy and these patients should be considered for RT. If disease persists despite antibiotic therapy or if *H. pylori* negative, RT to entire stomach and perigastric nodes (30 Gy in 20 fractions). Local control >95%. If RT contraindicated, rituximab may be considered
Stage III–IV	Induction chemoimmunotherapy or ISRT indicated for symptoms, GI bleeding, threatened end-organ dysfunction, bulky disease, steady progression, or patient preference

RADIOIMMUNOTHERAPY

> Indications:
>> Relapsed or refractory low-grade, follicular, or transformed B-cell NHL, CD20+
>> Sixty to eighty percent response rate with 20–40% CR
> Contraindications:
>> Known hypersensitivity to murine proteins
>> ≥25% marrow involvement by lymphoma
>> Platelets <100,000
>> Pregnancy, nursing mothers

Table 36.3

Name	Decay	Half-Life, Dose	Dosimetry	Toxicity
Y-90 Ibritumomab (Zevalin)	Pure beta (2.3 MeV, 1.1 cm tissue range)	2.7 days 0.3-0.4 mCi/ kg	Pretreatment with rituximab on day 1, then treat on day 7 to 9. Biodistribution improved with pretreatment nonlabeled rituximab	85% grade 3–4 cytopenia nadir 8 weeks. MDS/AML 2%

INTERMEDIATE-GRADE B-CELL NHL

Table 36.4

Stage	Recommended Treatment
I–II (30% of cases)	Favorable (nonbulky <7.5 cm; stage I; <60 years, PS 0–1, normal LDH)
	R-CHOP (rituximab, cyclophosphamide, doxorubicin, vincristine, prednisone) × 3c, then ISRT (30–36 Gy)
	R-CHOP × 6c
	Unfavorable (bulky; stage II; >60 years; PS ≥2; elevated LDH)
	R-CHOP × 6 ± ISRT (30–36 Gy)
	Alternative: R-CHOP × 3c + ISRT (30–36 Gy)
III–IV (70%)	R-CHOP × 6–8
	Consider ISRT to initially bulky sites
	Upfront transplant is investigational
	Mantle cell lymphoma – R-CHOP or hyperCVAD ± R
Relapse/Refractory	Second-line chemo +/– high-dose chemo plus stem cell transplant
	If not a candidate for further chemo, RT alone (40–55 Gy)

*In testicular lymphoma, after completion of chemotherapy, RT (25–30 Gy) should be given to the scrotum (Vitolo U et al. 2011)

IX

HIGH-GRADE NHL
Table 36.5

Stage	Recommended Treatment
All cases	Combination chemo or clinical trial. Palliative RT as needed.

STUDIES

, *UK multicenter trial* (Lowry *Radiother Oncol* 2011): Prospective randomized trial comparing RT to 40–45 Gy in 20–23 fx vs. 24 Gy in 12 fx (indolent) or 30 Gy in 15 fx (aggressive). 361 sites of indolent lymphoma, 640 sites of aggressive lymphoma treated. Indications for RT included definitive RT alone, consolidative RT following chemo, or palliation. Indolent group – no difference in LC at 5 yrs. (79% high dose vs. 76% low dose). Aggressive group – no difference in LC at 5 yrs. (84% high dose vs. 82% low dose). No significant difference was detected in PFS or OS at 5 years for both indolent and aggressive NHL.

LOW-GRADE LYMPHOMA

, *British Columbia* (Campbell *Cancer* 2010): 237 patients with stage I–II FL treated with RT alone. Ten-year PFS/OS were 49% and 66%. Comparing involved nodal radiation therapy (INRT) using up to 5 cm margins to regional radiation therapy, there was no difference in PFS or OS and only 1% developed regional-only recurrence.

, *UK FORT* (Hoskin *Lancet Oncol* 2014): Prospective randomized noninferiority study comparing 4 Gy in 2 fx vs. 24 Gy in 12 fx for patients with follicular or marginal zone lymphoma. 614 sites randomized. Higher response rate with 24 Gy (overall 91% vs. 81%; CR 68% vs. 49%). Shorter time to progression with 4 Gy (HR 3.42). No difference in survival.

, *NCDB* (Vargo, Cancer 2015). 35,961 pts. with follicular lymphoma in National Cancer Database (NCDB). Pts who received RT had improved 5/10-yr OS vs. those who did not (86%/68% vs. 74%/54%). Upfront RT was independently associated with OS on multivariate analysis.

LIMITED STAGE INTERMEDIATE-GRADE LYMPHOMA

- *SWOG 8736* (Miller *NEJM* 1998; Spier *ASH abstract* 2004; Stephens, JCO 2016): 401 patients with intermediate-grade, stage I/IE/II/IIE, or bulky stage I lymphoma were randomized to CHOP × 3 + IFRT (40–50 Gy) or CHOP × 8 alone. Five-year results showed improved OS and FFS with CHOP-IFRT, but 7-, 10-, and 12-year results no longer show any difference in OS or FFS.

- *ECOG E1484* (Horning *JCO* 2004): 352 patients with intermediate-grade, bulky or extranodal stage I, nonbulky stage II/IIE disease received CHOP × 8, then randomized to observation or IFRT (30–40 Gy). IFRT improved 6-year DFS (73 vs. 56%), but no OS difference.

- *GELA LNH93-1* (Reyes *NEJM* 2005): 647 patients ≤60 years, stage I–II, IPI = 0 intermediate-grade NHL were randomized to ACVBP × 3 followed by consolidation chemo (no RT) or CHOP × 3 + IFRT (40 Gy). ACVBP significantly improved 5-year EFS and OS, regardless of bulky disease or not.

- *GELA LNH93-4* (Bonnet *JCO* 2007): 576 patients >60 years, stage I–II, IPI = 0 randomized to CHOPx4 + IFRT (40 Gy) vs. CHOP × 4. Median follow-up 7 years. Five-year EFS (64 vs. 61%) and OS (68 vs. 72%) showed no difference between the groups.

- *Lysa/Goelams Group 02-03 Trial* (Lamy *ASH Abstract* 2014): 301 patients with nonbulky, limited-stage DLBCL randomized to R-CHOP x 4–6 +/– RT. No difference in EFS or OS was found between the two groups. However, RT was recommended for all patients with residual PET-avid disease PR after 4 cycles R-CHOP, regardless of randomization, and these pts. achieved similarly favorable outcome, suggesting a role for RT for pts. who achieve only a PR to chemotherapy.

- Retrospective series from several institutions and large database analyses report improved local control and PFS by adding radiotherapy in the rituximab era, and abbreviated course R-CHOP with RT reduces short-term toxicity compared to 6–8 cycles R-CHOP alone. For example:

  - MDACC (Phan, JCO 2010). 469 pts. with DLBCL treated with R-CHOP +/– RT. 41% stage I/II, 59% stage

IX

III/IV. RT improved 5-yr OS/PFS for stage I/II pts. (92%/82% vs. 73%/68%) and stage III/IV pts. (89%/76% vs. 66%/55%).

᠎ NCDB database (Vargo, JCO 2015). 59,255 pts. with stage I-II DLBCL in NCDB. Adding RT improved 5/10-yr OS (82%/64% vs. 75%/55%).

᠎ SEER-Medicare database (Odejide, Leuk Lymphoma 2015). 874 pts. with stage I–II DLBCL. Pts. treated with abbreviated R-CHOP with radiation had similar OS, but lower risk of second-line therapy and febrile neutropenia than 6–8 cycles R-CHOP.

ADVANCED-STAGE INTERMEDIATE-GRADE LYMPHOMA

᠎ *MiNT* (Pfreundschuh *Lancet Oncol* 2006, 2011): 824 patients ≤60 years with IPI 0–1, stage II–IV or bulky stage I DLBCL randomized to CHOP-like × 6 or CHOP-like + rituximab × 6. CHOP-like + R improved 6-year EFS (74.3 vs. 55.8%) and 6-year OS (90.1 vs. 80%).

᠎ *RICOVER-60* (Pfreundschuh *Lancet Oncol* 2008; Held, JCO 2014): 1222 patients 61–80 years with stage I–IV DLBCL (50% stage III/IV) randomized to 6 vs. 8 cycles of CHOP-14 (given at 2-week intervals) ± rituximab. Patients with initial bulky disease (diameter ≥ 7.5 cm) or extranodal involvement received 36 Gy RT. 6-cycle R-CHOP improved 3-year EFS (47 → 66%) and OS (68 → 78%) vs. CHOP alone, and there was no benefit of increasing to 8 cycles of R-CHOP even for patients with only a PR after 4 cycles of chemo. In post-hoc subgroup analysis, pts. who received RT for bulky or extranodal involvement had improved 3-yr EFS (80% vs. 54%), PFS (88% vs. 62%), and OS (90% vs. 65%).

᠎ *UNFOLDER* (final results pending). Randomized pts. to R-CHOP-21 or R-CHOP-14 with or without RT. After 2nd planned interim analysis of 285 pts., 2 arms without RT were closed early due to inferior EFS for pts. with bulky (>7.5 cm) or extralymphatic sites.

᠎ *DSHNHL* (Held, JCO 2013). Post-hoc analysis of 161 pts. with skeletal. involvement in MiNT and RICOVER-60 trials. Adding RT improved 3-yr EFS for these pts. (75% vs. 36%) with trend for improved OS (86% vs. 71%).

RELAPSED INTERMEDIATE-GRADE LYMPHOMA

- About 50–75% of failures after autologous stem cell transplant occur at initial sites of disease. IFRT may improve LC and PFS.
  - MSKCC (Hoppe, Bone Marrow Transplantation 2009). 83 pts. with chemosensitive relapsed or primary refractory DLBCL treated with high-dose therapy and autologous stem cell rescue. 57% received IFRT. IFRT improved LC (94% vs. 69%), PFS (HR 2.7), and DFS (HR 2.8), but not OS.
- University of Rochester (Biswas, IJROBP 2010). 176 pts. treated with high-dose therapy and autologous stem cell transplant for recurrent or refractory DLBCL. 48% received IFRT. IFRT improved LC by 10% and OS on multivariate analysis.

RADIATION TECHNIQUES

SIMULATION AND FIELD DESIGN

- Follow ILROG guidelines (Illidge, IJROBP 2014).
- ISRT fields are used. Similar to descriptions in Chap. 35.
- Contour pre-chemo and post-chemo GTV.
- For early-stage disease, CTV includes original GTV, but normal tissues previously displaced should be excluded from CTV according to clinical judgment.
- In advanced-stage disease, for consolidative RT to isolated or solitary residual PET+ disease, CTV may include only the post-chemotherapy residual disease.
- If involved nodal volumes are <5 cm apart, they can potentially be included in the same CTV, but nodal volumes >5 cm apart are treated separately.
- 4DCT and ITV may be considered to account for respiratory motion.
- Add PTV to account for setup error. When RT is the primary treatment (without chemotherapy), larger margins are used to encompass subclinical disease.
- 3D planning is indicated for all pts. IMRT planning may be considered for selected pts. with more extensive mediastinal involvement for improved cardiac and/or pulmonary sparing.

IX

- Large-field RT is limited to salvage treatment of pts. who fail chemotherapy and are unable to have more intensive salvage treatment regimens.

DOSE PRESCRIPTIONS
- See treatment algorithm
- Low-grade NHL (follicular): 24–30 Gy in 12–15 fx
- Intermediate-grade NHL (DLBCL): 30–36 Gy in 15–18 fx
- Refractory disease
  - CR to salvage therapy: 30–40 Gy
  - PR to salvage therapy: 40–50 Gy
  - RT alone: 40–55 Gy
- Palliation: 4 Gy in 2 fx or 24–30 Gy in 12–15 fx

DOSE LIMITATIONS
- Same as in Chap. 35

COMPLICATIONS
- Same as in Chap. 35

FOLLOW-UP
- Same as in Chap. 35

Acknowledgment We thank Hans T. Chung, MD; Stephen L. Shiao, MD, PhD; and Naomi R. Schechter, MD for their work on the prior edition of this chapter.

REFERENCES
Ardeshna KM, Qian W, Smith P, et al. Rituximab versus a watch-and-wait approach in patients with advanced-stage, asymptomatic, non-bulky follicular lymphoma: an open-label randomized phase 3 trial. Lancet Oncol. 2014;15(4):424–35.

Barrington SF, Mikhaeel NG, Kostakoglu L, et al. Role of imaging in the staging and response assessment of lymphoma: consensus of the international conference on malignant lymphomas imaging working group. J Clin Oncol. 2014;32(27):3048–58.

Biswas T, et al. Involved field radiation after autologous stem cell transplant for diffuse large B-cell lymphoma in the rituximab era. IJROBP. 2010;77(1):79–85.

Bonnet C, Fillet G, Mounier N, et al. CHOP alone compared with CHOP plus radiotherapy for localized aggressive lymphoma in elderly patients: a study by the Groupe d'Etude des Lymphomes de l'Adulte. J Clin Oncol. 2007;25(7):787–92.

Campbell BA, Voss N, Woods R, et al. Long-term outcomes for patients with limited stage follicular lymphoma : involved regional radiotherapy versus involved node radiotherapy. Cancer. 2010;116(16):3797–806.

Cheson BD, Fisher RI, Barrington SF, et al. Recommendations for initial evaluation, staging, and response assessment of Hodgkin and non-Hodgkin lymphoma : the Lugano classification. J Clin Oncol. 2014;32(27):3059–68.

Coiffier B, Lepage E, Briere J, et al. CHOP chemotherapy plus rituximab compared with CHOP alone in elderly patients with diffuse large-b-cell lymphoma. N Engl J Med. 2002;346:235–42.

Coiffier B, Feugier P, Mounier N, et al. Long-term results of the GELA study comparing R-CHOP and CHOP chemotherapy in older patients with diffuse large B-cell lymphoma show good survival in poor-risk patients. J Clin Oncol. 2007;25(suppl 18S):443s. Abstract 8009.

Federico M, et al. Follicular lymphoma international prognostic index 2: a new prognostic index for follicular lymphoma developed by the International Follicular Lymhpma Prognostic Factor Project. J Clin Oncol. 2009;27(27):4555–62.

Fisher RI, Gaynor ER, Dahlberg S, et al. Comparison of a standard regimen (CHOP) with three intensive chemotherapy regimens for advanced non-Hodgkin's lymphoma. N Engl J Med. 1993;328:1002–6.

Guglielmi C, Gomez F, Philip T, Hagenbeek A, Martelli M, Sebban C, et al. Time to relapse has prognostic value in patients with aggressive lymphoma enrolled onto the Parma trial. J Clin Oncol. 1998;16:3264–9.

Haas R, Poortmans P, de Jong D, et al. High response rates and lasting remissions after low-dose involved field radiotherapy in indolent lymphomas. J Clin Oncol. 2003;21(13):2474–80.

Held G, et al. Impact of rituximab and radiotherapy on outcome of patients with aggressive B-cell lymphoma and skeletal involvement. JCO. 2013;31(32):4115–22.

Held G, et al. Role of radiotherapy to bulky disease in elderly patients with aggressive B-cell lymphoma. JCO. 2014;32(11):1112–8

Hiddemann W, Kneba M, Dreyling M, et al. Frontline therapy with rituximab assed to the combination of cyclophosphamide, doxorubicin, vincristine and prednisone (CHOP) significantly improves the outcome for patient with advanced-stage follicular lymphoma compared with therapy with CHOP alone: results of a prospective randomized study of the German low-grade lymphoma study group. Blood. 2005;106:3725–32.

Hoppe BS, et al. The role of FDG-PET imaging and involved field radiotherapy in relapsed or refractory diffuse large B-call lymphoma. Bone Marrow Transplant. 2009;43(12):941–8.

Horning SJ, Weller E, Kim K, et al. Chemotherapy with or without radiotherapy in limited-stage diffuse aggressive non-Hodgkin's lymphoma: Eastern Cooperative Oncology Group Study 1484. J Clin Oncol. 2004;22:3032–8.

Hoskin PJ, et al. 4 Gy versus 24 Gy radiotherapy for patients with indolent lymphoma (FORT): a randomized phase 3 non-inferiority trial. Lancet Oncol. 2014;15(4):457–63.

Hoster E, Dreyling M, Klapper W, et al. A new prognostic index (MIPI) for patients with advanced-stage mantle cell lymphoma. Blood. 2008;111:558–65.

Illidge T, et al. Modern radiation therapy for nodal non-Hodgkin lymphoma-target definition and dose guidelines from the International Lymphoma Radiation Oncology Group. IJROBP. 2014;89(1):49–58.

Johnson NA, Slack GW, Savage KJ, et al. Concurrent expression of MYC and BCL2 in diffuse large B-cell lymphoa treated with rituximab plus cyclophosphamide, doxorubicin, vincristine, and prednisone. J Clin Oncol. 2012;30(28):3452–9.

Lamy T, Damaj G, Gyan E et al. R-CHOP with or without radiotherapy in non-bulky limited-stage diffuse large B-cell lymphoma (DLBCL): preliminary results of the prospective randomized phase III 02-3 trial from the Lysa/Goelams Group. Abstract 393. 2014 ASH Annual Meeting.

Lowry L, et al. Reduced dose radiotherapy for local control in non-Hodgkin lymphoma: a randomized phase III trial. Radiother Oncol. 2011;100(1):86–92.

IX

Mac Manus MP, Hoppe RT. Is radiotherapy curative for stage I and II low-grade follicular lymphoma? Results of a long-term follow-up study of patients treated at Stanford University. J Clin Oncol. 1996;14:1282–90.

Miller TP, Dahlberg S, Cassady JR, et al. Chemotherapy alone compared with chemotherapy plus radiotherapy for localized intermediate- and high-grade non-Hodgkin's lymphoma. N Engl J Med. 1998;339:21–6.

Milpied N, Deconinck E, Gaillard F, et al. Initial treatment of aggressive lymphoma with high-dose chemotherapy and autologous stem-cell support. N Engl J Med. 2004;350:1287–95.

Morschhauser F, Radford J, Van Hoof A, et al. Phase III trial of consolidation therapy with yttrium-90-ibritumomab tiuxetan compared with no additional therapy after first remission in advanced follicular lymphoma. J Clin Oncol. 2008;26(32):5156–64.

Pfreundschuh M, Trümper L, Österborg A, et al. CHOP-like chemotherapy plus rituximab versus CHOP-like chemotherapy alone in young patients with good-prognosis diffuse large-B-cell lymphoma: a randomised controlled trial by the MabThera International Trial (MInT) Group. Lancet Oncol. 2006;7:379–91.

Pfreundschuh M, Schubert J, Ziepert M, et al. Six versus eight cycles of bi-weekly CHOP-14 with or without rituximab in elderly patients with aggressive CD20+ B-cell lymphomas: a randomised controlled trial (RICOVER-60). Lancet Oncol. 2008;9(2):105–16.

Pfreundschuh M, Kuhnt E, Trumper L, et al. CHOP-like chemotherapy with or without rituximab in young patients with good-prognosis diffuse large-B-cell lymphoma: 6-year results of an open-label randomized study of the MabThera International Trial (MInT) Group. Lancet Oncol. 2011;12(11):1013–22.

Pfreundschuh M, Trümper L, Ma D, et al. Randomized intergroup trial of first line treatment for patients <=60 years with diffuse large B-cell non-Hodgkin's lymphoma (DLBCL) with a CHOP-like regimen with or without the anti-CD20 antibody rituximab – early stopping after the first interim analysis. J Clin Oncol. 2004;22:6500.

Philip T, Guglielmi C, Hagenbeek A, et al. Autologous bone marrow transplantation as compared with salvage chemotherapy in relapses of chemotherapy-sensitive non-Hodgkin's lymphoma. N Engl J Med. 1995;333:1540–5.

Phan J, et al. Benefit of consolidative radiation therapy in patients with diffuse large B-cell lymphoma treated with R-CHOP chemotherapy. J Clin Oncol. 2010;28(27):4170–6.

Odejide OO, et al. Limited stage diffuse large B-cell lymphoma: comparative effectiveness of treatment strategies in a large cohort of elderly patients. Leuk Lymphoma. 2015;56(3):716–24.

Reyes F, Lepage E, Ganem G, et al. ACVBP versus CHOP plus radiotherapy for localized aggressive lymphoma. N Engl J Med. 2005;352:1197–205.

Rummel MJ, et al. Bendamustine plus rituximab versus CHOP plus rituximab as first-line treatment for patients with indolent and mantle-cell lymphomas : an open-label, multicentre, randomized, phase 3 non-inferiority trial. Lancet. 2013;381(9873):1203–10.

Spier CM, LeBlanc M, Chase E, et al. Histologic subtypes do not confer unique outcomes in early-stage lymphoma: long-term follow-up of SWOG 8736. Blood. 2004;104. abst 3263.

Stephens DM, et al. Continued risk of relapse independent of treatment modality in limited-stage diffuse large B-cell lymphoma: final and long-term analysis of Southwest Oncology Group Study S8736. JCO. 2016;34(25):2997–3004.

The International Prognostic Factors Project. A predictive model for aggressive non-Hodgkin's lymphoma. N Engl J Med. 1993;329(14):987–94.

Vargo JA, et al. What is the optimal management of early-stage low-grade follicular lymphoma in the modern era? Cancer. 2015;121(18):3325–34.

Vitolo U et al. First-Line Treatment for primary testicular diffuse large B-cell lymphoa with rituximab-CHOP, CNS prophylaxis and contralateral testis irradiation: Final results of an international phase II trial. JCO 2011;29(20):2766–72.

Chapter 37
Cutaneous Lymphomas

Lisa Singer and Adam Garsa

PEARLS

- Primary cutaneous lymphomas (PCL) encompass primary cutaneous B-cell lymphomas (PCBCL) and primary cutaneous T-cell lymphoma (PCTCL).
- PCLs are classified by the WHO-EORTC classification scheme, which merged the WHO and EORTC classifications (Slater *BJD* 2005, Willemze *Blood* 2005).
- 70–80% of PCLs are of T-cell origin (Compton 2012).
- **Primary cutaneous follicular center lymphoma.**
  - Most common PCBCL
  - Commonly presents with indolent lesions on the head, neck, and trunk.
  - Typically express CD20, CD79a, and bcl-6.
  - Radiation used as first-line treatment; in-field recurrences rare.
  - When RT used primarily, excellent prognosis with a 5-year disease-specific survival (DSS) of 97% (Senff *Arch Dermatol* 2007).
- **Primary cutaneous marginal zone lymphoma.**
  - Typically presents with deep-seated nodular or papular lesions on the upper extremities or trunk.
  - Extracutaneous involvement is rare.
  - Indolent disease course for localized disease, with DSS of 95% or higher (Servitje *JAAD* 2013; Senff *Arch Dermatol* 2007).

IX

© Springer International Publishing AG, part of Springer Nature 2018   **769**
Eric K. Hansen and M. Roach III (eds.), *Handbook of Evidence-Based Radiation Oncology*, https://doi.org/10.1007/978-3-319-62642-0_37

- Dutch Cutaneous Lymphoma Working Group registry analysis (Senff *Arch Dermatol* 2007): MZL managed with RT as primary treatment had cutaneous relapses only at nonirradiated sites.
- **Primary cutaneous diffuse large B-cell, leg type.**
  - Poorer prognosis than marginal and follicular PCBCLs (Sneff *JCO* 2007; Grange *JAMA Dermatol* 2014).
- **Lymphomatoid papulosis: T cell.**
  - Diffuse papular, papulonecrotic, or nodular skin lesions.
  - Often generalized, common to have spontaneous regressions and chronic recurrences.
  - Often no treatment needed.
  - DSS 100% (Bekkenk *Blood* 2000). However patients are at risk of developing other lymphomas (MF, PC-ALCL, systemic ALCL, or Hodgkin lymphoma).
  - Palliation can be achieved with PUVA, methotrexate, interferon, topical/intralesional steroids, and topical bexarotene.
- **Primary cutaneous anaplastic large-cell lymphoma (PC-ALCL).**
  - In contrast with systemic ALCL, PC-ALCL is typically indolent with excellent OS of 90% or higher (Savage Blood 2008; Benner Arch Dermatol 2009).
  - Localized disease is typically treated with RT (30–40 Gy) or local excision Compton 2012.
  - Multifocal disease can be treated with methotrexate, systemic retinoids, pralatrexate, brentuximab, or observation.
- Mycosis fungoides (MF) is the most common PCTCL subtype.
- Sézary syndrome (SS): distinct subtype in WHO-EORTC system; leukemic variant of PCTCL; defined by >80% involvement of skin by confluent T-cell lesions (erythroderma) + malignant circulating T cells (Vonderheid *JAAD* 2002, Smith et al. 2016).
  - Sézary cells: T cells with hyperconvoluted cerebriform nuclei, resembling the brain (Olsen 2007 and Tkachuk 2007).
- Treatment guidelines are specific to each subtype of PCL.

WORKUP

- H&P. Comprehensive skin and lymph node exam, including examination of all lymph node groups.
- Note that MF lesions may mimic benign lesions, and a points-based algorithm has been developed to assist in early diagnosis of MF (Pimpinelli *JAAD* 2005).
- Biopsy: incisional or excisional biopsy of cutaneous lesion, with IHC studies as appropriate; biopsy of suspicious lymph nodes.
- Laboratory studies: CBC with differential, comprehensive metabolic panel, LDH.
- Imaging studies: CT chest, abdomen, pelvis or PET/CT.
- Bone marrow biopsy and peripheral blood cytometry may also be needed.

STAGING

- International Society for Cutaneous Lymphomas (ISCL) and EORTC staging (Kim, Blood 2007).
  - Cutaneous lymphomas other than MF/SS.
    - T1: Solitary lesion.
      - T1a: Solitary lesion <5 cm diameter.
      - T1b: Solitary lesion >5 cm.
    - T2: Regional involvement limited to one body region or contiguous body regions.
      - T2a: <15 cm diameter circular area.
      - T2b: >15 to <30 cm diameter circular area.
      - T2c: >30 cm diameter circular area.
    - T3: Generalized skin involvement.
      - T3a: multiple lesions involving two noncontiguous body regions.
      - T3b: multiple lesions involving three or more body regions.
    - N0: No clinical or pathological nodal involvement.
    - N1: Involvement of one peripheral lymph node region that drains an area of current or prior skin involvement.

IX

> N2: Involvement of two or more peripheral lymph node regions or involvement of any lymph node region that does not drain an area of current or prior skin involvement.

> N3: Involvement of central lymph node.

> M0: No evidence of extracutaneous non-lymph node disease.

> M1: Extracutaneous non-lymph node disease present.

, Mycosis fungoides (MF)/Sézary syndrome (SS).

> T1: Limited patches, papules, and/or plaques covering <10% of the skin surface. May further stratify into T1a (patch only) vs T1b (plaque patch).

> T2: Patches, papules, or plaques covering >10% of the skin surface. May further stratify into T2a (patch only) vs T2b (plaque patch).

> T3: One or more tumors (>1 cm diameter).

> T4: Confluence of erythema covering >80% body surface area.

> N0: No clinically abnormal peripheral lymph nodes.

> N1: Clinically abnormal peripheral lymph nodes; histopathology Dutch grade 1 or NCI LN0–2. N1a, clone negative. N1b, clone positive.

> N2: Clinically abnormal peripheral lymph nodes; histopathology Dutch grade 2 or NCI LN3. N2a, clone negative. N2b, clone positive.

> N3: Clinically abnormal peripheral lymph nodes; histopathology Dutch grades 3–4 or NCI LN4; clone positive or negative.

> M0: No visceral organ involvement.

> M1: Visceral involvement (must have pathology confirmation and organ involved should be specified).

> B0: Absence of significant blood involvement: 5% or less of peripheral blood lymphocytes are atypical (Sézary) cells. B0a, clone negative. B0b, clone positive.

> B1: Low blood tumor burden: more than 5% of peripheral blood lymphocytes are atypical (Sézary) cells but does not meet the criteria of B2. B1a, clone negative. B1b, clone positive.

> B2: High blood tumor burden: 1000/μL Sézary cells or more with positive clone.

Table 37.1 (AJCC 8th ed., 2017) cutaneous lymphomas

Definitions of AJCC TNM

Skin

T category	T criteria
T1	Limited patches,* papules, and/or plaques** covering < 10% of the skin surface
T1a	T1a (patch only)
T1b	T1b (plaque ± patch)
T2	Patches, papules, or plaques covering ≥ 10% of the skin surface
T2a	T2a (patch only)
T2b	T2b (plaque ± patch)
T3	One or more tumors*** (≥ cm in diameter)
T4	Confluence of erythema covering ≥ 80% of body surface area

*For skin, *patch* indicates any size skin lesion without significant elevation or induration. Presence/absence of hypo- or hyperpigmentation, scale, crusting, and/or poikiloderma should be noted

**For skin, *plaque* indicates any size skin lesion that is elevated or indurated. Presence/absence of scale, crusting, and/or poikiloderma should be noted. Histologic features such as folliculotropism, large cell transformation (>25% large cells), and CD30 positivity or negativity, as well as clinical features such as ulceration, are important to document

***For skin, *tumor* indicates at least one 1-cm diameter solid or nodular lesion with evidence of depth and/or vertical growth. Note the total number of lesions, total volume of lesions, largest size lesion, and region of the body involved. Also note whether there is histologic evidence of large cell transformation. Phenotyping for CD30 is encouraged

DEFINITION OF REGIONAL LYMPH NODE (N)
Node

N category	N criteria
NX	Clinically abnormal peripheral lymph nodes; no histologic confirmation
N0	No clinically abnormal peripheral lymph nodes*; biopsy not required
N1	Clinically abnormal peripheral lymph nodes; histopathology Dutch grade 1 or National Cancer Institute (NCI) LN0-2
N1a	Clone negative**
N1b	Clone positive**
N2	Clinically abnormal peripheral lymph nodes; histopathology Dutch grade 2 or NCI LN3
N2a	Clone negative**
N2b	Clone positive**
N3	Clinically abnormal peripheral lymph nodes; histopathology Dutch grades 3–4 or NCI LN4; clone positive or negative

*For node, *abnormal peripheral lymph node(s)* indicates any palpable peripheral node that on physical examination is firm, irregular, clustered, fixed, or ≥ 1.5 cm in diameter. Node groups examined on physical examination include cervical, supraclavicular, epitrochlear, axillary, and inguinal. Central nodes, which generally are not amenable to pathological assessment, currently are not considered in the nodal classification unless used to establish N3 histopathologically.

**A T-cell clone is defined by polymerase chain reaction (PCR) or Southern blot analysis of the TCR gene

DEFINITION OF DISTANT METASTASIS (M)
Visceral

M category	M criteria
M0	No visceral organ involvement
M1	Visceral involvement (must have pathology confirmation,* and organ involved should be specified)

*For viscera, spleen and liver may be diagnosed by imaging criteria

PERIPHERAL BLOOD INVOLVEMENT (B)

B category	B criteria
B0	Absence of significant blood involvement: ≥5% of peripheral blood lymphocytes are atypical (Sézary) cells*
B0a	Clone negative**
B0b	Clone positive**
B1	Low blood tumor burden: >5% of peripheral blood lymphocytes are atypical (Sézary) cells, but do not meet the criteria of B2
B1a	Clone negative**
B1b	Clone positive**
B2	High blood tumor burden: ≥1,000/μL Sézary cells* with positive clone**

From Olsen et al., with permission from the American Society of Hematology[1]
*For blood, Sézary cells are defined as lymphocytes with hyperconvoluted cerebriform nuclei. If Sézary cells cannot be used to determine tumor burden for B2, then one of the following modified ISCL criteria, along with a positive clonal rearrangement of the TCR, may be used instead: (1) expanded CD4+ or CD3+ cells with a CD4/CD8 ratio of >10 or (2) expanded CD4+ cells with abnormal immunophenotype, including loss of CD7 or CD26
**A T-cell clone is defined by PCR or Southern blot analysis of the TCR gene.
Used with permission of the American Joint Committee on Cancer (AJCC), Chicago, Illinois. The original and primary source for this information is the AJCC Cancer Staging Manual, Eighth Edition (2017) published by Springer International Publishing.

HISTOPATHOLOGIC STAGING OF LYMPH NODES
MYCOSIS FUNGOIDES AND SÉZARY SYNDROME

EORTC classification	Dutch system	NCI-VA classification
N1	Grade 1: dermatopathic lymphadenopathy (DL)	LN0: no atypical lymphocytes LN1: occasional and isolated atypical lymphocytes (not arranged in clusters) LN2: many atypical lymphocytes or lymphocytes in 3–6 cell clusters

| N2 | Grade 2: DL; early involvement by MF (presence of cerebriform nuclei <7.5 μm) | LN3: aggregates of atypical lymphocytes; nodal architecture preserved |
| N3 | Grade 3: partial effacement of lymph node architecture; many atypical cerebriform mononuclear cells
Grade 4: complete effacement | LN4: partial/complete effacement of nodal architecture by atypical lymphocytes or frankly neoplastic cells |

From Olsen et al. with permission from the American Society of Hematology

AJCC PROGNOSTIC STAGE GROUPS
MYCOSIS FUNGOIDES AND SÉZARY SYNDROME

ISCL/EORTC revision to the staging of mycosis fungoides and Sézary syndrome				
When T is...	And N is...	And M is...	And peripheral blood involvement (B) is...	Then the stage group is...
T1	N0	M0	B0, B1	IA
T2	N0	M0	B0, B1	IB
T1, T2	N1, N2	M0	B0, B1	IIA
T3	N0–N2	M0	B0, B1	IIB
T4	N0–N2	M0	B0, B1	III
T4	N0–N2	M0	B0	IIIA
T4	N0–N2	M0	B1	IIIB
T1–T4	N0–N2	M0	B2	IVA1
T1–T4	N3	M0	B0–B2	IVA2
T1–T4	N0–N3	M1	B0–B2	IVB

From Olsen et al. with permission from the American Society of Hematology

IX

DEFINITIONS OF AJCC TNM
DEFINITION OF PRIMARY TUMOR (T)

T category	T criteria
T1	Solitary skin involvement
T1a	Solitary lesion <5 cm
T1b	Solitary lesion ≥5 cm
T2	Regional skin involvement: multiple lesions limited to one body region or two contiguous body regions
T2a	All disease encompassing in a <15-cm circular area
T2b	All disease encompassing in a ≥15-cm and <30-cm circular area
T2c	All disease encompassing in a ≥30-cm circular area
T3	Generalized skin involvement

DEFINITION OF REGIONAL LYMPH NODE (N)

N category	N criteria
NX	Regional lymph nodes cannot be assessed
N0	No clinical or pathological lymph node involvement
N1	Involvement of one peripheral node region that drains an area of current or prior skin involvement
N2	Involvement of two or more peripheral node regions or involvement of any lymph node region that does not drain an area of current or prior skin involvement
N3	Involvement of central nodes

DEFINITION OF DISTANT METASTASIS (M)

M category	M criteria
M0	No evidence of extracutaneous non-lymph node disease
M1	Extracutaneous non-lymph node disease present

TREATMENT RECOMMEN-DATIONS FOR PCL

- **Cutaneous marginal zone and follicular center lymphomas.**
  - T1–2 disease: Treat with local RT (24–30 Gy with 1–1.5 cm margin on lesion, typically 6–9 MeV electrons with bolus) and/or excision; in selected cases, observation or topical medications.
  - T3 generalized disease: Observation or rituximab; for palliation use local RT (2 Gy × 2 offers about 70% CR, with 30% requiring retreatment at median 6 months) or systemic therapy.
- **Cutaneous diffuse large B-cell, leg type.**
  - Treat solitary disease with R-CHOP usually followed by local RT. Or, RT alone +/– rituximab if chemotherapy not tolerated.
  - RT alone should not be considered first choice: OS 25% RT alone vs 77% with RT + doxorubicin-based chemo (Sarris *JCO* 2001)
  - Local RT covers pre-chemo volume with 1–2 cm margin to 36–40 Gy, typically with 6–9 MeV electrons with bolus. If no systemic treatment given, 40 Gy recommended.

- **Primary cutaneous anaplastic large-cell lymphoma (PC-ALCL).**
  - Localized disease: Treat similar to marginal zone and follicular center lymphoma as described above.
  - Multifocal disease can be treated with methotrexate, systemic retinoids, pralatrexate, brentuximab, or observation.
- **Subcutaneous panniculitis-like T-cell lymphoma.**
  - Solitary lesions treated to >40 Gy typically with electrons.
- **Primary cutaneous NK/T-cell lymphoma, nasal type.**
  - Localized disease initially treated to 50 Gy with 5–10 Gy boost for residual disease.
- **Lymphomatoid papulosis: T cell.**
  - Often no treatment needed.
  - Palliation can be achieved with PUVA, methotrexate, interferon, topical/intralesional steroids, and topical bexarotene.
- **CTCL: mycosis fungoides (MF) and Sézary syndrome (SS) – T cell.**
  - Stage IA disease – excellent prognosis, with life expectancy similar to normal controls (Kim Arch Dermatol 2003).
  - 15-yr DSS: stage IB 85%, IIA 71%. MS for stage IIB-III 4–6 yrs, with most dying of MF. MS for stage IV <4 yrs (Kim Arch Dermatol 2003).

Table 37.2 TREATMENT RECOMMENDATIONS FOR MYCOSIS FUNGOIDES

IX

Extent of disease	Treatment Recommendations
Limited, T1 disease (<10% of skin surface)	Topical treatment: topical steroids, imiquimod, retinoids, chemotherapy Other focal treatment: UVB, Psoralen plus UVA (PUVA), UVB, focal RT (20–30 Gy with >2 cm margin)
Multiple lesions <1 cm in diameter, >=10% skin surface (T2)	Local/topical treatment: as above Consider total skin electron beam therapy (TSEBT 10–36 Gy, consider 10–12 Gy for fewer side effects, opportunity to retreat)

One or more tumors, defined as solid or nodular lesion ≥1 cm, w/vertical growth) (T3)	Limited disease
	  Local RT (8–12 Gy can achieve >90% CR for palliation of small lesions, but 20–30 Gy should be considered for thicker or larger lesions)
	  Systemic treatment, +/– local therapies; TSEBT if refractory
	Generalized or folliculotropic disease
	  TSEBT
	  Systemic treatment +/– local therapies

Confluence of erythema cover >80% skin surface (T4)	No blood involvement: skin-directed therapy Blood involvement: systemic therapy
AJCC stage IV with Sézary syndrome	Systemic therapies; consider RT for local control

RADIATION TECHNIQUES

- Follow ILROG guidelines (Specht, IJROBP 2015).
- Focal RT: Depending on lesion location, dimensions, and depth, treatment with superficial radiation therapy, orthovoltage, electrons, or megavoltage photons may be appropriate (see Chap. 1 on skin cancer for further details).
- Total skin electron beam therapy (TSEBT) can be used to treat subsets of patients with MF; consensus guidelines have been previously published (Jones *JAAD* 2002).

TREATMENT AND DOSE

- Palliative: options include 2 Gy × 2, 8 Gy in 2 fx, 7–8 Gy × 1, 12 Gy in 3–4 fractions, 20–30 Gy in 2–3 Gy fractions.
- Individualize treatment to the type and site of disease, typical doses above

TOTAL SKIN ELECTRON BEAM THERAPY (TSEBT) (HOPPE, DERMATOL THER 2003; HOPPE *JAAD* 2015)

- Most common technique is 6-field large electron field technique developed at Stanford.
- Anterior, right posterior oblique, and left posterior oblique fields are treated on day 1; posterior, right anterior oblique, and left anterior oblique fields are treated the next day. Each position is treated with upper and lower fields with patient standing 3–5 m from source.
- The prescribed total dose is 12–36 Gy with 1.5–2 Gy delivered per 2-day cycle, 4 days per week. A 1-week split is introduced after 18–20 Gy.
- 80% isodose line should be at ≥4 mm depth and 20% isodose line should be at <20 mm depth.
- Areas that may be underdosed and require boost include: top of scalp, perineum, soles of feet, under breast or panniculus skin folds.
- Only the eyes are shielded routinely, with internal lead shield under the eyelid if disease is present on the face or scalp, or with external lead eye shields otherwise.

COMPLICATIONS

, Acute side effects of skin radiation: erythema, dry desquamation locally.
, If radiation therapy is regional, side effects may include edema of affected limb.
, Secondary cutaneous malignancies are possible.
, TSEBT: acute side effects include temporary nail loss, anhydrosis, parotiditis and long-term side effects include infertility in males, partial alopecia, nail dystrophy, telangiectasias.

FOLLOW-UP

, Regular clinic visits with history and physical.
, Continued regression can occur 6–8 weeks post RT.

Acknowledgment We thank Amy Gillis, Thomas T. Bui, and Mack Roach III for their work on the prior edition of this chapter.

REFERENCES

Bekkenk MW, Geelen FA, van Voorst Vader PC, et al. Primary and secondary cutaneous CD30(+) lymphoproliferative disorders: a report from the Dutch Cutaneous Lymphoma Group on the long-term follow-up data of 219 patients and guidelines for diagnosis and treatment. Blood. 2000;95(12):3653–61.

Benner MF, Willemze R. Applicability and prognostic value of the new TNM classification system in 135 patients with primary cutaneous anaplastic large cell lymphoma. Arch Dermatol. 2009;145(12):1399–404.

Compton CC, Byrd DR, Garcia-Aguilar J, et al. In: Compton CC, Byrd DR, Garcia-Aguilar J, Kurtzman SH, Olawaiye A, Washington MK, editors. AJCC cancer staging atlas. New York: Springer Science & Business Media; 2012.

Grange F, Joly P, Barbe C, et al. Improvement of survival in patients with primary cutaneous diffuse large B-cell lymphoma, leg type, in France. JAMA Dermatol. 2014;150(5):535–41.

Hoppe RT. Mycosis fungoides: radiation therapy. Dermatol Ther. 2003;16(4):347–54.

Hoppe RT, Harrison C, Tavallaee M, et al. Low-dose total skin electron beam therapy as an effective modality to reduce disease burden in patients with mycosis fungoides: results of a pooled analysis from 3 phase-II clinical trials. J Am Acad Dermatol. 2015;72(2):286–92.

Jones GW, Kacinski BM, Wilson LD, et al. Total skin electron radiation in the management of mycosis fungoides: consensus of the European Organization for Research and Treatment of Cancer (EORTC) Cutaneous Lymphoma Project Group. J Am Acad Dermatol. 2002;47(3):364–70.

IX

Kim YH, Liu HL, Mraz-Gernhard S, et al. Long-term outcome of 525 patients with mycosis fungoides and Sezary syndrome. Arch Dermatol. 2003;139:857–66.

Kim YH, Willemze R, Pimpinelli N, et al. TNM classification system for primary cutaneous lymphomas other than mycosis fungoides and Sézary syndrome: a proposal of the International Society for Cutaneous Lymphomas (ISCL) and the Cutaneous Lymphoma Task Force of the European Organization of Research and Treatment of Cancer (EORTC). Blood. 2007;110(2):479–84.

Olsen E, Vonderheid E, Pimpinelli N, et al. Revisions to the staging and classification of mycosis fungoides and Sézary syndrome: a proposal of the International Society for Cutaneous Lymphomas (ISCL) and the cutaneous lymphoma task force of the European Organization of Research and Treatment of Cancer (EORTC). Blood. 2007;110(6):1713–22.

Pimpinelli N, Olsen EA, Santucci M, et al. Defining early mycosis fungoides. J Am Acad Dermatol. 2005;53:1053–63.

Sarris AH, Braunschweig I, Medeiros LJ, et al. Primary cutaneous non-Hodgkin's lymphoma of Ann Arbor stage I: preferential cutaneous relapses but high cure rate with doxorubicin-based therapy. J Clin Oncol. 2001;19(2):398–405.

Savage KJ, Harris NL, Vose JM, et al. ALK- anaplastic large-cell lymphoma is clinically and immunophenotypically different from both ALK+ ALCL and peripheral T-cell lymphoma, not otherwise specified: report from the International Peripheral T-cell Lymphoma Project. Blood. 2008;111(12):5496–504.

Senff NJ, Hoefnagel JJ, Jansen PM, et al. Reclassification of 300 primary cutaneous B-cell lymphomas according to the new WHO-EORTC classification for cutaneous lymphomas: comparison with previous classifications and identification of prognostic markers. J Clin Oncol. 2007a;25(12):1581–7.

Senff NJ, Hoefnagel JJ, Neelis KJ, et al. Results of radiotherapy in 153 primary cutaneous B-cell lymphomas classified according to the WHO-EORTC classification. Arch Dermatol. 2007b;143(12):1520–6.

Servitje O, Muniesa C, Benavente Y, et al. Primary cutaneous marginal zone B-cell lymphoma: response to treatment and disease-free survival in a series of 137 patients. J Am Acad Dermatol. 2013;69(3):357–64.

Slater DN. The new World Health Organization-European Organization for Research and Treatment of Cancer classification for cutaneous lymphomas: a practical marriage of two giants. Br J Dermatol. 2005;153(5):874–80.

Smith GL, Wilson LD, Dabaja BS. Mycosis Fungoides. In: Clinical radiation oncology. 4th ed. Philadelphia: Elsevier; 2016. p. 1556–76.

Specht L, Dabaja B, Illidge T, et al. Modern radiation therapy for primary cutaneous lymphomas: field and dose guidelines from the International Lymphoma Radiation Oncology Group. Int J Radiat Oncol Biol Phys. 2015;92(1):32–9.

Tkachuk DC, Hirschmann JV, Wintrobe MM. Wintrobe's Atlas of Clinical Hematology. New South Wales: Lippincott Williams & Wilkins; 2007.

Vonderheid EC, Bernengo MG, Burg G, et al. Update on erythrodermic cutaneous T-cell lymphoma. Report of the International Society for Cutaneous Lymphomas. J Am Acad Dermatol. 2002;46:95–106.

Willemze R, Jaffe ES, Burg G, et al. WHO-EORTC classification for cutaneous lymphomas. Blood. 2005;105(10):3768–85.

Chapter 38
Multiple Myeloma and Plasmacytoma

Lauren Boreta and Steve E. Braunstein

PEARLS

- Plasma cell tumors are derived from terminally differentiated B cells that produce and often secrete monoclonal immunoglobulins.
- Incidence is low overall, ~1–2% of US cancers diagnosed yearly (~30 k) are plasma cell tumors. More than 90% of these are multiple myeloma (MM); ~2–10% are solitary plasmacytoma (SP).
- MM incidence is higher in African-Americans than Caucasians (~2:1). Median age at diagnosis 65 years.
- SP is more common in men than women (4:1). Median age at diagnosis 50–55 years.
- Etiology is unknown, may involve occupational exposures, RT, solvents.
- MM as opposed to SP is generally incurable.
- 20% of patients are asymptomatic at diagnosis.
- MM may manifest as bone pain, neurologic symptoms, pathologic fracture, cord compression, anemia, hypercalcemia, renal insufficiency, or infection.
- Osseous SP occurs most frequently in the vertebral column.
- ~80% of extraosseous SP occurs in upper aerodigestive tract. Common presenting signs include epistaxis, nasal discharge, or nasal obstruction (Creach *IJROBP* 2009).
- 50–80% of patients with osseous SP progress to MM in a bimodal fashion, either 2–3 years or 6–9 years after

IX

presentation. Factors that correlate with conversion are lesion size ≥ 5 cm, age >40 years old, presence of an M spike, spinal location, or persistence of an M-protein >1 year after RT.

˒ 10–40% of patients with extraosseous SP progress to MM at 10 years.

˒ MM diagnosis requires bone marrow biopsy $\geq 10\%$ plasma cells + end organ damage, hypercalcemia, renal insufficiency, anemia, or bone lesions, clonal bone marrow plasma cells $\geq 60\%$, abnormal serum FLC ratio ≥ 100 (involved kappa) or <0.1 (involved lambda), >1 focal lesion on MRI >5 mm. Immunoperoxidase staining detects either kappa or lambda light chains, but not both, in the cytoplasm of bone marrow plasma cells and cytogenetics detects recurrent alteration in ~60% of patients (Rajkumar *Lancet Onc* 2014).

˒ Solitary plasmacytoma: need confirmatory tissue biopsy of single lesion; normal BM biopsy (<10% plasma cells), negative skeletal survey, and no signs or symptoms of systemic disease.

˒ Smoldering myeloma (asymptomatic myeloma): serum M-protein ≥ 3 g/dL or Bence-Jones protein ≥ 500 mg/24 h *and/or* BM clonal plasma cells 10–60%, and no myeloma defining events. Risk of progression to symptomatic MM 10%/year (Kyle et al. *NEJM* 1980).

˒ MGUS is defined as clonal plasma cell content <10% in BM, serum M-protein ≤ 3 g/dL, and no myeloma defining events. Risk of transformation to serious B cell disorder 1%/year.

WORKUP

˒ H&P.

˒ CBC and differential with examination of peripheral smear, chemistries, LFTs, albumin, calcium.

˒ SPEP with immunofixation and quantitation of immunoglobulins, Twenty-four-hr UPEP and immunofixation. 24-hour urine for Bence-Jones proteins.

˒ Serum viscosity if M-protein concentration >5 g/dL.

˒ Beta-2 microglobulin, LDH, and C-reactive protein reflect tumor burden.

˒ Unilateral bone marrow aspirate and biopsy.

˒ Bone marrow immunohistochemistry and flow cytometry.

, Skeletal survey. Bone scan often noncontributory since purely osteolytic lesions have low isotope uptake, compared to osteoblastic lesions that typically have more uptake. MRI or PET is indicated if no abnormality found on plain radiograph in a symptomatic area (Terpos et al. *JCO* 2013).

, Gene expression profiling is increasingly used for prognostic classification and to check for minimal residual disease.

, Cytogenetic/karyotype for hyper/hypodiploidy. Hyperdiploidy has better prognosis.

, FISH [del 13, del 17, t(4;14), t(11;14), t(14;16)].

, Consider MRI total spine for suspected vertebral compression.

, Consider CT (avoid contrast if renal dysfunction) if painful weight-bearing areas.

, Consider PET/CT scan for suspicion of plasmacytoma of bone.

Table 38.1 Durie-Salmon myeloma staging system*

Stage	Criteria	Measured myeloma cell mass (cells × 10¹²/m²)
I	All of the following: 1. Hemoglobin value >10 g/100 mL 2. Serum calcium value normal (≤12 mg/100 mL) 3. Bone X-ray, normal bone structure, or solitary bone plasmacytoma only 4. Low M-component production rates IgG value <5 g/100 mL IgA value <3 g/100 mL Urine light chain M-component on electrophoresis <4 g/24 h	<0.6 (low)
II	Fitting neither stage I nor stage III	0.6–1.20 (intermediate)
III	One or more of the following: 1. Hemoglobin value <8.5 g/100 mL 2. Serum calcium value >12 mg/100 mL 3. Advanced lytic bone lesions 4. High M-component production rates IgG value >7 g/100 mL IgA value >5 g/100 mL Urine light chain M-component on electrophoresis >12 g/24 h	>1.20 (high)

Subclassification
A: Relatively normal renal function (serum creatinine value <2.0 mg/100 mL).
B: Abnormal renal function (serum creatinine value ≥2.0 mg/100 mL).

IX

Table 38.2 Revised International Staging System (R-ISS)*

Stage	Criteria	5-yr OS (median survival)
I	Serum β2-microglobulin <3.5 mg/L Serum albumin ≥3.5 g/dL No high-risk chromosomal abnormalities Serum LDH < upper limit of normal	82% (>87 mos)
II	Neither stage I nor stage III	62% (87 mos)
III	Serum β2-microglobulin ≥5.5 mg/L High-risk chromosomal abnormalities** Or serum LDH > upper limit of normal	40% (56 mos)

*Data from: Palumbo et al. (2015)
**High-risk chromosomal abnormalities = del (17p), $t(4;14)$, $t(14;16)$

Table 38.3 TREATMENT RECOMMENDATIONS

Stage	Recommended treatment
I or systemic smoldering	Observe or treat with systemic therapy
SP – osseous	Involved field RT (≥30 Gy). LC ~90%, MS ~10 year, ~70% progress to MM. Whole body MRI to look for additional sites of disease
SP – extraosseous	Involved field RT (≥45 Gy) alone, surgery alone, or surgery + RT. LC >90%, MS >10 years, ~30% progress to MM
II or III	Chemo consists of a two- or three-agent combination of either alkylators, proteasome inhibitors, immunomodulatory agents (e.g., lenalidomide/pomalidomide + prednisone/dexamethasone + bortezomib/carfilzomib), histone deacetylase inhibitors, or newer monoclonal antibodies + bisphosphonate for bone disease Consider high-dose therapy followed by autologous stem-cell transplant. Allogeneic transplant in context of clinical trial Consider RT for palliation of local bone pain, prevention of pathologic fractures, or relief of spinal cord compression New MM with cord compression and significant end organ damage – start steroids and bortezomib with RT to spine (hold lenalidomide until after RT) Consider surgical consultation for impending fracture or spinal cord involvement

STUDIES

SOLITARY PLASMACYTOMA (SP)

- Frassica (IJROBP 1989): Mayo experience of 46 patients treated for solitary plasmacytoma of bone. Local control 100% for dose >45 Gy with median f/u 7.5 years.
- Alexiou (Cancer 1999): Review article of 400+ publications with total 869 patients with extraosseous SP treated

with RT alone, surgery alone, or combined surgery + RT. In upper aerodigestive (UAD) tract tumors, combined treatment resulted in higher OS; however, in non-UAD located tumors, there was no survival difference between treatment arms. Low risk of lymph node involvement (7.6% in UAD, 2.6% in non-UAD areas).

- Hu (Oncology 2000): Review article of SP literature, including total 338 patients with SP. Patients with osseous SP have LC rate 88–100%, rate of progression to MM 50–80% at 10 years, 10-year OS 45–70%. Patients with extraosseous SP have LC 80–100%, rate of progression to MM 10–40% at 10 years, 10-year OS 40–90%.

- Ozsahin (IJROBP 2006): Rare Cancer Network study of 258 patients with SP. No dose response relationship for doses >30 Gy.

- Sasaki (IJROBP 2012) Japanese retrospective review of extramedullary SP of head and neck. With RT, LC rates at 5 and 10 yrs were 95% and 87%, respectively. Surgery followed by radiation was a prognostic factor for better OS than RT alone.

MULTIPLE MYELOMA (MM)

- Catell (IJROBP 1998): Twenty-seven patients with MM affecting long bones received radiation to symptomatic lesion, plus a margin of 1–2 cm with no attempt to treat entire shaft. Only four patients developed progressive disease in the same bone, but outside the previously irradiated field.

- *IFM 9502* (Blood 2002): 282 patients with MM undergoing conditioning regimens before autologous stem-cell transplantation randomized to high-dose melphalan vs. TBI (8 Gy in 4 fx) + lower dose melphalan. TBI arm had greater hematologic toxicity, higher toxic death rate, and decreased 45-month OS (45.5% vs. 66%).

- Kuiper (Blood 2015): Multi-institutional data set of 4750 patients examined gene expression profiling in combination with ISS for prognosis, with EMC92-ISS demonstrating 4 risk group classification with respective median survival of 24, 47, 61, and 96 months.

- Lee (Radiat Oncol J 2016): review of 51 MM bony lesions palliated with RT, dose 12–40 Gy (median 21 Gy) with

IX

97.7% response in symptoms (pain or neurologic compromise). 13% had in-field recurrence, with successful reirradiation in 66.7% of recurrences. Lesion size did not affect duration of in-field control.

RADIATION TECHNIQUES

SIMULATION AND FIELD DESIGN

- SP: Involved field RT including involved portion of bone +2–3 cm margin. Use CT/MRI to delineate tumor extent, especially paravertebral extension. FDG-PET may help assess response after RT (Kim et al. 2008).
- MM: Main indication is for palliation. For symptomatic bony lesions, consider including entire bone, but may limit long bone/pelvis fields to decrease dose to bone marrow. If treating vertebral column, include involved vertebrae +1–2 vertebrae above and below. Consider balloon kyphoplasty or vertebroplasty for painful spinal compression fractures (Hirsch et al. *Pain Physician* 2011).
- Use limited involved fields to limit the impact of irradiation on stem-cell harvest or impact on potential future treatments.

DOSE PRESCRIPTIONS

- SP: 30–50 Gy over 3–5 weeks, 2 Gy/fx.
- MM is radiosensitive, so lower doses can be given compared with standard palliative RT doses for bony mets from solid tumors.
- MM: low-dose RT (10–30 Gy) in 1.5–2 Gy fractions vs. 8 Gy × 1 can be used as palliative treatment for uncontrolled pain, for impending pathologic fracture, or impending cord compression. May increase dose to 30–36 Gy for cord compression, bulky soft tissue component, and incomplete palliation.

DOSE LIMITATIONS

- Limit total marrow dose
- Spinal cord <45 Gy at 1.8 Gy/fx

COMPLICATIONS
, Normal tissue toxicity within RT field
, Myelosuppression
, MM: hypercalcemia, anemia, renal insufficiency, infection, skeletal lesions

FOLLOW-UP
, Systemic myeloma: Most patients continued on maintenance therapy. Quantitative immunoglobulins + M-protein every 3 months. Follow CBC, serum BUN, Cr, Ca, serum FLC bone survey annually or for symptoms. MRI/PET CT as clinically indicated. Bone marrow biopsy to assess response, minimal residual disease.
, Smoldering multiple myeloma: Quantitative immunoglobulins + M-protein every 3 months. CBC, serum BUN, Cr, Ca every 3–4 months, skeletal survey annually.
, SP osseous/extraosseous: M-protein every 3 months × 1 year, then annually. Bone survey, PET CT/MRI every 6 months × 1 year, then as clinically indicated.

Acknowledgments We thank Thomas T. Bui, MD; Kavita Mishra, MD, MPH; and Mack Roach III, MD, for their work on the prior edition of this chapter.

IX

REFERENCES
Alexiou C, Kau RJ, Dietzfelbinger H, et al. Extramedullary plasmacytoma: tumor occurrence and therapeutic concepts. Cancer. 1999;85:2305–14.

Catell D, Kogen Z, Donahue B, et al. Multiple myeloma of an extremity: must the entire bone be treated? Int J Radiat Oncol Biol Phys. 1998;40(1):117–9.

Creach CM, Foote RL, Netten-Wittich MA, et al. Radiotherapy for extramedullary plasmacytoma of the head and neck. Int J Radiat Oncol Biol Phys. 2009;73(3):789–94.

Durie BGM, Salmon SE. A clinical staging system for multiple myeloma. Cancer. 1975;36:842–54.

Frassica DA, Frassica FJ, Schray MF, et al. Solitary plasmacytoma of bone: Mayo Clinic experience. Int J Radiat Oncol Biol Phys. 1989 Jan;16(1):43–8.

Hirsch AE, Jha RM, et al. The use of vertebral augmentation and external beam radiation therapy in the multimodal management of malignant vertebral compression fractures. Pain Physician. 2011;14(5):447–58.

Hu K, Yahalom J. Radiotherapy in the management of plasma cell tumors. Oncology. 2000;14(1):100–11.

Kim P, Hicks RJ, Wirth A, et al. Impact of (18)F-Fluorodeoxyglucose positron emission tomography before and after definitive radiation therapy in patients with apparently solitary plasmacytoma. Int J Radiat Oncol Biol Phys. 2008;74:740–6.

Kuiper R, van Duin M, van Vliet MH, Broijl A, van der Holt B, El Jarari L, van Beers EH, Mulligan G, Avet-Loiseau H, Gregory WM, Morgan G, Goldschmidt H, Lokhorst HM, Sonneveld P. Prediction of high- and low-risk multiple myeloma based on gene expression and the international staging system. Blood. 2015 Oct 22;126(17):1996–2004.

Kyle RA, Greipp PR. Smoldering multiple myeloma. N Engl J Med. 1980;302:1347.

Lee JW, Lee JE. Local radiotherapy for palliation in multiple myeloma patients with symptomatic bone lesions. Radiat Oncol J. 2016;34(1):59–63.

Moreau P, Facon T, Attal M, et al. Comparison fo 200mg/m2 mephalan and 8 Gy Tbi plus 140 mg/m2 mephalan as conditioning regiments for peripheral blood stem cell transplantation in patients with newly diagnosed multiple myeloma: Final analysis of the Intergroupe Francophone du Myelome 9502 randomized trial. Blood. 2002;99(3):731–5.

Myeloma Aredia Study Group. Efficacy of pamidronate in reducing skeletal events in patients with advanced multiple myeloma. N Engl J Med. 1996;334:488–93.

Nau K, Lewis W. Multiple myeloma: diagnosis and treatment. Am Fam Physician. 2008;78(7):853–9. 860

Ozsahin M, Tsang RW, Poortmans P, et al. Outcomes and patterns of failure in solitary plasmacytoma: a multicenter Rare Cancer Network study of 258 patients. Int J Radiat Oncol Biol Phys. 2006;64(1):210–7.

Palumbo A, Avet-Loiseau H, Oliva S, et al. Revised international staging system for multiple myeloma: a report from the IMWG. J Clin Oncol. 2015;33:2863–9.

Terpos E, et al. International Myeloma Working Group recommendations for the treatment of multiple myeloma related bone disease. J Clin Oncol. 2013;20(June):2347–57.

Rajkumar V, et al. International Myeloma Working Group updated criteria for the diagnosis of multiple myeloma. Lancet Oncol. 2014;15:e538–48.

Sasaki R, Yasuda K, Abe E, et al. Multi-institutional analysis of solitary extramedullary plasmacytoma of the head and neck treated with curative radiotherapy. Int J Radiat Oncol Biol Phys. 2012 Feb 1;82(2):626–34.

Part X

Musculoskeletal Sites

Chapter 39
Bone Tumors

Lauren Boreta and Steve E. Braunstein

PEARLS

- Diaphysis = shaft; epiphysis = growth plate and end of bone; metaphysis = conical portion between diaphysis and epiphysis.
- Prevalence: osteosarcoma > chondrosarcoma > Ewing's > undifferentiated pleomorphic sarcoma (UPS) of the bone [aka malignant fibrous histiocytoma (MFH) of the bone].
- Primary bone tumors account for <0.2% of all cancers.
- 60% of the cases occur between 10 and 20 years of age (most active age of skeletal growth).
- 80% of the cases in long bones until epiphyseal closure (then occur with appendicular skeleton).
- Osteosarcoma: malignant osteoid is hallmark (not seen in chondrosarcoma). Most common bone tumor in children. 75% present in metaphyses of long bones with local pain/swelling. 85% are grades 3–4.
    - Associated with Li-Fraumeni syndrome (p53) and retinoblastoma. In patients >60 years, >50% of the cases arise from other conditions (i.e., Paget's disease, fibrous dysplasia) and demonstrate poor chemo response.
    - 3 histologic subtypes: intramedullary (80%), surface juxtacortical (5%), extraskeletal.

X

- Most common in the femur > tibia > humerus. DM most common in the lung > bone/BM.
- 20% have metastatic disease at presentation.
- Chondrosarcoma: ~25% of all primary bone cancers. Most common in the femur. Frequent local recurrence, DM less common than osteosarcoma.
  - 1/3 are high grade. 50% are related to IDH1/IDH2 mutations.
  - Prognostic factors: primary vs. secondary (worse), peripheral vs. central (worse), grade, and size.
- MFH: very aggressive locally with frequent DM. Often presents with fracture.
- Fibrosarcoma: high grade and behaves like osteosarcoma. Often presents with fracture.
- Chordoma: physaliferous cell ("bubbly cell") is histologic hallmark. S-100 and EMA positive. Associated with increased expression of brachyury (ch6q27). Arises from notochordal tissue. Most often in sacrococcygeal area (50–60%), base of the skull (25–35%), and spine (15%). Presentation is location specific.
  - 3 histologic subtypes – conventional (77%), chondroid (15%), and dedifferentiated (8%).
  - 10-year OS: negative margins 61 vs. 17% with positive margins.
- Giant cell tumors: giant multinucleated osteoclast cells. Only 8–15% are malignant. Cyst formation, hemorrhage, and necrosis are important with regard to radiosensitivity. Frequent LR (45–60%).
- Lung metastases common in osteosarcoma, chondrosarcoma, MFH.

WORKUP

- H&P.
- CBC, chemistries, urinalysis, ESR, alkaline phosphatase, LDH.

Table 39.1 Differentiating Ewing's from osteosarcoma

Ewing's	Osteosarcoma
Lytic, destructive lesion	Sclerotic lesion
Diaphysis	Metaphysis
Onion skin effect	Sunburst pattern (periosteal new bone formation)

- Plain films (primary region and CXR) – Codman's triangle, periosteal bone spicules, 1° tumor often seen as cloud-like density.
- CT and MRI (primary area and chest) to evaluate soft tissue extension and distant metastases. Especially important for chordoma.
- Bone scan to evaluate for intramedullary skip metastases. Consider PET scan.
- Staging scans should be complete before biopsy is performed.
- Incisional or percutaneous core biopsy is recommended, and biopsy should be placed in area to be excised or radiated. High risk of seeding scar tract.

STAGING: BONE TUMORS

Editors' note: All TNM stage and stage groups referred to elsewhere in this chapter reflect the 2010 AJCC staging nomenclature unless otherwise noted as the new system below was published after this chapter was written.

Table 39.2 (AJCC 7TH ED., 2010)

Primary tumor (T)

TX:	Primary tumor cannot be assessed
T0:	No evidence of primary tumor
T1:	Tumor 8 cm or less in greatest dimension
T2:	Tumor more than 8 cm in greatest dimension
T3:	Discontinuous tumors in the primary bone site

Regional lymph nodes (N)

NX:	Regional lymph nodes cannot be assessed
N0:	No regional lymph node metastasis
N1:	Regional lymph node metastasis

Note: Because of the rarity of lymph node involvement in bone sarcomas, the designation NX may not be appropriate and cases should be considered N0 unless clinical node involvement is clearly evident

continued

Table 39.2 (continued)

Distant metastasis (M)	
M0:	No distant metastasis
M1:	Distant metastasis
M1a:	Lung
M1b:	Other distant sites

Anatomic stage/prognostic groups	
IA:	T1 N0 M0 G1,2 low grade, GX
IB:	T2 N0 M0 G1,2 low grade, GX
T3:	N0 M0 G1,2 low grade, GX
IIA:	T1 N0 M0 G3,4 high grade
IIB:	T2 N0 M0 G3,4 high grade
III:	T3 N0 M0 G3,4
IVA:	Any T N0 M1a any G
IVB:	Any T N1 any M any G
	Any T any N M1b any G

Used with the permission of the American Joint Committee on Cancer (AJCC), Chicago, Illinois. The original source for this material is the *AJCC Cancer Staging Manual, Seventh Edition (2010)* published by Springer Science + Business Media

Table 39.3 (AJCC 8TH ED., 2017)

Definitions of AJCC TNM	
Definition of Primary Tumor (T)	
Appendicular Skeleton, Trunk, Skull, and Facial Bones	
T category	**T criteria**
TX	Primary tumor cannot be assessed
T0	No evidence of primary tumor
T1	Tumor ≤8 cm in greatest dimension
T2	Tumor >8 cm in greatest dimension
T3	Discontinuous tumors in the primary bone site
Spine	
T category	**T criteria**
TX	Primary tumor cannot be assessed
T0	No evidence of primary tumor
T1	Tumor confined to one vertebral segment or two adjacent vertebral segments
T2	Tumor confined to three adjacent vertebral segments
T3	Tumor confined to four or more adjacent vertebral segments, or any nonadjacent vertebral segments
T4	Extension into the spinal canal or great vessels
T4a	Extension into the spinal canal
T4b	Evidence of gross vascular invasion or tumor thrombus in the great vessels
Pelvis	
T category	**T criteria**
TX	Primary tumor cannot be assessed
T0	No evidence of primary tumor

Table 39.3 (continued)

T1	Tumor confined to one pelvic segment with no extraosseous extension
T1a	Tumor ≤8 cm in greatest dimension
T1b	Tumor >8 cm in greatest dimension
T2	Tumor confined to one pelvic segment with extraosseous extension or two segments without extraosseous extension
T2a	Tumor ≤8 cm in greatest dimension
T2b	Tumor >8 cm in greatest dimension
T3	Tumor spanning two pelvic segments with extraosseous extension
T3a	Tumor ≤8 cm in greatest dimension
T3b	Tumor >8 cm in greatest dimension
T4	Tumor spanning three pelvic segments or crossing the sacroiliac joint
T4a	Tumor involves sacroiliac joint and extends medial to the sacral neuroforamen
T4b	Tumor encasement of external iliac vessels or presence of gross tumor thrombus in major pelvic vessels

Definition of Regional Lymph Node (N)

N category	N criteria
NX	Regional lymph nodes cannot be assessed.
	Because of the rarity of lymph node involvement in bone sarcomas, the designation NX may not be appropriate, and cases should be considered N0 unless clinical node involvement clearly is evident.
N0	No regional lymph node metastasis
N1	Regional lymph node metastasis

Definition of Distant Metastasis (M)

M category	M criteria
M0	No distant metastasis
M1	Distant metastasis
M1a	Lung
M1b	Bone or other distant sites

X

AJCC PROGNOSTIC STAGE GROUPS
APPENDICULAR SKELETON, TRUNK, SKULL, AND FACIAL BONES

When T is...	And N is...	And M is...	And grade is...	Then the stage group is...
T1	N0	M0	G1 or GX	IA
T2	N0	M0	G1 or GX	IB
T3	N0	M0	G1 or GX	IB
T1	N0	M0	G2 or G3	IIA
T2	N0	M0	G2 or G3	IIB
T3	N0	M0	G2 or G3	III
Any T	N0	M1a	Any G	IVA
Any T	N1	Any M	Any G	IVB
Any T	Any N	M1b	Any G	IVB

HISTOLOGIC GRADE (G)

G	G definition
GX	Grade cannot be assessed
G1	Well differentiated, low grade
G2	Moderately differentiated, high grade
G3	Poorly differentiated, high grade

Used with permission of the American Joint Committee on Cancer (AJCC), Chicago, Illinois. The original and primary source for this information is the *AJCC Cancer Staging Manual, Eighth Edition (2017)* published by Springer International Publishing

- A two-grade, three-grade, or four-grade system may be used.
- If a grading system is not specified, generally the following system is used:
  - GX Grade cannot be assessed.
  - G1 Well differentiated – low grade.
  - G2 Moderately differentiated – low grade.
  - G3 Poorly differentiated.
  - G4 Undifferentiated.
- Note: Ewing's sarcoma is classified as G4.

TREATMENT RECOMMENDATIONS

- In general, limb-sparing strategies are preferred, which may involve a combination of neoadjuvant chemo, RT, and surgery.
- Input of orthopedic oncologist is essential in determining whether limb sparing is possible. Final limb function may sometimes be better with prosthesis than with partially resected and/or irradiated limb. In children, RT has added implications on growth of the limb and future function.
- Suggested total doses in table above depend on location and adjacent normal tissue tolerance.
- Aneurysmal bone cyst: surgery. RT 25–30 Gy for recurrent disease and surgically inaccessible (e.g., vertebral).
- Ewing's sarcoma – see Chap. 41.

Table 39.4 TREATMENT RECOMMENDATIONS

Pathology	Treatment recommendations	Dose	5-yr OS	Follow-up
Osteosarcoma	WLE, amputation vs. limb sparing surgery. Metastectomy for pulmonary, visceral metastases improves survival. Neoadjuvant chemotherapy for high-grade, localized disease or metastatic disease Consider RT for positive margin, subtotal resection, or unresectable Consider SBRT for unresectable oligometastatic disease Consider Radium-223 or Sm-EDTMP for metastatic disease Consider clinical trial Consider intra-arterial chemo for pelvic tumors	Post-op: R0 55–60 Gy R1 64–66 Gy R2 68–70 Gy Unresectable: 60–70 Gy	Localized 60–75% (vs. 20% if M1)	Exam and imaging q3–6 mos (including chest imaging) for 5 years, annually to 10 years
Chondrosarcoma	WLE is the primary treatment RT for inadequate margins, unfavorable location, palliation	Post-op: 60–70 Gy IORT: 15–30Gy Unresectable: >70 Gy	50–70%	Exam and imaging q3–6 mos (including chest imaging) for 5 years, annually to 10 years
Chordoma	WLE or en bloc resection is the primary treatment, followed by RT Consider proton or particle beam Preoperative RT may be effective RT alone for unresectable disease EGFR inhibitors can be added to surgery/RT for recurrent disease	SBRT 40Gy in 5 Fr (UCSF) 66–70 Gy standard fractionation Proton:74 Gy RBE	75–80%	Exam and imaging (including chest) q6 mos for 5 years, then annually
UPS/MFH	Treat similar to osteosarcoma	60–70 Gy	15–70%	Exam and imaging q3 mos
Giant cell tumor	Stage I–II: Intralesional curettage Stage III: WLE RT for unresectable, recurrent disease or inadequate margins Denosumab, interferon	>40 Gy	80–100% 30% for malignant	Exam and imaging q6 mos x 2 years, annually thereafter

STUDIES

OSTEOSARCOMA

- Randomized trials have established that neoadjuvant and adjuvant chemo helps to prevent relapse or recurrence in patients with localized resectable primary tumors (Link NEJM 1986; Eilber JCO 1987).
- Cooperative German/Austrian Osteosarcoma Study Group (Ozaki JCO 2003): subset analysis of 67 patients with nonmetastatic, high-grade pelvic osteosarcomas. RT improved survival for patients with intralesional excision and unresectable tumors.
- DeLaney (IJROBP 2005): review of 41 patients with osteosarcoma who were either unresectable or had close or + margins and were treated with RT. No definitive dose-response, although doses >55 Gy had higher LC ($p = 0.11$). RT more effective for patients with microscopic or minimal residual disease.
- Machak (Mayo Clin Proc 2003): 31 patients with nonmetastatic osteosarcoma who refused surgery were treated with induction chemotherapy followed by RT, median dose 60 Gy. OS, PFS, and metastases-free survival (MFS) at 5 years were a mean of 61%, 56%, and 62%, respectively. Patients who were responders had OS and MFS at 5 years of 90% and 91%, respectively, vs. nonresponders 35% and 42%, respectively ($p = 0.005$ and $p = 0.005$, respectively). PFS among nonresponders was 31% at 3 years and 0% at 5 years.
- Wagner (IJROBP 2009): 48 patients had solid bone tumors (52% chordoma, 31% chondrosarcoma, 8% osteosarcoma, 4% Ewing's sarcoma) and were treated with preoperative RT, 20 Gy, followed by resection and then postoperative RT, median dose of 50.4 Gy. Five-year OS, DFS, and LC were 65%, 53.8%, and 72%, respectively. No differences according to histology. This approach appears to inhibit tumor seeding and allows for dose escalation without high-dose preoperative RT or large-field postoperative RT.

CHORDOMA/CHONDROSARCOMA

- Delaney (J Surg Oncol 2014): phase II trial of 50 patients with chordoma/chondrosarcoma receiving high-dose photon/proton RT in pre- or postoperative setting. LC at 8-yr was 81% primary vs. 74% for all tumors. Late grade 3–4 RT-related toxicity was 13%.
- Catton (Radiotherapy Oncology, 1996): Princess Margaret series of 48 patients who received post-op photon RT for microscopic or gross residual chordoma. RT dose 50 Gy in 25 fractions or 40 Gy in 44 fractions over 14 days. Median OS 5.2 years. 5-yr PFS 23%, 10-yr 15%. Median time to progression ~3 years. No difference daily vs. hyperfractionated photon RT.
- Carpentier (Neurosurg 2002): review of patients treated with surgery + RT up front vs. radiation at time of recurrence. RT at the time of surgery had improved outcomes, with 5-year survival 65% vs. 50% and 10-year survival 50% vs. 0.
- Yamada (Neurosurg 2013): 24 patients with unresectable spine/sacral chordoma treated with high-dose SRS (24 Gy × 1). At 24 mos, 95% had stable or reduced disease.
- Imai (IJROBP 2010): retrospective analysis of 38 patients with unresectable sacral chordoma treated with carbon ions to median dose 70.4 Gy RBE. 5-year OS was 86%, LC 89%. Majority of patients were ambulatory after treatment.
- Di Maio (J Neurosurg 2011): literature review of 807 skull base chordoma patients. 5-yr PFS 87% if complete resection vs. 50% if incomplete resection. No significant difference in PFS between radiotherapy techniques (linac fractionated, radiosurgery, protons, carbon ion).
- Bloch (Skull Base 2010): literature review of 560 cranial chondrosarcoma patients. 5-yr recurrence rate reduced with adjuvant RT vs. surgery alone (9% vs. 44%), regardless of extent of resection in subset analysis. 5-yr recurrence rate 19% for 46 patients treated with RT alone.

X

RADIATION TECHNIQUES

SIMULATION AND FIELD DESIGN
CONVENTIONALLY FRACTIONATED PHOTON RADIOTHERAPY

- Spare 1.5–2 cm strip of the skin in extremity XRT, if possible, to prevent edema.
- Include entire surgical bed + scar + 2 cm margin, if possible.
- Bolus on scar may be considered as indicated.
- CT/MRI data for treatment planning.
- Try to exclude the skin over anterior tibia, if possible, due to poor vascularity.
- Physical therapy instituted as early as possible during treatment to improve functional outcome.

SBRT

- Pre-op: CTV to include region of microscopic disease up to 1 cm from GTV
- Post-op: CTV 0–1 cm expansion of GTV/surgical bed based on the extent of resection and location adjacent to critical structures
- PTV: 2–3 mm on CTV with modern immobilization/IGRT

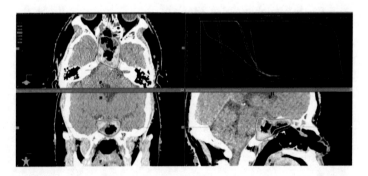

Fig. 39.1 Sample postoperative SBRT plan for clival chordoma, 40 Gy in 5 fractions

DOSE LIMITATIONS

- >20 Gy can prematurely close epiphysis.
- >40 Gy will ablate bone marrow.
- ≥50 Gy to bone cortex significantly increases risk of fracture.
- 30 Gy Dmax for 5-fraction SBRT to the brainstem or spinal cord.
- Conventionally fractionated RT Dmax spinal cord 45–50 Gy; Dmax brainstem 59.4 Gy.

COMPLICATIONS

- Abnormal bone and soft tissue growth and development, permanent weakening of the affected bone, scoliosis, decreased range of motion due to fibrosis or joint involvement, vascular changes resulting in greater sensitivity to infection, fracture, lymphedema, skin discoloration or telangiectasia, osteoradionecrosis
- Increased risk of 2° cancers (leukemia, sarcomas)

Acknowledgment We thank Tania Kaprealian MD; Brian Lee MD, PhD; and Jean L. Nakamura MD for their work on the prior edition of this chapter.

REFERENCES

Bloch OG, Jian BJ, Yang I, et al. Cranial Chondrosarcoma and recurrence. Skull Base. 2010;20:149–56.

Catton C, O'Sullivan B, et al. Chordoma: long term follow-up after radical photon irradiation. Radiother Oncol. 1996;41(1):p67–72.

Carpentier A, et al. Suboccipital and cervical chordomas: the value of aggressive treatment at first presentation of the disease. J Neurosurg. 2002;97(5):1070–7.

DeLaney TF, Park L, Goldberg SI, et al. Radiotherapy for local control of osteosarcoma. Int J Radiat Oncol Biol Phys. 2005;61:492–8.

DeLaney TF, et al. Long term results of phase II study of high dose photon/proton radiotherapy in the management of spine chordomas, chondrosarcomas and other sarcomas. J Surg Oncol. 2014;110(2):115–22.

Di Maio S, Temkin N, Ramanathan D, Sekhar L. Current comprehensive management of cranial base chordomas: 10-year meta-analysis of observational studies. J Neurosurg. 2011;115:1094–105.

Eilber F, Giuliano A, Eckardt J, et al. Adjuvant chemotherapy for osteosarcoma: a randomized prospective trial. J Clin Oncol. 1987;5:21–6.

Imai R, Kamada T, et al. Effect of carbon ion radiotherapy for sacral chordoma: results of a phase I-II and phase II clinical trials. Int J Radiat Oncol Biol Phys. 2010;77(5):1470–6.

X

Link MP, Goorin AM, Miser AW, et al. The effect of adjuvant chemotherapy on relapse-free survival in patients with osteosarcoma of the extremity. N Engl J Med. 1986;314:1600–6.

Machak GN, Tkachev SI, Solovyev YN, et al. Neoadjuvant chemotherapy and local radio-therapy for high-grade osteosarcoma of the extremities. Mayo Clin Proc. 2003;78:147–55.

Ozaki T, Flege S, Kevric M, et al. Osteosarcoma of the pelvis: experience of the coopera-tive osteosarcoma study group. J Clin Oncol. 2003;21:334–41.

Wagner TD, Kobayashi W, Dean S, et al. Combination short-course preoperative irradia-tion, surgical resection, and reduced-field high-dose postoperative irradiation in the treatment of tumors involving the bone. Int J Radiat Oncol Biol Phys. 2009;73:259–66.

Yamada Y, Laufer I, et al. Preliminary results of high dose single fraction radiotherapy for the management of chordomas of the spine and sacrum. Neurosurgery. 2013;73(4):673–80.

Chapter 40
Soft-Tissue Sarcoma

Lauren Boreta and Alexander R. Gottschalk

PEARLS

- ~12,300 cases/year and ~5000 deaths/year in the United States (additional 5000 cases GIST/year) Gastrointestinal stromal tumors (GIST)
- Heterogeneous with >50 subtypes
- Median age 40–60 years
- Slight male predominance, more frequent among African-Americans
- Genetics: NF-1, retinoblastoma, Gardner's syndrome, Li-Fraumeni syndrome, Carney Stratakis syndrome
- Environmental risk factors: ionizing radiation, herbicides, thorotrast, chlorophenols, vinyl chloride, arsenic
- Extremities (45%) > trunk (30%) > visceral (19%) > retroperitoneal (15%)H&N (8%)
- Extremity = liposarcoma, MFH (malignant fibrous histiocytoma/undifferentiated pleomorphic sarcoma), synovial, fibrosarcoma, myxoid liposarcoma (upper medial thigh)
- Retroperitoneal = liposarcoma (fewer diabetes mellitus (DM)) > leiomyosarcoma (increased DM)
- H&N = MFH, usually high grade (except myxoid MFH = intermediate grade)
- Frequency: MFH (20–30%), liposarcoma (10–20%), leiomyosarcoma (10–15%), fibrosarcoma (5–10%), synovial

X

© Springer International Publishing AG, part of Springer Nature 2018
Eric K. Hansen and M. Roach III (eds.), *Handbook of Evidence-Based Radiation Oncology*, https://doi.org/10.1007/978-3-319-62642-0_40

cell sarcoma (5–10%), rhabdomyosarcoma (5–10%), malignant peripheral nerve sheath tumor/malignant schwannoma (5%)

- Rhabdomyosarcoma most common sarcoma in children
- Synovial sarcoma = usually high grade, near (but not within) joints in tendon sheaths, bursae, and joint capsules
- GIST: stomach (60%) > small intestine (30%) > duodenum or rectum (10%)
- Grade based on cellularity, differentiation, pleomorphism, necrosis, #mitoses

CYTOGENETICS

- Many sarcoma types harbor characteristic genetic aberrations, including single base pair substitutions, deletions and amplifications, and translocations. For example:
- cKIT or PDGFRA activating mutation→ GIST.
- CTNNBI mutation (beta-catenin pathway)→ Desmoid.

PRESENTATION

- Painless mass. Typically 4–6 months from symptoms to diagnosis.
- Stewart–Treves syndrome = chronic lymphedema of upper extremity → lymphangiosarcoma.
- Approximately 10% have metastases at diagnosis. Extremity → lung, retroperitoneal → liver (Ferguson Cancer 2011).
- Increased risk of lymph node (LN) spread: SCARE = synovial (14%), clear cell (28%), angiosarcoma (11%), rhabdomyosarcoma (15%), epithelioid (20%).

Table 40.1 Common chromosomal translocations in Sarcoma

Sarcoma	Ewings	Rhabdomyosarcoma	Synovial	Myxoid liposarcoma	Alveolar	Dermato fibrosarcoma Protuberans
Fusion gene	t(11;22)	t(2;13)	t(x;18)	t(12;16)	t(x;17)	t(17;22)

WORKUP

, H&P, CBC, BUN/Cr, ESR, LDH, CT/MRI of primary, CT chest. If myxoid liposarcoma, include CT abdomen because it frequently metastasizes to retroperitoneum. MRI brain for alveolar type. PET scan may be useful for monitoring treatment response.

, Always perform imaging prior to biopsy or surgery. Perform biopsy at institution where surgery will be performed.

, Incisional biopsy or core needle biopsy preferred. Core biopsy predicts type and grade 90% of time. Incision for biopsy should be oriented so that it can be excised during the definitive surgery. Excisional biopsy often contaminates surrounding tissue.

, Cytogenetic analysis of tissue to look for characteristic chromosomal translocations.

PROGNOSIS

, Adverse factors for local recurrence: + margins, >50 years age, deep location, fibrosarcoma type including desmoid, malignant peripheral nerve sheath tumors.

, Adverse factors for distant metastasis: high grade (5 y DM<10% for low grade versus 50% for high grade), increasing size, deep location, leiomyosarcoma, or malignant peripheral nerve sheath tumor, high Ki-67.

STAGING: SOFT-TISSUE SARCOMA

Editors' note: All TNM stage and stage groups referred to elsewhere in this chapter reflect the 2010 AJCC staging nomenclature unless otherwise noted as the new system below was published after this chapter was written (Table 40.2).

Table 40.2   AJCC 7TH ED., (2010)

Primary tumor (T)	
TX:	Primary tumor cannot be assessed
T0:	No evidence of primary tumor
T1:	Tumor 5 cm or less in greatest dimension*
T1a:	Superficial tumor
T1b:	Deep tumor
T2:	Tumor more than 5 cm in greatest dimension*
T2a:	Superficial tumor
T2b:	Deep tumor

Note: Superficial tumor is located exclusively above the superficial fascia without the invasion of the fascia; deep tumor is located either exclusively beneath the superficial fascia, superficial to the fascia with invasion of or through the fascia, or both superficial yet beneath the fascia

Regional lymph nodes (N)	
NX:	Regional lymph nodes cannot be assessed
N0:	No regional lymph node metastasis
N1**:	Regional lymph node metastasis

**Note*: Presence of positive nodes (N1) in M0 tumors is considered Stage III

Distant metastasis (M)	
M0:	No distant metastasis
M1:	Distant metastasis

Anatomic stage/prognostic groups	
IA:	T1a N0 M0 G1, GX
T1b N0 M0 G1, GX	
IB:	T2a N0 M0 G1, GX
T2b	N0 M0 G1, GX
IIA:	T1a N0 M0 G2, G3
T1b	N0 M0 G2, G3
IIB:	T2a N0 M0 G2
T2b	N0 M0 G2
III:	T2a, T2b N0 M0 G3
Any T N1 M0 any G	
IV:	Any T any N M1 any G

Used with the permission from the American Joint Committee on Cancer (AJCC), Chicago, Illinois. The original source for this material is the AJCC Cancer Staging Manual, Seventh Edition (2010), published by Springer Science + Business Media

HISTOLOGIC GRADE (G) (FRENCH FNCLCC SYSTEM PREFERRED)

, The FNCLCC grade is determined by three parameters: differentiation (histology specific), mitotic activity, and extent of necrosis. Grades 1, 2, or 3

> Note: Kaposi's sarcoma, fibromatosis (desmoid tumor), and sarcomas arising from the dura mater, brain, parenchymatous organs, or hollow viscera are not included (Tables 40.3 and 40.4).

Table 40.3   AJCC 8TH ED., (2017)
Soft Tissue Sarcoma of the Head & Neck

Definitions of AJCC TNM

Definition of primary tumor (T)

T category	T criteria
TX	Primary tumor cannot be assessed
T1	Tumor ≤2 cm
T2	Tumor >2 to ≤4 cm
T3	Tumor >4 cm
T4	Tumor with invasion of adjoining structures
T4a	Tumor with orbital invasion, skull base/dural invasion, invasion of central compartment viscera, involvement of facial skeleton, or invasion of pterygoid muscles
T4b	Tumor with brain parenchymal invasion, carotid artery encasement, prevertebral muscle invasion, or central nervous system involvement via perineural spread

DEFINITION OF PRIMARY TUMOR (T)
Soft Tissue Sarcoma of the Trunk & Extremities

T category	T criteria
TX	Primary tumor cannot be assessed
T0	No evidence of primary tumor
T1	Tumor 5 cm or less in the greatest dimension
T2	Tumor more than 5 cm and less than or equal to 10 cm in the greatest dimension
T3	Tumor more than 10 cm and less than or equal to 15 cm in the greatest dimension
T4	Tumor more than 15 cm in the greatest dimension

DEFINITION OF REGIONAL LYMPH NODE (N)
Head and Neck and Trunk and Extremities

N category	N criteria
N0	No regional lymph node metastases or unknown lymph node status
N1	Regional lymph node metastasis

DEFINITION OF DISTANT METASTASIS (M)

M category	M criteria
M0	No distant metastasis
M1	Distant metastasis

X

TUMOR DIFFERENTIATION

Differentiation score	Definition
1	Sarcomas closely resembling normal adult mesenchymal tissue (e.g., low-grade leiomyosarcoma)
2	Sarcomas for which histology typing is certain (e.g., myxoid/round cell liposarcoma)
3	Embryonal and undifferentiated sarcomas, sarcomas of doubtful type, synovial sarcomas, soft tissue osteosarcoma, Ewing sarcoma/primitive neuroectodermal tumor (PNET) of soft tissue

MITOTIC COUNT

Mitotic count score	Definition
1	0–9 mitoses per 10 HPF
2	10–19 mitoses per 10 HPF
3	≥20 mitoses per 10 HPF

TUMOR NECROSIS

Necrosis score	Definition
0	No necrosis
1	<50% tumor necrosis
2	≥50% tumor necrosis

FNCLCC HISTOLOGIC GRADE

G	G definition
GX	Grade cannot be assessed
G1	Total differentiation, mitotic count, and necrosis score of 2 or 3
G2	Total differentiation, mitotic count, and necrosis score of 4 or 5
G3	Total differentiation, mitotic count, and necrosis score of 6, 7, or 8

AJCC PROGNOSTIC STAGE GROUPS

When T is...	And N is...	And M is...	And grade is...	Then the stage group is...
T1	N0	M0	G1,GX	IA
T2, T3, T4	N0	M0	G1,GX	IB
T1	N0	M0	G2, G3	II
T2	N0	M0	G2, G3	IIIA
T3, T4	N0	M0	G2, G3	IIIB
Any T	N1	M0	Any G	IV
Any T	Any N	M1	Any G	IV

TREATMENT RECOMMENDATIONS

TABLE 40.4 TREATMENT RECOMMENDATIONS

Stage	Recommended Treatment
I extremity	Surgery alone, unless close (<1 cm) or +margin, re-resect or post-op RT. ~5-year LC 90–100%, OS 90%
II–III extremity	Pre-op RT → surgery or surgery → post-op RT. consider neoadjuvant/adjuvant chemo for large deep high-grade tumors since ~50% develop metastases. ~5-year LC 90%, OS 80% for stage II, 60% for stage III. For LR, amputation can salvage ~75%
IV	For controlled primary, with ≤4 lung lesions and/or extended disease-free interval, consider surgical resection and metastatectomy. ~5-year OS ~25%.Otherwise, best supportive care, chemo, and/or palliative surgery or RT. ~5-year OS 10%
Unresectable	Definitive RT (70-80Gy), chemo (Doxorubicin + ifosfamide), or chemoRT. Surgery if becomes resectable.
Retroperitoneal	Surgery + IORT (12–15 Gy) → post-op EBRT 45–50 Gy. Alternatively, pre-op RT +/– chemo → resection +/– IORT boost. ~5-year LC 50%, DM 20–30%, OS 50%
GIST	If resectable, surgery → imatinib (consider observation vs. imatinib if completely resected). If marginally or unresectable, imatinib → consider surgery → imatinib
Desmoid tumors	Surgery. R0 resection: Observe. R1 resection: Re-resect or observe R2 resection or inoperable: RT (54–58 Gy). ~5-year LC 60–70% Consider chemo/hormonal/targeted therapy for R2 or inoperable cases as ~1/3 can have stable disease or a response

X

SURGERY

- Prefer wide en bloc resection with ≥2 cm margin in all directions. Biopsy site should be removed at the time of surgery.
- A radical resection removes entire anatomic compartment including neurovascular structures (LC >90%).
- Wide excision removes cuff of normal tissue (LC 40–70%).
- Excisional biopsy = marginal excision "shellout" of pseudocapsule only (LC <20%).
- Intralesional biopsy = inside pseudocapsule. Surgical scars should be oriented longitudinally, so circumferential RT can be avoided.
- Re-resection indicated for positive margins– 38% LR at 6 years versus 12% with negative margins (Alananda Acta Onc 2013).
- Recommend clip placement to assist RT planning.

CHEMO

- Approximately 50% of patients with high-grade tumors will die of DM, despite LC of primary.
- Most active single chemo agent = anthracycline, ifosfamide (15–30% response).
- Contradictory results in trials comparing single versus combination chemo. No clear OS benefit to combination chemo.
- Postop chemo controversial. If used, based on meta-analysis (doxorubicin/ifosfamide) or Italian study (epirubicin/ifosfamide).
- Chemo is generally not used in low-grade sarcoma, superficial lesions, high grade<5 cm, or intermediate grade 5–10 cm that have been fully resected.
- Consider neoadjuvant chemo → surgery for high-grade or unresectable tumors.

TARGETED THERAPY

- Pazopanib: TKI approved to treat STS after prior chemotherapy (nonadipocytic only) (van der Graaf Lancet 2012).
- Imatinib: TKI approved as first line for unresectable/metastatic GIST.
- Palbociclib: CDK4/6 inhibitor is shown to have improved PFS in CDK amplified liposarcoma (Dickson JCO 2013).
- Bevacizumab is an investigational treatment for advanced angiosarcoma (Agulnik Ann Onc 2013).

STUDIES

- Postop brachy or EBRT may improve LC.
  - Pisters (JCO 1996): 160 patients with extremity and superficial trunk sarcoma s/p WLE. Randomized to brachytherapy (Ir-192 42–45 Gy over 4–6 d) or observation. RT to tumor +2 cm margin. Brachytherapy increased LC for high-grade lesions (65–90%), but not for low-grade lesions (~70%). No difference in DSS (80%) and DM.
  - NCI (Yang, JCO 1998): 140 patients with extremity sarcoma treated with WLE. Low-grade randomized to observation versus postop EBRT. High-grade randomized to postop chemo versus postop chemo-RT. RT = large field to 45 Gy → boost to 63 Gy. RT increased LC for low grade (60% vs. 95%) and high grade (75% vs. 100%). No difference in OS (70%) or DMFS (75%).
- Preop RT increases early wound complications, but has less late fibrosis, versus postop RT with no LC or OS difference.
  - NCIC (O'Sullivan, JCO 2002; Davis, Radiother Oncol 2005): 190 patients with extremity STS randomized preop RT (50 Gy) versus postop RT (66 Gy). If +margins, preop got 16 Gy boost. No difference in LC (93%), DM (25%), and PFS (65%). Initially, better OS with pre-op due to deaths other than sarcoma in post-op arm, but on 6-year follow-up, no difference in OS. More wound-healing problems with pre-op (35% vs. 15%), but increased late fibrosis with post-op RT (48% vs. 31%, $p = 0.07$).

X

- Sophisticated EBRT planning can improve therapeutic ratio.
  - Folkert (JCO 2014a) Retrospective comparison of 319 patients with extremity STS treated with 3D and IMRT given pre- or postoperatively following limb sparing surgery. Despite higher risk features, IMRT improved LC on multivariate analysis. IMRT also reduced dermatitis and edema.
  - VORTEX (Robinson, ASTRO 2016 abstract 2). 216 patients with extremity STS randomized after surgery to 50 Gy to CTV1 (GTV + 5 cm craniocaudal and 2 cm axial margin) followed by 16 Gy boost to CTV2 (GTV + 2 cm) versus 66 Gy in 33 fractions to CTV2 alone. No significant difference in 5-yr LR (14% conventional vs. 16% reduced volume), OS (72% conventional vs. 67% reduced volume), or late toxicity, but because of small number of events cannot state noninferiority.
  - RTOG 0630 (Wang, JCO 2015). 98 patients with extremity STS treated with image-guided preoperative 3D or IMRT, 50 Gy in 25 fx. CTV = GTV + 3 cm longitudinal and 1.5 cm radial including suspicious MRI T2 edema for intermediate- to high-grade tumors >8 cm. CTV = GTV + 2 cm longitudinal and 1 cm radial margin including suspicious edema for low-grade tumors <8 cm. PTV = CTV + 0.5 cm. At 3.6-yr follow-up, 7% of patients had LR inside the CTV (60% of whom had +margins). Only 11% grade ≥2 toxicity.
- IORT may also improve LC.
  - *NCI* (Sindelar, Arch Surg 1993): 35 patients with resectable retroperitoneal STS randomized to surgery + IORT 20 Gy → postop 35–40 Gy versus surgery → postop 50–55 Gy. No difference in 5-year OS (35%), but nonsignificant increase in LC (20% vs. 60%). IORT increased neuropathy if >15 Gy, but lower GI complications.
  - Oertel (IJROBP 2006): 153 patients with primary or recurrent extremity STS treated with limb-sparing surgery + IORT 10–20 Gy → postoperative EBRT 36–50 Gy. Five-year OS 77%, DMFS 48%, and LC 78%. IORT dose >15 Gy improved LC, but EBRT <45 or ≥45 Gy not significant for LC. Seventeen percent acute wound-healing toxicity.

, Tinkle (Sarcoma 2015): UCSF experience of limb sparing surgery + IORT for locally recurrent extremity STS. 5-yr LC 58%, amputation-free survival 81%, OS 50%.

, Chemo may offer modest benefit, particularly for high-grade tumors.

  , Meta-analysis (Pervaiz, Cancer 2008): 1953 patients with resectable STS treated with WLE ± RT randomized to observation versus adjuvant doxorubicin-based chemo. Chemo improved LC (absolute 4%), DMFS (9%), RFS (10%), and OS (6%). Specifically doxorubicin/ifosfamide improved LC (absolute 5%, not significant), DMFS (10%), RFS (12%), and OS (11%).

  , French Sarcoma Group (Italiano, Ann Oncol 2010). 1513 patients with STS, adjuvant chemo improved 5-yr OS for grade 3 patients (58% vs. 45%) but not grade 2 patients.

  , RTOG 9514 (Kraybill, Cancer 2010): Phase II study of 66 patients with ≥8 cm high-grade STS of extremities or torso that were not amenable to R0 resection, treated with neoadjuvant chemo + RT (44 Gy in 2 split cycles), followed by surgery. 5-yr Local-Regional Failure (LRF) 22%, DM 28.1%, OS 71.2%. Very high rates of acute hemotologic toxicity.

RETROPERITONEAL

, Nussbaum (Lancet Onc 2016): Retrospective case-control study of 9068 patients from National Cancer Data Base with RP sarcoma treated with preop RT, postop RT, or no RT. Both preop and postop RT were associated with improved median OS compared to surgery alone (110 mo, 89 mo vs. 64 mo, respectively).

, Mendenhall (Cancer 2005): Reviewed literature on retroperitoneal STS. GTR feasible in ~50–67%, but most patients have close/+ margins. Major site of failure is local. With surgery and RT, 5-year LC is ~50%, 5-year DM ~20–30%, 5-year OS ~50%. Preop RT may increase resectability, allow normal tissues to be displaced by tumor, and decrease hypoxia. IORT may improve LC but not OS.

, NCI trial (1993, above) reported improved LC with postop IORT.

X

SBRT

- Dhakal (IJROBP 2012): Restrospective review of 15 patients treated with SBRT for pulmonary metastases (50 Gy, 5 fractions). 3-yr LC 82%, median OS 2.1 yrs versus 0.6 years for those who went untreated. No grade 3 or 4 toxicity.
- Folkert (IJROBP 2014a, b): Retrospective review of 88 patients with STS metastatic to spine treated with hypofractionated RT (24–36 Gy) or single fraction RT (18–24 Gy). At 12 mos, LC 87.9%, OS 60.6%, MS 17 mos. Single fraction provided better LC than multifraction (90.8 vs. 84.1).

RADIATION TECHNIQUES

POSTOPERATIVE EBRT

- Start 10–20 days after surgery for healing.
- 4–6 MV for extremities.
- Bolus scar and drain sites for first 50 Gy unless in tangential beam.
- Traditional postoperative field: CTV = tumor bed, scar, drainage sites +4 cm longitudinal and 1.5 cm perpendicular margin in initial field. After 50 Gy, reduce field to surgical bed (outlined by clips, scar) + 2 cm longitudinal and 1.5 cm radial margin. Add 1 cm PTV.
- Preliminary results of VORTEX study (above) suggest it may be safe to reduce postoperative target volume, but longer term study results are awaited.
- Dose 2 Gy/fx with negative margins or microscopic residual to 60 Gy, +margins to 66 Gy, gross disease to 70–76 Gy.
- Always spare 1.5–2 cm strip of skin. Try to exclude skin over anterior tibia, if possible, due to poor vascularity.
- Never treat whole circumference of extremity to >50 Gy.
- Spare 1/2 of cross-section of weight-bearing bone, entire or >1/2 of joint cavities, and major tendons (patellar, achilles).
- IMRT improves sparing of normal tissues and has been shown to provide superior local control compared to 3D (Folkert JCO 2014a), but careful planning with adequate margin and close attention to treatment set up are required to avoid marginal misses.
- Upper inner thigh best treated in frog-leg position.
- Buttock/post thigh best treated in prone position.
- Nodes: Gross nodes should be resected. No elective nodal radiation.

, For distal extremities, patients often have severe reaction with pain, edema, erythema. Usually heals within 1 month.

PRE-OP EBRT
, Dose = 2 Gy/fx to 50 Gy.
, Traditional field = GTV = tumor (MRI T1 postcontrast, but not T2). CTV = GTV + 4 cm longitudinal margin and 1.5 cm radial margin (not beyond surface of adjacent bone& fascia unless involved) plus suspicious peritumoral edema (MRI T2). PTV add 1 cm. No conedown. Based on RTOG 0630 fields may be reduced per protocol.
, Surgery 3 weeks after RT.
, Postoperative boost with EBRT, IORT, or brachytherapy for close/+margins to 65–66 Gy, gross disease to 75 Gy.

POST-OP BRACHYTHERAPY
, As monotherapy for high-grade tumors with negative surgical margins: 45–50 Gy LDR or HDR equivalent.
, Postoperatively after preop EBRT 50 Gy:
  , R1: 16–18 Gy LDR or 14–16 Gy at 3–4 Gy BID HDR.
  , R2: 20–26 Gy LDR or 18–24 Gy HDR.
, Brachytherapy target: tumor bed +2 cm longitudinal margin +1–1.5 cm circumferential margin.
, Catheters placed in OR 1 cm apart. Load catheters on or after the sixth postop day to allow time for wound healing.
, Do not include scar or drainage site.

POST-OP IORT
, Dose = 10–12.5 Gy for microscopic residual and 15 Gy for gross residual.

UNRESECTABLE EBRT
, 50 Gy to large field, conedown to 60 Gy, then to 70–76 Gy.
, Consider decreasing RT total dose and dose/fx (1.8 Gy) if doxorubicin given.
, Delay RT >3 days from doxorubicin.
, Use gonadal shield to preserve fertility.
, Physical therapy instituted as early as possible during treatment to improve functional outcome.

X

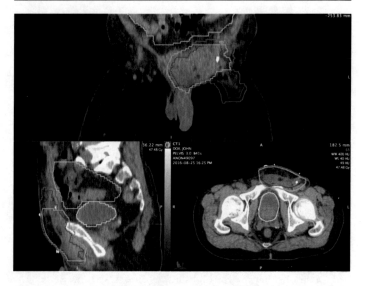

Fig. 40.1 pT2bN0M0G3 stage III L inguinal node liposarcoma, post-op IMRT contours. *Red* CTV, *pink* PTV, *turquoise* boost. Dose to PTV = 50 Gy in 25 fractions, boost = 10 Gy in 5 fractions. Also received IORT 15 Gy at time of resection

DOSE LIMITATIONS

- >20 Gy can prematurely close epiphysis.
- ≥40 Gy ablates bone marrow.
- ≥50 Gy to bone cortex can cause fracture and healing problems. Risk may be reduced by limiting bone V40Gy < 64%, mean bone dose <37 Gy, and bone Dmax <59 Gy (Dickie, IJROBP 2009).
- Exclude joint space after 40–45 Gy to avoid fibrotic constriction.

COMPLICATIONS

- Wound healing complications: 5–15% with postop RT versus 25–35% with preop RT.
- Abnormal bone and soft-tissue growth and development.
- Limb length discrepancy (2–6 cm managed with shoe lift, otherwise needs surgical correction).

, Permanent weakening of affected bone with highest risk for fracture within 18 months of RT.
, Decreased range of motion secondary to fibrosis.
, Lymphedema.
, Dermatitis and recall reaction with doxorubicin and dactinomycin.
, Skin discoloration, telangiectasia.
, 5% of patients may develop secondary malignancy.

FOLLOW-UP

, Exam with functional status, MRI of primary, CT chest every 3 months × 2 years, then every 6 months for an additional 2–3 years, then annually thereafter.
, Ultrasound can be used to follow more superficial lesions.
, Consider bone scan or PET, if clinically indicated.

Acknowledgments We thank Brian Lee MD, PhD and Stuart Y. Tsuji MD, PhD for their work on the prior edition of this chapter.

REFERENCES

Agulnik M, Yarber JL, Okuno SH, et al. An open-label, multicenter, phase II study of bevacizumab for the treatment of angiosarcoma and epithelioid hemangioendotheliomas. Ann Oncol. 2013;24:257–63.

Alamanda VK, Crosby SN, Archer KR, et al. Predictors and clinical significance of local recurrence in extremity soft tissue sarcoma. Acta Oncol. 2013;52:793–802.

Alektiar KM, Hu K, Anderson L, et al. High-dose-rate intraoperative radiation therapy (HDR-IORT) for retroperitoneal sarcomas. Int J Radiat Oncol Biol Phys. 2000;47:157–63.

Davis AM, O'Sullivan B, et al. Late radiation morbidity following randomization to preoperative versus postoperative radiotherapy in extremity soft tissue sarcoma. Radiother Oncol. 2005;75:48–53.

Dhakal S, et al. Stereotactic body radiotherapy for pulmonary metastases from soft tissue sarcomas: excellent local lesion control and improved patient survival. Int J Radiat Oncol Biol Phys. 2012;82(2):940–5.

Dickie CI, Parent AL, et al. Bone fractures following EBRT an limb preservation surgery for lower extremity soft tissue sarcoma: relationship to irradiated bone length, volume, tumor location and dose. IJROBP. 2009;75(4):1119–24.

Dickson MA, Tap WD, Keohan ML, et al. Phase II trial of the CDK4 inhibitor PD0332991 in patients with advanced CDK4-amplified well- differentiated or dedifferentiated liposarcoma. J Clin Oncol. 2013;31(16):2024–8.

Ferguson PC, Deheshi BM, Chung P, et al. Soft tissue sarcoma presenting with metastatic disease: outcome with primary surgical resection. Cancer. 2011;117:372–9.

X

Folkert M, Bilsky M, et al. Outcomes and toxicity or hypofractionated and singe fraction image guided stereotactic radiosurgery for sarcomas metastasizing to the spine. Int J Radiat Oncol Biol Phys. 2014a;88(5):1085–91.

Folkert M, Singer S, et al. Comparison of local recurrence with conventional and IMRT for primary soft tissue sarcomas of the extremity. J Clin Oncol. 2014b;32(29):3236–41.

Italiano A, Delva F, et al. Effect of adjuvant chemotherapy on survival in FNCLCC grade 3 soft tissue sarcomas: a multivariate analysis of the French Sarcoma Group Database. Ann Oncol. 2010;21(12):2436–41.

Mendenhall WM, Zlotecki RA, Hochwald SN, et al. Retroperitoneal soft tissue sarcoma. Cancer. 2005;104:669–75.

Nussbaum D, Rushing C, et al. Preoperative or postoperative radiotherapy vs surgery alone for retroperitoneal sarcoma: a case control, propensity score matched analysis of a nationwide clinical oncology database. Lancet Oncol. 2016;17(7):966–75.

O'Sullivan B, Davis AM, Turcotte R, et al. Preoperative versus postoperative radiotherapy in soft-tissue sarcoma of the limbs: a randomised trial. Lancet. 2002;359:2235–41.

O'Sullivan B, Chung P, Euler C, et al. Soft tissue sarcoma. In: Gunderson LL, Tepper JE, editors. Clinical radiation oncology. 2nd ed. Philadelphia: Elsevier; 2007. p. 1519–49.

Oertel S, Treiber M, Zahlten-Hinguranage A, et al. Intraoperative electron boost radiation followed by moderate doses of external beam radiotherapy in limb-sparing treatment of patients with extremity soft-tissue sarcoma. Int J Radiat Oncol Biol Phys. 2006;64:1416–23.

Pervaiz N, Colterjohn N, Farrokhyar F, et al. A systematic meta-analysis of randomized controlled trials of adjuvant chemotherapy for localized Resectable soft-tissue sarcoma. Cancer. 2008;113:573–81.

Pisters PW, Harrison LB, Leung DH, et al. Long-term results of a prospective random-ized trial of adjuvant brachytherapy in soft tissue sarcoma. J Clin Oncol. 1996;14:859–68.

Pollack A, Zagars GK, Goswitz MS, et al. Preoperative vs. postoperative radiotherapy in the treatment of soft tissue sarcomas: a matter of presentation. Int J Radiat Oncol Biol Phys. 1998;42:563–72.

Robinson MH, Gaunt P, et al. Vortex trial : a randomized controlled multicenter phase 3 trial of volume of postoperative radiation therapy given to adult patients with extremity soft tissue sarcoma. Int J Radiat Oncol Biol Phys. 2016;96(2):S1.

Roeder F, Lehner B, et al. Excellent local control with IORT and postoperative EBRT in high grade extremity sarcoma: results from a subgroup analysis of a prostpective trial. BMC Cancer. 2014;14:350.

Sindelar WF, Kinsella TJ, Chen PW, et al. Intraoperative radiotherapy in retroperitoneal sarcomas. Final results of a prospective, randomized, clinical trial. Arch Surg. 1993;128:402–10.

Tinkle C, Weinberg V, et al. Intraoperative radiotherapy in the management of locally recurrent extremity soft tissue sarcoma. Sarcoma. 2015;2015(3):1–8. 913565

van der Graaf WT, Blay JY, Chawla SP, et al. Pazopanib for metastatic soft-tissue sar-coma (PALETTE): a randomised, double- blind, placebo-controlled phase 3 trial. Lancet. 2012;379:1879–86.

Wang D, Burton LE, et al. Significant reduction of late toxicities in patients with extrem-ity sarcoma treated with IGRT to a reduced target volume: results of RTOG 0630 trial. J Clin Oncol. 2015;33(20):2231–8.

Yang JC, Chang AE, Baker AR, et al. Randomized prospective study of the benefit of adjuvant radiation therapy in the treatment of soft tissue sarcomas of the extremity. J Clin Oncol. 1998;16:197–203.

PART XI
Pediatric (Non-CNS)

Chapter 41
Pediatric (Non-CNS) Tumors

David R. Raleigh, Daphne A. Haas-Kogan, and Steve E. Braunstein

GENERAL PEARLS

- This chapter will discuss Wilms' tumor, neuroblastoma, rhabdomyosarcoma, Ewing's sarcoma, pediatric Hodgkin's disease, and retinoblastoma.
- The number one cause of death in children is accidents (38%), followed by cancer (18%), congenital abnormalities (14%), homicide (9%), and heart disease (5%).
- Of childhood cancers, leukemias (20%) and CNS neoplasms (20%) are the most common, followed by lymphomas (11%), neuroblastoma (7%), Wilms' tumor (6%), osteosarcoma (3%), rhabdomyosarcoma (3%), nonrhabdomyosarcoma soft-tissue sarcomas (3%), Ewing's sarcoma (2%), retinoblastoma (2%), and others.
- Of pediatric CNS neoplasms, gliomas are most common (low-grade gliomas 15%, malignant gliomas 23%), followed by embryonal tumors (12%), pituitary tumors (10%), neuronal and mixed neuronal glial tumors (7%), ependymal tumors (5%), craniopharyngioma (4%), germ cell tumors (<5%), and meningioma (3%). These are discussed in Chap. 2.
- Whenever possible, we recommend that children be enrolled in cooperative group protocols.

XI

WILMS' TUMOR

PEARLS

- Primitive embryonal renal tumor that presents as a solid or cystic mass, often displacing the collecting system.
- Approximately 450 cases per year in the USA.

PRESENTATION

- Presents with abdominal mass, pain, hematuria, hypertension, fever, and/or malaise.
- Seventy-five percent of cases present before age 5. Median age at diagnosis is 3–4 or 2.5 years for bilateral tumors (only 7% of cases).
- Calcifications are uncommon (10%) in contrast to neuroblastoma (90%).

HISTOLOGY

- Ninety percent of cases are favorable histology (FH; no anaplastic or sarcomatous components), while 10% are unfavorable histology (anaplastic [focal vs. diffuse], clear cell sarcoma, or rhabdoid tumor).
- FH is associated with triphasic mesenchymal, epithelial, and blastemal histology.
- Difference between focal and diffuse anaplasia is strongly significant for stage II–IV 4-year OS (90–100% vs. 4–55%).
- Clear cell sarcoma and rhabdoid tumors may not be true subtypes of Wilms' tumor, but they were included in early NWTS trials.

GENETICS

- Congenital anomalies associated with Wilms' tumor (10%) include WAGR syndrome (Wilms', aniridia, genitourinary malformations, retardation due to del 11p13 and WT1 gene), Denys-Drash syndrome (pseudohermaphroditism, renal mesangial sclerosis, renal failure due to WT1 gene mutation) and Beckwith-Wiedemann syndrome (hemihypertrophy, macroglossia, GU abnormalities, gigantism due to 11p15 abnormality near WT2 gene).
- FH patients with gain of 1q, LOH of 1p, and/or 16q have poorer RFS and OS.

WORKUP

- ˒ H&P; abdominal US, CT, or MRI of primary; CXR and/or CT chest; CBC; UA; BUN/Cr; LFTs.
- ˒ For clear cell variant, add bone scan, MRI brain, and bone marrow aspiration with biopsy due to propensity for bone, bone marrow, and brain metastases.
- ˒ For rhabdoid variant, add MRI of brain because 10–15% of patients have synchronous embryonal neoplasm of the cerebellum or pineal regions.
- ˒ Do not biopsy unless unresectable or bilateral.

STAGING

Table 41.1 COG staging system

I:	Tumor limited to kidney, completely resected. Renal capsule intact. Tumor not ruptured or biopsied prior to resection. Vessels of renal sinus not involved. Margins negative.
II:	Tumor extends beyond kidney, but is completely excised with negative margins. Penetration of renal capsule or extensive invasion of the soft tissue of the renal sinus or involvement of blood vessels within nephrectomy specimen outside renal parenchyma, including renal sinus.
III:	Abdominal or pelvic LN+; penetration of peritoneal surface or peritoneal implants; +margins (gross or microscopic); unresectable due to infiltration of vital structures; tumor was biopsied before removal; tumor spillage either before or during surgery; tumor removed in >1 piece. *(Note: Biopsy or tumor spillage confined to the flank was formerly stage II in NWTS-5, while diffuse peritoneal spillage was stage III. All are now classified stage III.)*
IV:	Hematogenous mets (except for adrenal gland) or LN mets outside of abdomen or pelvis.
V:	Bilateral renal tumors at diagnosis. Stage each side separately.

NWTS 3 AND 4 10-YEAR OVERALL SURVIVAL

- ˒ Favorable histology: I 97%, II 93%, III 90%, IV 80%, and V 78%
- ˒ Anaplastic histology: II–III 49% and IV 18%
- ˒ Clear cell sarcoma: 77%
- ˒ Rhabdoid tumor: 28%

XI

TREATMENT RECOMMENDATIONS

, In the USA, surgery with radical nephrectomy is the standard of care for all cases of unilateral Wilms' tumor (when possible). Ninety to ninety-five percent are resectable at diagnosis. Nodes must be sampled; liver and contralateral kidney should be evaluated. Clips should be placed in residual disease to guide radiotherapy. If unresectable, perform biopsy and give neoadjuvant therapy ultimately to be followed by resection, if possible.

, Chemotherapy agents include vincristine (V), actinomycin (A), doxorubicin (D), cyclophosphamide (C), etoposide (E), carboplatin (P), and irinotecan (I). Actinomycin not given during RT.

Table 41.2 TREATMENT RECOMMENDATIONS

Tumor-risk classification		Treatment
Very low-risk FH	I, <2 years, and tumor <550 g	Nephrectomy and observation, only if central pathology review and LN sampling performed
Low-risk FH	I, ≥2 years, tumor ≥550 g II no LOH (both 1p and 16q)	Nephrectomy → VA. No RT
Standard-risk FH	I–II with LOH 1p and 16q (except very low-risk group)	Nephrectomy → VAD. No RT
	III, no LOH	Nephrectomy → RT → VAD
	IV, no LOH, rapid responders of lung mets at week 6 from VAD	Nephrectomy → RT → VAD. No whole lung radiation
Higher-risk FH	III with LOH 1p and 16q	Nephrectomy → RT → VAD/C/E
	IV with LOH 1p and 16q IV, no LOH, slow responders (lung and nonpulm mets)	Nephrectomy → RT → VAD/ C/E + whole lung RT, and RT to mets
High-risk UH	I–IV focal anaplasia I diffuse anaplasia	Nephrectomy → RT → VAD
	I–III clear cell	Nephrectomy → RT → alternating VDC/CE

Table 41.2 (continued)

Tumor-risk classification		Treatment
Highest risk	II–IV diffuse anaplasia	Nephrectomy → RT → alternating VDC/ CPE → RT to mets
	IV clear cell	
	I–IV rhabdoid	

Bilateral Wilms: Stage each side separately. Initial nephron-sparing resection only if >2/3 of each kidney can be preserved. Otherwise, induction chemotherapy followed by surgery, if possible. Flank radiation indicated for I–II FH, only if unresectable disease after chemotherapy, residual tumor, or positive surgical margins. Other stages and UH: RT given as above

Table 41.3 COG RT summary

General RT points	Start RT by day 9 post-op (day of surgery = day 0) CT plan to contour normal structures, but typically treat with APPA fields with 4–6 MV photons Fraction size is 1.8 Gy (except for whole abdomen and whole lung = 1.5 Gy)
Stage I–II FH	None
Stage III FH, I–III focal anaplasia, I–II diffuse anaplasia, I–III clear cell	10.8 Gy to flank Whole abdomen RT indicated if diffuse tumor spillage, pre-op or intraperitoneal tumor rupture, peritoneal tumor seeding, and cytology + ascites. Gross residual disease after surgery should receive 10 Gy boost
Stage III diffuse anaplasia, I–III rhabdoid	19.8 Gy (infants 10.8 Gy) to flank Whole abdomen RT indicated if diffuse tumor spillage, pre-op or intraperitoneal tumor rupture, peritoneal tumor seeding, and cytology + ascites Gross residual disease after surgery should receive 10 Gy boost
Recurrent abdominal tumor	12.6–18 Gy (for <12 months) or 21.6 Gy, if previous RT dose ≤10.8 Gy. Boost dose up to 9 Gy to gross residual tumor after surgery
Lung mets	12 Gy whole lung RT in 8 fx
Brain mets	30.6 Gy whole brain RT in 17 fx or 21.6 Gy whole brain RT + 10.8 Gy IMRT or stereotactic boost
Liver mets	19.8 Gy whole liver RT in 11 fx
Bone mets	25.2 Gy to lesion +3 cm margin
Unresected lymph node mets	19.8 Gy

XI

TRIALS

- *NWTS 1* (Cancer 1976) demonstrated that RT is not needed for group 1 patients <2 years old if chemotherapy is given. No radiation dose response is seen for 10–40 Gy, although RT should be started within 9 days of surgery. VCR/AMD is better than either alone for groups 2 and 3, and preoperative chemotherapy is not helpful for group 4.

- *NWTS 2* (Cancer 1981) demonstrated that RT is unnecessary for all group 1 patients. Only 6 months of VCR/AMD are necessary for group 1, but adding ADR for groups 2 and 3 improves OS.

- *NWTS 3* (Cancer 1989, Cancer 1991) demonstrated that RT is unnecessary for stage II when chemotherapy is given; 10 Gy (instead of 20 Gy) is adequate for stage III if ADR is used. Only 11 weeks of chemotherapy are necessary for stage I; ADR is unnecessary for stage II, but is necessary for stage III; and CY did not benefit stage IV.

- *NWTS 4* (JCO 1998) demonstrated that pulse-intensive chemotherapy has less hematologic toxicity and is less expensive than standard chemotherapy and that it should be used in stage I–IV patients with favorable histology.

- *NWTS 5* (JCO 2001; JCO 2005; JCO 2006) investigated treatment of stage I FH patients <2 years old and tumor <550 g with nephrectomy alone. Seventy-five patients entered, and 11 patients relapsed with 2-year DFS 87% with OS 100%. Among all FH patients, loss of heterozygosity (LOH) at chromosomes 1p and 16q is associated with increased risk of relapse and death. Patients with LOH 16q and/or 1p need treatment intensification. Stage I UH patients initially treated with only VCR/AMD have worse OS and EFS vs. similarly treated stage I FH (83 vs. 98%, 70 vs. 92%). For stage II–IV UH, addition of etoposide improves OS compared to NWTS 3–4.

- Dome (JCO 2015): Overview of COG and SIOP approaches to Wilms' tumor. Current therapy and clinical trial design based on an increasingly complex risk stratification system based on patient age; tumor stage, histology, and volume; response to chemotherapy; and loss of heterozygosity at chromosomes 1p and 16q.

RADIATION TECHNIQUES

- The treatment volume is determined by preoperative CT/MRI including the renal fossa/kidney and the tumor plus a 1–2 cm margin.
- When crossing midline, treat all of the vertebral body to avoid scoliosis.
- For para-aortic nodes, treat bilateral para-aortic chains to 10.8 Gy.
- Whole abdomen RT borders: dome of the diaphragm superiorly, bottom of the obturator foramen inferiorly, and flash laterally with blocking of the femoral heads.
- Whole lung RT borders: flash the supraclavicular fossa bilaterally, extend 1 cm beyond the ribs laterally, and extend below the posterior aspect of the diaphragm inferiorly (usually to L1). Patients treated with whole lung RT should receive TMP/SMX for PCP prophylaxis.

NWTS-5 DOSE LIMITATIONS

- Contralateral kidney: D100% ≤14.4 Gy
- Liver: uninvolved liver, D50% ≤19.8 Gy; with liver metastases, D75% ≤30.6 Gy
- Bilateral whole lungs: 9 Gy (age <1.5 years) or 12 Gy (age >1.5 years)

COMPLICATIONS

- Scoliosis, kyphosis, soft-tissue hypoplasia, small-bowel obstruction, iliac wing hypoplasia, liver/kidney hypoplasia, renal failure, pneumonitis, congestive heart failure (related to doxorubicin), subsequent high-risk pregnancy, and second malignancy.

XI

NEUROBLASTOMA

PEARLS

- Neuroblastoma is the most common extracranial solid tumor in children and the most common malignancy in infants <1 year old. The median age at diagnosis is 17 months.
- Neuroblastoma, a small round blue cell tumor (along with lymphoma, all other "blastomas," small cell carcinoma of the lung, PNET and Ewing's sarcoma, and rhabdomyosarcoma), arises from primitive neural crest cells of the spinal ganglion, dorsal spinal nerve roots, and adrenal medulla.
- Homer-Wright pseudorosettes are found in 15–50% of cases.
- Shimada classification divides neuroblastoma into favorable (FH) and unfavorable (UH) histology based on age, amount of Schwann cell stroma, nodular vs. diffuse pattern, degree of differentiation, and mitotic index.
- Cytogenetic abnormalities associated with poorer prognosis include LOH 1p, 11q, or isolated 17p; gain of 1q or 17q; N-myc proto-oncogene amplification; diploid tumors (DNA index 1); increased telomerase activity through TERT promoter rearrangement; and ALK copy number gain and gene amplification.
- Screening does not change the mortality rate of neuroblastoma, as confirmed in international trials. The high spontaneous regression rate led to overdiagnosis of clinically insignificant disease.
- Neuroblastoma most commonly arises in the adrenal gland, followed by the abdomen and thorax.
- MIBG scan sensitivity is 97% for neuroblastoma and 94% for pheochromocytoma with specificity of 92%.
- Sixty percent of patients <1 year present with localized disease, while 70% of patients >1 year present with metastases.
- London (JCO 2005): Retrospective analysis of 3666 patients on POG and CCG studies from 1986 to 2001

demonstrated prognostic contribution of age to outcome is continuous; 460-day cutoff selected to maximize the outcome difference between younger and older patients.
, Classic signs include the blueberry muffin sign (nontender blue skin nodules), raccoon eyes (orbital mets with proptosis and bruising), and opsoclonus-myoclonus-truncal ataxia (a paraneoplastic syndrome of myoclonic jerking and random eye movements that is associated with early stage and may persist after cure).
, Molecular and immunotherapy for chemotherapy-resistant marrow minimal residual disease.

WORKUP
, H&P.
, Labs include urine catecholamines, vanillylmandelic acid, and homovanillic acid, CBC, BUN/Cr, and LFTs.
, Imaging includes CT/MRI of primary, MIBG scan, and CXR. If CXR is concerning for metastases, order CT chest. Primary tumor is calcified on X-ray in 80–90% of cases (vs. 5–10% in Wilms'). Obtain bone scan if primary tumor is not MIBG+.
, Biopsy the primary or involved nodes.
, All patients should have a bilateral bone marrow biopsy and aspirate.
Note: The International Neuroblastoma Risk Group (INRG) classification system is used to develop pretreatment risk stratification to help standardize patients enrolled on trial. The International Neuroblastoma Staging System (INSS) is based on surgicopathologic findings.
, Five-year EFS cutpoints for the INRG pretreatment risk groups:
, Very low: >85%
, Low: 75–85%
, Intermediate: 50–75%
, High: <50%

XI

Table 41.4 INRG image-defined risk factors (IDRF)

Ipsilateral tumor extension within two body compartments	Neck-chest, chest-abdomen, or abdomen-pelvis
Neck	Encasing carotid and/or vertebral artery and/or internal jugular vein. Extending to the base of skull. Compressing the trachea
Cervicothoracic junction	Encasing brachial plexus roots. Encasing subclavian vessels and/or vertebral and/or carotid artery. Compressing the trachea
Thorax	Encasing the aorta and/or major branches. Compressing the trachea and/or principal bronchi. Lower mediastinal tumor, infiltrating the costovertebral junction between T9 and T12
Thoracoabdominal	Encasing the aorta and/or vena cava
Abdomen/pelvis	Infiltrating porta hepatis and/or the hepatoduodenal ligament. Encasing branches of the SMA at the mesenteric root. Encasing the origin of the celiac axis and/or the SMA. Invading one or both renal pedicles. Encasing aorta and/or vena cava. Encasing iliac vessels. Pelvic tumor crossing the sciatic notch
Intraspinal tumor extension	More than one-third of the spinal canal in the axial plane is invaded, and/or the perimedullary leptomeningeal spaces are not visible, and/or the spinal cord signal is abnormal
Infiltration of adjacent organs/ structures	Pericardium, diaphragm, kidney, liver, duodeno-pancreatic block, and mesentery

Conditions to be recorded, but *not* considered IDRFs, include multifocal primary tumors; pleural effusion, with or without malignant cells; and ascites, with or without malignant cells

Table 41.5 International Neuroblastoma Risk Group staging system

L1	Localized tumor without any IDRFs
L2	Locoregional tumor with the presence of one or more IDRFs
M	Distant metastatic disease (except stage MS), analogous to INSS stage 4
MS	Metastatic disease in children <18 months with metastases confined to skin, liver, and/or bone marrow (no cortical bone involvement), analogous to INSS stage 4S

Table 41.6 INRG pretreatment risk groups

INRG stage	Age (months)	Histologic category	Grade of tumor differentiation	MYCN	11q aberration	Ploidy	Pretreatment risk group
L1/L2		GN maturing; GNB intermixed					Very low
L1		Any, except GN maturing or GNB intermixed		NA			Very low
				Amp			High
L2	<18	Any, except GN maturing or GNB intermixed		NA	No		Low
				NA	Yes		Intermediate
	≥18	GNB nodular neuroblastoma	Differentiating	NA	No		Low
			Differentiating	NA	Yes		Intermediate
			Poorly differentiated or undifferentiated	NA			
				Amp			High
M	<18			NA		Hyperdiploid	Low
	<18			NA		Diploid	Intermediate
	<18			Amp			High
	≥18						High
MS	<18			NA	No		Very low
				NA	Yes		High
				Amp			

GN ganglioneuroma; *GNB* ganglioneuroblastoma; *Amp* amplified

XI

Table 41.7 INSS staging

1:	Localized tumor with GTR ± microscopic residual. Adherent LN may be positive but nonadherent ipsilateral LN must be negative
2A:	Localized tumor with incomplete gross resection; ipsilateral nonadherent nodes negative
2B:	Localized tumor with ipsilateral nonadherent LN involvement, but contralateral nodes negative
3:	Unresectable tumor or tumor extends across midline (defined as opposite side of vertebral body) or contralateral LN involvement or a midline tumor with bilateral extension
4:	Metastases to distant lymph nodes, bone, bone marrow, liver, skin, or other organs.
4S:	Age <1 year with an otherwise 1–2B primary tumor with metastases limited to skin, liver, and/or <10% of bone marrow (MIBG scan, if performed, should be negative in bone marrow)

COG risk groups (based on INSS stage)

Low risk (3-year OS >90%)
Any stage I
Stage 2 <1 year
Stage 2 >1 year without N-myc amplification
Stage 2 >1 year with N-myc amplification and FH
Stage 4S <1 year without N-myc amplification but with FH and hyperdiploid

Intermediate risk (3-year OS 70–90%)
Stage 3 <1 year without N-myc amplification
Stage 3 >1 year without N-myc amplification with FH
Stage 4 <18 months without N-myc amplification
Stage 4S <1 year without N-myc amplification but with UH or diploid

High risk (3-year OS 30%)
Stage 2 >1 year with N-myc amplification and UH
Stage 3 <1 year with N-myc amplification
Stage 3 >1 year with N-myc amplification or UH
Stage 4 <18 months with N-myc amplification
Stage 4 ≥18 months
Stage 4S <1 year with N-myc amplification

Table 41.8 TREATMENT RECOMMENDATIONS

Risk group	Recommended treatment
Low risk	Surgery → observation if GTR. If STR, unresectable, or recurrence after GTR → chemo for 6–12 weeks. Chemotherapy regimens consist of carboplatin, VP-16, CY, ADR, and/or topotecan and cyclophosphamide. However, if patient has severe symptoms from spinal cord compression, respiratory compromise, or GI/GU obstruction, start chemotherapy immediately (consider early radiation in symptomatic/progressive cases) → surgery
	RT (1.5/21 Gy) is used for symptoms that do not respond to chemotherapy or for massive hepatomegaly causing respiratory distress (1.5/4.5 Gy). RT also used for rare local recurrences after chemotherapy and surgery.
	For clinically stable stage 4S low-risk patients, observe after biopsy unless massive hepatomegaly causes respiratory distress (then treat with chemotherapy ± RT). Biopsy only necessary as resection does not affect outcome

Table 41.8 (continued)

Risk group	Recommended treatment
Intermediate risk	Maximal safe resection with lymphadenectomy → chemotherapy for 12–24 weeks depending on biology. Chemotherapy regimens consist of carboplatin, VP-16, CY, ADR, and/or topotecan and cyclophosphamide. Unresectable tumors may require preoperative chemotherapy to convert them to resectable status. Radiation controversial in intermediate-risk disease If PR to chemotherapy → second-look surgery. If viable residual disease present → RT to primary (1.5/24 Gy) If stage 4S with respiratory distress → RT to liver (1.5/4.5 Gy)
High risk	High-dose induction chemotherapy (same drugs, although often with ifosfamide and cisplatin) including 131 I-MIBG → attempt maximal safe resection. After surgery → high-dose chemotherapy and tandem transplant. All patients then get RT (1.8/21.6 Gy) to the postchemotherapy, presurgical extent of tumor +/− 1.8/14.4 Gy boost to gross residual disease (boost is current study question) → *cis*-retinoic acid +/− antibody therapy for 6 months. If available, IORT may be used at the time of operation, although this is not standard of care

STUDIES
Low Risk
 ˌ *POG 8104* (Nitschke, JCO 1988): 101 patients with POG A (INSS 1) disease treated with gross total resection → observation; 2-year DFS 89%.
 ˌ *CCG 3881* (Perez, JCO 2000): 374 patients treated with Evans I–II (INSS 1–2B) treated with surgery alone (plus RT for spinal cord compression). 4-year EFS and OS were 93 and 99% for stage I and 81 and 98% for stage II, respectively. Recurrences managed successfully with surgery or multimodality therapy. Stage II patients with N-myc amplification or ≥2 years old with either UH or involved lymph nodes identified as patients at higher risk of death when treated with surgery alone.

XI

INTERMEDIATE RISK
 ˌ *Castleberry, POG* (Castleberry, JCO 1991): 62 patients >1 year old with POG C (INSS 2B-3) randomized to post-op chemotherapy ± concurrent RT → second-look surgery → chemotherapy. RT was to the primary and regional nodes (1.5/24 Gy for <2 years old or 1.5/30 Gy for >2 years old). Chemo-RT improved DFS (31 → 58%) and CR rate (45 → 67%).

, *POG 8742 & 9244 (Eur J Cancer* 1997): 49 patients >1 year old with INSS 2B-3 treated with surgery → chemotherapy × 5c → second-look surgery → RT for viable residual tumor → chemo-RT was 1.5/24 Gy for age 1–2 years, 1.5/30 Gy for age >2 years. Two-year EFS was 85% after GTR vs. 70% after STR and 92% for FH vs. 58% for UH.

HIGH RISK

, *CCG 3891* (NEJM 1999; IJROBP 2003; JCO 2009): 539 high-risk patients treated with chemotherapy × 5 months → surgery, followed by 10 Gy RT for gross residual disease → randomized to myeloablative chemotherapy, 10 Gy TBI, and ABMT vs. intensive chemotherapy without TBI. Disease-free patients then randomized to observation vs. 6 months of *cis*-retinoic acid. ABMT + TBI improved 5-year EFS (19 → 30%), and *cis*-retinoic acid trended toward an improved 5-year EFS (31 → 42%), with a trend toward improved OS for both.

, *ANBL0532* (Park, ASCO 2016): 652 patients with high-risk NB receiving induction chemotherapy and surgery with randomization to single vs. tandem ASCT with three-year EFS favoring tandem ASCT (48.4% vs. 61.4%, p = 0.0081). OS 83.7% vs. 74.4% (p = 0.032) observed in single vs. tandem arms receiving anti-GD2 antibody with isotretinoin (vs. isotretinoin alone) in second randomization.

, Gross residual disease (Caussa, IJROBP 2011; Paulino, Pediatr Hematol Oncol 2003; Hogsdon, PRO 2015): Retrospective studies suggest dose response in palliative setting, with metastatic sites, and residual disease at the primary site. For postoperative gross residual disease, the benefit of a boost of 14.4 Gy to a total dose of 36 Gy is a study question (ANBL0532).

RADIATION TECHNIQUES

Simulation and Field Design

, CT and/or MRI used for planning 3DCRT or IMRT plans.

, Treat the postchemotherapy, presurgical tumor extent with a 1–1.5 cm margin, adjusted for pushing borders. If lymph node involvement is suspected or proven, cover involved LN. Do not give elective nodal RT because of morbidity and lack of benefit.

, Always cover full width of vertebrae to avoid scoliosis.

, After induction chemo, give RT to metastases if persistent active disease. For widespread disease, 131I-MIBG scan, chemotherapy, or bone marrow transplantation could be considered.

DOSE PRESCRIPTIONS
, Intermediate risk = 1.5/24 Gy (controversial)
, High risk = 1.8/21.6 Gy plus 1.8/14.4 Gy boost to gross residual disease as indicated
, 4S liver involvement = 1.5/4.5 Gy

DOSE LIMITATIONS
, Ipsilateral kidney: D25% <18 Gy, D100% <14.4 Gy
, Contralateral kidney: D75% <18 Gy
, Liver: mean <15 Gy, D85% <30 Gy
, Lung: ipsilateral D70% <20 Gy, contralateral D10% <20 Gy
, Vertebral bodies: min 18 Gy if overlaps with PTV
, Spine: 36 Gy after induction with bleomycin and mitomycin

COMPLICATIONS
, Disturbances of growth, infertility, neuropsychological sequelae, endocrinopathies, cardiac effects, pulmonary effects, bladder dysfunction, second malignancy.

RHABDOMYOSARCOMA

PEARLS
, Rhabdomyosarcoma accounts for 3% of childhood cancers.
, The most common primary sites are the head and neck (40% [parameningeal (25%), orbit (9%) and nonparameningeal sites (6%)]), genitourinary tract (30%), extremity (15%), and trunk (15%).
, Primary sites are categorized as favorable or unfavorable (see table below).
, Most cases are sporadic, but predisposing conditions include Li-Fraumeni syndrome (germline p53 mutation), neurofibromatosis type 1, and Beckwith-Wiedemann syndrome (more commonly associated with Wilms' tumor).
, The classic histologic subtypes include embryonal (60–70%), alveolar (20–40%), botryoid (10%), undifferentiated (5%), and spindle cell (<5%).

XI

- Embryonal tumors typically arise in the orbit, head and neck, or genitourinary tract (OS 66%).
- Botryoid tumors often arise in the vagina, bladder, nasopharynx, and biliary tract (OS 95%).
- Spindle cell tumors most frequently occur in paratesticular sites (OS 88%).
- Alveolar tumors most commonly arise in the extremity, trunk, or retroperitoneum of adolescents (OS 54%).
- Like alveolar tumors, undifferentiated rhabdomyosarcoma has a poor prognosis (OS 40%).
- Alveolar tumors are often associated with LOH on 11p15.5. Other cytogenetic markers include t(2;13) (70%) and t(1;13) (20%), which influence multiple genes including FKHR (chromosome 13), PAX3 (chromosome 2), and PAX7 (chromosome 1).

WORKUP
- H&P: EUA may be required for pelvic tumors; cystoscopy should be performed for GU sites.
- Labs include CBC, LFTs, BUN/Cr, and LDH.
- Imaging includes CT/MRI of primary, CT of the chest and abdomen, and bone scan.
- If parameningeal site → lumbar puncture; obtain neuraxis MRI for positive CSF cytology.
- Bone marrow biopsy.

STAGING

Table 41.9 IRS preoperative staging system (dictates induction chemotherapy)

Stage 1:	Favorable site, any T, N0–1, M0
Stage 2:	Unfavorable site, T1a/T2a, N0 M0
Stage 3:	Unfavorable site, T1b/T2b, N0 M0, or any T, N1 M0
Stage 4:	Any M1

Favorable sites: Orbit, nonparameningeal H&N (scalp, parotid, OPX, oral cavity, larynx), GU nonbladder-prostate (paratestes, vagina, vulva, uterus), and biliary tract
Unfavorable sites: Parameningeal (NPX, nasal cavity, paranasal sinuses, middle ear, mastoid, pterygopalatine fossa, infratemporal fossa), bladder, prostate, extremity, and others (trunk, retroperitoneum, etc.)

T1:	Tumor is confined to site/organ of origin (a ≤5 cm, b >5 cm)
T2:	Tumor extends beyond site/organ of origin (a ≤5 cm, b >5 cm)
N1:	Regional lymph node involvement
M1:	Distant metastases at diagnosis

Table 41.9 (continued)

IRS surgical-pathologic grouping system (dictates adjuvant RT)	
I:	Localized disease, completely resected (~13% of all patients)
A:	Confined to organ or muscle of origin
B:	Infiltration outside organ or muscle of origin
II:	Gross total resection (~20% of all patients)
A:	Microscopic residual disease, but no regional LN involvement
B:	Resected regional LN
C:	Both microscopic residual disease and resected regional LN
III:	Incomplete resection with gross residual disease (~48% of all patients)
A:	Biopsy only
B:	Subtotal resection (>50%)
IV:	Distant metastases at diagnosis (~18% of all patients)

IRS risk groups

Low risk: Localized embryonal or botryoid histology at favorable sites (stage 1, Groups I–III) or at unfavorable sites with completely resected or microscopic residual disease (stages 2–3, Groups I–II)

Intermediate risk: Embryonal or botryoid histology at unfavorable sites with gross residual disease (stages 2–3, Group III); patients 2–10 years with metastatic embryonal histology (stage 4); nonmetastatic alveolar or undifferentiated histology (stages 1–3)

High risk: Any stage 4/Group IV (except for patients 2–10 years with embryonal histology)

~3-year OS by risk group	~5-year OS by histology	~5-year OS by site
Low >90–95%	Botryoid 95%	Orbit >90%
Intermediate 55–70%	Spindle cell 88%	Parameningeal 75%
High 30–50%	Embryonal 66%	H&N nonparameningeal: 80%
	Alveolar 54%	Genitourinary sites 82%
	Undifferentiated 40%	Paratesticular 69–96%
		Gynecologic sites 90–98%
		Extremity 70%

IRS TREATMENT

˒ All patients require multimodality therapy consisting of surgery (if possible) followed by chemo ±RT. Treatment is based on stage, group, and primary site.

˒ Chemotherapy agents include VCR, AMD, CY, topotecan, and irinotecan.

˒ VA = VCR/AMD; VAC = VCR/AMD/CY; VTC = VCR/topotecan/CY; VCPT = VCR/irinotecan.

XI

Table 41.10 IRS-V treatment scheme

Stage/group	IRS-V treatment
Low risk	
Stage 1–3 Group I	Surgery → chemotherapy (VA or VAC). No RT
Stage 1 Group II	Surgery → chemotherapy (VA) + RT at week 3 (36 Gy for N0 or 41.4 Gy for N1)
Stage 1 Group III	Surgery (biopsy only for orbit) → chemotherapy (VA) + RT (50.4 Gy except for orbit which is 45 Gy). Most get RT at week 3, but primary sites at vulva, uterus, biliary tract, and certain nonparameningeal H&N get RT at week 12 to allow for possible second-look surgery; vaginal primaries get RT at week 12 (N1) or 28 (N0)
Stage 2 Group II	Surgery → chemotherapy (VAC) + RT at week 3 (36 Gy)
Stage 3 Group II	Surgery → chemotherapy (VAC) + RT at week 3 (36 Gy for N0 or 41.4 Gy for N1)
Intermediate risk	
Embryonal stages 2–3, Group III; embryonal stage 4, age 2–10 years; alveolar/undifferentiated stages 1–3	Surgery → chemotherapy (VAC or VAC alternating with VTC) At week 12, perform second-look surgery or definitive RT if unresectable RT doses depend on extent of resection and site, but, in general, 0–36 Gy for complete resection, 36 Gy for microscopic residual and N0, 41.4 Gy for microscopic residual and N1, and 50.4 Gy for gross residual
High risk	Chemotherapy (VCPT → VAC or VAC alternating with VCPT depending on response) RT at week 15 to primary and metastatic sites, except for patients with intracranial extension, spinal cord compression, or other indications for emergent RT (day 0). Definitive RT dose is 50.4 Gy except for the orbit which is 45 Gy. If second-look surgery is performed, postoperative RT doses are the same as for intermediate-risk disease
Site-specific recommendations	
Orbit	Biopsy to establish diagnosis → chemotherapy → RT. RT target is tumor +2 cm margin. Dose depends on stage and group as above (45 Gy for stage 1, Group III). Orbital exenteration is reserved for salvage
Head and neck (nonparameningeal sites)	Follow stage/group guidelines above. For Group III, perform second-look surgery or definitive RT if unresectable at week 12 with RT doses as above

Table 41.10 (continued)

Stage/group	IRS-V treatment
Parameningeal sites	If intracranial extension or cranial neuropathy present, RT is given first. Otherwise, RT is given at week 12 or week 15 if a second-look surgery is performed. For focal intracranial extension, include a 2 cm margin. If extensive intracranial involvement, treat the whole brain
Biliary tract	Follow stage/group guidelines above. For Group III, perform second-look surgery or definitive RT if unresectable at week 12. Postoperative dose is 36 Gy for complete resection and microscopic residual and 50.4 Gy for gross residual
Extremity	Wide local excision with *en bloc* removal of a cuff of normal tissue and nodal sampling → chemotherapy → local treatment as described in stage/group guidelines above
Trunk, retroperitoneum, perineum, GI	Follow stage/group guidelines above
Bladder/prostate	Follow stage/group guidelines above. Because one goal is bladder preservation, an initial biopsy is often performed followed by chemotherapy + RT, with surgery reserved for residual disease
Paratesticular	Inguinal orchiectomy with resection of entire spermatic cord and ipsilateral lymph node dissection including high and low infrarenal and bilateral iliac nodes for all patients ≥10 and for those <10 with radiographic involvement (except Group I and III biopsy-only patients) If scrotal violation, give RT to hemiscrotum. Contralateral testicle can be transposed into thigh prior to RT and later reimplanted. RT dose depends on stage and group as above (50.4 Gy for stage 1, Group III)
Uterus, cervix	Follow stage/group guidelines above. For Group III, perform second-look surgery or definitive RT if unresectable at week 12 with doses as above
Vulva	Follow stage/group guidelines above. For Group III, perform second-look surgery or definitive RT if unresectable at week 12 with doses as above
Vagina	Follow stage/group guidelines above, but local treatment is at week 12 (N1) or week 28 (N0) followed by reassessment with biopsy. If biopsy is negative, no further local treatment. If biopsy is positive, resect or initiate RT if unresectable with doses as above

XI

Table 41.11 IRS VI treatment (IRS VI trial currently open)

Stage/group	IRS-VI treatment
	All patients require multimodality therapy consisting of surgery (if possible) followed by chemo ± RT. Chemotherapy agents include VCR, AMD, CY, irinotecan, Doxo, etoposide

Overall IRS-VI summary

Chemo

Low risk: VAC × 22–46 weeks (46 weeks for stage III or Group III nonorbit)

Intermediate risk (all alveolar, Group III unfavorable embryonal): VAC vs. VAC/VI × 42 weeks

High risk (met): Alternating between V/Irinotecan, VDC, IE, and VAC

Timing of RT

Direct extension into brain or cord compression or loss of vision: day 0

Intermediate risk (Group III unfavorable sites and all alveolar): week 4

Low risk: week 13

Base of skull invasion or CN palsy: week 15

High risk (metastatic): week 20

Vagina Group II–III: week 25

AMD is given just before, but not during RT. No doxo during RT

RT volumes

GTV = prechemo, presurgical tumor, and mets at diagnosis

CTV = GTV + 1 cm. If planning 50.4 Gy, cone down to GTV + 0.5 cm after 36–41.4 Gy

If LN+, include entire LN chain

For orbit, CTV does not extend beyond bony orbit

If pushing border, do not need to cover displaced normal tissues that return to normal position after chemo. Do include entire pretreatment extent of disease

PTV = CTV + 0.5 cm

RT dose

Stage 1–3 Group I = No RT, except alveolar = 36 Gy

Stage 1–3 Group II = 36 Gy N0, 41.4 Gy N+

Stage 1 Group III = 45 Gy (orbit only). Otherwise, 50.4 Gy

IV = 50.4 Gy unless resected initially, as above. If second-look surgery margin, 36 Gy

If >1 lung met = whole lung RT 1.5/15 Gy

RT dose limitations

Optic nerve/chiasm: 46.8 Gy

Lacrimal gland: 41.4 Gy

Small bowel, spinal cord: 45 Gy

Lung: <50% >18 Gy

Kidney: <14.4 Gy

Liver: whole <23.4 Gy

Heart: whole <30.6

Table 41.11   (continued)

Stage/group	IRS-VI treatment
Low risk Stage 1 Group I–III Stage 2 Group I–II Stage 3 Group I–II	All patients get surgery first (except orbit and vagina biopsy only) → VAC chemo × 22–46 weeks; 46-week chemo is given for stage III or Group III nonorbit *Timing of RT* RT at week 13 for most patients, except Group I disease or node-negative Group III uterine/cervix primaries that are completely resected at week 13 (who do not receive RT), and patients with node-negative vaginal primaries (who begin RT following surgery at week 24) Patients with Group III disease may undergo second-look surgery at week 13, followed by response-adjusted RT dosing (see Appendix VI of ARST 0331 protocol) *Volumes* GTV = prechemo, presurgical tumor at diagnosis CTV = GTV + 1 cm. If Group III and CR to chemo, give 36 Gy to 1 cm margin, and then cone down to 0.5 cm margin to complete 50.4 Gy. If LN+, include entire LN chain. There are special modifications of GTV and CTV for certain sites (see protocol) PTV = CTV + 0.5 cm *Dose* Stage 1–3 Group I = No RT Stage 1–3 Group II = 36 Gy N0, 41.4 Gy N+ Stage 1 Group III = 45 Gy (orbit only). Otherwise, 50.4 Gy
Intermediate risk Stage 2–3, Group III embryonal unfavorable site; Nonmetastatic, Group I–III alveolar	Surgery → chemo × 42 weeks (randomized to VAC vs. VAC alternating with VI for total of 14 cycles) *Timing of RT* Simulation before week 4, RT begins at week 4 Symptomatic spinal cord compression RT may begin during week 1 No second-look surgery for unfavorable site Group III or alveolar *Volumes* Same as low risk *Dose* Stage 1–3 Group I alveolar = 36 Gy Stage 2–3 Group II = 36 Gy N0, 41.4 Gy N+ Group III = 45 Gy (orbit only). Otherwise, 50.4 Gy. For patients receiving total dose of 50.4 Gy, cone down is permitted after 36 Gy. Volume reduction not recommended for invasive tumors

XI

continued

Table 41.11 (continued)

Stage/group	IRS-VI treatment
High risk (metastatic patients, patients with parameningeal paraspinal, or intracranial extension)	Chemo for 51 weeks (alternating between V/Irinotecan, VDC, IE, and VAC)
	Timing of RT
	RT begins at week 20 to the primary and metastatic sites
	Exceptions
	Intracranial extension consisting of direct extension into the brain, or emergent RT for spinal cord compression or loss of vision, begins week 1, day 0, with RT to other metastatic sites at week 20
	Volumes
	Same as low risk, include all sites of metastases
	Patients with >1 lung met or pleural effusion receive bilateral whole lung RT
	Dose
	All patients 50.4 Gy to primary and met sites
	Orbit limited to 45 Gy
	Whole lung RT for >1 met = 1.5/15 Gy. Boost residual if possible to 50.4 Gy
	If initial surgery, resected margins negative, embryonal = 0 Gy, alveolar = 36 Gy. Microscopic residual LN– 36 Gy, microscopic residual LN + 41.4 Gy
	If second-look surgery, same except all patients with negative margins get 36 Gy

TRIALS

, *IRS-I* (Cancer 1988): 1972–1978, 686 patients. All patients got chemotherapy for 2 years. RT was given initially for Groups I and II and, at week 6, for Groups III and IV. RT dose was 40–60 Gy (<3 years = 40 Gy; <6 years and <5 cm = 50 Gy; >6 years or >5 cm = 55 Gy; >6 years and >5 cm = 60 Gy). Group I patients randomized to RT vs. no RT and no difference in OS/DFS for embryonal/botryoid. However, there was a benefit of postoperative RT for Group I alveolar/undifferentiated histologies. Orbit and GU sites had the best prognosis, and retroperitoneal and alveolar histology had the worst prognosis. DM was much more common than LF.

, *IRS-II* (Cancer 1993): 1978–1984, 990 patients. RT to tumor plus a 5 cm margin was modified from IRS-I with initiation at week 0 for Group II versus week 6 for Groups III and IV. Patients with CN palsies, base of skull (BOS) involvement, or intracranial disease got whole brain RT ± intrathecal chemotherapy to prevent meningeal relapse (which improved outcomes relative to IRS-I). RT doses were Group I = 0, Group II = 40–45 Gy, and Group III = 40–45 Gy if <6 years and <5 cm, 45–50 Gy if >6 years or >5 cm, or 50–55 Gy if both. LC for all patients receiving >40 Gy was 93%. LC for Groups I and II was 90 vs. 80% for Group III. Worse LC and OS for patients with unfavorable histology and tumors >5 cm. Local-regional relapse was more common than distant relapse except for stage IV patients.

- *IRS-III* (*JCO* 1995): 1984–1991, 1062 patients. All patients got postoperative RT except Group I favorable histology and Group III special pelvic sites in CR after chemotherapy. RT was given at day 0 for CN palsy, BOS erosion, and intracranial extension; week 2 for Group II favorable sites and Group III orbit and H&N; and otherwise at week 6. RT target included tumor plus a 2 cm margin. RT doses were Group I unfavorable site or Group II = 41.4 Gy. Group III = 41.4 Gy if <6 years and <5 cm, 50.4 Gy if ≥6 years and ≥5 cm, and 45 Gy for older children or large tumors. Five-year OS was superior in IRS-III (71%) compared to IRS-II (63%) and IRS-I (55%). LC was 90% for Group I and II patients, but only ~80% for Group III.

- *IRS-IV* (*JCO* 2001, J Pediatr Hematol Oncol 2001): 1991–1997, 1000 patients. Pretreatment staging assigned chemotherapy, and clinical grouping assigned RT. Most patients got surgery followed by chemotherapy on day 0 and RT at week 9. RT was again given at day 0 for CN palsy, BOS erosion, or intracranial extension; at week 3 for orbit and paratesticular; at week 18.5 for stage 4. RT target was presurgery, prechemotherapy tumor +2 cm margin. Whole brain RT omitted for patients with parameningeal primaries except when CSF+. Group I stages I–II did not get RT. Group I stage III and all Group II got 41.4 Gy. All Group III got 50.4 Gy in qd fractions vs. 1.1 Gy b.i.d. to 59.4 Gy. Orbital tumors were usually Group III due to biopsy only, so it got 50.4 Gy.

XI

Table 41.12 Treatment approaches and survival rates

Group/stage	Treatment	3-year OS	Findings
I paratesticular	VA	90%	No difference from IRS III
I orbit	VA	100%	No difference from IRS III
II orbit	VA + RT	100%	No difference from IRS III
I, stage 1–2	VAC vs. VAI vs. VIE; no RT	84–88%	No difference between chemo regimens
I, stage 3; all II	VAC vs. VAI vs. VIE + RT	84–88%	No difference between chemo regimens
III	VAC vs. VAI vs. VIE, + RT (qd vs. b.i.d.)	72–83% (3-year FFS)	No difference between chemo regimens. b.i.d. RT did not improve LC (~87%) or OS vs. qd RT
IV	VM vs. IE → VAC, + RT	27 vs. 55%	IE improved FFS, OS vs. VM chemo

› *COG D9803 Intermediate-risk protocol (IRS-V)* (Arndt, JCO 2009): 617 patients with intermediate-risk disease randomized to 39 weeks of VAC vs. VAC alternating with VTC. Local therapy after week 12 as per IRS-V. Patients with parameningeal disease and intracranial extension received VAC and immediate RT. Treatment strata: stage 2/3 Group III embryonal (33%) and Group IV embryonal <10 years (7%) and stage 1 Group I alveolar or undifferentiated (17%), alveolar or undifferentiated (27%), and parameningeal extension (16%). No significant difference in 4-year FFS (73% VAC vs. 68% VAC/VTC) across risk groups or in frequency of second malignancies. No difference in 4-year LF (16.5–18.5%), regional failure (4.5–4.8%), or DM (10.5–13%).

RADIATION TECHNIQUES
Simulation and Field Design
› Many patients may require pediatric anesthesia.
› Excellent immobilization is required, and 3DCRT or IMRT is encouraged to limit doses to normal structures.
› In IRS-V RT, volumes were to the prechemotherapy, presurgical tumor plus a 2 cm margin with inclusion of involved lymph nodes (prophylactic nodal RT not used). For Group III patients requiring 50.4 Gy, the volume is reduced to the prechemotherapy, presurgical tumor plus a 0.5 cm margin at 36 Gy for N0 patients or at 41.4 Gy for N1 patients.

, The timing of RT is described in the IRS-V treatment summary table above and always given at 1.8 Gy/day.
, Dose limitations are as follows: kidney <14.4 Gy, whole liver <23.4 Gy, bilateral lungs <15 Gy in 1.5 Gy fractions, optic nerve and chiasm <46.8 Gy, spinal cord <45 Gy, GI tract <45 Gy, whole abdomen 24 Gy in 1.5 Gy fractions, heart <30.6 Gy, lens <14.4 Gy, and lacrimal gland and cornea <41.4 Gy.
, Uninvolved ovaries or testicles should be shielded or moved in patients with pelvic or paratesticular primaries.

COMPLICATIONS

, Complications are site dependent.
, Chemotherapy complications include nausea, vomiting, mucositis, alopecia, and hematopoietic suppression. Ifosfamide and etoposide can cause renal and electrolyte imbalance. CY can cause hemorrhagic cystitis. ADR can cause cardiomyopathy. Cisplatin can cause hearing impairment. Topoisomerase inhibitors can cause second malignancies, particularly AML.
, AMD and ADR can accentuate radiation "recall" reaction if given during or immediately after RT.

FOLLOW-UP

, H&P and CXR every 2 months for first year with repeat imaging studies that were positive at diagnosis every 3 months, then H&P and CXR every 4 months for second and third years, then H&P annually for years 5–10, and annual visit or phone contact after 10 years.

XI

EWING'S SARCOMA

PEARLS

, Ewing's sarcoma is the second most common bone cancer of children, following osteosarcoma.
, Approximately 200 cases per year in the USA; rarely affecting African Americans and Asians.
, Boys are affected more than girls (1.5–2:1). The median age at presentation is 14 years (usually 8–25 years).

- Ewing's family of tumors includes Ewing's sarcoma (bone 87%), extraosseous Ewing's sarcoma (8%), peripheral PNET (5%), and Askin's tumor (PNET of chest wall).
- Ewing's sarcoma commonly presents in the lower extremity (femur 15–20%, tibia or fibula 5–10%), pelvis (20–30%), upper extremity (humerus 5–10%), ribs (9–13%), and spine (6–8%).
- Seventy-five to eighty percent of patients present with localized disease, but 20–25% have gross metastases to the lung, bone, or bone marrow, and nearly all patients have micrometastases at diagnosis, so all patients require chemotherapy.
- More than 90% of patients have t(11;22) [or t(21;22)] involving the EWS gene on chromosome 22, and c-Myc proto-oncogene is frequently expressed.

WORKUP

- H&P and labs including CBC, LFTs, LDH, and ESR.
- X-rays frequently show "moth-eaten," lytic diaphysis lesion, but blastic or "onion-skinning" findings can also occur.
- Imaging includes CT and/or MRI of primary, bone scan, CT chest, and ±PET scan.
- Tissue diagnosis with biopsy of primary lesion and bone marrow biopsy.
- Negative prognostic factors include metastases, pelvic, or truncal primaries, proximal (vs. distal) extremity primaries, large tumors (>8 cm or >100–200 ml), age > 17 years, high LDH or ESR, poor response to induction chemotherapy, and no surgery.

STAGING

- There is no uniform staging system for Ewing's sarcomas. The AJCC staging systems for bone or soft-tissue sarcomas may be used. Please refer to the chapters on bone tumors and soft-tissue sarcomas for more details on staging.

Table 41.13 Ewing's sarcoma outcomes

Long-term overall survival	
Localized disease	60–70% (10–25% local failure after definitive RT)
Lung and pleural metastases	30%
Bone and bone marrow metastases	15%
Local treatment without chemotherapy	10%

TREATMENT RECOMMENDATIONS

, Induction chemotherapy (VDC(A) alternating with IE) × 48 weeks with local treatment (surgery or RT with concurrent multiagent chemotherapy) at week 12–18.

, Response rate to induction chemotherapy is up to 90%.

, Adding IE to VDCA does not improve survival for patients with metastatic disease at diagnosis.

, Chemotherapy agents = vincristine (V), doxorubicin (D), cyclophosphamide (C), actinomycin-D (A), ifos-famide (I), and etoposide (E).

, Limb-salvage surgery is preferred over amputation or radiotherapy, but adequate margins for surgery are >1 cm for bone, >0.5 cm for soft tissue, and >0.2 cm for fascia.

, Postoperative RT is given for gross residual disease (55.8 Gy), positive microscopic margins (45 Gy), or poor histologic response to induction chemotherapy in the resected specimen.

, Definitive RT is used for skull, face, vertebral, or pelvic primaries and for unresectable disease (45 Gy to the pre-chemotherapy GTV + 2 cm margin with a boost to 55.8 Gy to the initial bony GTV plus the postchemotherapy soft-tissue extent). Recent data indicate 1 cm margin may be sufficient.

, For rib primary with malignant pleural effusion, RT is given to the hemithorax (1.5/15 Gy) with RT to the primary as described above.

, For lung metastases, whole lung RT (1.5/15 Gy) is given with boost to 45 Gy for gross metastases post-whole lung RT. Resection should be considered for oligometastatic pulmonary disease.

XI

STUDIES

Chemotherapy

- *IESS-1* (JCO 1990): Nonrandomized comparison of 342 patients with localized disease treated with VAC + D vs. VAC vs. VAC + prophylactic bilateral whole lung RT plus noncontrolled local intervention. 5-year RFS was best with VAC + D (60%) vs. VAC (24%) vs. VAC + RT (44%).

- *IESS-2* (JCO 1991): 214 patients with localized nonpelvic primaries randomized to high-dose, intermittent VAC + D vs. moderate dose continuous VAC + D. Local treatment was surgery ± postoperative RT or RT alone (whole bone to 45 Gy with primary boost to 55 Gy). High-dose VAC + D improved OS (63 → 77%); no difference in OS for local control modalities.

- *IESS-3/INT 0091* (NEJM 2003): 518 patients with localized or metastatic disease randomized to VDCA vs. VDCA alternating with IE. Local treatment was given at week 9–15 with RT, surgery, or both. Adding IE improved 5-year OS (61 → 72%) for localized disease, but not for metastatic disease (25%).

LOCAL THERAPY

No randomized trials have directly compared RT to surgery for LC of Ewing's sarcoma.

- *CESS 86 (JCO 2001)*: 177 patients with localized Ewing's treated with chemotherapy and nonrandomized local control arms of surgery alone, surgery plus 45 Gy RT, or 60 Gy RT alone (definitive radiotherapy randomized to qd vs. b.i.d.). RT used 5 cm proximal/distal margins and 2 cm lateral/deep margins. 5-year OS was 69% with no differences in OS or RFS according to local therapy. Local control was 100% for surgery, 95% for surgery plus RT, and 86% for RT alone (no difference for qd vs. b.i.d. RT).

- *POG 8346 (IJROBP 1998)*: 178 patients treated with chemotherapy and surgery or RT; for 44 patients, RT volume was randomized to (1) whole bone (39.6 Gy) with a boost to the initial tumor plus 4 cm margin to 55.8 Gy vs. (2) involved-field to boost volume alone for 55.8 Gy. Remaining patients treated with involved-field RT. No difference in LC or EFS when RT done properly. Five-year

EFS was highest for distal extremity and central site (63–65%) vs. proximal extremity (46%) and pelvic/sacral (24%).

, *CESS 81, CESS 86, EICESS 92* (IJROBP 2003; JCO 2008): Reviewed 1058 patients treated on trial for localized disease. After surgery, LF was 7.5% with or without postoperative RT and 5.3% after preoperative RT. After definitive RT, LF was 26.3%, but patients treated with definitive RT were negatively selected with unfavorable tumor sites. Compared to surgery alone, postoperative RT improved LC after intralesional resections or with poor histologic response to systemic therapy. After marginal resections, postoperative RT had similar LC to surgery alone despite poorer histologic response.

, Talleur (IJROBP 2016): St. Judes phase II trial of 45 EWS patients stratified to received 55.8 vs. 64.8 Gy based on tumor size <8 vs. ≥8 cm, respectively. All patients treated with 1 cm margins on gross tumor. LF rate 4.4% at 10 year.

RADIATION TECHNIQUES

, Radiation fields customized depending on primary site, and MRI is recommended for treatment planning in all cases. General dose and target volume recommendations are presented, which should be interpreted with respect to dose limitations of adjacent critical structures. Avoid bladder RT with CY or ifosfamide.

, Definitive RT for bone tumors with no soft-tissue involvement: Prechemotherapy GTV plus a 2 cm margin to 55.8 Gy.

, Definitive RT for bone tumors with a soft-tissue component: Prechemotherapy GTV plus a 2 cm margin to 45 Gy, with a boost to 55.8 Gy to the initial bony GTV plus the postchemotherapy soft-tissue extent with a minimal margin.

, For postoperative RT, treat the pretreatment GTV plus a 2 cm margin to 45 Gy with a boost to any postoperative gross residual disease plus 2 cm margin to 55.8 Gy.

, For node-positive disease, treat the nodal bed to 50.4 Gy if resected or 55.8 Gy for gross residual disease.

XI

DOSE LIMITATIONS

- Depends on primary site.
- More than 18 Gy can prematurely close epiphysis.
- For extremity lesions, spare a 1–2 cm strip of skin to prevent lymphedema. 20–30 Gy usually can be given to the entire circumference of an extremity, if necessary.

COMPLICATIONS

- Dermatitis and recall reaction may occur with ADR and dactinomycin.
- Abnormal bone and soft-tissue growth and development. Most of leg growth occurs at the distal femur and proximal tibia. Limb length discrepancy of 2–6 cm can be managed with a shoe lift; otherwise, surgery is needed.
- Permanent weakening of affected bone. The highest risk for fracture is within 18 months of RT, during which time patients should avoid contact and high-impact sports.
- Decreased range of motion secondary to soft-tissue and/or joint fibrosis.
- Skin discoloration.
- Lymphedema.
- Cystitis (especially with CY or ifosfamide).

FOLLOW-UP

- H&P + CXR every 3 months for 2 years. X-ray primary every 3 months (and/or MRI every 6 months) for 2 years. After 2 years, may increase follow-up intervals, but should obtain CBC annually.

PEDIATRIC HODGKIN'S LYMPHOMA

PEARLS

- Hodgkin's lymphoma constitutes ~6% of childhood cancers and has many biological and clinical aspects in common with adult Hodgkin's lymphoma.
- Due to morbidity from RT, lower-dose RT with chemotherapy or chemotherapy alone is used to treat children.

, Hodgkin's lymphoma is most common among children >10 years (male:female incidence = 3–4:1) and rare among children <4 years (male:female incidence = 1.3:1).

, Nodular sclerosing histology is the most common subtype in all age groups, but is less common among children (44%) than among adolescents and adults (72–77%).

, Mixed cellularity histology is more common in children (33%) than in adolescents or adults (11–17%).

, Lymphocyte-predominant histology is relatively more common in children <10 years (13%), whereas lymphocyte-depleted subtype is rare.

, Approximately 80–85% of children present with stage I–III disease, 80% have cervical lymphadenopathy, ~25–30% have B symptoms, and ~20% have bulky mediastinal adenopathy.

WORKUP

, History (including B symptoms, pruritis, and respiratory symptoms) and physical exam with labs including CBC, LFTs, BUN/Cr, alkaline phosphatase, and ESR.

, Imaging includes CXR; CT of chest, abdomen, and pelvis; and PET scan. Bone scan is ordered only for patients with bone pain or elevated alkaline phosphatase.

, Pathologic diagnosis is obtained by excisional biopsy (FNA distorts critical architectural features). Bone marrow biopsy is obtained for patients with B symptoms or stage III–IV disease.

, Adverse prognostic factors include stage IIB–IV disease, B symptoms, male sex, WBC >11,500/mm3, and hemoglobin ≤11 g/dL.

XI

STAGING

, *Ann Arbor Staging System* used.

, Ten-year OS is ≥90% for stages I–III and 75–80% for stage IV.

Table 41.14 TREATMENT RECOMMENDATIONS

Stage	Recommended treatment
Low risk: IA, IIA favorable (no bulky disease, no extranodal disease, ≤3 sites)	Chemo × 2–4c → IFRT 15–25 Gy AHOD0431 investigating whether patients with CR after chemotherapy can bypass IFRT
Intermediate risk: stage I or II (not low risk); IIIA	Chemo × 4–6c → IFRT 15–25 Gy, except for rapid early responders who achieve a CR per AHOD0031
High risk: IIIB, IVA/B, selected IIB with adverse associated features (e.g., bulky disease)	Chemo × 6–8c → IFRT 15–25 Gy
Relapse	For patients with low-risk disease at diagnosis with relapse confined to an area of initial involvement after chemotherapy and no RT, use salvage chemotherapy and IFRT For postpubertal patients, standard-dose RT may be used. For all other patients, induction chemo and high-dose chemotherapy with peripheral blood stem cell rescue is used. Recently closed COG study (AHOD 0121) offered hyperfractionated RT, 21 Gy/ 1.5 b.i.d. to involved sites not previously treated plus ASCT
Chemotherapy	Hybrid regimens that utilize lower cumulative doses of alkylators, doxorubicin, and bleomycin are used [e.g., COPP/ABV, OEPA (males), OPPA (females), etc.]. Drugs include: cyclophosphamide (C), procarbazine (P), vincristine (O) and/or vinblastine (V), prednisone (P) or dexamethasone, doxorubicin (A) or epirubicin, bleomycin (B), dacarbazine (D), etoposide (E), methotrexate (M), and cytosine arabinoside

TRIALS

- *CCG 5942* (JCO 2002): 501 patients with a CR to risk-adapted combination chemotherapy randomized to IFRT or observation. In an as-treated analysis, 3-year EFS was increased with IFRT (85 → 93%) but OS was the same (98–99%).
- Hudson (JCO 2004): 159 unfavorable patients (I/II bulky or B symptoms, III, IV) were treated with alternating VAMP/COPP, then response-based IFRT. Five-year OS 93%, EFS 76%. Trial stopped early due to poor EFS. Poor result due either to chemotherapy regimen or omitting RT.
- Donaldson (JCO 2007): 110 low-risk patients were treated with VAMP × 4 + IFRT (15 Gy for CR, 25.5 Gy for PR). Ten-year OS 96%, EFS 89%. Toxicity: hypothyroidism in 42%. One patient developed cardiac dysfunction; two patients developed secondary malignancies.

- *GPOH-HD 95* (JCO 2013): 925 patients were treated with risk-adapted chemotherapy (2–6 cycles) and RT. No RT was given for a CR as assessed by CT or MRI. PR of >75% tumor regression: 20 Gy; for PR <75%: 30 Gy; residual mass > 50 mL: 35 Gy. 10-year PFS was similar for low-risk patients with or without RT (97% vs. 92%), but superior with RT for intermediate-risk patients (69% vs. 91%).

- *AHOD0031* (JCO 2014): 1721 patients with pediatric intermediate-risk HL treated with 2 cycles of ABVE-PC. Rapid early responders (RERs) received 2 additional cycles, and those who achieved CR were randomly assigned to IFRT vs. no additional therapy. Slow early responders (SERs) randomly assigned to 2 additional cycles of ABVE-PC with or without DECA. RERs without a CR and all SERs received IFRT. 4-year EFS and OS were 87% and 99% for RER and 77% and 95% for SER (SS). No difference in outcomes for RERs with CR with and without RT or SERs with and without DECA.

- *AHOD0431* (Keller Klin Padiatr 2014): Nonrandomized trial of 278 stage IA/IIA, low-risk, cHL patients treated with AV-PC × 3. If CR on PET after 3 cycles, no RT; otherwise, IFRT (21 Gy in 14 fx). 4-year EFS and OS 80% and 99.6%, respectively. 48% of subjects successfully treated without RT. Preliminary results suggest early responders who have a negative PET scan after 1 cycle may have an improved outcome without adjuvant RT.

- *AHOD1331* (study open): Randomized phase III study of ABVE-PC vs. brentuximab vedotin plus AVEPC for newly diagnosed high-risk cHL in children and adolescents. Target accrual 600 patients. 5 cycles of chemotherapy for all patients, with RT for those without a rapid response after 2 cycles of chemotherapy, and for all patients with bulky mediastinal disease.

XI

RADIATION TECHNIQUES
Simulation and Field Design

- Use immobilization for reproducibility and 6 MV photons for better dose distribution.
- Involved fields are protocol specific, but generally include the initially involved lymph nodes (prechemotherapy GTV) and initially involved sites that remain abnormal

after chemo (postchemotherapy GTV). The CTV should reflect postchemotherapy reduction in target volume in noninvolved tissues (e.g., lung). ITV may be used to account for target motion during breathing.

, See ILROG guidelines (Hodgson, Pract Radiat Oncol 2015) for contemporary radiation therapy planning concepts.

, Supradiaphragmatic fields may be simulated with the arms up over the head or akimbo. Arms up pulls the axillary nodes away from the lungs, allowing greater lung shielding, but the nodes are closer to the humeral heads. Attempts should be made to exclude as much lung, humeral head, and breast tissue as possible.

, For children <5 years, some consider bilateral RT to avoid growth asymmetry. However, with low doses, unilateral fields are usually appropriate.

DOSE PRESCRIPTIONS

, In general, RT dose is 15–25 Gy depending on the protocol. Occasionally, a 5 Gy boost is used for poor responders following initial chemotherapy. Dose may be determined by response to initial chemotherapy.

DOSE LIMITATIONS

, Shield femoral head. Doses >25 Gy increase the risk of slipped capital femoral epiphysis, and doses >30–40 Gy increase the risk of avascular necrosis.

, Dental abnormalities may occur with doses of 20–40 Gy.

, Mean heart dose <15 Gy and cardiac shielding limit cardiac sequelae.

, Thyroid abnormalities are more common with doses >26 Gy.

, Pneumonitis is uncommon with V24Gy <30% except when used in combination with bleomycin.

, Shield testes to limit oligospermia or infertility.

, Consider oophoropexy for girls to preserve ovarian function.

COMPLICATIONS

, Chemotherapy complications include bleomycin (pulmonary fibrosis/pneumonitis), doxorubicin (cardiomyopathy), alkylators and etoposide (AML and myelodysplasia), procarbazine (male infertility), and prednisone (avascular necrosis).

, Acute side effects of mantle RT include epilation, dermatitis, dysgeusia, xerostomia, odynophagia, and esophagitis. Para-aortic RT may cause acute nausea or vomiting.

, Subacute and late effects of RT include musculoskeletal hypoplasia, sterility, hypothyroidism, radiation pneumonitis, increased risk for myocardial atherosclerotic heart disease, and increased risk of second malignancy.

, The rate of second malignancies is ~8–15% at 20 years. Breast cancer is the most common solid 2nd malignancy following treatment.

RETINOBLASTOMA

PEARLS

, Retinoblastoma (RB) is the most common intraocular tumor of childhood, accounting for ~4% of all pediatric malignancies; ninety-five percent of cases occur in children <5 years.

, The RB1 tumor suppressor gene on chromosome 13 causes RB only when both alleles are "hit" (40% germline, 60% sporadic).

, Although autosomal recessive, RB is inherited in an autosomal dominant pattern due to second hit penetrance approaching 100%.

, Genetic counseling should be given to all patients with RB and siblings should be examined.

, With germline RB, 15–35% of nonirradiated patients and 50–70% of irradiated patients develop second tumors by 50 years after diagnosis, mainly sarcomas or melanomas.

, 65–80% of cases are unilateral (mostly sporadic) and 20–35% are bilateral (mostly due to germline mutations).

, Trilateral RB refers to bilateral RB and midline CNS neuroblastic tumors, frequently of the pinoblastoma or other suprasellar embryonal tumors.

XI

- In the developing world, patients present with proptosis, orbital mass, or metastases. In the USA, the most common presentation is leukocoria, strabismus, painful glaucoma, irritability, failure to eat, and low-grade fever.
- Five patterns of spread: contiguous spread through the choroid/sclera/orbit; extension along the optic nerve into the brain; invasion of the subarachnoid space/leptomeninges; hematogenous spread to the bone, liver, or spleen; and lymphatic spread from the conjunctiva.

WORKUP

- H&P includes external ocular examination, slit lamp biomicroscopy, and binocular indirect ophthalmoscopy (often under anesthesia for mapping).
- Labs: CBC, chemistries, BUN, Cr, and LFTs.
- Imaging: fluorescein angiography, bilateral US (A&B mode), and MRI.
- Bone scan and/or lumbar puncture for symptoms or suspected metastatic disease.
- Risk factors for metastatic disease include optic nerve invasion, uveal invasion, orbital invasion, and choroidal involvement.

STAGING

- The most commonly used system is the Reese-Ellsworth system, which predicts the chance of visual preservation but not survival. The Abramson-Grabowski system addresses both intraocular and extraocular RB. The International Classification ("ABCDE") system for intraocular RB is under modification and is used in recent clinical protocols. The AJCC TNM system is new as of 2017.

Table 41.15 Reese-Ellsworth staging system

Group I:	Very favorable (refers to chance of salvaging the affected eye)
	A: Solitary tumor, <4 disc diameters (DD) in size, at or behind the equator
	B: Multiple tumors, none over 4 DD in size, all at or behind the equator
Group II:	Favorable
	A: Solitary tumor, 4–10 DD in size, at or behind the equator
	B: Multiple tumors, 4–10 DD in size, behind the equator
Group III:	Doubtful
	A: Any lesion anterior to the equator
	B: Solitary tumors larger than 10 DD behind the equator
Group IV:	Unfavorable
	A: Multiple tumors, some larger than 10 DD
	B: Any lesion extending anteriorly to the ora serrata
Group V:	Very unfavorable
	A: Massive tumors involving over half the retina
	B: Vitreous seeding

INTERNATIONAL CLASSIFICATION SYSTEM FOR INTRAOCULAR RETINOBLASTOMA

GROUP A
Small intraretinal tumors away from foveola and disc
   All tumors are 3 mm or smaller in greatest dimension, confined to the retina *and* located further than 3 mm from the foveola *and* 1.5 mm from the optic disc.

GROUP B
All remaining discrete tumors confined to the retina
   ، All other tumors confined to the retina not in Group A.
   ، Tumor-associated subretinal fluid <3 mm from the tumor with no subretinal seeding.

XI

GROUP C

Discrete local disease with minimal subretinal or vitreous seeding

‚ Tumor(s) are discrete.

‚ Subretinal fluid, present or past, without seeding involving up to 1/4 retina.

‚ Local fine vitreous seeding may be present close to discrete tumor.

‚ Local subretinal seeding <3 mm (2 DD) from the tumor.

GROUP D

Diffuse disease with significant vitreous or subretinal seeding

‚ Tumor(s) may be massive or diffuse.

‚ Subretinal fluid present or past without seeding, involving up to total retinal detachment.

‚ Diffuse or massive vitreous disease may include "greasy" seeds or avascular tumor masses.

‚ Diffuse subretinal seeding may include subretinal plaques or tumor nodules.

GROUP E

Presence of any one or more of these poor prognosis features

‚ Tumor touching the lens

‚ Tumor anterior to anterior vitreous face involving ciliary body or anterior segment

‚ Diffuse infiltrating retinoblastoma

‚ Neovascular glaucoma

‚ Opaque media from hemorrhage

‚ Tumor necrosis with aseptic orbital cellulites

‚ Phthisis bulbi

STAGING: RETINOBLASTOMA

Editors' note: All TNM stage and stage groups referred to elsewhere in this chapter reflect the 2010 AJCC staging nomenclature unless otherwise noted as the new system below was published after this chapter was written.

Table 41.16 (AJCC 7TH ED., 2010)

Clinical classification (cTNM)

Primary tumor (T)

TX: Primary tumor cannot be assessed

T0:   No evidence of primary tumor

T1:   Tumors no more than 2/3 the volume of the eye with no vitreous or subretinal seeding

T1a: No tumor in either eye is >3 mm in largest dimension or located closer than 1.5 mm to the optic nerve or fovea

T1b: At least one tumor is greater than 3 mm in largest dimension or located closer than 1.5 mm to the optic nerve or fovea. No retinal detachment or subretinal fluid beyond 5 mm from the base of the tumor

T1c: At least one tumor is >3 mm in largest dimension or located closer than 1.5 mm to the optic nerve or fovea, with retinal detachment or subretinal fluid beyond 5 mm from the base of the tumor

T2:   Tumors no more than 2/3 the volume of the eye with vitreous or subretinal seeding. Can have retinal detachment

T2a: Focal vitreous and/or subretinal seeding of fine aggregates of tumor cells is present, but no large clumps or "snowballs" of tumor cells

T2b: Massive vitreous and/or subretinal seeding is present, defined as diffuse clumps or "snowballs" of tumor cells

T3:   Severe intraocular disease

T3a: Tumor fills more than 2/3 of the eye

T3b: One or more complications present, which may include tumor-associated neovascular or angle closure glaucoma, tumor extension into the anterior segment, hyphema, vitreous hemorrhage, or orbital cellulitis

T4:   Extraocular disease detected by imaging studies

T4a: Invasion of optic nerve

T4b: Invasion into the orbit

T4c: Intracranial extension not past chiasm

T4d: Intracranial extension past chiasm

Regional lymph nodes (N)

NX: Regional lymph nodes cannot be assessed

N0:   No regional lymph node involvement

N1:   Regional lymph node involvement (preauricular, cervical, submandibular)

N2:   Distant lymph node involvement

XI

Metastasis (M)

M0:   No metastasis

M1:   Systemic metastasis

M1a: Single lesion to sites other than CNS

M1b: Multiple lesions to sites other than CNS

M1c: Prechiasmatic CNS lesion(s)

M1d: Postchiasmatic CNS lesion(s)

M1e: Leptomeningeal and/or CSF involvement

continued

Table 41.16 (continued)

Pathologic classification (pTNM)

Primary tumor (pT)

pTX:	Primary tumor cannot be assessed
pT0:	No evidence of primary tumor
pT1:	Tumor confined to eye with no optic nerve or choroidal invasion
pT2:	Tumor with minimal optic nerve and/or choroidal invasion
pT2a:	Tumor superficially invades optic nerve head but does not extend past lamina cribrosa *or* tumor exhibits focal choroidal invasion
pT2b:	Tumor superficially invades optic nerve head, but does not extend past lamina cribrosa *and* exhibits focal choroidal invasion
pT3:	Tumor with significant optic nerve and/or choroidal invasion
pT3a:	Tumor invades optic nerve past lamina cribrosa, but not to surgical resection line, *or* tumor exhibits massive choroidal invasion
pT3b:	Tumor invades optic nerve past lamina cribrosa, but not to surgical resection line, *and* exhibits massive choroidal invasion
pT4:	Tumor invades optic nerve to resection line or exhibits extraocular extension elsewhere
pT4a:	Tumor invades optic nerve to resection line, but no extraocular extension identified
pT4b:	Tumor invades optic nerve to resection line and extraocular extension identified

Regional lymph nodes (pN)

pNX:	Regional lymph nodes cannot be assessed
pN0:	No regional lymph node involvement
pN1:	Regional lymph node involvement (preauricular, cervical)
N2:	Distant lymph node involvement

Metastasis (pM)

cM0 no metastasis	
pM1:	Metastasis to sites other than CNS
pM1a:	Single lesion
pM1b:	Multiple lesions
pM1c:	CNS metastasis
pM1d:	Discrete mass(es) without leptomeningeal and/or CSF involvement
pM1e:	Leptomeningeal and/or CSF involvement

Table 41.17 (AJCC 8TH ED., 2017)

Definition of AJCC TNM	
Clinical classification (cTNM)	
Definition of primary tumor (cT)	
cT category	**cT criteria**
cTX	Unknown evidence of intraocular tumor
cT0	No evidence of intraocular tumor
cT1	Intraretinal tumor(s) with subretinal fluid ≤5 mm from the base of any tumor
cT1a	Tumors ≤3 mm and further than 1.5 mm from disc and fovea
cT1b	Tumors >3 mm or closer than 1.5 mm from disc or fovea
cT2	Intraocular tumor(s) with retinal detachment, vitreous seeding, or subretinal seeding
cT2a	Subretinal fluid >5 mm from the base of any tumor
cT2b	Vitreous seeding and/or subretinal seeding
cT3	Advanced intraocular tumor(s)
cT3a	Phthisis or pre-phthisis bulbi
cT3b	Tumor invasion of choroid, pars plana, ciliary body, lens, zonules, iris, or anterior chamber
cT3c	Raised intraocular pressure with neovascularization and/or buphthalmos
cT3d	Hyphema and/or massive vitreous hemorrhage
cT3e	Aseptic orbital cellulitis
cT4	Extraocular tumor(s) involving orbit, including optic nerve
cT4a	Radiology evidence of retrobulbar optic nerve involvement or thickening of optic nerve or involvement of orbital tissues
cT4b	Extraocular tumor clinically evident with proptosis and/or an orbital mass

DEFINITION OF REGIONAL LYMPH NODE (CN)

cN category	cN criteria
cNX	Regional lymph nodes cannot be assessed
cN0	No regional lymph node involvement
cN1	Evidence of preauricular, submandibular, and cervical lymph node involvement

XI

DEFINITION OF DISTANT METASTASIS (M)

cM category	cM criteria
cM0	No signs or symptoms of intracranial or distant metastasis
cM1	Distant metastasis without microscopic confirmation
cM1a	Tumor(s) involving any distant site (e.g., bone marrow, liver) on clinical or radiology tests

continued

cM1b	Tumor involving the CNS on radiology imaging (not including trilateral retinoblastoma)
pM1	Distant metastasis with microscopic confirmation
pM1a	Pathological evidence of tumor at any distant site (e.g., bone marrow, liver, or other)
pM1b	Pathological evidence of tumor in the cerebrospinal fluid or CNS parenchyma

DEFINITION OF HERITABLE TRAIT (H)

H category	H criteria
HX	Unknown or insufficient evidence of a constitutional *RB1* gene mutation
H0	Normal *RB1* alleles in blood tested with demonstrated high-sensitivity assays
H1	Bilateral retinoblastoma, retinoblastoma with an intracranial primitive neuroectodermal tumor (i.e., trilateral retinoblastoma), patient with family history of retinoblastoma, or molecular definition of a constitutional *RB1* gene mutation

PATHOLOGICAL CLASSIFICATION (PTNM)

DEFINITION OF PRIMARY TUMOR (PT)

pT category	pT criteria
pTX	Unknown evidence of intraocular tumor
pT1	No evidence of intraocular tumor
pT1	Intraocular tumor(s) without any local invasion, focal choroidal invasion, or pre- or intralaminar involvement of the optic nerve head
pT2	Intraocular tumor(s) with local invasion
pT2a	Concomitant focal choroidal invasion and pre- or intralaminar involvement of the optic nerve head
pT2b	Tumor invasion of stroma of iris and/or trabecular meshwork and/or Schlemm's canal
pT3	Intraocular tumor(s) with significant local invasion
pT3a	Massive choroidal invasion (>3 mm in the largest diameter, or multiple foci of focal choroidal involvement totaling >3 mm, or any full-thickness choroidal involvement)
pT3b	Retrolaminar invasion of the optic nerve head, not involving the transected end of the optic nerve
pT3c	Any partial-thickness involvement of the sclera within the inner two thirds

pT3d	Full-thickness invasion into the outer third of the sclera and/or invasion into or around emissary channels
pT4	Evidence of extraocular tumor: tumor at the transected end of the optic nerve, tumor in the meningeal spaces around the optic nerve, full-thickness invasion of the sclera with invasion of the episclera, adjacent adipose tissue, extraocular muscle, bone, conjunctiva, or eyelids

DEFINITION OF REGIONAL LYMPH NODE (PN)

pN category	pN criteria
pNX	Regional lymph node involvement cannot be assessed
pN0	No lymph node involvement
pN1	Regional lymph node involvement

DEFINITION OF DISTANT METASTASIS (M)

M category	M criteria
cM0	No signs or symptoms of intracranial or distant metastasis
cM1	Distant metastasis without microscopic confirmation
cM1a	Tumor(s) involving any distant site (e.g., bone marrow, liver) on clinical or radiology tests
cM1b	Tumor involving the CNS on radiology imaging (not including trilateral retinoblastoma)
pM1	Distant metastasis with histopathologic confirmation
pM1a	Histopathologic confirmation of tumor at any distant site (e.g., bone marrow, liver, or other)
pM1b	Histopathologic confirmation of tumor in the cerebrospinal fluid or CNS parenchyma

AJCC PROGNOSTIC STAGE GROUPS

CLINICAL STAGE (CTNM)

When cT is...	And N is...	And M is...	And H is...	Then the clinical stage group is...
cT1, cT2, cT3	cN0	cM0	Any	I
cT4a	cN0	cM0	Any	II
cT4b	cN0	cM0	Any	III
Any	cN1	cM0	Any	III
Any	Any	cM1 or pM1	Any	IV

XI

PATHOLOGICAL STAGE (PTNM)

When pT is...	And N is...	And M is...	And H is...	Then the pathological stage group is...
pT1, pT2, pT3	pN0	cM0	Any	I
pT4	pN0	cM0	Any	II
Any	pN1	cM0	Any	III
Any	Any	cM1 or pM1	Any	IV

HISTOLOGIC GRADE (G)

G	G definition
GX	Grade cannot be assessed
G1	Tumor with areas of retinoma (fleurettes or neuronal differentiation)
G2	Tumor with many rosettes (Flexner-Wintersteiner or Homer Wright)
G3	Tumor with occasional rosettes (Flexner-Wintersteiner or Homer Wright)
G4	Tumor with poorly differentiated cells without rosettes and/or with extensive areas (more than half of tumor) of anaplasia

Used with permission of the American Joint Committee on Cancer (AJCC), Chicago, Illinois. The original and primary source for this information is the *AJCC Cancer Staging Manual*, Eighth Edition (2017) published by Springer International Publishing

TREATMENT RECOMMENDATIONS

Table 41.18 TREATMENT RECOMMENDATIONS

Stage	Treatment recommendation
Unilateral, intraocular	Laser therapy alone or chemoreduction × 6c → focal therapy Chemotherapy agents include vincristine, carboplatin, and etoposide. Focal therapy options include: EBRT (35–46 Gy) for small tumors located within macula, with diffuse vitreous seeding or multifocality Cryotherapy is used in addition to EBRT or in place of photocoagulation for lesions <4 DD in the anterior retina Photocoagulation is used for posteriorly located tumors <4 DD distinct from the optic nerve head and macula and occasionally for small tumors, often in addition to EBRT Episcleral plaque brachytherapy is used for either focal unilateral disease or recurrent disease following prior EBRT Enucleation if the tumor is massive or if the eye is unlikely to have useful vision after treatment
Bilateral	Each eye is assessed individually. If there is potential vision preservation in both eyes, bilateral chemoreduction ± EBRT with close follow-up for focal treatment may be used
Extraocular	Orbital EBRT + chemotherapy for palliation. High-dose chemotherapy with stem cell rescue may also be attempted in select cases. Intrathecal chemo may be given for patients with CNS or meningeal disease
Trilateral retinoblastoma	Treat eyes as above. Neurosurgical resection, chemotherapy, with cranial RT or CSI. MS is only 11 months, but as high as 24 months if caught early

RESULTS

, Five-year DFS: Intraocular >90%, extraocular (T4, N1 or M1) <10%.
, Eye preservations rates range from ~60–90% when using EBRT and depend on extent of disease. Group E patients have eye preservation rates of only 2%.

RADIATION TECHNIQUES
EBRT

, Indicated for small tumors involving the macula, associated with diffuse vitreous seeding, multifocal tumors, or for those that failed prior chemotherapy and local therapy.
, Simulate patient supine with thermoplastic head mask immobilization; pediatric anesthesia may be required.
, 3DCRT is recommended (or IMRT if at an experienced center) using CT and/or MRI for planning and photons (4–6 MV).
, For unilateral RB, four anterior oblique noncoplanar fields may be used (superior, inferior, medial, and lateral).
, For bilateral RB when both eyes require treatment, 3DCRT (or IMRT) is used with opposed lateral fields and anterior oblique fields.
, Depending on stage and anatomy, 0.5 cm bolus may be required.
, At a minimum, the entire retina is treated including 5–8 mm of the optic nerve.
, Dose is 42–45 Gy in 1.8–2 Gy fractions.
, Critical structures to limit RT dose to include the opposite globe (including lens and retina), lacrimal glands, optic chiasm, pituitary gland, brainstem, posterior mandibular teeth, and upper C-spine.

XI

EPISCLERAL PLAQUE BRACHYTHERAPY

, Refer to the chapter on orbital tumors for details of brachytherapy for orbital melanoma; many techniques similar for RB.

₃ Treatment volume covers the tumor plus radial (~2 mm) and deep (1–2 mm) margins.

₃ Dose to the tumor apex is 40 Gy with 100–200 Gy to the base.

₃ Dose rate is 0.7–1.0 Gy/h, requiring ~2–4 days of treatment.

COMPLICATIONS

₃ EBRT complications include dermatitis; depigmentation; telangiectasias; ectropion or entropion of the eyelid; loss of hair of the scalp, eyebrow, or eyelid; facial/temporal bone hypoplasia; decreased tear production due to radiation damage to the lacrimal gland; direct corneal injury; cataracts; vitreous hemorrhage; retinopathy; hypopituitarism; and second tumors in radiation field.

₃ With plaque brachytherapy, the risk of orbital bone hypoplasia is low, but long-term retinopathy, cataract, maculopathy, papillopathy, and glaucoma are possible.

FOLLOW-UP

₃ H&P every 3 months for 1 year, every 4 months for second year, every 6 months for third and fourth years, and then annually. Patients with bilateral or familial RB advised to have screening for CNS midline neuroblastic tumors with biannual CT or MRI of the brain until 5 years of age. In addition, they need screening of the contralateral eye every 2–4 months for up to 7 years.

Acknowledgment We thank Stuart Y. Tsuji MD, PhD, and Linda W. Chan, MD, for their work on the prior edition of this chapter.

REFERENCES

WILMS' TUMOR

Dome JS, Graf N, Geller JI, et al. Advances in wilms tumor treatment and biology: progress through international collaboration. JCO. 2015;33(27):2999–3005.

NEUROBLASTOMA

Bresler SC, Weiser DA, Huwe PJ, et al. ALK mutations confer differential oncogenic activation and sensitivity to ALK inhibition therapy in neuroblastoma. Cancer Cell. 2014;26(5):682–94.

Castleberry RP, Kun LE, Shuster JJ, et al. Radiotherapy improves the outlook for patients older than 1 year with Pediatric oncology group stage C neuroblastoma. J Clin Oncol. 1991;9:789–95.

Caussa L, Hijal T, Michon J, et al. Role of palliative radiotherapy in the management of metastatic pediatric neuroblastoma: a retrospective single-institution study. Int J Radiat Oncol Biol Phys. 2011;79:214–9.

Chen Y, Takita J, Choi YL, et al. Oncogenic mutations of ALK kinase in neuroblastoma. Nature. 2008;455(7215):971–4.

Cheung NV, Cheung IY, Kushner BH, et al. Murine anti-GD2 monoclonal antibody 3F8 combined with granulocyte-macrophage colony-stimulating factor and 13-cis-retinoic acid in high-risk patients with stage 4 neuroblastoma in first remission. J Clin Oncol. 2012;30(26):3264–70.

Jacobson AF, Deng H, Lombard J, et al. 123I-meta-iodobenzylguanidine scintigraphy for the detection of neuroblastoma and pheochromocytoma: results of a meta-analysis. J Clin Endocrinol Metab. 2010;95(6):259–2606.

London WB, Castleberry RP, Matthay KK, et al. Evidence for an age cutoff greater than 365 days for neuroblastoma risk group stratification in the children's oncology group. J Clin Oncol. 2005;23:6459–65.

McCabe MG, Backlund LM, Leong HS, et al. Chromosome 17 alterations identify good-risk and poor-risk tumors independently of clinical factors in medulloblastoma. Neurooncol. 2010;13(4):376–83.

Nitschke R, Smith EI, Shochat S, et al. Localized neuroblastoma treated by surgery: a pediatric oncology group study. J Clin Oncol. 1988;6:1271–9.

Park JR, Kreissman SG, London WB, et al. A phase 3 randomized clinical trial of tandem myeloablative autologous stem cell transplant using peripheral blood stem cell as consolidation therapy for high-risk neuroblastoma: a children's oncology group study. 2016 ASCO Annual Meeting. Abstract LBA3. 2016.

Paulino AC. Palliative radiotherapy in children with neuroblastoma. Pediatr Hematol Oncol. 2003;20:111–7.

Peifer M, Hertwig F, Roeis F, et al. Telomerase activation by genomic rearrangements in high-risk neuroblastoma. Nature. 2015;526(7575):700–4.

Perez CA, Matthay KK, Atkinson JB, et al. Biologic variables in the outcome of stages I and II neuroblastoma treated with surgery as primary therapy: a children's cancer group study. J Clin Oncol. 2000;18:18–26.

Pinto NR, Applebaum MA, Volchenboum SL, et al. Advances in risk classification and treatment strategies for neuroblastoma. J Clin Oncol. 2015;33(27):3008–17.

XI

RHABDOMYOSARCOMA

Arndt CA, Stoner JA, Hawkins DS, et al. Vincristine, actinomycin, and cyclophosphamide compared with vincristine, actinomycin, and cyclophosphamide alternating with vincristine, topotecan, and cyclophosphamide for intermediate-risk rhabdomyosarcoma: children's oncology group study D9803. J Clin Oncol. 2009;27(31):5182–8.

EWING'S SARCOMA

Talleur AC, Navid F, Spunt SL, McCarville MB, Wu J, Mao S, Davidoff AM, Neel MD, Krasin MJ. Limited margin radiation therapy for children and young adults with Ewing sarcoma achieves high rates of local tumor control. Int J Radiat Oncol Biol Phys. 2016;96(1):119–26.

PEDIATRIC HODGKIN'S LYMPHOMA

Donaldson SS, Link MP, Weinstein HJ, et al. Final results of a prospective clinical trial with VAMP and low-dose involved-field radiation for children with low-risk Hodgkins disease. J Clin Oncol. 2007;25:332–7.

Dorffel W, Ruhl U, Luders H, et al. Treatment of children and adolescents with Hodking lympha without radiotherapy for patients in complete remission after chemotherapy: final results of the multinational trial GPOH-HD95. J Clin Oncol. 2013;31:1562–8.

Friedman DL, Chen L, Wolden S, et al. Dose-intensive response-based chemotherapy and radiation therapy for children and adolescents with newly diagnosed intermediate-risk Hodgkin lymphoma: A report from Children's Oncology Group Study AHOD0031. J Clin Oncol. 2014;32(32):3651–8.

Hodgson DC, Dieckmann K, Terezakis S, et al. Implementation of contemporary radiation therapy planning concepts for pediatric Hodgkin lymphoma: guidelines from the International Lymphoma Radiation Oncology Group. Pract Radiat Oncol. 2015;5(2):85–92.

Hudson MM, Krasin N, Link MP, et al. Risk-adapted, combined-modality therapy with VAMP/COPP and response-based, involved-field radiation for unfavorable pediatric Hodgkins disease. J Clin Oncol. 2004;22:4541–50.

Keller F, Castellino S, Constine L, et al. Intensive therapy free survival (ITFS) for early-stage Hodgkin lymphoma (cHL) including chemotherapy and radiation therapy (IFRT) for recurrence after chemotherapy alone. Klin Padiatr. 2014;226:O_09

PART XII
Palliation

Chapter 42
Palliation and Benign Conditions

Lauren Boreta, Yao Yu, and Steve E. Braunstein

INTRODUCTION

- This chapter will cover brain metastases, bone metastases, spinal cord compression, liver metastases, airway obstruction, superior vena cava obstruction, and gynecologic bleeding.

PALLIATION OVERVIEW

- Palliative care should be integrated earlier in cancer care than at end-of-life because it may improve patient and caregiver outcomes (ASCO guideline, Ferrell, JCO 2017).
- ENABLE III trial comparing early vs delayed palliative care showed significant 1-year OS benefit to early intervention (63% vs 48%).

BRAIN METASTASES

PEARLS

- Most common type of intracranial tumor (incidence ~200,000/year in the USA).
- Approximately 20–30% of all cancer patients develop brain metastases.

XII

© Springer International Publishing AG, part of Springer Nature 2018   **871**
Eric K. Hansen and M. Roach III (eds.), *Handbook of Evidence-Based Radiation Oncology*, https://doi.org/10.1007/978-3-319-62642-0_42

⌐ Primary cancers most likely to metastasize to brain are lung, breast, and melanoma.
⌐ Hemorrhagic metastases: renal cell carcinoma, choriocarcinoma, and melanoma.

WORKUP

⌐ H&P with detailed neurologic exam
⌐ Brain MRI: T1 pre- and post-contrast. T2 FLAIR
⌐ For new cancer diagnosis, staging workup for identification of primary, evaluation of systemic disease burden, and tissue biopsy

PROGNOSTIC FACTORS

⌐ RTOG Recursive Partitioning Analysis (Gaspar IJROBP 1997; IJROBP 2000) was based upon RTOG brain metastases trials 1979–1993. Class I (MS 7.1 mo): KPS 70–100, primary controlled, age <65, brain metastases only. Class III (MS 2.3 mo): KPS <70. Class II (MS 4.2 mo): all others.
⌐ More recent multi-institutional series, including original disease-specific graded prognostic index (DS-GPA) and updates, report improved outcomes in more modern era with improved imaging and systemic therapies. (Sperduto IJROBP 2010; JCO 2012; IJROBP 2016).
⌐ Specific indices are available for NSCLC, Melanoma, Breast Cancer, Renal Cell Carcinoma, and GI cancers at www.brainmetgpa.com.

TREATMENT RECOMMENDATIONS
GENERAL

⌐ Steroids can improve neurologic symptoms, including headaches.
⌐ Antiepileptics are recommended for patients with seizures. There is no benefit to prophylactic antiepileptic use in patients without seizure history (Sirven Mayo Clin Proc 2004, Tremont-Lukats Cochrane Rev 2008).
⌐ Multidisciplinary coordination is needed between medical oncology, neurosurgery, and radiation oncology for optimal care.
⌐ Treatment should be tailored to the patient, taking into account: clinical scenario, tumor histology, extracranial

disease burden, intracranial disease burden, performance status, life expectancy, cancer-directed treatment options, and patient preferences.

, Consider memantine for neuroprotection with whole brain radiotherapy.

, Hippocampal-sparing radiation is investigational pending NRG-CC001 results.

, Use of SRS alone is associated with increased risk of distant brain failure compared to whole brain radiotherapy, so close follow-up with surveillance MRIs is recommended to maximize opportunity for salvage treatment(s).

, Concurrent administration of systemic agents and brain radiation should be carefully reviewed and discussed with the medical oncologist (Table 42.1).

Table 42.1 TREATMENT RECOMMENDATIONS

Clinical scenario	Treatment recommendation
Acute decompression required	Surgery plus: Adjuvant SRS (small cavity) or fractionated SRT (large cavity) for limited brain metastases Adjuvant WBRT for leptomeningeal or diffuse brain metastases
Single large (>3 cm) metastasis, surgical candidate	Surgery + adjuvant SRS (small cavity), or adjuvant FSRT (large cavity) Adjuvant WBRT may be considered if SRS or FSRT is not available or for patient preference
Single large metastasis (>3 cm), not surgical candidate	Fractionated SRT (preferred). Single-session SRS is associated with increased risk of local failure and toxicity WBRT ± SRS boost
Single small metastasis, good prognosis	SRS or surgery + adjuvant SRS. LC for small tumors with SRS is excellent
Limited metastases, good prognosis	SRS and close observation, reserving WBRT or additional SRS for salvage
Diffuse metastases, good prognosis	WBRT
Prior brain radiation	For limited volume brain metastases, SRS Repeat WBRT for selected cases (good PS, absent or limited and controlled extracranial disease, prolonged disease-free interval) Systemic therapy
Poor performance status	Best supportive care or WBRT
Leptomeningeal disease	Prognosis is poor and options are limited WBRT or focal RT to bulky disease Intrathecal chemotherapy Shunting if CSF obstruction suspected (communicating or noncommunicating)

XII

STUDIES
WBRT VERSUS BEST SUPPORTIVE CARE

- QUARTZ (Mulvenna Lancet 2016): Phase III non-inferiority study of 538 patients with NSCLC brain metastases not considered suitable for resection or radiosurgery were randomized to optimal supportive care (OSC) vs WBRT (20 Gy/5 fx) + OSC. More patients undergoing WBRT developed drowsiness, hair loss, nausea, or dry/itchy scalp. There was no difference in MS (8.5 vs 9.2 wks), QOL, or dexamethasone use between groups. 56% RPA 2, 38% RPA 3. 83% DS-GPA 0–2. Patients <60 yrs had better OS with WBRT, and a similar trend was observed for good GPA, and good performance status. No data on cause of death (neurologic vs other). Patients with poor prognosis (GPA) may not benefit from WBRT.

WBRT WITH OR WITHOUT SURGERY

- Patchell (NEJM 1990): 54 patients with documented cancer and newly diagnosed solitary brain lesion randomized to resection + WBRT (36 Gy/12 fx) vs WBRT alone. Patients with supratentorial lesions on WBRT alone arm underwent biopsy. 11% of brain tumors were not metastases (3 gliomas, 2 abscesses, 1 inflammatory). Surgery reduced local failures (crude: 20% vs 52%), and increased median survival (40 vs 15 wks), time to neurologic death (62 vs 26 weeks), and time with functional independence (38 vs 8 wks).

SURGERY WITH OR WITHOUT WBRT

- Patchell (JAMA 1998): 95 pts with single brain metastases s/p GTR were randomized to postoperative WBRT (50.4 Gy/28 fx) vs observation. WBRT reduced in-brain failure (crude, 18% vs 70%), local failure (crude 10% vs 46%), likelihood of neurologic death (14% vs 44%), and increased time to local failure (>57 vs 27 wks). No effect on OS (48 vs 43 weeks) or functional independence.
- *EORTC 22952–26001* (Kocher JCO 2011): 359 pts with WHO PS 0–2, 1–3 brain mets treated with surgery (GTR, N = 160), or SRS (20 Gy, N = 199) randomized to WBRT (30 Gy/10 fx) vs observation. 71% linac-based SRS. 96% of surgery pts had 1 brain metastasis, compared with 73% of

SRS pts. WBRT decreased 2-year distant brain failure (27% vs 59%), local failure (surgery, 23% vs 42%; SRS, 33% vs 48%), and neurologic death (28% vs 44%). There was no difference in OS (10.9 vs 10.7 mo), or preservation of performance status (10 vs 9.5 mo).

SURGERY + ADJUVANT/SALVAGE RADIOSURGERY

- Mahajan (ASTRO 2016 abstr 3). 131 pts with 1–3 brain mets with complete resection of at least one randomized to observation vs SRS to resection cavity (12–14–16 Gy assigned by cavity volume at time of SRS). SRS improved 1-yr LC (72% vs 45%). 1-yr distant brain met rate was 43% after SRS, 33% after observation (nonsignificant). MS was 17 mo in both arms. Perioperative tumor >3 cm had worse LC.
- N107C/CEC.3 (Brown, ASTRO 2016a LBA-1). 194 pts with 1–4 brain mets randomized to cavity SRS (12–20 Gy volume-based prescription) vs WBRT (37.5 Gy) after resection of one lesion. SRS had less 6-month cognitive deterioration (54% vs 86%) and better QOL with no survival difference (MS 11.8 vs 11.5 mo) despite more surgical bed LF by 1 yr (44% vs 22%) and worse overall intracranial tumor control (55% vs 79%).
- JCOG 0504 (Kayama, ASCO 2016 abstr.). 271 pts with 1–4 brain mets with only one lesion >3 cm having been resected randomized within 21 days after surgery to WBRT vs salvage SRS for residual or recurrent tumors. No difference in MS (15.6 mo). WBRT had better intracranial PFS (10.4 mo vs 4 mo) but more grade 2–4 cognitive dysfunction at 90 days (16.4% vs 7.7%).
- A number of other institutional series report 1-year LC on the order of 70–90% with adjuvant SRS or FSRT after resection, similar to whole brain radiation (Brennan IJROBP 2014, Jensen JNS 2011).
- Distant brain failures occur in about 40–60% of pts, however.
- Pts with large tumors or resection cavity volume may benefit from fractionated SRT vs single session SRS. One commonly used scheme is 27 Gy in 3 fractions (Minniti, IJROBP 2013).
- PTV margin of 2 mm may be considered with linac-based radiation (Soltys et al., IJROBP 2008).

XII

WBRT VERSUS WBRT + SRS BOOST

  » *RTOG 9508* (Andrews Lancet 2004): 331 pts with 1–3 brain mets and KPS ≥70 were randomized to WBRT (37.5 Gy/15 fx) +/− SRS (dose per RTOG 9005). 19% dropout rate in SRS group. SRS improved 1-year local control (82% vs 71%), increased likelihood of stable/improved KPS at 6 mo (43% vs 27%). In a prespecified subgroup analysis for pts with a single metastasis, SRS improved MS (6.5 vs 4.9 mo). Unplanned subset analyses showed survival advantage in RPA class 1 pts (11.6 vs 9.6 mo), and those with tumors >2 cm (6.5 vs 5.3 mo).

SRS VERSUS SRS + WBRT

  » *Multi-institutional* (Sneed IJROBP 1999; IJROBP 2002): Multi-institutional retrospective reviews of SRS vs SRS + WBRT. No difference in OS by RPA class (I = 14–15 months, II = 7–8 months, III = 5 months). Brain FFP worse without WBRT, but brain FFP allowing for first salvage not different.

  » *JROSG 99–1* (Aoyama JAMA 2006): 132 pts with 1–4 mets and KPS ≥70 randomized to SRS (18–25 Gy) +/− WBRT (30 Gy/10 fractions). No difference in OS (8.0 vs 7.5 mo), neurologic or KPS preservation, or MMSE. WBRT reduced rate of new mets (63.7% vs 41.5%), and improved 1-year LC (72.5% vs 88.7%).

  » *MDACC* (Chang Lancet Oncol 2009): 58 pts with 1–3 mets and KPS ≥70 randomized to SRS (15–24 Gy) +/− WBRT (30 Gy/12 fractions). Pts treated with SRS + WBRT had worse neurocognitive decline at 4 months (24% vs 52%) by Hopkins Verbal Learning Test, despite better 1-year LC (SRS 67% vs SRS + WBRT 100%) and 1-year distant brain tumor control (45% vs 73%). SRS alone had better MS (15.2 vs 5.7 months). SRS alone pts received more salvage therapy, but 61% did not have WBRT by 1 yr.

  » See EORTC 22952–26001 above.

  » *Meta-analysis* (Sahgal IJROBP 2009): Meta-analysis of three phase III randomized trials (JROSG 99–1, MDACC, EORTC 22952) comparing SRS ± WBRT, with individual patient data. Pts ≤ 50 yrs old had better survival with SRS alone. These pts also had similar rates of distant brain failure with or without WBRT. Pts older than 50 had no different survival, and WBRT reduced distant brain failure. Pts with single metastases had better survival and lower rates of distant brain failure than those with multiple metastases.

- *NCCTG* (Brown JAMA 2016b): 213 pts with 1–3 brain metastases randomized to receive SRS alone (20–24 Gy) or SRS (18–22 Gy) + WBRT (30 Gy/12 fx). The primary endpoint was neurocognitive decline. SRS alone resulted in less cognitive decline at 3 months (63.5% vs 91.7%) and 12 months (60% vs 94.4%), and better quality of life. The 12-mo local control (72.8% vs 90.1%) and distant brain control (69% vs 92%) were lower with SRS alone, but there was no difference in MS (7.6 vs 5.9 mo), and salvage therapy was more likely with SRS alone (32% vs 7.8%).

DOSE AND FRACTIONATION CONSIDERATIONS

- *WBRT fractionation* (Tsao, PRO 2012b; Tsao, Cochrane 2012a): Multiple fractionation regimens have been evaluated. No difference in OS or symptom control has been demonstrated among commonly prescribed schemes, including 30 Gy/10 fx, 20 Gy/5 fx. Other common schemes include 37.5 Gy/15 fx or 40 Gy/20 fx. Treatment with 10 Gy × 1 and 7.5 Gy × 2 have less durable responses, and can result in serious toxicity.

- *SRS dose RTOG 9005* (Shaw IJROBP 2000): Dose escalation protocol of single-fraction radiosurgery for pts with previously treated primary brain tumors and recurrent brain metastases. Pts were stratified based upon tumor diameter. Maximum tolerated doses for tumors with diameter 0–2 cm, 2.1–3 cm, and 3.1–4 cm were 24 Gy, 18 Gy, and 15 Gy, respectively. Actuarial risk of radionecrosis was 11% at 2 years. Pts treated with linac-based SRS had higher risk of progression. Pts with larger tumors had higher risk of radionecrosis.

- *UCSF* (Sneed JNS 2015): Retrospective review of 435 pts and 2200 brain metastases on a per lesion basis. Treatment failure, adverse radiation effect (ARE), and treatment failure + ARE occurred in 9.2%, 5.4%, and 1.4% of pts. ARE occurred 3–18 months after radiation, and 76% improved within 18 months. ARE risk was correlated with lesion size, brain radiation (20% prior SRS, 8% concurrent

XII

WBRT), kidney primary, connective tissue disorder, and capecitabine use.

NUMBER OF METASTASES

, *JKLG 0901* (Yamamoto Lancet Oncol 2014): Multi-institutional, prospective study. Pts with 1–10 brain metastases (largest <10 ml, largest <3 cm diameter, cumulative volume < 15 ml) and KPS ≥ 70 were treated with SRS. Median survival was 13.9, 10.8, and 10.8 mo for pts with 1, 2–4, and 5–10 tumors (no difference 2–4 vs 5–10 mets). The proportion of pts with adverse events did not differ based upon number of mets.

NEUROPROTECTION

, *RTOG 0614* (Brown Neuro Oncol 2013): 554 pts with brain metastases treated with WBRT were randomized to memantine (20 mg/d) vs placebo for 24 weeks. Memantine did not meet primary endpoint of improving 24-week delayed recall (p = 0.059), but the trial only had 35% statistical power due to greater than expected patient loss rates. Memantine was well tolerated, and improved time to cognitive decline, executive function, processing speed, and delayed recognition at various time-points.

, *RTOG 0933* (Gondi JCO 2014): 100 pts with brain metastases were treated with WBRT with hippocampal avoidance (HA-WBRT). Compared with historical control, HA-WBRT improved cognitive outcomes as measured by the Hopkins Verbal Learning Test.

, *NRG-CC001* is randomizing pts to WBRT (30 Gy/10 fx) and memantine with or without hippocampal avoidance.

WHOLE BRAIN REIRRADIATION

, Heidelberg (Scharp Radiat Oncol 2014): 134 pts with brain metastases received whole brain reirradiation (20 Gy/10 fx) with 13.4-month median interval after initial course (30 Gy/10 fx). Median OS after second course was 2.8 months, and 39% had clinical improvement. Small cell lung carcinoma, low KPS, and uncontrolled primary tumor were associated with worse survival.

- MGH (Son IJROBP 2012): 17 pts with brain metastases receiving whole brain reirradiation with 15.3 month median interval between courses. Re-RT median dose was 21.6 Gy in 12 fractions. Median OS after second course was 5.2 months.
- Multi-institutional (Logie, ASTRO 2015 abstr. 139). 92 pts at 5 centers received whole brain reirradiation. Pts with KPS > 80, stability of primary, or absence of extracranial disease had longer survival.

SPECIAL CIRCUMSTANCES

- Systemic agents have historically been ineffective for treatment of brain metastases, in part due to poor CNS penetration due to the blood brain barrier. Studies of novel systemic agents for metastatic disease often exclude pts with brain metastases.
- *ALK/ROS1-positive NSCLC:* Brain metastases are a common mode of failure for ALK-positive NSCLC treated with Crizotinib. Treatment of oligoprogressive brain metastases can prolong duration of TKI use and potentially improve survival (Weickhardt J Thor Onc 2012). These pts have favorable prognosis with pts surviving several years. Consideration should be given to quality of life and delayed toxicities. Certain TKIs may have CNS penetrance; however randomized comparisons with radiation are limited (Johung JCO 2016, Rusthoven JCO 2016).
- *EGFR-mutated NSCLC:* Current TKIs active against EGFR mutant NSCLCs (erlotinib, gefitinib) have CNS penetrance; however response rates are typically less than with radiation (Magnuson JCO 2017). As with ALK/ROS1 positive NSCLC, these pts have favorable prognosis compared to nontargetable NSCLC. TKI therapy may be a viable alternative for pts with TKI-sensitive EGFR-mutated tumors with brain metastases if the morbidity of radiation is high and the risk of progressive disease is modest (e.g., asymptomatic tiny brain metastases or prior WBRT) (Iuchi Lung Cancer 2013).
- *Melanoma:* SRS is preferred over WBRT for pts with good performance status and limited metastases due to relative radioresistance of melanoma brain metastases. Discontinue BRAF-inhibitors 3 days prior to WBRT, or 1 day prior to SRS to avoid dermatologic toxicity (Anker IJROBP 2016). Immunotherapies are discussed below.

XII

, *Immune therapy:* Immunotherapies, including checkpoint inhibitors, may have activity for CNS metastases from a variety of primary tumors (Margolin Lancet Onc 2012; Goldberg Lancet Onc 2016; Knisely JNS 2012). Published experience with concurrent immunotherapy and SRS/SBRT is rapidly evolving (Kroeze, Cancer Treat Rev 2017).

, *Leptomeningeal Disease:* Median OS is only 10–30 weeks based on histology and KPS. MRI of the craniospinal axis is important to assess disease burden. Steroids may relieve some symptoms, including CSF obstruction. Pts with bulky disease may benefit from RT to affected areas, selectively followed by IT-MTX. Craniospinal RT may be considered, but has significant toxicity and life expectancy must be considered. Intrathecal chemotherapy after RT can be used to address non-bulky disseminated disease; however this is also associated with adverse effects (Atalar IJROBP 2013).

TECHNIQUES
WBRT
, Opposed laterals, flash anterior/posterior/superior (Fig. 42.1).
, Bottom of field at foramen magnum, inferior to C1, or inferior to C2.
, Use eye block.
, Acceptable fractionation schemes include 30 Gy/10 fx (most common), 20 Gy/5 fx, 37.5 Gy/15 fx, and 40 Gy/20 fx.
, Choose fractionation based on performance status, life expectancy, and histology.
, More sophisticated RT delivery techniques including VMAT and IMRT may reduce hair loss but without reported benefit to QOL (De Puysseleyr Rad Onc 2014).

STEREOTACTIC RADIATION
, Consider double-dose gadolinium for eligible pts to improve sensitivity of MRI for tiny metastasis.
, Dexamethasone may be given prior to single-fraction radiosurgery to reduce acute edema particularly for pts with preexisting edema before treatment.
, SRS vs FSRT depends on number, size, and location of lesion(s).

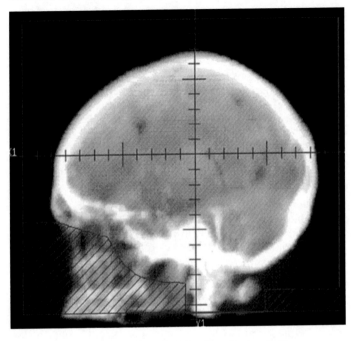

Fig. 42.1 Lateral DRR of a whole brain radiation field

- SRS dose: RTOG 9005 doses were 24 Gy for 0–2 cm, 18 Gy for 2.1–3 cm, and 15 Gy for 3.1–4 cm, all in the setting of prior radiotherapy. See contemporary review on dose selection in SRS (Flickinger et al., Prog Neurol Surg 2013).
- FSRT: A number of dose schemes have been published. One common regimen is 9 Gy × 3 fractions (Minniti et al., J Neurooncol 2014; Navarria et al., Radiat Oncol 2016).
- We recommend individualizing dose based on location, size/volume, histology, and other factors.

XII

COMPLICATIONS
- Neurocognitive deficits can occur early after WBRT.
- Somnolence syndrome is a rare complication characterized by extreme sleepiness at 1–6 months following WBRT.
- Radionecrosis can occur following CNS radiation. Treatments include steroids, surgery, bevacizumab.

FOLLOW-UP

˒ Brain MRI with and without contrast as often as every 3–4 months initially, then less frequent depending on clinical situation.

˒ Steroid taper as tolerated.

˒ Differentiation between tumor progression, adverse radiation effect, or both on imaging can be challenging. Careful radiology review is needed.

BONE METASTASES

PEARLS

˒ Common cause of severe cancer pain.

˒ Pain relief after RT can be expected in 60–90% of pts.

˒ Good pain control may improve OS, QOL.

˒ Sites of mets: spine (lumbar > thoracic) > pelvis > ribs > femur > skull.

˒ Primary cancers most likely to metastasize to bone are breast, prostate, thyroid, kidney, and lung.

˒ ~1% of bone mets fracture. 40% of pathologic fractures occur in the femur.

˒ Pathologic fracture can be due to osteolytic/blastic or mixed lesions.

WORKUP

˒ Bone scan is the primary imaging modality.

˒ Plain films should be used to look for fracture or impending fracture, but are not sensitive for diagnosis as cortical involvement occurs late.

˒ MRI is the procedure of choice when evaluating for spinal cord compression or nerve root compromise.

˒ Biopsy and/or PET scan are not routinely needed, but should be considered if radiographic studies are equivocal or if histology has not been established.

TREATMENT RECOMMENDATIONS
SURGERY

˒ Required for pathologic fracture or impending fracture that would cause instability, loss of function, or neurologic compromise (Nousianinen 2009).

, Mirels (Clin Orthop 1989): 12-point scoring system estimates risk of pathologic fracture based on the site of disease (upper extremity, lower extremity, peritrochanteric), amount of pain (mild, moderate, functional), type of lesion (blastic, mixed, lytic), and size (<1/3, 1/3–2/3, >2/3 diameter of the bone involved). Scores of 10–12 have 72–100% chance of fracture.

, Van der Linden (J Bone Joint Surg Br 2004): Data show that axial cortical involvement >30 mm and/or circumferential cortical involvement >50% predict for high rates of fracture.

, Spinal Instability Neoplastic Score (SINS): classification for spinal instability based on patient and imaging factors. Scores ≥7 are potentially unstable, ≥13 are unstable.

EBRT

, See ASTRO evidence-based guideline (Lutz, PRO 2017) for current consensus statements on interdisciplinary management of bone metastases.

, Local field RT is recommended for discrete painful lesions. Avoid uninvolved sensitive tissues when possible.

, Doses: 8 Gy/1 fx, 20 Gy/5 fx, 24 Gy/6 fx, or 30 Gy/10 fx offer equivalent chance of pain relief, including spinal sites.

, Pts with persistent or recurrent pain more than 1 month after initial palliative RT may be offered retreatment, respecting normal tissue dose constraints.

, Wide-field ("hemibody") RT is no longer used for diffuse bone mets.

SPINE SBRT

, Delivers higher BED with greater conformality than EBRT.

, Generally reserved for disease confined to 1–2 spinal segments.

, Spine SBRT may be considered for primary treatment of radioresistant histology (e.g., renal cell, melanoma), salvage treatment in previously irradiated spine, or after marginal miss.

, Ideal pts have good to excellent PS, oligometastatic disease, no more than 3 spinal levels involved, no or minimal spinal instability (SINS score 0–6), no or minimal

XII

epidural disease (Bilsky 0–1), radioresistant histology, no prior EBRT, or prior EBRT >5 mo prior.

˛ Contraindications include poor PS, widely metastatic or progressive disease, limited life expectancy, >3 contiguous spinal levels involved or diffuse spine disease, spine instability (SINS 13–18), high-grade epidural disease (Bilsky 3), prior EBRT <3 mo, inability to tolerate near-rigid supine immobilization, unable to have full spine MRI and/or CT myelogram.

˛ Excellent LC and pain response has been reported in a number of series with low-reported toxicity and risk of myelopathy, despite a range of dose and fractionation schedules and its use in cases of reirradiation and/or post-resection (Jabbari, Cancer J 2016).

˛ There is no current consensus standard dose fractionation schedule. We recommend meticulous adherence to published techniques and dose constraints and/or enrollment on clinical trial.

VERTEBROPLASTY/KYPHOPLASTY

˛ Vertebral compression fractures are common and can be due to the cancer itself, treatment (hormonal therapies → osteoporosis, osteonecrosis from radiosurgery), or underlying osteoporosis.

˛ Open surgery typically reserved for pts with neurologic compromise.

˛ Vertebroplasty: percutaneous injection of cement into compromised vertebral body.

˛ Balloon kyphoplasty: minimally invasive technique in which an intravertebral cavity is opened and filled with PMMA cement. Restores vertebral height.

˛ In a multinational randomized trial (CAFE), pts with compression fracture were randomized to kyphoplasty vs nonsurgical treatment. Pts treated with kyphoplasty had improved QOL, KPS, and increased activity at 1 month (Berenson Lancet Onc 2011).

˛ No consensus on utility of kyphoplasty prior to radiation therapy.

RADIOPHARMACEUTICAL THERAPY

˛ Best for pts with multiple lesions that show uptake on bone scan.

- Should not be used for fractures, spinal cord compression, nerve root compression, or lesions with large extra osseous component.
- Pts must have adequate blood counts, and typically no myelosuppressive chemotherapy for 4 weeks before and 6–8 weeks after treatment.
- Radium-223 (α-emitter) significantly improved OS, delayed progression of disease, and decreased PSA in men with metastatic castrate-resistant prostate cancer.
- Strontium-89 (β-emitter) response rates 40–95%, pain relief at 1–4 weeks, lasts up to 18 months. Improved response rate and duration with low-dose platinum (Porter IJROBP 1993, Sciuto JNM 2002).
- Samarium-153 (β- and γ-emitter) response rates 70–95%, pain relief at 1–2 weeks, lasts up to 4 months.

PHARMACOLOGIC THERAPIES AND SUPPORTIVE CARE

- Denosumab: monoclonal antibody that binds to the receptor of RANKL, which is a mediator of osteoclast activity. In randomized trials comparing denosumab to zoledronic acid in pts with breast and prostate cancer, denosumab significantly delayed in time to skeletal-related events (Stopeck JCO 2010).
- Bisphosphonates also are effective in reducing skeletal-related events.
- Endocrine therapy can be very effective in breast and prostate cancer.
- Pain management is important (NSAIDs, narcotics, steroids, anticonvulsants, tricyclic antidepressants, electric stimulation, nerve blocks).
- Mechanical assistance with bracers and walkers.

STUDIES
EBRT DOSE

XII

- Updated ASTRO review (Lutz, PRO 2017) of high-quality data continues to show equivalent pain relief between shorter and longer fractionation schemes, but retreatment rates are increased in pts with prolonged survival.
- Meta-analysis (Chow, Clin Oncol 2012) of 25 randomized trials of single-fraction vs multiple-fraction palliative RT regimens. No difference in response rates (CR 23–24%). Trend for reduced risk of spinal cord compression with multifraction RT. There is a 2.6× increased retreatment rate with single-fraction RT.

> *RTOG 9714* (Hartsell, JNCI 2005; Howell ASCO 2009): 898 pts with breast or prostate cancer and KPS ≥40 randomized to 8 Gy in 1 fx vs 30 Gy in 10 fractions. Higher acute toxicity with 30 Gy (17% vs 10%). Pain CR/PR rates at 3 months were equivalent, 15%/50% for 8 Gy and 18%/48% for 30 Gy, but higher retreatment at 3 years for 8 Gy (18% vs 9%). Same conclusions in subgroup with vertebral body mets.

SBRT

> International Spine Radiosurgery Consortium (Cox IJROBP 2012, Redmond IJROBP 2017): Consensus guidelines for target delineation in spine radiosurgery for metastases in definitive and postoperative settings.

> Jabarri (Cancer J 2016) provides one of several contemporary literature reviews describing evidence for spine SBRT including outcomes, side effects, and technological requirements.

> Gerszten (Spine 2007): Prospective single-arm study of 393 pts (500 lesions) treated with SBRT (12.5–25 Gy in 1 fraction). 344 lesions had received prior EBRT. Long-term improvement in 86% of pts treated for pain. For pts treated for imaging progression, LC was 90%, 88% for primary and salvage SBRT. No episodes of radiation myelopathy.

> Risk of vertebral compression fracture following spine SBRT dependent upon percent lytic vertebral body disease ≥11.6%, preexisting vertebral collapse, and dose/fraction ≥20 Gy (Thibault IJROBP 2017).

SPINAL CORD COMPRESSION

PEARLS

> Most important prognostic factor is ambulatory status.
> Pain precedes neurologic dysfunction and is the most common presenting symptom. Evaluate for sensory/motor changes, urinary/fecal incontinence.
> Etiology: epidural extension of disease causing local mass effect, vertebral body disease with bony retropulsion, or leptomeningeal disease.
> Pathogenesis: compression venous obstruction vasogenic edema ischemia and demyelination.

WORKUP

- MRI scan of entire spine to determine location and extent of disease and to rule out other sites of cord compression.
- Biopsy required if metastatic disease has not been previously documented or if patient does not have proven cancer diagnosis.

TREATMENT RECOMMENDATIONS
STEROIDS

- Start steroids immediately and then taper as tolerated. 10 mg IV × 1 loading dose, then 4 mg q6h thereafter. Give concurrent proton pump inhibitor for gastric prophylaxis.
- Used for symptom relief (improved neurologic function, reduced pain).

SURGERY AND RT

- Maximum safe debulking surgery with appropriate spine stabilization followed by post-op RT is treatment of choice for pts with single region of cord compression and life expectancy >3 months.
- Pts with fracture or high spinal instability neoplastic score (SINS) or retropulsion of bone fragments should have surgical stabilization followed by RT.
- Laminectomy is not an equal alternative to maximal safe debulking and stabilization because studies have reported minimal neurologic benefit; frequently the tumor lies ventral to the thecal sac, which makes meaningful decompression difficult or impossible; and laminectomy can cause or worsen preexisting spinal instability.
- If patient has multiple levels of compression or is not medically fit for surgery, then give immediate RT.

XII

TRIALS

- Patchell (Lancet 2005): Prospective randomized trial of surgery with post-op RT to 30 Gy vs RT alone to 30 Gy. Surgery pts regained ability to walk more often (62% vs 19%), retained ability to walk longer (122 vs 13 days), and required less steroid and pain medication. Improved survival with surgery (126 vs 100 days).

- Rades (IJROBP 2011a): Prospective nonrandomized trial of 265 pts with metastatic spinal cord compression treated with short (8 Gy/1 fx or 20 Gy/5 fx) vs long (30 Gy/10 fx, 37.5 Gy/15 fx, or 40 Gy/20 fx) course RT. Long-course RT achieved higher 1-year LC 61% vs 81%. Motor function improvement (37–39%) and OS (23–30%) similar. Better OS with better KPS, no visceral mets, 1–3 vertebral mets, ability to ambulate, and use of bisphosphonates.
- Rades (Strahlenther Onkol 2011b). 191 pts with cord compression with favorable survival prognosis treated with 30 Gy/10 fx vs higher dose (37.5 Gy/15 fx or 40 Gy/20 fx). Higher dose increased 2-yr LC (92% vs 71%), PFS (90% vs 58%), and OS (68% vs 53%), including on multivariate analysis.
- ARO 2009/01 (Rades, JCO 2016). 203 pts with cord compression with poor to intermediate expected survival randomized to 30 Gy/10 fx vs 20 Gy/5 fx. No significant difference through 6 months in response rate, improvement, stability, progression, or ambulatory status. 6 mo local PFS 20 Gy 75% vs 30 Gy 82% ($p = 0.51$).
- Rades (Cancer 2008): Retrospective review of 124 pts reirradiated for in-field recurrence of metastatic cord compression. Motor function improved in 36%, stable in 50%. No radiation myelopathy at 11 months median follow-up with 24% of pts receiving cumulative BED <100 Gy, including both courses of RT. [BED = $n*d*(1 + d/\alpha\beta)$; n = # of fractions; d = dose per fraction; $\alpha\beta$ = 2].
- ACR (Lo J Palliat Med 2015) has published evidence-based appropriateness criteria for EBRT and SBRT for spinal cord compression and recurrent spinal metastases. SBRT may be considered for selected cases or recurrences after prior radiation, but it is critical to consider tolerance of the normal tissues. It is generally recommended that 6 months or more time elapses between treatment courses when reirradiating.

TECHNIQUES
- EBRT
  - AP/PA gives more homogenous dose distribution and is the preferred technique for T/L spine, opposed laterals for C-spine.

- 1–2 vertebral bodies above/below target are included as margin for clinical setup.
- Consider beam splitting to aid in matching or reducing overlap in previously treated field.
- Dose: 30 Gy/10 fx, 20 Gy/5 fx, 8 Gy/1 fx, 37.5 Gy/15 fx, 40 Gy/20 fx.
- SBRT
  - See International Spine Radiosurgery Consortium consensus guidelines (Cox IJROBP 2012; Redmond IJROBP 2017) for target delineation in spine radiosurgery for metastases in definitive and postoperative settings.
  - There is no current consensus standard dose fractionation schedule. We recommend meticulous adherence to published techniques and dose constraints and/or enrollment on clinical trial.

LIVER METASTASES

PEARLS
- MS typically 5–10 months without intervention.
- Colorectal primary is most common with 50,000 cases of colorectal liver mets per year in the USA.
- Liver has remarkable ability for regeneration and can grow back after 50% resection in just 3 weeks.

WORKUP
- Triphasic CT is primary imaging modality used for diagnosis and follow-up.
- MRI scan can distinguish benign from malignant disease and can provide specific information about involvement of biliary tree.

TREATMENT RECOMMENDATIONS
SURGERY
- Surgery with curative intent possible in ~10% of pts.
- MS after complete resection is ~30 months with small number of pts surviving >10 years.
- Contraindications for liver resection:
  - Presence of extrahepatic disease (although carefully selected pts with limited pulmonary and liver mets are

XII

candidates for surgical resection of both sites of disease).

˻ Complete resection not possible (unacceptable LF rates with + margins).

˻ Second resections can be performed for liver-only failures that meet criteria for surgery. Long-term survival after second resection is also possible.

CHEMOTHERAPY

˻ Systemic chemotherapy for unresectable mets is palliative.

˻ Neoadjuvant chemotherapy can be used to shrink disease and increase resectability.

˻ Adjuvant chemotherapy (including hepatic arterial chemotherapy) can be used to reduce LR rates and possibly improve survival.

RADIOFREQUENCY ABLATION, CRYOABLATION, IR EMBOLIZATION, ETHANOL INJECTION

˻ Alternative therapies for pts who are not surgical candidates.

˻ See Hepatobiliary Chapter 21.

˻ Favorably located lesions <3 cm often achieve LC.

EBRT

˻ Whole liver RT (3 Gy × 7) may be considered for symptomatic pts with multiple small lesions who are not candidates for other therapies.

˻ 3DCRT ± hepatic artery chemo is preferred over whole liver RT for pts with good KPS and limited metastatic disease.

SBRT

˻ SBRT may be considered as a noninvasive alternative local therapy for lesions not amenable to surgery or ablative techniques such as radiofrequency ablation (e.g., larger size, situated close to large vessels).

˻ A number of retrospective and prospective studies of SBRT for liver metastases have reported LC rates 60–90% using a variety of dose regimens with grade 3–4 toxicity 1–10%.

, Motion management is recommended with liver SBRT, including respiratory gating with fiducial marker placement or breath-hold technique and conebeam CT imaging. Ideal lesions are >8 mm from visceral organs at risk. Normal tissue tolerance should always take priority over PTV coverage for metastatic pts.

, Nausea prophylaxis should be given prior to treatment, such as ondansetron 1 h before treatment and q8h thereafter prn.

STUDIES

, McCarter (Semin Surg Oncol 2000): Good review of surgical data.

, Rusthoven (JCO 2009): Phase I/II trial of 47 pts (63 lesions) with 1–3 liver metastases, each <6 cm, treated with SBRT escalated from 36 to 60 Gy in 3 fractions. Two-year LC 92%. For 38 lesions treated to 60 Gy, LC 100% for ≤3 cm, 77% for >3 cm. OS 20.5 months. No radiation-induced liver disease, 2% incidence grade ≥3 toxicity.

, Aiken (Clin Oncol 2015) provide a contemporary review of SBRT for liver metastases.

, See Hepatobiliary section for other studies.

RADIATION TOLERANCE/COMPLICATIONS

, See Hepatobiliary Chapter 21.

, Pan (IJROBP 2010): Overview of radiation-induced liver injury and critical dose constraints.

FOLLOW-UP

, Liver function tests 2–3 weeks after treatment

, Exam and CT and/or MRI every 3–6 months or sooner for recurrent symptoms

XII

AIRWAY OBSTRUCTION

, Presents with stridor, dyspnea, cough, hemoptysis, postobstructive atelectasis or pneumonia.

, Emergency: Bronchoscopy with stent placement.

, Radiation effect takes median of 7 days.

, EBRT.

» ASTRO guideline (Rodrigues, PRO 2011): Accepted dose and fractionation schedules include: 10 Gy × 1, 8.5 Gy × 2 (1 week apart), 4 Gy × 5, 3 Gy × 10, 2.5 Gy × 15. 30 Gy/10 fx or greater equivalent preferred over shorter courses for pts with good PS.

» If large fields will be necessary, use caution. Do not want to induce radiation pneumonitis in pts needing palliation for shortness of breath.

» Do not exceed spinal cord tolerance when using large fraction sizes.

» Intraluminal brachytherapy.

  » Use caution in previously treated areas near major vessels.

  » Cochrane review (Reveiz 2012) concluded that EBRT alone is more effective than endobronchial brachy alone and that there are no conclusive results that adding endobronchial brachy to EBRT improves symptom relief.

SUPERIOR VENA CAVA SYNDROME

» Most frequently seen in lung cancer pts (NSCLC 50%, SLCL 25%, NHL 10%).

» Presents with cough, dyspnea, dysphagia, swelling or discoloration of the neck, face, upper extremities.

» Pleural effusions associated in 60% of cases due to backflow.

» Biopsy required to evaluate for benign conditions and sensitive tumors.

» Treatment includes percutaneous stent placement, supportive care, steroids, diuretics, and elevation of the head and torso.

» Accepted external beam radiation therapy dose and fractionation schedules include 3 Gy × 10, 4 Gy × 5, 2.5 Gy × 15.

» Expect relief in 3–14 days, depending on histology.

» Wilson (NEJM 2007) – review of anatomy, physiology, and management of SVC syndrome.

GYNECOLOGIC BLEEDING

‚ Treatment options:
  ‚ Vaginal packing.
  ‚ Cauterization.
  ‚ IR embolization.
  ‚ Hysterectomy.
  ‚ EBRT options: 30 Gy/10 fx, 20 Gy/5 fx, 37.5 Gy/15 fx, or "Quad Shot" 3.7 Gy b.i.d. × 2 days (= 14.8 Gy) repeated 2–4 weeks later up to total dose 44.4 Gy (RTOG 8502, Spanos, IJROBP 1994). Use CT planning to determine field borders.
  ‚ Bleeding typically stops 12–48 h after initiating RT.
  ‚ Intracavitary brachytherapy may also be considered.

Acknowledgment We thank Stuart Y. Tsuji MD, PhD, and William M. Wara MD for their work on the prior edition of this chapter.

REFERENCES

Aiken KL, Hawkins MA. Stereotactic body radiotherapy for liver metastases. Clin Oncol. 2015;27:307–15.

Andrews DW, Scott CB, Sperduto PW, et al. Whole brain radiation therapy with or without stereotactic radiosurgery boost for patients with one to three brain metastases: phase III results of the RTOG 9508 randomised trial. Lancet. 2004;363:1665–72.

Anker CJ, Grossmann KF, Atkins MB, et al. Avoiding severe toxicity from combined BRAF inhibitor and radiation treatment: consensus guidelines from the eastern cooperative oncology group (ECOG). Int J Radiat Oncol Biol Phys. 2016;95:632–46.

Aoyama H, Shirato H, Tago M, et al. Stereotactic radiosurgery plus whole-brain radiation therapy vs stereotactic radiosurgery alone for treatment of brain metastases: a randomized controlled trial. JAMA. 2006;295(21):2483–91.

Atalar B, Modlin LA, Choi CYH, et al. Risk of leptomeningeal disease in patients treated with stereotactic radiosurgery targeting the postoperative resection cavity for brain metastases. Int J Radiat Oncol Biol Phys. 2013;87:713–8.

Berenson J, Pflugmacher R. Balloon kyphoplasty vs nonsurgical fracture management for treatment of painful vertebral body compression fractures in patients with cancer: a multicenter raondomized controlled trial. Lancet Oncol. 2011;12(3):225–35.

Blitzer PH. Reanalysis of the RTOG study of the palliation of symptomatic osseous metastasis. Cancer. 1985;55:1468–72.

Borgelt B, Gelber R, Kramer S, et al. The palliation of brain metastases: Final results fo the first two studies by the radiation therapy oncology group. Int J Radiat Oncol Biol Phys. 1980;6:1–9.

Borgelt B, Gelber R, Larson M, et al. Ultra-rapid high dose irradiation schedules for the Palliarion of brain metastases: Final results of the first two studies by the radiation therapy oncology group. Int J Radiat Oncol Biol Phys. 1981;7:1633–8.

XII

Brennan C, Yang TJ, Hilden P, et al. A phase 2 trial of stereotactic radiosurgery boost after surgical resection for brain metastases. Int J Radiat Oncol Biol Phys. 2014;88:130–6.

Brown PD, Pugh S, Laack NN, et al. Memantine for the prevention of cognitive dysfunction in patients receiving whole-brain radiotherapy: a randomized, double-blind, placebo-controlled trial. Neuro-Oncol. 2013;15:1429–37.

Brown PD, Ballman KV, Cerhan J, et al. N107C/CEC.3: A phase III trial of postoperative stereotactic radiosurgery compared with whole brain radiotherapy for resected metastatic brain disease. ASTRO Annual Meeting, Boston, MA; Sept 2016a, LBA-1.

Brown PD, Jaeckle K, Ballman KV, et al. Effect of radiosurgery alone vs radiosurgery with whole brain radiation therapy on cognitive function in patients with 1 to 3 brain metastases: a randomized clinical trial. JAMA. 2016b;316:401–9.

Chang EL, Wefel JS, Hess KR, et al. Neurocognition in patients with brain metastases treated with radiosurgery or radiosurgery plus whole-brain irradiation: a randomised controlled trial. Lancet Oncol. 2009;10:1037–44.

Choi CYH, Chang SD, Gibbs IC, et al. Stereotactic radiosurgery of the postoperative resection cavity for brain metastases: prospective evaluation of target margin on tumor control. Int J Radiat Oncol Biol Phys. 2012;84:336–42.

Chow E, Zheng L, et al. Update on the systematic review of palliative radiotherapy trials for bone metastases. Clin Oncol. 2012;24(2):112–24.

Cox BW, et al. International spine radiosurgery consortium consensus guidelines for target volume definition in spinal stereotactic radiosurgery. IJROBP. 2012;83(5):e597–605.

De Puysseleyr A, Van De Velde J, Speleers B, et al. Hair-sparing whole brain radiotherapy with volumetric arc therapy in patients treated for brain metastases: dosimetric and clinical results of a phase II trial. Radiat Oncol. 2014;9:170.

Ferrell BR, Temel JS et al. Integration of palliative care into standard oncology care: american society of clinical oncology clinical practice guideline update. Journal of Clinical Oncology 2017 35:1, 96–112

Flickinger JC, Kano H, Niranjan A. Dose selection in stereotactic radiosurgery. Prog Neurol Sur. 2013;27:49–57.

Gaspar L, Scott C, Rotman M, et al. Recursive partitioning analysis (RPA) of prognostic factors in three radiation therapy oncology group (RTOG) brain metastases trials. Int J Radiat Oncol Biol Phys. 1997;37:745–51.

Gaspar LE, Scott C, Murray K, Curran W. Validation of the RTOG recursive partitioning analysis (RPA) classification for brain metastases. Int J Radiat Oncol Biol Phys. 2000;47:1001–6.

Gerszten PC, Burton SA, Ozhasoglu C. Radiosurgery for spinal metastases: clinical experience in 500 cases from a single institution. Spine. 2007;32:193–9.

Goldberg SB, Gettinger SN, Mahajan A, Chiang AC, Herbst RS, Sznol M, et al. Pembrolizumab for patients with melanoma or non-small-cell lung cancer and untreated brain metastases: early analysis of a non-randomised, open-label, phase 2 trial. Lancet Oncol. 2016;17:976–83.

Gondi V, Pugh SL, Tome WA, et al. Preservation of memory with conformal avoidance of the hippocampal neural stem-cell compartment during whole-brain radiotherapy for brain metastases (RTOG 0933): a phase II multi-institutional trial. J Clin Oncol. 2014;32:3810–6.

Hartsell WF, Scott CB, Bruner DW, et al. Randomized trial of short-versus long-course radiotherapy for palliation of painful bone metastases. J Natl Cancer Inst. 2005;97:798–804.

Howell DD, James JL, Hartsell WF, et al. Randomized trial of short-course versus long-course radiotherapy for palliation of painful vertebral bone metastases: a retrospective analysis of RTOG 97-14. J Clin Oncol. 2009;27:7s. ASCO 2009, abstract

Iuchi T, Shingyoji M, Sakaida T, et al. Phase II trial of gefitinib alone without radiation therapy for Japanese patients with brain metastases from EGFR-mutant lung adenocarcinoma. Lung Cancer. 2013;82:282–7.

Jabbari S, Gerszten P, Ruschin M, et al. Stereotactic body radiotherapy for spinal metastases: practical guidelines, outcomes, and risks. Cancer J. 2016;22(4):280–9.

Jensen CA, Chan MD, McCoy TP, et al. Cavity-directed radiosurgery as adjuvant therapy after resection of a brain metastasis. J Neurosurg. 2011;114:1585–91.

Johung KL, Yeh N, Desai NB, et al. Extended survival and prognostic factors for patients with ALK-rearranged non-small-cell lung cancer and brain metastasis. J Clin Oncol. 2016;34:123–9.

Kayama T, Sato S, Sakurata K, et al. JCOG0504: a phase III randomized trial of surgery with whole brain radiation therapy versus surgery with salvage stereotactic radiosurgery in paitnets with 1 to 4 brain metastases. Abstract only. J Clin Oncol. 2016;34:Suppl abst 2003.

Knisely JPS, Yu JB, Flanigan J, et al. Radiosurgery for melanoma brain metastases in the ipilimumab era and the possibility of longer survival. J Neurosurg. 2012;117:227–33.

Kocher M, Soffietti R, Abacioglu U, et al. Adjuvant whole-brain radiotherapy versus observation after radiosurgery or surgical resection of one to three cerebral metastases: results of the EORTC 22952-26001 study. J Clin Oncol. 2011;29:134–41.

Kondziolka D, Patel A, Lunsford LD, et al. Stereotactic radiosurgery plus whole brain radiotherapy versus radiotherapy alone for patients with multiple brain metastases. Int J Radiat Oncol Biol Phys. 1999;45:427–34.

Kroeze SG, Fritz C, Hoyer M, et al. Toxicity of concurrent stereotactic radiotherapy and targeted therapy or immunotherapy: a systematic review. Cancer Treat Rev. 2017;53:25–37.

Ling DC, Vargo JA, Wegner RE, et al. Postoperative stereotactic radiosurgery to the resection cavity for large brain metastases. Neurosurgery. 2015;76:150–7.

Lo SS, Ryu S, Chang EL, et al. ACR appropriateness criteria: metastatic epidural spinal cord compression and recurrent spinal metastases. J Palliative Med. 2015;8:573–84.

Logie N, Jimenez RB, Pulenzas RB, et al. Recursive partitioning analysis to predict survival for patients receiving cranial re-irradiation for brain metastases. IJROBP. 2015;93(3 supp):S62–3.

Lutz SJ, Balboni T, Jones J, Lo S, Petit J, et al. Palliative radiation therapy for bone metastases: update of an ASTRO evidence-based guideline. Prac Radiat Oncol. 2017;7(1):4–12.

Magnuson WJ, Lester-Coll NH, Wu AJ, et al. Management of Brain Metastases in tyrosine kinase inhibitor-Naïve epidermal growth factor receptor-mutant non-small-cell lung cancer: a retrospective multi-institutional analysis. J Clin Oncol. 2017;35(10):1070–7.

Mahajan A, Ahmed S, McAleer MF, et al. Postoperative stereotactic radiosurgery versus observation for completely resected brain metastases: results of a prostpective randomized study. Abstract only. IJROBP. 2016;96-2:s2.

Mak KS, Gainor JF, Niemierko A, Oh KS, Willers H, Choi NC, et al. Significance of targeted therapy and genetic alterations in EGFR, ALK, or KRAS on survival in patients with non-small cell lung cancer treated with radiotherapy for brain metastases. Neuro-Oncol. 2015;17:296–302.

Margolin K, Ernstoff MS, Hamid O, et al. Ipilimumab in patients with melanoma and brain metastases: an open-label, phase 2 trial. Lancet Oncol. 2012;13:459–65.

McCarter MD, Fong Y. Metastatic liver Tumors. Semin Surgl Oncol. 2000;19:177–88.

Minniti G, Esposito V, Clarke E, et al. Multidose stereotactic radiosurgery (9 Gy × 3) of the postoperative resection cavity for treatment of large brain metastases. Int J Radiat Oncol Biol Phys. 2013;86:623–9.

Minniti G, D'Angelillo RM, Scaringi C, et al. Fractionated stereotactic radiosurgery for patients with brain metastases. J Neuro-Oncol. 2014;117(2):295–301.

XII

Mirels H. Metastatic disease in long bones. A proposed scoring system for diagnosing impending pathologic fractures. Clin Orthop Relat Res. 1989;249:256–64.

Mulvenna P, Nankivell M, Barton R, et al. Dexamethasone and supportive care with or without whole brain radiotherapy in treating patients with non-small cell lung cancer with brain metastases unsuitable for resection or stereotactic radiotherapy (QUARTZ): results from a phase 3, non-inferiority, randomised trial. Lancet. 2016;388:2004–14.

Navarria P, Pessina F, Cozzi L, et al. Hypo-fractionated stereotactic radiotherapy alone using volumetric modulated arc therapy for patients with single, large brain metastases unsuitable for surgical resection. Radiat Oncol. 2016;11:76.

Nousianinen M. Surgical management of bone metastases. In: Bone metastases, a translational and clinical approach, vol. 12. Dordrecht: Springer; 2009. p. 263–86.

Ou S-HI, Jänne PA, Bartlett CH, et al. Clinical benefit of continuing ALK inhibition with crizotinib beyond initial disease progression in patients with advanced ALK-positive NSCLC. Ann Oncol. 2014;25:415–22.

Pan C, Kavanagh B, et al. Radiation associated liver injury. IJROBP. 2010;76(3):S94–S100.

Patchell RA, Tibbs PA, Walsh JW, et al. A randomized trial of surgery in the treatment of single metastases to the brain. N Engl J Med. 1990;322:494–500.

Patchell RA, Tibbs PA, Regine WF, et al. Postoperative radiotherapy in the treatment of single metastases to the brain. JAMA. 1998;280:1485–9.

Patchell RA, Tibbs PA, Regine WF, et al. Direct decompressive surgical resection in the treatment of spinal cord compression caused by metastatic cancer: a randomised trial. Lancet. 2005;366:643–8.

Park SJ, Kim HT, Lee DH, et al. Efficacy of epidermal growth factor receptor tyrosine kinase inhibitors for brain metastasis in non-small cell lung cancer patients harboring either exon 19 or 21 mutation. Lung Cancer. 2012;77:556–60.

Porter AT, McEwan AJ, Powe JE, et al. Results of a randomized phase III trial to evaluate the efficacy of strontium-89 adjuvant to local field external beam irradiation in the Management of Endocrine Resistant Metastatic Prostate Cancer. Int J Radiat Oncol Biol Phys. 1993;25:805–13.

Rades D, Rudat V, Veninga T, et al. Prognostic factors for functional outcome and survival after Reirradiation for in-field recurrences of metastatic spinal cord compression. Cancer. 2008;113:1090–6.

Rades D, Lange M, Veniga T, et al. Final results of a prospective study comparing the local control of short course and long course radiotherapy for metastatic spinal cord compression. IJROBP. 2011a;79(2):524–30.

Rades D, Stalpers LJA, Hulshof MC, et al. Comparison of 1 x 8 Gy and 10 x 3 Gy for functional outcome in patients with metastatic spinal cord compression. Int J Radiat Oncol Biol Phys. 2005;62:514–8.

Rades D, Panzner A, Rudat V, et al. Dose escalation of radiotherapy for metastatic spinal cord compression in patients with relativel favorable survival prognosis. Strahlenther Onkol. 2011b;187(11):729–35.

Rades D, Segedin B, Conde-Moreno A, et al. Radiotherapy with 4 Gy x 5 versus 3 Gy x 10 for metastatic epidural spinal cord compression: Final results of the SCORE-2 trial (ARO2009/01). J Clin Oncol. 2016;34(6):597–602.

Redmond KJ, Robertson S, Lo S, Soltys S, et al. Consensus contouring guidelines for postoperative stereotactic body radiation therapy for Metastastic solid tumor malignancies to the spine. Int J Radiat Oncol Biol Phys. 2017;97(1):64–74.

Reveiz L, et al. Palliative endobroncial brachytherapy for non-small cell lung cancer. Cochrane Review. 2012;12:CD004284.

Rodrigues G et al. Palliative thoracic radiotherapy in lung cancer: an american society for radiation oncology evidence-based clinical practice guideline. *Practical Radiation Oncology* 1.2 (2011): 60–71.

Rusthoven CG, Doebele RC. Management of Brain Metastases in ALK-positive non-small-cell lung cancer. J Clin Oncol. 2016;34:2814–9.

Rusthoven KE, Kavanagh BD, Cardenes H, et al. Multi-institutional phase I/II trial of stereotactic body radiation therapy for liver metastases. J Clin Oncol. 2009;27(10):1572–8.

Sahgal A, Ames C, Chou D, et al. Stereotactic body radiotherapy is effective salvage therapy for patients with prior radiation of spinal metastases. Int J Radiat Oncol Biol Phys. 2009;74(3):723–31.

Scharp M, Hauswald H, Bischof M, et al. Re-irradiation in the treatment of patients with cerebral metastases of solid tumors: retrospective analysis. Radiat Oncol. 2014;9:4.

Sciuto R, Festa A, Rea S, et al. Effects of low-dose cisplatin on ^{89}Sr therapy for painful bone metastases from prostate cancer: a randomized clinical trial. J Nucl Med. 2002;43:79–86.

Shaw E, Scott C, Souhami L, et al. Single dose Radiosurgical treatment of recurrent previously irradiated primary brain Tumors and brain metastases: Final report of RTOG protocol 90-05. Int J Radiat Oncol Biol Phys. 2000;47:291–8.

Sirven JI, Wingerchuk DM, Drazkowski JF, et al. Seizure prophylaxis in patients with brain tumors: a meta-analysis. Mayo Clin Proc. 2004;79:1489–94.

Sneed PK, Lamborn KR, Forstner JM, et al. Radiosurgery for brain metastases: is whole brain radiotherapy necessary? Int J Radiat Oncol Biol Phys. 1999;43:549–58.

Sneed PK, Suh JH, Goetsch SJ, et al. A multi-institutional review of radiosurgery alone vs. radiosurgery with whole brain radiotherapy as the initial management of brain metastases. Int J Radiat Oncol Biol Phys. 2002;53:519–26.

Sneed PK, Mendez J, Vemer-van den Hoek JGM, Seymour ZA, Ma L, Molinaro AM, et al. Adverse radiation effect after stereotactic radiosurgery for brain metastases: incidence, time course, and risk factors. J Neurosurg. 2015;123:373–86.

Soltys SG, Adler JR, Lipani JD, et al. Stereotactic radiosurgery of the postoperative resection cavity for brain metastases. Int J Radiat Oncol Biol Phys. 2008;70:187–93.

Son CH, Jimenez R, Niemierko A, et al. Outcomes after whole brain reirradiation in patients with brain metastases. Int J Radiat Oncol Biol Phys. 2012;82:e167–72.

Spanos WT et al. Late effect of multiple daily fraction palliation schedule for advanced pelvic malignancies (RTOG 8502), IJROBP 29:5, 1994, P 961–967.

Sperduto PW, Berkey B, Gaspar LE, et al. A new prognostic index and Comparison to three other indices for patients with brain metastases: an analysis of 1,960 patients in the RTOG database. Int J Radiat Oncol Biol Phys. 2008;70:510–4.

Sperduto PW, Chao ST, Sneed PK, et al. Diagnosis-specific prognostic factors, indexes, and treatment outcomes for patients with newly diagnosed brain metastases: a multi-institutional analysis of 4,259 patients. Int J Radiat Oncol Biol Phys. 2010;77:655–61.

Sperduto PW, Kased N, Roberge D, et al. Summary report on the graded prognostic assessment: an accurate and facile diagnosis-specific tool to estimate survival for patients with brain metastases. J Clin Oncol. 2012;30:419–25.

Stopeck AT. Denosumab compared with zoledronic acid for the treatment of bone metastases in patients with advanced breast cancer: a randomized, double blind study. JCO. 2010;28(35):5132–9.

Thibault I, Whyne C, Zhou S, Campbell M, et al. Volume of lytic vertebral body metastatic disease quantified using computer tomography-based image segmentation predicts fracture risk after spine stereotactic body radiation therapy. Int J Radiat Oncol Biol Phys. 2017;97(1):75–81.

Tremont-Lukats IW, Ratilal BO, Armstrong T, et al. Antiepileptic drugs for preventing seizures in people with brain tumors. Cochrane Database Syst Rev 2008;(16):CD004424.

Tsao MN, Lloyd N, Wong RKS, et al. Whole brain radiotherapy for the treatment of newly diagnosed multiple brain metastases. Cochrane Database Syst Rev 2012a;(18):CD003869.

Tsao MN, Rades D, Wirth A, et al. Radiotherapeutic and surgical management for newly diagnosed brain metastases: an amarican society for radiation oncology evidence based guideline. Prac Radiat Oncol. 2012b;2(3):210–25.

XII

Van der Linden YM, Dijkstra PD, Kroon HM, et al. Comparative analysis of risk factors for pathological fracture with femoral metastases. J Bone Joint Surg Br. 2004;86:566–73.

Wang TJC, Saad S, Qureshi YH, et al. Does lung cancer mutation status and targeted therapy predict for outcomes and local control in the setting of brain metastases treated with radiation? Neuro-Oncol. 2015;17:1022–8.

Weber JS, Amin A, Minor D, et al. Safety and clinical activity of ipilimumab in melanoma patients with brain metastases: retrospective analysis of data from a phase 2 trial. Melanoma Res. 2011;21:530–4.

Weickhardt AJ, Scheier B, Burke JM, et al. Local ablative therapy of oligoprogressive disease prolongs disease control by tyrosine kinase inhibitors in oncogene-addicted non-small-cell lung cancer. J Thorac Oncol. 2012;7:1807–14.

Wilson L, et al. Superior vena cava syndrome with malignant causes. NEJM. 2007;356:1862–9.

Yamamoto M, Serizawa T, Shuto T, et al. Stereotactic radiosurgery for patients with multiple brain metastases (JLGK0901): a multi-institutional prospective observational study. Lancet Oncol. 2014;15:387–95.

Part XIII
Radiobiology and Physics

Chapter 43
Clinical Radiobiology and Physics

Serah Choi, Yao Yu, Eleanor A. Blakely, and John Murnane

RADIOBIOLOGY PEARLS

The Four Rs of Radiobiology (rationale for fractionation of radiation)

- *Repair* – refers to DNA repair in response to sublethal or potentially lethal radiation damage. Fractionation of radiation allows normal tissues time to repair.
- *Reassortment* – refers to the redistribution of cells into a more radiosensitive phase of the cell cycle due to cell cycle checkpoints after a fraction of radiation.
- *Repopulation* – refers to tumor cell proliferation during the course of radiation therapy; this can be problematic with prolonged radiation treatment durations.
- *Reoxygenation* – refers to the oxygenation of hypoxic cells after a fraction of radiation. Tumors consist of a mixture of oxygenated and hypoxic cells. The oxygenated cells are more radiosensitive, and therefore oxygenation of hypoxic cells during fractionated therapy increases the sensitivity of tumors to ionizing radiation.

A Fifth R has been added to account for in vivo differences in tissue sensitivity

- *Radiosensitivity* – accounts for differences in cell metabolism, maturity, and microenvironment of cells *in vivo* that when combined explain the differences in the sensitivities of different tissues.

XIII

© Springer International Publishing AG, part of Springer Nature 2018   **901**
Eric K. Hansen and M. Roach III (eds.), *Handbook of Evidence-Based Radiation Oncology*, https://doi.org/10.1007/978-3-319-62642-0_43

DNA DAMAGE AND IONIZING RADIATION

﹐ DNA is the critical target for radiation-induced cell lethality.

﹐ Photons produce their effects through direct action (~1/3) and indirect action (~2/3). Direct action refers to the direct interaction of a secondary electron (resulting from absorption of an X-ray photon) with DNA. Indirect action refers to DNA damage caused by free radicals produced through the ionization of H_2O by a secondary electron.

﹐ DNA damage to the cell can come in several forms:

  ﹐ Base damage: repaired via base excision repair, not a major contributor to radiosensitivity, except in the case of XRCC1 deficiency.

  ﹐ Single-strand breaks (SSBs): repaired via single-strand break repair, not a major contributor to radiosensitivity.

  ﹐ Double-strand breaks (DSBs): repaired via homologous recombination repair (in late S/G_2, when a DNA template is available), which is accurate; or nonhomologous end-joining, which is error-prone. DSBs are the most important radiation-induced lesions in terms of cell killing.

  ﹐ Chromosomal and chromatid aberrations: result from unrepaired or misrepaired DSBs. Symmetric translocations and small deletions tend to be nonlethal, but are frequently involved in carcinogenesis. Lethal aberrations include acentric fragments, rings, dicentric chromosomes, and anaphase bridges.

﹐ *LET* (linear energy transfer) – refers to the average energy transferred to tissue per unit length of an ionizing particle (in keV/μm). Generally, heavy particles like alpha particles or iron ions have high LET, while photons and protons have lower LET.

﹐ *RBE* (relative biological effectiveness) = (dose of 250 keV X-rays or ^{60}Cobalt or ^{137}Cesium gamma rays required for a given effect)/(dose from a different type of radiation to yield the same effect). The greatest RBE for cell killing occurs when LET reaches 100 keV/μm since this is the diameter of a DNA double helix.

CELL SURVIVAL CURVES

ˌ A cell survival curve is a graph of the relationship between radiation dose and the surviving fraction of cells that retained their reproductive integrity (clonogenic). Dose is plotted on a linear scale (x-axis) and surviving fraction on a logarithmic scale (y-axis).

ˌ The *multitarget model* describes survival curves in terms of an initial slope, D_1, which results from single-event killing and a final slope, D_0, which results from multiple-event killing where the curve approximates a straight line at higher doses. D_1 and D_0 are the reciprocals of the initial and final slopes and represent the doses of radiation that induce an average of one lethal event per cell, leaving 37% of the cells still viable. The extrapolation number (n) and quasithreshold dose (D_q) are measures of the width of the shoulder of the curve. D_q is the dose below which there is minimal effect. The multitarget model was largely discarded because it is not consistent with our current understanding of cell killing by ionizing radiation.

ˌ For a typical mammalian cell, the D_0 is between 1 and 2 Gy and results in >1000 damaged bases, ~1000 SSBs, and 40 DSBs per cell.

ˌ The D_{10} is the dose required to kill 90% of the population = $2.3 \times D_0$.

ˌ The *linear–quadratic model (LQM)* describes radiation-induced cell killing as a linear–quadratic function of dose. At low doses, DSBs are likely to be caused by a single photon or particle, and aberrations are directly proportional to dose (linear). At higher doses, DSBs are likely to be caused by two separate photons or particles, and are proportional to the square of the dose (quadratic). The linear–quadratic model is more consistent with our current understanding of cell killing by ionizing radiation.

ˌ According to the LQM, $S = e^{-\alpha D - \beta D^2}$, where S = surviving fraction, and α and β represent the linear and quadratic components of cell killing, respectively. The initial slope is determined by α, while the β causes the curve to bend at higher doses.

XIII

ˌ The *universal survival model (USM)* has recently been proposed to account for the fact that the *LQM* does not accurately predict radioresponse at higher doses per fraction due to the continuous slope in the predicted curve. The *USM* is a combination of the *LQM* and the multitarget model at higher doses per fraction, with D_T (6 Gy) as the transition point.

- Most tumors and early-responding tissues (e.g., mucosa) have a high α/β ratio (~10), whereas some tumors (e.g., prostate) and late-responding tissues (e.g., spinal cord) have a low α/β ratio (~3).

- When treatments are fractionated, sublethal damage (SLD) can be repaired between treatments. This allows the "shoulder" of the survival curve to be repeated, thereby sparing late-responding tissues. This is the basis for hyperfractionation during which treatments are given twice per day or more to mitigate late effects.

- The *biological equivalent dose (BED)* refers to the effective total absorbed dose (in Gy) for a given fractionation scheme if it were given by standard fractionation (1.8–2.0 Gy/day).

- For the *LQM*:
    BED = $nd[1 + d/(\alpha/\beta)]$, where n = number of fractions and d = the dose per fraction.

- For the *USM*:
    Below D_T(6Gy): BED = $nd[1 + d/(\alpha/\beta)]$, same as *LQM*.
    Above D_T(6Gy): BED = $([1/\alpha \times D_o] \times [(D - n) \times D_q])$, where D_o is the final slope of the survival curve, and D_q is the quasithreshold dose.

MECHANISMS OF RADIATION-INDUCED CELL DEATH

- Mitotic cell death: cellular death while attempting to divide due to damaged chromosomes; the most common cell death mechanism following radiation in cancer cells; death can occur in the first or subsequent divisions following radiation.

- Apoptosis: programmed cell death; occurs in some normal tissues (lymphocytes, embryonic development) and can occur in some tissues after radiation; dominant cell death mechanism in lymphoid cells following radiation; characterized by cytoplasmic condensation, cell shrinkage, apoptotic bodies, chromatin condensation, and DNA fragmentation.

, Necrosis: can be either non-programmed cell death by autolysis, or programmed through a process called necroptosis.

, Autophagic cell death: evolutionarily conserved self-digestive process regulated by autophagy-related genes (Atgs). It involves the sequestration of portions of the cytoplasm into double membrane vesicles called autophagosomes, which fuse with lysosomes, leading to degradation of proteins and organelles.

, Cellular senescence: a programmed cellular stress response to the accumulation of damage to a cell that results in irreversible cell cycle arrest.

THE CELL CYCLE AND DNA REPAIR

, The cell cycle for mammalian cells can be divided into G_1 (initial growth phase) $\rightarrow$ S (DNA replication phase) $\rightarrow$ G_2 (additional growth phase) $\rightarrow$ M (mitotic phase during which chromosomes are evident). In general, M phase is the most radiosensitive, and late S/early G_2 phase the most radioresistant portion of the cell cycle.

, Transition through the cell cycle is governed by cyclins and cyclin-dependent kinases (CDKs). The important cell cycle checkpoints include:

, $G_1 \rightarrow S$ is governed by cyclin D1/CDK4/6 and cyclin E/CDK2.

, S is governed by cyclin A/CDK2.

, $G_2 \rightarrow M$ is governed by cyclin B/CDK1.

, DNA damage activates cell cycle checkpoint pathways, which inhibit the progression of cells through the cell cycle, allowing for DNA repair before mitosis.

, Retinoblastoma (pRb) is a tumor suppressor protein that restricts $G_1 \rightarrow S$. When a cell is ready to divide, the CDK–cyclin kinase complex phosphorylates pRb, releasing pRb's inhibition of E2F, a transcription factor that binds

XIII

to the promoter region of genes whose protein products are essential for S phase.

, p21 (CIP1/WAF1) protein is a CDK inhibitor (CKI) that regulates G1 → S; it binds to and inhibits cyclin D-CDK6, cyclin D-CDK4, and cyclin E-CDK2 complexes. p21 can also mediate cellular senescence.

, p16^Ink4a(*CDKN2A*) is a tumor suppressor protein that inhibits S phase by binding to CDK4/6, inhibiting cyclin D–CDK4/6 complex formation and CDK4/6-mediated phosphorylation of Rb family members.

, ATM, ATR, and DNA-PK$_{CS}$ are members of the phosphatidylinositol 3-kinase-related kinase (PIKK) family, are activated by DNA DSBs, and function as kinases that regulate DNA repair and cell cycle proteins.

, p53 is a tumor suppressor protein that functions in cell cycle regulation, DNA repair, and apoptosis. It is a transcription factor that activates the expression of several genes, including p21 (*CDKN1A*), *GADD45*, and apoptotic genes. In unstressed cells, p53 is negatively regulated by MDM2, an E3 ubiquitin ligase that targets p53 for proteasomal degradation. DNA DSBs activate ATM (or ATR if DSBs are at the replication fork), resulting in the phosphorylation of p53, thereby preventing its degradation by MDM2.

, DSBs are repaired by either nonhomologous end-joining (NHEJ), which involves proteins DNA-PK$_{CS}$, Ku70, Ku80, Artemis, XRCC4, PNK, XLF, and DNA ligase IV; or homologous recombination repair (HRR, also known as HDR, homology directed repair), which involves proteins MRE11, Rad50, NBS1, RPA, BRCA1, RAD51, BRCA2, RAD52, and RAD54. 53BP1 inhibits homologous recombination. NHEJ is inaccurate, but can occur anytime in the cell cycle, while HRR is accurate, but can only occur in late S/early G$_2$.

, Most DSBs (80–90%) are repaired within 1–2 hours, while the remaining DSBs take many hours to repair. Some DSBs (multiply damaged sites or in heterochromatin) are much more difficult to repair than others, and along with HRR account for the DSBs that are slow to be repaired.

, Base damage is repaired by base excision repair, which involves a glycosylase, AP endonuclease (creating a SSB), PNKP and then polβ, DNA ligase III, XRCC1 for short-patch BER or RFC, PCNA, polβ/polδ/polε, FEN1, and DNA ligase I for long-patch BER.

- Nucleotide excision repair (NER) removes bulky DNA adducts, such as pyrimidine dimers. It consists of two pathways: global genome repair (GG-NER) and transcription coupled repair (TC-NER), which differ in the detection of the lesion: XPC-XPE for GG-NER; and RNA polymerase I/II, CSA, and CSB for TC-NER. The rest of the pathways involve TFIIH, XPA, RPA, XPG, XPF-ERCC1, RFC, PCNA, and polδ/polε.

- Mismatch repair removes base–base and small insertion/deletion mismatches and involves MSH2-MSH6, MSH2-MSH3 or MLH1-PMS2 and MLH1-PMS1 or MLH1-MLH3 and EXO1, RFC, PCNA, and polδ/polε.

- DNA crosslink repair is repaired by a combination of NER and homologous recombination repair pathways.

- Telomeres protect the ends of chromosome and consist of TTAGGG repeats that are shortened after each cell division. After ~40 to 60 somatic cell divisions, the telomeres become so shortened that cells cannot further divide and undergo senescence (Hayflick limit). Telomerase is a reverse transcriptase that adds telomere repeat sequence to the 3′ end of telomeres to offset telomere shortening, but is turned off in most somatic human cells. Virtually all cancers must reacquire the ability to maintain telomeres for continuous cell division, either through the expression of telomerase (90%) or through an alternative mechanism (ALT) that involves recombination.

- DNA damage can be categorized as:
  - Potentially lethal damage (PLD) – would ordinarily cause cell death, but can be modified by postirradiation environmental conditions – demonstrated by the fact that nondividing cells are more resistant than cells that divide soon after radiation exposure.
  - Sublethal damage (SLD) – can be repaired in hours unless additional SLD is added – demonstrated by the increased survival shown in split-dose experiments, where cells are more resistant to conventional X-rays and gamma radiation if the dose is split in two with time for repair in between doses. For maximal effect in the clinic, the time between doses must be at least 6 hours.
  - Lethal damage – irreversible damage that leads to cell death.

XIII

⌙ Dose-rate effect refers to repair of SLD that occurs during radiation exposure at a low dose rate. Below 1 Gy per minute, cells can repair DNA sufficiently to avoid lethal damage, similar to a split-dose experiment.

COMMON DNA DAMAGE ASSAYS

⌙ *In vitro* clonogenic survival assay – the gold standard to test cell survival after a short- or long-term treatment with a DNA damaging agent. Cells are plated in plastic dishes, exposed to the agent(s) of interest, and allowed to grow into colonies for several days to weeks. As a control, untreated cells are plated to determine the plating efficiency: (# colonies counted/cells plated × 100%). To determine the surviving fraction after exposure to an agent: (# colonies counted)/(cells seeded × (plating efficiency/100)).

   ⌙ *In vivo* clonogenic assays include skin colony assay, jejunal crypt stem cell assay, testes stem cell assay, bone marrow stem cell assay, and kidney tubules assay.

⌙ Pulsed-field gel electrophoresis (PFGE): used to detect DNA DSBs. Irradiated cells are embedded in agarose plugs, lysed and DNA fragments are separated by size using an electric field. The fraction of DNA released from the agarose plug is proportional to radiation dose.

⌙ Comet assay (single-cell electrophoresis): irradiated cells are embedded in an agarose plug and lysed under neutral buffer conditions to quantify DNA DSBs or lysed with an alkaline buffer to assess for DNA SSBs. The migration of DNA (comet's tail) in the agarose is proportional to the extent of DNA damage.

⌙ Radiation-induced nuclear foci assay: cells/tissues are incubated with antibodies against DNA damage signaling or repair proteins that localize to sites of nuclear DNA DSBs (e.g., γH2AX, 53BP1, ATM, RPA, RAD51, and BRCA1). The antibodies are tagged with fluorescent molecules, which can be visualized and quantified by fluorescence microscopy.

Chromosome aberrations in human lymphocytes: cytogenetic assay used as a biomarker of radiation exposure. Lymphocytes from blood samples obtained days to weeks after exposure to total body irradiation are stimulated to divide with phytohemagglutinin and arrested at metaphase. The frequency of long-lived symmetric aberrations (translocations) in the lymphocytes reflects the dose received. The assay can detect radiation exposure as low as 0.25 Gy.

HEREDITARY DNA REPAIR SYNDROMES

- Ataxia-telangiectasia (AT): autosomal recessive disease, caused by mutations in *ATM* resulting in loss of protein kinase function, which results in radiosensitivity, progressive cerebellar ataxia, immunodeficiency, telangiectasias, genome instability, and a high incidence of cancers.
- Ataxia-telangiectasia-like disorder (ATLD): autosomal recessive disease, due to mutations in *MRE11*, which results in radiosensitivity (MRE11 is required for activation of ATM), progressive cerebellar ataxia, and genome instability.
- Nijmegen breakage syndrome (NBS): autosomal recessive disease, due to mutations in *NBS1*, which results in radiosensitivity (NBS1 is required for activation of ATM), microcephaly, short stature, cognitive impairment, genome instability, and an increased risk of cancers.
- Seckel syndrome: autosomal recessive disease, caused by hypomorphic mutations in the *ATR* gene, which results in microcephaly and growth and developmental delay; not radiosensitive because cells still possess some ATR activity.
- Li-Fraumeni syndrome: autosomal dominant disease caused by mutations in *TP53* and associated with mutations in *CHEK2*. Loss of p53 function leads to loss of cell cycle regulation following DNA damage, allowing cells with DNA damage to continue to divide, and results in genome instability and an increased risk of sarcoma and cancers of the breast, brain, and adrenal glands.

XIII

, Athabascan severe combined immunodeficiency syndrome (SCIDA): autosomal recessive disease, caused by mutations in *DCLRE1C* (Artemis), which results in NHEJ defects, radiosensitivity, and immunodeficiency (absence of T and B cells).

, Hereditary *BRCA1* or *BRCA2* mutations: autosomal dominant inheritance, which results in defects in HRR and an increased risk of breast, ovarian, and other cancers.

, Fanconi anemia: autosomal recessive (majority) and X-linked recessive, caused by mutations in at least 15 genes (*BRCA2, BRIP1, FANCA, FANCB, FANCC, FANCD2, FANCE, FANCF, FANCG, FANCI, FANCL, FANCM, PALB2, RAD51C, SLX4*), which result in HRR defects, radiosensitivity, increased cancer risk (acute myelogenous leukemia), bone marrow failure, short stature, developmental defects, chromosomal aberrations (radial chromosomes), and sensitivity to DNA crosslinking agents.

, Bloom syndrome: autosomal recessive disease caused by mutations in the *BLM* helicase gene, which result in HRR defects, high incidence of cancers, sun-exposed skin rash, dwarfism, hypogonadism, immunodeficiency, and increased sister chromatid exchanges.

, Werner syndrome: autosomal recessive disease caused by mutations in the *WRN* helicase gene, which result in HRR defects, premature aging (progeria), and increased cancer risk.

, Rothmund-Thomson syndrome (RTS): autosomal recessive disease caused by mutations in the *RECQL4* helicase gene, which result in HRR defects, poikiloderma, photosensitivity, juvenile cataracts, congenital bone defects, hair growth problems, and increased risk of osteosarcomas.

, Cockayne syndrome: autosomal recessive disease caused by mutations in *CSA* (*ERCC8*) or *CSB*(*ERCC6*) genes, which result in TC-NER defects, microcephaly, neurodegeneration, failure to thrive, growth defects, sensitivity to UV radiation, and premature aging.

, Xeroderma pigmentosa (XP): autosomal recessive disease caused by mutations in genes that encode for NER proteins (DDB2, ERCC2, ERCC3, ERCC4, ERCC5, POLH, XPA, XPC), which result in NER defects, extreme sensitivity to UV radiation, and an increased risk of skin cancers.

, Lynch syndrome (HPNCC): autosomal dominant disease caused by mutations in the *MLH1, MSH2, MSH6, PMS2,* and *EPCAM* genes, which result in mismatch repair defects, increased microsatellite instability, and increased risk of colorectal, endometrial and other cancers.

EFFECTS OF OXYGEN

, Oxygen is required to "fix" the indirect damage to DNA caused by free radicals, and therefore hypoxic cells are resistant to low LET ionizing radiation. Because of the short half-life of free radicals, oxygen must be present in the target at the time of irradiation for this effect to be observed.

, OER (oxygen enhancement ratio) = (dose required for biological effect under anoxic conditions)/(dose required for the same biological effect under aerobic conditions). At low LET (such as for X-rays or γ-rays), the OER is 2.5–3.0. At high LET, OER approaches 1.0 since the damage produced is mostly direct, which is oxygen-independent.

, Damage from high LET radiation is mostly direct and not through free radicals and therefore does not require oxygen to "fix" the damage. Hypoxic cells are therefore less resistant to high LET radiation compared to low LET radiation.

, ~2% oxygen concentration results in maximum radiosensitization. Some areas of tumors are chronically or acutely hypoxic and therefore are resistant to ionizing radiation, while most normal tissues have 5% oxygen, so are fully sensitized to low LET radiation.

, In addition to rendering cells more radioresistant, both chronic and acute hypoxia also contribute to malignant and metastatic progression.

, In animal models, there is a wide range of percentage of hypoxic cells in tumors, with an average of ~15%. After a fraction of radiation in which tumor cells in aerobic conditions are killed, the remaining hypoxic cells tend to become reoxygenated. In this way, fractionation of

XIII

radiation can improve tumor cell kill in the subsequent dose fraction.

, Under normoxic conditions, HIF-1α is hydroxylated by the oxygen-dependent 4-prolyl hydroxylases (PHDs), allowing HIF-1α binding to von Hippel-Lindau (VHL) protein, which targets HIF-1α for proteasomal degradation. Under hypoxic conditions, HIF-1α becomes stabilized since the PHDs are unable to hydroxylate HIF-1α without oxygen. HIF-1α can then bind to the HIF-1β subunit in the nucleus, promoting the transcription of genes involved in angiogenesis (e.g., VEGF), erythropoiesis (e.g., EPO), and glycolysis.

, Hypoxic radiosensitizers (oxygen substitutes that can penetrate into poorly vascularized areas of tumors since they are not as rapidly metabolized as oxygen) include metronidazole, misonidazole, etanidazole, nimorazole, and nicotinamide.

, Hypoxic cytotoxins (bioreductive drugs that are reduced preferentially in hypoxic cells to cytotoxic agents) include quinone antibiotics (e.g., mitomycin C), nitroaromatic compounds, benzotriazine di-N-oxides (e.g., tirapazamine), dinitrobenzamide modified nitrogen mustard, and 2-nitroimidazole attached to dibromo isophosphoramide.

EFFECTS OF HYPERTHERMIA

, Hyperthermia (~41 to 45 °C) has additive and synergistic cytotoxic effects with radiation. Methods: microwaves, radiofrequency-induced currents, and ultrasound.

, Hyperthermia induces cellular damage, preferentially damages tumor vasculature, and increases normal tissue vessel wall permeability so that there is a differential temperature increase in tumors versus normal tissues. Mild hyperthermia can also enhance antitumor immunity.

, Cell survival curves for heat are similar in shape to those obtained for X-rays (shoulder with exponential region of cell kill), but resistance tails develop at lower temperatures due to thermotolerance.

, Cells treated with hyperthermia die by apoptosis and the damage is expressed more quickly than damage from radiation.

, Thermotolerance: induced resistance of a tumor cell to a second fraction of heat, which coincides with the increased expression of heat shock proteins.

, Arrhenius plot describes the relationship between treatment time and temperature for a biologic isoeffect: x-axis is $1/T$ and y-axis is $1/D_0$, where T is the absolute temperature and D_0 is the time at a given temperature to reduce the surviving fraction to 37%. There is a breakpoint in the curve at ~43 °C in human cells. Below 43 °C, thermotolerance can develop during heating and the heating time required to produce a given level of cell killing is halved for every 1 °C temperature rise. Above 43 °C, thermotolerance develops after heating and the heating time must be reduced by a factor of 4–6 for each 1 °C temperature rise.

, Thermal enhancement ratio (TER): the ratio of doses of X-rays required to produce a given level of biologic damage with and without the application of heat. TER is between 1.15 and 1.5 in previous clinical studies.

, Cells in late S phase are the most sensitive to hyperthermia (and most resistant to X-rays). Cells in G_1 and early S are the most heat resistant.

, Hypoxia does not protect cells from hyperthermia.

, Lower pH environment and nutrient deficiency increases sensitivity to hyperthermia.

EFFECTS OF ACUTE TOTAL BODY IRRADIATION

, Clinical effects from acute radiation syndrome have been observed in the survivors of atomic bombings of Hiroshima and Nagasaki, as well as various nuclear installation accidents.

, The LD50 (lethal dose in 50% of recipients) for humans who do not receive treatment for an acute, whole-body dose exposure is ~4 Gy. With antibiotics and careful

XIII

nursing, the LD50 can be increased to 7–8 Gy. Acute doses of ≥10 Gy are uniformly fatal; however, people receiving doses between 8 and 10 Gy may benefit from bone marrow transplantation.

، Temporally acute effects of radiation exposure can be divided into the following:

 ، Prodromal radiation syndrome (20+ Gy can be severe, <20 Gy variable): timing depends on dose but can occur ~5 min–days; symptoms include fatigue, anorexia, and nausea/vomiting; symptoms if supralethal doses received include fever, hypotension, and immediate diarrhea.

 ، Cerebrovascular syndrome (50–100 Gy): death occurs in 24–48 h; thought to primarily result from damage to intracranial blood vessels; symptoms include severe nausea/vomiting, ataxia, respiratory distress, coma, and seizures.

 ، Gastrointestinal syndrome (5–12 Gy): death occurs in 3–10 days; thought to result from death of intestinal crypt stem cells and/or apoptosis of vascular endothelial cells; symptoms include nausea/vomiting and prolonged diarrhea.

 ، Hematopoietic syndrome (3–8 Gy): peak deaths at 30 days and continues for 60 days, which results from death of hematologic stem cells resulting in eventual pancytopenia.

EFFECTS OF RADIATION ON THE EMBRYO/FETUS

 ، Preimplantation period (0–9 days): 0.05–0.15 Gy prenatal death.

 ، Organogenesis (10 days to 6 weeks): congenital malformations with increased risk for neonatal death, peak incidence of teratogenesis.

 ، Fetal period (6 weeks to birth): microcephaly (0–15 weeks), mental retardation (~40%/Sv at 8–15 weeks; 10%/Sv at 15–25 weeks), carcinogenesis (excess absolute risk ~6%/Gy).

RADIATION SAFETY

Table 43.1   Effective dose limits

Occupational effective dose (ED) for whole body (not permitted for persons <18 years old)	Annual limit: 50 mSv/yr Cumulative limit: 10 mSv*age in yrs
Occupational ED for individual organs	500 mSv/yr
Occupational ED for the lens of the eye	20 mSv/yr, averaged over 5 yrs; no single yr >50 mSv
Occupational ED for declared pregnant workers (fetus)	0.5 mSv/mo
General public ED, frequent/continuous exposure	1 mSv/yr
General public ED, infrequent exposure	5 mSv/yr
General public ED, children (<18 years old)	1 mSv/yr

Note:

1 rem = 0.01 Sv

Effective dose was previously called effective dose equivalent

Background radiation in the San Francisco Bay Area is in the range 2–2.5 mSv/yr Dose equivalent flying from San Francisco to New York round trip is <0.06 mSv. This is comparable to standing 24 h at a 1 m distance from a patient recently treated for prostate cancer with a permanent implant

Table 43.2   Release criteria for patients treated with brachytherapy

Isotope	Activity at or below which pts. may be released with instructions (mCi)	Dose rate at 1 m at or below which pts. may be released with instructions	Activity at or below which pts. may be released without instructions (mCi)	Dose rate at 1 m at or below which pts. may be released without instructions
I-125	9	0.01 mSv/hr	2	0.002 mSv/hr
Pd-103	40	0.03 mSv/hr	8	0.007 mSv/hr
Ir-192	2	0.008 mSv/hr	0.3	0.002 mSv/hr
I-131	33	0.07 mSv/hr		

Release criteria can be based on any of these measures. For patients who exceed these levels, they can still be released with instructions if a calculation can be provided which proves no member of family or general public could receive more than 5 mSv (0.5 rem) as a result of exposure from the patient or if lead shielding is provided (e.g., lead cap for brain patients) to reduce the dose rate level at 1 m.

XIII

PHYSICS PEARLS

ATOMIC STRUCTURE AND NUCLEAR DECAY

- Atoms consist of a small central core or nucleus of protons and neutrons surrounded by a cloud of electrons in orbit; the vast majority of atomic mass lies in the nucleus.
- Elements and isotopes are denoted with the following abbreviation $_{Z}^{A}X$, where X is the element on the periodic table, A = mass number = neutrons + protons, Z = atomic number = protons = electrons.
- Gamma rays are produced intranuclearly (e.g., radioactive decay) and X-rays are produced extranuclearly (e.g., linear accelerator).
- Proton mass = neutron mass = 1.01 atomic mass units (amu); mass-energy equivalence is described by Einstein's famous $E = mc^2$; therefore, 1 amu = 931.5 MeV (electron volt) defined as the kinetic energy acquired by passing an electron through a potential difference of 1 V.
- Arrangement of electrons is in orbits or shells denoted by K (innermost), L, M, N, O, etc. Maximum number of electrons per orbit is $2n^2$ (where n depends on shell, $K = 1$, $L = 2$, etc.).
- Four fundamental forces of nature in order of decreasing strength are strong nuclear, electromagnetic, weak nuclear, and gravity.
- The binding energy of electrons refers to the magnitude of force (in Coulombs) between the electrons and nucleus; high Z atoms have greater binding energies because of greater nuclear charge; if inner orbital electrons are ejected from the atom, they will be filled by higher orbital electrons resulting in characteristic X-ray production.
- Nuclei are most stable at certain numbers of nucleons (neutrons + protons): 2, 8, 20, 82, 126. Also nuclei with odd numbers of protons and neutrons are less stable than those with even numbers of both.

, The rate of nuclear decay (or radioactivity) is described by $N = N_0 e^{-\lambda t}$, where N is activity at time (t) and N_0 is initial activity and λ is the rate decay constant; activity can be described in curies (Ci) where 1 Ci = 3.7×10^{10} dps (disintegrations/sec); 1 dps = 1 Becquerel (Bq) = 2.7×10^{-11} Ci.

, When $N = 0.5(N_0)$, the half-life ($T_{1/2}$) of a radioisotope has been reached; this can also be described as $T_{1/2} = 0.693/\lambda$; the mean life (T_{ave}) or average lifetime for decay of a radioactive nucleus can be described as $T_{ave} = 1/\lambda = 1.44 * T_{1/2}$.

, *Radioactive equilibrium* refers to the ratio between the activity of the parent isotope and its daughter product.

, In *transient equilibrium*, the $T_{1/2}$ of the parent is not too much greater than the $T_{1/2}$ of the daughter.

, In *secular equilibrium*, the half-life of the parent isotope is much longer than that of the daughter.

Table 43.3 Modes of radioactive decay

Type	Formula	Notes
Alpha decay	$_{Z}^{A}X \rightarrow {_{Z-2}^{A-4}}Y + {_{2}^{4}}He + Q$	Q = energy released
Positron decay (β plus decay)	$_{Z}^{A}X \rightarrow {_{Z-1}^{A}}Y + {_{+1}^{0}}\beta + v + Q$	v = neutrino; Q = energy released; produces positrons (useful in nuclear medicine)
Negatron decay (β minus decay)	$_{Z}^{A}X \rightarrow {_{Z+1}^{A}}Y + {_{-1}^{0}}\beta + \tilde{v} + Q$	$\tilde{v}$ = antineutrino; Q = energy released; common in reactor-produced isotopes (e.g., ^{60}Co)
Electron capture	$_{1}^{1}P + {_{-1}^{0}}\beta \rightarrow {_{0}^{1}}Y + \tilde{v} + Q$	An orbital electron (usually from K shell) is captured by nuclear proton which is converted to neutron; competitive with positron decay in nuclei with neutron deficiencies
Internal conversion	$_{Z}^{A}X + {_{0}^{0}}\gamma \rightarrow {_{Z}^{A}}Y + {_{-1}^{0}}\beta$	A gamma ray is ejected from the nucleus and in turn, ejects an orbital electron; the gamma ray is completely absorbed; the orbital vacancy is filled by an outer shell electron resulting in emission of a characteristic X-ray

XIII

PHOTONS AND THEIR INTERACTIONS

، The photon is a chargeless basic quantum particle that exhibits wave–particle duality.

، In linear accelerators (linacs), electrons are accelerated through an electric field and are rapidly decelerated in a target material such as tungsten. This results in the production of X-rays of varying energies. The basic unit of X-rays is photons.

، X-ray production can be achieved by two major mechanisms. In Bremsstrahlung radiation, an accelerated electron changes direction when it comes into the proximity of a positively charged nucleus, resulting in photon production. Characteristic X-rays are produced when an accelerated electron knocks an inner orbital electron out of its shell. This causes an outer shell electron to fill in the vacancy which subsequently results in photon production. The energy of this photon is the difference in binding energies of the two electrons.

، Photon beams are attenuated as they pass through matter and the degree of attenuation depends on both the thickness (x) and the linear attenuation coefficient (μ) of the material. This relationship can be described by $I(x) = I_0 e^{-\mu x}$. I_0 represents the intensity of the beam prior to attenuation, μ has units of (distance)$^{-1}$ and it represents the fraction of incoming photons that are removed from the beam per unit thickness of material.

Table 43.4 Common photon energies and attenuation properties

Energy	~Tissue attenuation/cm (%)	~D_{max} (cm)
Co-60 (1.25 MV)	5	0.5
6 MV	3.5	1.5
18 MV	2.4	3.0

, The mass attenuation coefficient (μ_m) is equal to μ/ρ where ρ is the density of the material (in gm/cm^3). Unlike the linear attenuation coefficient, the mass attenuation coefficient does not vary much for different materials for photons in the therapeutic range.

, Derived from the above equation, the half-value layer [HVL] (e.g., the thickness of a given material required to attenuate the beam intensity to one-half) can be expressed as $I_0 = I_0 e^{-\mu(\text{HVL})}$. Solving for HVL yields, $HVL = \dfrac{0.693 \cdot}{\mu}$

, If all photons are of the same energy (monoenergetic), the first HVL is identical to subsequent HVLs. However, for polyenergetic photons, the first HVL is smaller than subsequent HVLs because of beam hardening. In other words, more material is required to remove the remaining higher energy photons.

Table 43.5 Summary of major photon interactions

	Photoelectric effect	Compton scattering	Pair production
Brief description	Accelerated electron knocks inner orbital electron out of its shell; this leads to outer orbital electron filling in vacancy and production of characteristic X-ray	A photon hits an outer orbital electron causing it to be ejected from an atom; the photon is itself scattered	A photon hits the nucleus and produces an electron and positron
Prevalent at which energies in tissue?	$E < 30$ keV (diagnostic radiology)	30 keV $< E < 25$ MeV (Linacs)	$E > 5$ MeV (present)$E > 25$ MeV (dominant)
Dependence of mass attenuation coefficient on atomic number	Z^3 (attenuation is variable based on Z of material; this results in good contrast between air, tissue, and bone)	Nearly independent of Z (proportional to electron density and provides poor contrast)	Z

XIII

BRACHYTHERAPY

, Brachytherapy is a form of radiation therapy where the radioactive sources are placed near or in the target to be treated.

, Brachytherapy can be categorized in different ways: by the source type, the anatomical site, the applicator type, the type of implants, or by the dose rate, HDR or LDR. None of these categories is complete by itself.

, There are three major types of brachytherapy implants: (1) molds/plaques, used for superficial lesions where radioactive sources are placed over the skin or orbital lesions; (2) interstitial implants, radioactive sources incased in wire or seeds and inserted in tumor (e.g., prostate); and (3) intracavitary implants, sealed radioactive sources placed inside a body cavity (e.g., cervix). Temporary seed insertion and removal are now performed with computerized afterloaders.

, High dose rate (HDR) implants use dose rates of >20 cGy/min. Lower than this is generally termed low dose rate (LDR).

, Note that the photon energies used in brachytherapy sources are far lower than for external beam. But more importantly, the sources are placed in or very close to

Table 43.6 Major radionuclides used in brachytherapy

Radionucleotide	Half-life	Photon energy (MeV)	HVL (mm Pb)	Clinical use
I-125	59.4 days	0.0028 avg	0.025	Permanent prostate implant
Pd-103	17.0 days	0.021 avg	0.008	Permanent prostate implant
Cs-131	9.7 days	0.029–0.034	0.030	Permanent prostate implant
Au-198	2.7 days	0.412	2.5	Permanent head and neck implant
Cs-137	30 yrs.	0.662	5.5	Temporary intracavitary implants
Ir-192	73.8 days	0.38 avg	2.5	Temporary intracavitary or interstitial implants (HDR) for prostate, breast, cervix. Also used for skin
Co-60	5.26 yrs.	1.25 avg	13.07	Older source for teletherapy
Ra-226	1622 yrs.	0.83 avg	12	Historical interest
Rn-222	3.83 days	0.83 avg	12	Temporary implant

the tumor. The inverse square law is of paramount importance in brachytherapy treatment planning. Briefly, this law states that the energy absorbed at a given distance from a point source is inversely proportional to the square of the distance of the source. This is denoted by $1/r^2$.

, There are three ways of quantifying radioactivity: (1) mCi (see above), (2) mg-Ra (milligram equivalent of radium) (obsolete), or (3) air-kerma strength (the current standard). Air-kerma strength is the dose rate in air at a specified distance in units of $(Gy)(m^2)/h$.

, Various systems exist for placing interstitial implants including:

   , Quimby system: radioactive sources are distributed uniformly over volume of tissue leading to nonuniform dose.

   , Manchester system: radioactive sources are distributed nonuniformly with the goal of ±10% dose uniformity.

   , Paris system: developed for linear sources of iridium wire; sources are distributed uniformly for a planar implant, but follow a particular pattern for volume implants.

, All these systems have an important historical purpose, but have been replaced entirely by computerized dose planning. At UCSF, all HDR treatments are planned with inverse planning using IPSA, an image-based anatomy-driven dose optimization tool. This is the equivalent of IMRT for brachytherapy.

, Modern implants are placed temporarily into a volume with the use of surgically placed catheters or intracavitary applicators. By positioning sources at a given position for variable periods of time (called dwell times), one can produce conformal dose distributions.

XIII

PHOTON DOSE DISTRIBUTIONS AND PLANNING FORMULAS

- In order to perform photon dose calculations, three key variables are important: (1) attenuation (see above) in tissue, (2) inverse square law (see above) or the distance from the radiation source, and (3) photon scattering due to the Compton effect (see above).
- Generally, radiation doses are given in the unit Gray (Gy), which represents absorbed dose (specifically 1 J/kg of tissue). However, in clinical practice, this is difficult to measure, so we instead use monitor units (MUs). A MU represents a specific amount of charge collected in one of the beam monitoring ionization chambers.
- A *depth-dose curve* is a graphical illustration of photon attenuation as it passes through matter. Note that since photons exert their effects primarily through indirect action, the maximum dose is not at the surface. The fact that the maximum dose (D_{max}) is not at the skin gives photons their *skin sparing* effect. Note that the depth-dose curve for protons is notable for the *Bragg peak*. This refers to the dose of protons being distributed over a narrow range, unlike photons.
- Useful photon planning formulas:
  - *Equivalent square formula*: used to convert rectangular fields into square equivalents for ease of calculation; E = 2XY/(X + Y), where E = equivalent square field size, and X and Y are the initial field dimensions.
  - *Wedge/hinge angle formula*: used to estimated necessary wedge angle when two beams are arranged at a particular hinge angle to each other in order to produce a more uniform dose distribution; *wedge angle = 90° – (hinge angle/2)*.
  - *Skin gap formula for matching fields*: used to calculate the separation between two field edges (e.g., the gap) on the skin when they are matched at a given depth in tissue:

$$\text{Skin Gap} = \frac{L1}{2} \frac{d}{\text{SSD1}} + \frac{L2}{2} \frac{d}{\text{SSD2}}$$

Fig. 43.1
Diagram for skin
gap formula

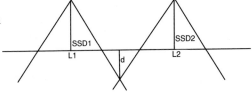

> L = length of the field, d = depth of match, SSD = source to surface distance; for isocentric setups, substitute SAD for SSD (Fig. 43.1).

ELECTRON DOSE DISTRIBUTIONS

> Unlike photons, electrons deposit most of their dose at the surface. Also unlike photons, as the energy of electrons increases, the percentage of dose deposited at the surface increases.

> The 4:3:2 rule for electrons refers to the fact that the 90% isodose line for electrons is generally $\simeq$MeV/4, the 80% isodose line is generally $\simeq$MeV/3, and the effective range of electrons is $\simeq$MeV/2.

> The amount of Pb shielding required for electrons may be estimated as MeV/2 (in mm).

ICRU DEFINITIONS

> Gross tumor volume (GTV): gross tumor by physical exam and/or imaging, including primary tumor, metastatic lymphadenopathy, or other metastases.

> Clinical target volume (CTV): tissue volume that contains GTV and area at risk of subclinical microscopic disease.

> Internal margin (IM): may be added to CTV to compensate for internal physiological movement and variation in size, shape, or position of the CTV, such as related to filling of bladder or respiratory movement.

> Internal target volume (ITV): volume encompassing the CTV and IM (ITV = CTV + IM).

> Planning target volume (PTV): PTV = CTV + IM + setup margin (SM) for setup uncertainty. The penumbra of the

XIII

beam(s) is not considered when delineating the PTV. However, when selecting beam sizes, the width of the penumbra has to be taken into account and the beam size adjusted accordingly.

꛳ Organs at risk (OAR): normal tissues whose radiation sensitivity may significantly influence treatment planning and/or the prescribed dose.

꛳ Planning organ at risk volume (PRV): analogous to PTV for OAR. PRV = OAR + IM + SM.

꛳ Treated volume: volume enclosed by an isodose surface (e.g., 95% isodose), selected and specified by radiation oncologist as being appropriate to achieve the purpose of treatment. Ideally, treated volume would be identical to PTV, but may also be considerably larger than PTV.

꛳ Irradiated volume: tissue volume receives a dose that is considered significant in relation to normal tissue tolerance. Dose should be expressed either in absolute values or relative to the specified dose to the PTV.

EXTERNAL BEAM TECHNIQUES

꛳ **3D conformal radiotherapy (3D CRT):** Beam angles and modulators are manually optimized (forward planned) to ensure dose conformality. Unmodulated arc therapy falls under this category.

꛳ **Intensity modulated radiotherapy (IMRT):** Beam intensity is modulated over the radiation field, often through the use of multi-leaf collimators.

꛳ **Volumetric modulated arc therapy (VMAT):** Variant of intensity-modulated radiotherapy or SBRT. Treatment is delivered via one or more modulated arcs, which can improve the speed of treatment delivery.

꛳ **Stereotactic radiosurgery (SRS):** Radiotherapy is delivered with reference to an established 3D coordinate system (stereotaxis). Treatment is typically highly conformal with steep dose gradients. Specialized immobilization, image-guidance, and quality-assurance measures are needed to ensure safe delivery. A number of treatment systems are specialized to deliver SRS, including Gamma Knife, CyberKnife, and linear-accelerator based systems. The term "radiosurgery" is typically reserved for single-fraction, intracranial delivery.

- **Stereotactic body radiotherapy (SBRT):** Stereotactic body radiotherapy refers to stereotactic radiotherapy delivered outside of the cranium. Treatments are typically delivered in 1–5 fractions. As with SRS, specialized immobilization, image-guidance, and quality-assurance systems are needed to ensure accurate delivery.

BRIEF TIMELINE OF RADIATION

1895: Roentgen discovers X-rays
1896: Radiation used to treat cancer
1896: Becquerel discovers natural radioactivity
1898: Marie Curie discovers radium
1943: Electron linear accelerators available
1946: Wilson proposes protons for medical therapy (HCL)
1950s: Medical linear accelerators in clinical use
1954: First proton treatment (Berkeley Radiation Laboratory)
1967: Stereotactic radiosurgery developed
1968: First Gamma Knife
1972: Clinical CT developed
1975: PET developed
1977: Clinical MRI developed
1980: Clinical CT scanners in widespread use
1987: First Gamma Knife in the US
1990s: IMRT development
2000s: IMRT in widespread use
2001: Cyberknife in widespread use
2001: PET/CT developed
2000s: Increased adoption of proton therapy

XIII

Acknowledgment: We thank Gautam Prasad MD, PhD, and Jean Pouliot PhD for their work on the prior edition of this chapter.

REFERENCES

Hall EJ, Amato JC. Radiobiology for the radiologist. 7th ed. Philadelphia: Lippincott Williams & Wilkins; 2011.

ICRP. Report No. 116 – Limitation of exposure to ionizing radiation; 1993.

ICRP. The 2007 recommendations of the international commission on radiological protection. ICRP Publication 103. Ann. ICRP 37 (2–4); 2007.

ICRP. Statement on tissue reactions; 2011.

ICRU. ICRU report 50 – prescribing, recording and reporting photon beam therapy. Med Phys. 1994;21(6):833–4.

ICRU. Prescribing, recording and reporting photon beam therapy (supplement to ICRU report 50), ICRU Report 62. Bethesda: ICRU; 1999a.

ICRU. Prescribing, Recording and Reporting Photon Beam Therapy (Supplement to ICRU Report 50), ICRU Report 62. Bethesda: ICRU, 1999b.

Kahn FM. The physics of radiation therapy. 3rd ed. Philadelphia: Lippincott Williams & Wilkins; 2003.

McDermott PN, Orton CG. The physics & technology of radiation therapy. Madison: Medical Physics Publishing; 2010.

NCRP. Limitation of exposure to ionizing radiation, report 116; 1999.

NCRP. Structural shielding design and evaluation for megavoltage X- and gamma-ray radiotherapy facilities, report 151; 2005.

NIH Genetics home reference. https://ghr.nlm.nih.gov. Last accessed 9/6/16.

Erratum to: Breast Cancer

Anna K. Paulsson, Tracy Sherertz,
and Catherine C. Park

Erratum to:
Chapter 17 in: Eric K. Hansen and M. Roach III (eds.),
Handbook of Evidence-Based Radiation Oncology,
https://doi.org/10.1007/978-3-319-62642-0_17

The tables in this chapter were inaccurate and the revised tables
have now been updated in the revised version of the book.

The updated online version of the original chapter can be found at
https://doi.org/10.1007/978-3-319-62642-0_17

Appendix A: Performance Status Scales

ECOG performance status	Karnofsky performance status[a]
0—Fully active, able to carry on all pre-disease performance without restriction	100—Normal, no complaints; no evidence of disease 90—Able to carry on normal activity; minor signs or symptoms of disease
1—Restricted in physically strenuous activity but ambulatory and able to carry out work of a light or sedentary nature, e.g., light house work, office work	80—Normal activity with effort, some signs or symptoms of disease 70—Cares for self but unable to carry on normal activity or to do active work
2—Ambulatory and capable of all self-care but unable to carry out any work activities; up and about more than 50% of waking hours	60—Requires occasional assistance but is able to care for most of personal needs 50—Requires considerable assistance and frequent medical care
3—Capable of only limited self-care; confined to bed or chair more than 50% of waking hours	40—Disabled; requires special care and assistance 30—Severely disabled; hospitalization is indicated although death not imminent
4—Completely disabled; cannot carry on any self-care; totally confined to bed or chair	20—Very ill; hospitalization and active supportive care necessary 10—Moribund
5—Dead	0—Dead

ECOG-ACRIN Cancer Research Group. Comparing the ECOG Performance Status to the Karnofsky Performance Status (2015) (Retrieved from http://ecog-acrin.org/resources/ecog-performance-status)
[a]Karnofsky DA. et al. The use of the nitrogen mustards in the palliative treatment of carcinoma. With particular reference to bronchogenic carcinoma. 1948;1(4):634–656 (licensed content date Jun 23, 2006) (Reprinted with permission from John Wiley and Sons)

© Springer International Publishing AG, part of Springer Nature 2018   **927**
Eric K. Hansen and M. Roach III (eds.), *Handbook of Evidence-Based Radiation Oncology*, https://doi.org/10.1007/978-3-319-62642-0

Appendix B: Commonly Prescribed Drugs

NOTE: Drug selection, method and duration of administration, and dosage should be verified by the reader with the most current product information provided by the manufacturer.

SKIN

- *Dry desquamation*
  - Moisturizing cream—avoid those containing alcohol, fragrances, dyes. Apply prn
  - Moisturizing ointment (e.g., Aquaphor, Radiacare gel, aloe vera, biaphene). Apply bid–tid
- *Pruritus*
  - Hydrocortisone ointment. 0.5–1%. Apply qid
  - Desonide (Tridesilon). 0.05% cream. Apply bid–tid
  - Diphenhydramine (Benadryl) topical 2% or oral 25–50 mg po q6h prn
  - Hydroxyzine (Vistaril). 25 mg po tid–qid prn
  - Dermoplast topical anesthetic. Spray or lotion. Apply tid
- *Moist desquamation*
  - Domeboro soaks. Dissolve one tablet or packet in 1 pint water. Moist soak 20 min tid–qid
  - Aquaphor/Xylocaine 5% ointment. Mix 1:1. Apply tid
  - Silvadene cream 1%. Apply tid Tube (20 or 85 g) or jar (50, 400, and 1000 g)
  - Zinc oxide cream if allergic to sulfa drugs
  - Non-adherent wound dressings (e.g., Telfa, Tegaderm). Apply prn.
  - Hydrogel wound dressings (e.g., Vigilon, Radicare, RadiaGel, Geliperm). Apply prn.
- *Ulceration*
  - Pentoxifylline (Trental). 400 mg po tid. Avoid if recent cerebral bleed or retinal hemorrhage. If GI or CNS side effects, decrease to 400 mg bid; if they persist, discontinue

˒ *Yeast infection*
  ˒ Clotrimazole topical 1%. Apply bid–tid for 2 weeks
  ˒ Nystatin powder. Apply q8–12 h for 2 weeks
  ˒ Fluconazole 200 mg po × 1, then 100 mg po qd × 13 days for extensive infection
˒ *Bacterial infection*
  ˒ Bacitracin ointment. Apply bid–tid
  ˒ Neosporin (neomycin, polymyxin B, bacitracin; OTC) ointment or cream. Apply bid–qid
˒ *Herpes*
  ˒ Acyclovir. 200 mg po 5×/day × 10 days for herpes infections. For zoster, 800 mg po 5×/day × 7–10 days.
  ˒ Valacyclovir. 500 mg po bid × 3 days (recurrent)

CNS

˒ *Cerebral edema*
  ˒ Dexamethasone. Severe: 10 mg IV x1, then 4–10 mg po/IV q6h. RT-induced: oral taper up/down for symptomatic response (e.g., 4 mg q6 h, 4 mg q8 h, 4 mg BID, 2 mg BID, 2 mg QD, 1 mg QD, 1 mg QOD)
˒ *Vertigo*
  ˒ Meclizine 25 mg po bid–tid
  ˒ Scopolamine patch apply behind ear, 1 patch q3 days
˒ *Seizure*
  ˒ Levetiracetam (Keppra). 500–1500 mg po q12h, start at 500 mg q12h. Max 3000 mg/day, taper gradually to discontinue
  ˒ Carbamazepine (Tegretol). 800–1200 mg po div bid–qid. Start 200–400 mg po bid. Monitor therapeutic levels
  ˒ Phenobarbital. 60 mg po bid–tid. Monitor therapeutic levels
˒ *Neuropathic pain*
  ˒ Gabapentin 300–1200 mg po TID

HEAD & NECK

˒ *Anesthesia for eyeshield*
  ˒ Proparacaine 0.5%. Topical anesthetic for conjunctiva. 1–2 gtts. Use care when manipulating eye because abrasions will not be felt

- *Conjunctivitis or keratitis (noninfectious)*
  - Cortisporin ophthalmic. Apply ointment or 1–2 gtts suspension q3–4 h. Contraindicated for viral infections or ulcerative keratitis and after foreign body removal. Do not use for more than 5–10 days. Caution if glaucoma
- *Dry eye*
  - Saline solutions. Apply prn
  - Ophthalmic ointment (e.g., Lacrilube). Apply qhs.
- *External otitis (noninfectious)*
  - Cortisporin otic suspension. 4 gtts OTIC q6h × 7–10 days
- *Decongestant*
  - Pseudoephedrine. 30–60 mg po q4–6 h prn. Max 240 mg/day
  - Phenylephrine. 10 mg PO q4h prn. Max 60 mg/day
- *Expectorant*
  - Guaifenesin. 200–400 mg po q4h prn. Max 2400 mg/day.
- *Mucositis*
  - Rinse 5–6x/day with 1/2 teaspoon (2.5 g) salt and 2 tablespoon (30 g) baking soda in 1 liter water
  - Gently brush teeth with very soft toothbrush 2–3x/day using non-detergent toothpaste
  - Supersaturated calcium phosphate solutions (e.g., Caphasol, NeutraSal)
  - Phenol (e.g., Chloraseptic, Ulcerease). Spray, rinse, or gargle prn. Do not swallow
  - Viscous lidocaine 2% (max 300 mg/dose, max 8 doses/day) typically combined 1:1:1 with diphenhydramine elixir 12.5 mg/5 mL and Maalox (calcium carbonate)
  - Sucralfate suspension 1 g/10 mL po BID-QID. Do not use within 30 min of lidocaine (interferes with binding)
  - Gelclair oral gel (hyaluronic acid, polyvinylpyrrolidone, and glycyrrhetinic acid), 1 packet TID or prn
  - Glutamine 15 g in glass of water, swish for 2 min then swallow BID
  - Benzydamine 0.15% mouthwash, 15 ml rinse or gargle prn
  - Doxepin 25 mg in 5 ml water rinse & spit prn
  - NSAIDs, opiates—see below
- *Oropharyngeal candidiasis*
  - Fluconazole, 200 mg po × 1, then 100 mg po QD × 6–13 days. For head/neck patients may consider prophylactic fluconazole 200 mg 2x/wk, at least 3 days apart starting 1st week of RT, continuing up to 15 weeks (30 doses). Many drug interactions.

- Nystatin suspension, 5 mL swish, and swallow qid. Continue 2 days post-symptom resolution
- *Secretions*
  - Antihistamines (e.g., diphenhydramine, loratadine) may dry mucous membranes
  - Decongestants [e.g., phenylephrine 10 mg po q4 h prn (max 60 mg/24 h) or pseudoephedrine 60 mg po q4–6 h prn (max 240 mg/24 h)]
  - Anticholinergic agents, such as scopolamine, glycopyrrolate, or atropine may be considered for severe secretions
  - Acetylcysteine as mucolytic: nebulizer via facemask, mouthpiece, or tracheostomy, 3–5 ml 20% solution or 6–10 ml 10% solution TID to QID, max 10 ml 20% or 20 ml 10% solution every 2 h. Give with bronchodilator
- *Parotitis*
  - Ibuprofen 600 mg po TID. Should resolve rapidly after first several treatments
- *Xerostomia*
  - Artificial saliva (e.g., Aquoral, Salivart, Xerolube, saliva substitute). Apply prn.
  - Amifostine. 200 mg/m^2 IV qd over 3 min, 15–30 min before RT. Monitor BP.
  - Pilocarpine (Salagen). 5–10 mg po tid. Requires some salivary function. Max 30 mg/day. Caution if asthma, glaucoma, liver dysfunction, cardiovascular disease, COPD
  - Cevimeline (Evoxac). 30 mg po tid. Max 90 mg/day. Similar cautions as pilocarpine

LUNG

- *Asthma*
  - Albuterol. 2 puffs q4h prn
- *Antitussive/expectorant*
  - Dextromethorphan/guaifenesin, 1–2 tablets po bid or 10 mL po q4h. Tablets 30/600 or solution 10/100/5 mL. Max 4 tablets/day or 60 mL/day
  - Benzonatate (Tessalon Perles). 100–200 mg po tid. Max 600 mg/day
  - Acetaminophen with codeine (300/30). 1–2 tablets po q4h prn. Max 12 tablets/day

- *Pneumonitis*
  - Prednisone, typically start 20 mg TID at diagnosis with slow taper over weeks.
  - Beclomethasone. 2 puffs qid or 4 puffs bid. May help reduce systemic steroid dose

GASTROINTESTINAL

- *Nausea*
  - Prochlorperazine 5–10 mg po q6–8 h
  - Promethazine 12.5–25 mg po/pr/IV q4–6 h
  - Metoclopramide 5–10 mg po/IV q6–8 h prn
  - Ondansetron 8 mg po q8h
  - Granisetron 2 mg po × 1 or 1 mg po q12h
  - Palonosetron 0.5 mg po × 1
  - Dolasetron 100 mg po × 1
  - Lorazepam. Anticipitory: 1–2 mg po 45 min before treatment. Adjunct: 0.5–1 mg po tid
- *Gastroparesis*
  - Metoclopramide 10 mg po qac, qhs
- *Esophagitis*
  - Viscous lidocaine 2% (max 300 mg/dose, max 8 doses/day) typically combined 1:1:1 with diphenhydramine elixir 12.5 mg/5 mL and Maalox (calcium carbonate). Swallow 5–15 min before meals and qhs
  - Sucralfate suspension 1 g/10 mL po BID-QID. Do not use within 30 min of lidocaine (interferes with binding)
- *Dyspepsia*
  - Famotidine 20 mg po BID
  - Omeprazole 20–40 mg po QD
  - Maalox
- *Esophageal candidiasis*
  - Fluconazole 200 mg po × 1, then 100 mg po qd × 13 days.
  - Nystatin suspension, 5 mL swish and swallow qid. Continue 2 days post-symptom resolution
- *Hiccups*
  - Baclofen 10 mg po BID
  - Gabapentin 100 mg po TID
  - Chlorpromazine. 25–50 mg IV (fluid preload to prevent or minimize hypotension)
  - Metoclopramide 10 mg q8 h

- *Appetite stimulant*
  - Megestrol. 400–800 mg po qd
  - Dronabinol. 2.5 mg po bid
- *Diarrhea*
  - Diet: restrict gluten, lactose, fried or spicy foods, raw vegetables, alcohol
  - Loperamide (Imodium). 4 mg × 1, then 2 mg po after each unformed stool. Max 16 mg/day
  - Atropine/diphenoxylate (Lomotil). 1–2 tablets po tid–qid prn. Max 8 tablets/day
- *Flatulence*
  - Simethicone. 80–120 mg po qac and qhs. Max 480 mg/day. Chew tablets before swallowing
- *Constipation*
  - Metamucil. 1–3 tsp. in juice qd with meals. Bulking agent
  - Miralax 17 g mixed in 4–8 oz. of water qd × 4 days prn
  - Colace 100 mg po BID. Stool softener
  - Senna. 2–4 tabs po QD-BID. Stool softener and laxative
  - Bisacodyl (Dulcolax). 10 mg po or pr. Laxative.
  - Fleet enema. 1–2 as directed
- *Proctitis*
  - Proctofoam HC 2.5%. Apply pr tid–qid
  - Hydrocortisone enema. 1 pr qhs, retain for 1 h
  - Anusol HC (hydrocortisone). 1–2.5%, apply qid25 mg

GENITOURINARY

- *Dysuria*
  - Phenazopyridine (Pyridium). 200 mg po tid–qid. Urine turns orange
- *Bladder spasm*
  - Tolterodine (Detrol). 2 mg po bid. Anticholinergic
  - Flavoxate (Urispas). 100–200 mg po tid–qid. Anticholinergic
  - Oxybutynin (Ditropan). 5 mg po bid–tid. Anticholinergic
- *BPH*
  - Finasteride (Proscar). 5 mg po qd. Type-2 alpha reductase inhibitor

- Dutasteride (Avodart). 0.5 mg po qd. Type-1 and type-2 alpha reductase inhibitor
- *Bladder outlet obstruction*
  - Doxazosin (Cardura). 1–8 mg po qd (start 1). Alpha-1 blocker
  - Terazosin (Hytrin). 1–10 mg po qhs (start 1). Alpha-1 blocker
  - Tamsulosin (Flomax). 0.4–0.8 mg po qd. Selective alpha-1a blocker
  - Alfuzosin (Uroxatral). 10 mg po qd. Selective alpha-1a blocker
- *Uncomplicated urinary tract infection*
  - Women: Trimethoprim/sulfamethoxazole 1 DS tablet po bid × 3 days, nitrofurantoin 100 mg po bid × 5 days, or Ciprofloxacin 250 mg po bid × 3 days
  - Men: Trimethoprim/sulfamethoxazole 1 DS tablet po bid × 7 days or ciprofloxacin 500 mg po bid × 7 days
- *Erectile dysfunction*
  - Sildenafil (Viagra). Start 25–50 mg po × 1. Max 100 mg. Contraindicated with nitrates. Caution if HTN, cardio-vascular disease
  - Tadalafil (Cialis). Start 10 mg po × 1. Lasts up to 36 h. Max 20 mg. Contraindicated with nitrates, alpha-blockers. Caution if HTN, cardiovascular disease
  - Vardenafil (Levitra). Start 5–10 mg po × 1. Max 20 mg. Contraindicated with nitrates, alpha-blockers. Caution if HTN, cardiovascular disease
- *Androgen deprivation*
  - Bicalutamide (Casodex). 50 mg po qd. Antiandrogen. Monitor LFTs at baseline, every month × 4
  - Flutamide. 250 mg po q8h. Antiandrogen. Monitor LFTs every month × 4
  - Leuprolide. 1 month, 3 months, 4 months, or 6 months depot. GnRH inhibitor
  - Goserelin. 1 month depot. GnRH inhibitor
  - Triptorelin (Trelstar). 1 month, 3 months, or 6 months depot. GnRH inhibitor
  - Degarelix (Firmagon). 1 month depot. GnRH antagonist
- *Hot flashes from androgen deprivation*
  - Medroxyprogesterone 20 mg daily
  - Venlafaxine 50–75 mg po qhs

GYNECOLOGIC

- *Vaginitis*
  - Replens vaginal moisturizer (OTC). One applicator full q2–3 days prn
  - Premarin vaginal cream. 1/2–2 g PV 1–3×/weeks for atrophic vaginitis. Conjugated estrogens
  - Vagifem 10 mcg PV daily x 14 days and then 2 times a week thereafter
  - Metronidazole 500 mg po bid × 7 days for bacterial vaginitis
- *Candidiasis*
  - Fluconazole. 150 mg po × 1; if refractory, 100 mg po qd × 14 days
  - Miconazole. 1 suppository qhs × 3 or cream qhs × 7 days

PSYCHIATRIC

- *Anxiety*
  - Lorazepam (Ativan). 0.5–2 mg po/IV q6–8 h prn
  - Alprazolam (Xanax). 0.25–0.5 mg po TID
- *Insomnia*
  - Melatonin 3–5 mg po qhs
  - Zolpidem (Ambien) 5–10 mg po qhs. Short-term treatment
  - Temazepam (Restoril) 7.5–30 mg po qhs. Short-term treatment
  - Trazodone 25–50 mg po qhs
  - Diphenhydramine 25–50 mg po qhs
- *Psychosis/agitation*
  - Haloperidol 0.5–5 mg po/IM q1–4 h

PAIN

- *Mild*
  - Acetaminophen. 325–1000 mg po q4–6 h prn. Max 1 g/dose, 3 g/day (2 g/day if cirrhosis)

- Ibuprofen. 200–800 mg po q4–6 h prn. Max 3200 mg/day
- Naproxen. 250–500 mg po bid. Max 1500 mg/day
- *Moderate*
  - Codeine/acetaminophen (Tylenol #2, #3, #4). 1–2 tablets po q4–6 h prn. 15, 30, or 60 mg/300 mg. Not to exceed 3 g acetaminophen/day from all sources
  - Hydrocodone/acetaminophen 5/325 tab or 10/300/15 ml elixir. 1–2 tablets po q4–6 h prn or 7.5–15 mL po q4–6 h prn. Not to exceed 3 g acetaminophen/day from all sources
  - Oxycodone/acetaminophen. 2.5/325, 5/325, 7.5/325, 10/325, 7.5/500, or 10/650 mg. 1–2 tablets po q4–6 h prn. Not to exceed 3 g acetaminophen/day from all sources
- *Severe*
  - Morphine. 10–30 mg po q3–4 h prn 2.5–10 mg IV q2–6 h prn. 10, 15, 30 mg tablets
  - MS Contin. 15–30 mg po q8–12 h prn. 15, 30, 60, 100, 200 mg tablets
  - Morphine elixir. 10–30 mg po q4h. 20 mg/mL solution
  - Oxycodone. 5–30 mg po q4h prn. 5, 15, 30 mg tablets
  - Oxycontin. 10–160 mg po bid prn. 10, 20, 40, 80 mg tablets
  - Fentanyl transdermal. 25–100 µg/h patch q72h
  - Fentanyl oral transmucosal. 1 unit (200 mcg) po × 1, may repeat ×1 after 30 min. Dissolve in mouth, do not chew or swallow. Max 2 doses/episode, 4 doses/day, wait >4 h before treating another episode
- *Muscle spasm*
  - Cyclobenzaprine. 5–10 mg po tid. Therapy should be limited to 3 weeks maximum
  - Baclofen. Start 5 mg po tid up to 20–80 mg/day. Taper gradually

ANAPHYLAXIS

- *Epinephrine*. 0.1–0.5 mg SC (1:1000) q10–15 min or 0.1–0.25 mg IV (1:10,000) over 5–10 min.
- *Diphenhydramine*. 25–50 mg PO/IV q6–8 h.

Appendix C: Intravascular Contrast Safety

We recommend following the latest American College of Radiology Manual on Contrast Media Recommendations.

http://www.acr.org/quality-safety/resources/contrast-manual

In general, identify patients at increased risk for adverse IV contrast reaction:

- History of prior contrast reaction
- Asthma
- Prior severe allergic reactions to other materials
- Patients with congestive heart failure, dysrhythmia, unstable angina, recent myocardial infarction, and pulmonary HTN
- Renal insufficiency (particularly with diabetes)
- Diabetes mellitus
- Metformin
- Multiple myeloma (due to paraprotein renal insufficiency)
- Sickle cell
- Pheochromocytoma
- Myasthenia gravis

Premedicate at-risk patients who require IV contrast:

- Encourage good oral or IV hydration for at least 12 h before and after injection.
- Prednisone 50 mg po at 13, 7, and 1 h before contrast medium injection.
- Diphenhydramine 50 mg po or IV 1 h before contrast medium injection.
- Emergency premedication: methylprednisolone 40 mg or hydrocortisone 200 mg IV every 4 h until contrast study plus diphenhydramine 50 mg 1 h prior to contrast injection

Management of acute reactions in adults

- *Urticaria*: Stop the injection. Give diphenhydramine 25–50 mg PO or IV slowly over 1–2 min. Alternative fexofenadine 180 mg PO. Preserve IV access if moderate to severe. Monitor vitals, pulse ox if moderate to severe

- *Facial or laryngeal edema*: Preserve IV access, monitor vitals, pulse oximeter, and give oxygen via mask. Start at 6–10 L/min. Consider calling emergency response. Give epinephrine IV 1 mL of 1:10,000 dilution (0.1 mg) into a running saline infusion. May repeat every 5–15 min up to 1 mL (1 mg) total.

- *Bronchospasm*: Preserve IV access, monitor vitals, and pulse oximeter, and give oxygen via mask. Start at 6–10 L/min. Give bronchodilator (e.g., Albuterol 2 puffs). If unresponsive to inhaler, consider calling emergency response. If moderate to severe, epinephrine IV 1 mL of 1:10,000 dilution (0.1 mg) into a running saline infusion. May repeat every 5–15 min up to 1 mL (1 mg) total.

- *Hypotension*: Preserve IV access, monitor vitals, and pulse oximeter, and give oxygen via mask. Start at 6–10 L/min. Elevate legs or Trendelenburg position. Administer 1 liter rapid IV fluid infusion (normal saline or Ringer's lactate). Consider calling emergency response. If hypotension with severe bradycardia, administer atropine 0.6–1 mg IV slowly into a running IV fluid infusion. If hypotension with tachycardia, give epinephrine IV 1 mL of 1:10,000 dilution (0.1 mg) into a running saline infusion.

- *Hypertension*: Preserve IV access, monitor vitals, and pulse oximeter, and give oxygen via mask. Administer labetalol 20 mg IV slowly over 2 min. If labetalol not available, give sublingual nitroglycerine 0.4 mg and furosemide 20–40 mg IV slowly over 2 min. Call emergency response team.

- *Seizures or convulsions*: Assess patient, turn patient on side to avoid aspiration, suction airway as needed, preserve IV access, monitor vitals, and pulse oximeter, and give oxygen by mask 6–10 L/min. Administer lorazepam 2–4 mg IV slowly. If unremitting, call emergency response team.

- *Pulmonary edema*: Preserve IV access, monitor vitals, and pulse oximeter, and give oxygen via mask. Elevate torso. Administer furosemide 20–40 mg IV slowly over 2 min. Call emergency response team.

If you've read this entire book, well done! I find personally editing all the chapters incredibly useful for my practice. I hope it will be for yours too. I welcome your feedback, positive or constructive. – Eric Hansen, ehansen@orclinic.com

Index

Printed in the United States
By Bookmasters